MAGILL'S MEDICAL GUIDE

HEALTH
AND
ILLNESS

MAGILL'S MEDICAL GUIDE

HEALTH
AND
ILLNESS

Volume I
Abdominal disorders — Epilepsy

A Magik Book
from the Editors of Salem Press

SALEM PRESS, INC.
Pasadena, California   Englewood Cliffs, New Jersey

Editor in Chief: Dawn P. Dawson

Project Editor: Tracy C. Irons   *Production Editor:* Joyce I. Buchea
Editorial Consultant, Reference Matter: *Proofreading Supervisor:* Yasmine A. Cordoba
L. Fleming Fallon, Jr., M.D., M.P.H.   *Layout:* James Hutson

Illustrations: Hans & Cassady, Inc., Westerville, Ohio

Note to Readers

The material presented in *Magill's Medical Guide: Health and Illness* is intended for broad informational and educational purposes. Readers who suspect that they suffer from any of the physical or psychological disorders,
diseases, or conditions described in this publication should contact a physician
without delay; this work should not be used as a substitute for professional
medical diagnosis or treatment. This publication is not to be considered definitive on the covered topics, and readers should remember that the field of
health care is characterized by a diversity of medical opinions and constant
expansion in knowledge and understanding.

Library of Congress Cataloging-in-Publication Data

Magill's medical guide : health and illness / the editors of Salem Press
    p.   cm.
  Includes bibliographical references and index.
  1. Medicine—Encyclopedias.   I. Salem Press.   II. Title: Medical guide.
RC41.M34   1995
610'.3—dc20   94-44709
ISBN 0-89356-712-4 (set)   CIP
ISBN 0-89356-713-2 (vol 1)

First Printing

PRINTED IN THE UNITED STATES OF AMERICA

CONTENTS

PUBLISHER'S NOTE

Magill's Medical Guide: Health and Illness is the first in a series of two reference publications planned to provide a general overview of the field of medicine from two perspectives: The current three volumes provide information on the major disorders of the human body in approximately 700,000 words divided into 375 essays. A second set in this series, slated for publication in 1996, will consider the institution of medicine itself, from the basic science of anatomy and physiology to the professional specializations and common procedures that form the basis for practice.

In the current set of volumes, *Health and Illness*, 98 writers from the fields of life science and medicine survey diseases, illnesses, infections, disorders, and life conditions—those with which many individuals will come in contact during their lives as well as those now rare in the industrialized world but continuing to plague areas of the so-called Third World that still lack access to basic medical care. Readers will find here articles that focus both on specific disorders, such as *Heartburn* and *Crohn's disease*, and articles that survey the range of afflictions attacking a particular system, such as *Gastrointestinal disorders* and *Liver disorders*. The majority of articles treat physical disorders—from more than 30 bacterial infections and 30 viral infections to a dozen types of cancer, two dozen genetic defects, and 35 heart and circulatory disorders. One will also find 39 entries on abdominal and gastrointestinal disorders, 25 on defects of bone and muscle, 44 on brain and nervous system problems, 6 on dental diseases, 19 on eating and nutritional disorders, 13 on endocrine disorders, 29 on conditions and disorders of the male and female reproductive systems, a dozen on immune disorders, 11 on problems of the kidneys and urinary system, 5 on liver disorders, 26 on respiratory diseases, 9 on sexually transmitted diseases, 28 on skin disorders, 3 on sleep disorders, 15 on trauma-related disorders, 15 on vector-borne diseases, and 9 on visual disorders. A large plate of entries also considers 29 psychic-emotional and learning disorders that have their basis in, or a significant impact on, the human body as well as the mind. Finally, some of the basic conditions of life—which while not "disorders" are nevertheless often the object of medical attention—are covered here, including *Aging*, *Pregnancy*, *Childbirth* and its complications, *Puberty and adolescence*, *Menopause*, and *Sexuality*.

The 375 articles devoted to this survey are arranged in an encyclopedic format—alphabetically from *Abdominal disorders* through *Zoonoses*. Lengths of the entries vary from brief definitions of 100 to 350 words (152 entries) to medium-length entries of 1,000 words (51 entries) to full, essay-length treatments of 2,500 to 3,500 words (172 entries). All of the entries begin with ready-reference top matter that identifies the bodily system or systems affected by the disorder under discussion, the primary specialists whom one afflicted with the disorder is likely to consult, and a brief definition of the disorder itself. In addition, the longer of the articles extract and define those "Key terms" that are at the center of the essay's discussion. Each of the longer entries is broken into major subsections of text appropriate to the topic at hand; given the focus of this set on illnesses and conditions, most of the entries are divided into sections entitled "Causes and Symptoms," "Treatment and Therapy," and "Perspective and Prospects," the latter of which places the topic in a larger context—historical or current or both. All but the shortest entries end with the author's byline, a listing of cross-references to other entries of interest, and a brief bibliography of sources to consult "For Further Information." In the case of the longer essays (nearly half of the total), these sources are annotated with the authors' comments on their usefulness.

In addition to the cross-references that appear at the end of each article, three listings will assist users of this reference work in locating articles of interest: "Alphabetical List of Contents," representing the entire contents of all three volumes; "Entries by Medical Specialization," a listing of the contents by those medical specialists who are involved in treatment of the disorder under discussion; and "Entries by System Affected," which arranges the disorders and conditions by the bodily system affected. In the case of the latter two listings, the disorders covered are listed as many times as necessary—that is, under all relevant categories. For the reader's convenience, these three lists are found at the end of each of the three volumes. In addition, volume III contains a "Glossary" of medical terms and a comprehensive subject index.

The editors are indebted to the contributors to this work, academicians from a variety of disciplines in the life sciences as well as health care professionals and faculty members at medical teaching institutions; they are listed in the front matter to volume I. We thank them for generously sharing their expertise as well as for their contributions to this publication. Special acknowledgment is extended to L. Fleming Fallon, Jr., M.D., M.P.H., of Jameson Hospital, New Castle, Pennsylvania, who reviewed the front matters to all entries and gave invaluable counsel during the editorial phase of production. Finally, the editors acknowledge the fine contributions of Hans & Cassady, Inc., of Westerville, Ohio, who supplied all of the drawings that appear in these three volumes.

LIST OF CONTRIBUTORS

L. Fleming Fallon, Jr.
Editorial Consultant, Reference Matter
Jameson Hospital, New Castle, Pennsylvania

Richard Adler
University of Michigan, Dearborn

E. Victor Adlin
Temple University School of Medicine

Bruce Ambuel
Medical College of Wisconsin

Iona C. Baldridge
Lubbock Christian University

John A. Bavaro
Slippery Rock University

Paul F. Bell
*The Medical Center, Beaver,
Pennsylvania*

Matthew Berria
Weber State University

Silvia M. Berry
*Englewood Hospital and Medical
Center, New Jersey*

Paul R. Boehlke
Dr. Martin Luther College

Barbara Brennessel
Wheaton College

John T. Burns
Bethany College

Louis A. Cancellaro
*Veterans Affairs Medical Center,
Mountain Home, Tennessee*

Byron D. Cannon
University of Utah

David L. Chesemore
California State University, Fresno

Leland J. Chinn
Biola University

Arlene R. Courtney
Western Oregon State College

Patrick J. DeLuca
Mt. St. Mary College

Katherine Hoffman Doman
Independent Scholar

Mark R. Doman
*Veterans Affairs Medical Center,
Mountain Home, Tennessee*

C. Richard Falcon
*Roberts and Raymond Associates,
Philadelphia*

L. Fleming Fallon, Jr.
*Jameson Hospital, New Castle,
Pennsylvania*

Mary C. Fields
Collin County Community College

K. Thomas Finley
State University of New York, Brockport

Katherine B. Frederich
Eastern Nazarene College

Jason Georges
Independent Scholar

Soraya Ghayourmanesh
City University of New York

Hans G. Graetzer
South Dakota State University

L. Kevin Hamberger
Medical College of Wisconsin

Ronald C. Hamdy
James H. Quillen College of Medicine

Peter M. Hartmann
York Hospital, Pennsylvania

H. Bradford Hawley
Wright State University

Robert M. Hawthorne, Jr.
Independent Scholar

Martha M. Henze
Boulder Community Hospital, Colorado

Carl W. Hoagstrom
Ohio Northern University

David Wason Hollar, Jr.
Rockingham Community College

Carol A. Holloway
Independent Scholar

Ryan C. Horst
Eastern Mennonite University

Howard L. Hosick
Washington State University

Katherine H. Houp
Midway College

Larry Hudgins
*Veterans Affairs Medical Center,
Mountain Home, Tennessee*

Tracy Irons
Independent Scholar

Vicki J. Isola
Independent Scholar

Louis B. Jacques
*Wayne State University School of
Medicine*

Karen E. Kalumuck
Cañada College

Armand M. Karow
Xytex Corporation

Hillar Klandorf
West Virginia University

Robert Klose
University of Maine

Craig B. Lagrone
Birmingham-Southern College

Victor R. Lavis
University of Texas, Houston

Jeffrey A. McGowan
West Virginia University

Wayne R. McKinny
*University of Hawaii
John A. Burns School of Medicine*

Laura Gray Malloy
Bates College

Charles C. Marsh
*University of Arkansas for Medical
Sciences*

Grace D. Matzen
Molloy College

Elva B. Miller
Independent Scholar

Roman J. Miller
Eastern Mennonite University

Randall L. Milstein
Oregon State University

Eli C. Minkoff
Bates College

Paul Moglia
St. Joseph's Medical Center, Yonkers, New York

Sharon Moore
Veterans Affairs Medical Center, Mountain Home, Tennessee

Rodney C. Mowbray
University of Wisconsin, LaCrosse

William L. Muhlach
Southern Illinois University

John Panos Najarian
William Paterson College

Victor H. Nassar
Emory University

Marsha M. Neumyer
Pennsylvania State University College of Medicine

William D. Niemi
Russell Sage College

J. Timothy O'Neill
Uniformed Services University of the Health Sciences

Sylvia Adams Oliver
Washington State University

Oliver Oyama
Duke/Fayetteville Area Health Education Center

Maria Pacheco
Buffalo State College

Joseph G. Pelliccia
Bates College

Carol Moore Pfaffly
Fort Collins Family Medicine Center

Kenneth A. Pidcock
Wilkes University

Nancy A. Piotrowski
University of California, San Francisco

George R. Plitnik
Frostburg State University

Layne A. Prest
University of Nebraska Medical Center

Connie Rizzo
Pace University

Eugene J. Rogers
Chicago Medical School

Robert Sandlin
San Diego State University

David K. Saunders
Emporia State University

Steven A. Schonefeld
Tri-State University

John Richard Schrock
Emporia State University

Martha Sherwood-Pike
University of Oregon

R. Baird Shuman
University of Illinois, Urbana-Champaign

Sanford S. Singer
University of Dayton

Jane A. Slezak
Fulton Montgomery Community College

Genevieve Slomski
Independent Scholar

Roger Smith
Linfield College

James R. Stubbs
University of South Alabama

Wendy L. Stuhldreher
Slippery Rock University

Gerald T. Terlep
Bon Secours Hospital System

Edith K. Wallace
Heartland Community College

Marc H. Walters
Portland Community College

Marcia Watson-Whitmyre
University of Delaware

David J. Wells
University of South Alabama Medical Center

Mark Wengrovitz
Hershey Medical Center

Russell Williams
University of Arkansas for Medical Sciences

Stephen L. Wolfe
University of California, Davis

Health
and
Illness

ABDOMINAL DISORDERS

SYSTEM AFFECTED: Gastrointestinal

SPECIALISTS: Colorectal surgeons, emergency physicians, family physicians, gastroenterologists, internists

DEFINITION: Disorders affecting the wide range of organs found in the torso of the body, including diseases of the stomach, intestines, liver, and pancreas.

KEY TERMS:

gastrointestinal: referring to the small and large intestines

pathogen: any microorganism that can cause infectious disease, such as bacteria, viruses, fungi, or other parasites

peritoneum: a membrane enclosing most of the organs in the abdomen

CAUSES AND SYMPTOMS

The main trunk, or torso, of the body includes three major structures: the chest cavity, contained within the ribs and housing the lungs and heart; the abdomen, containing the stomach, kidneys, liver, spleen, pancreas, and intestines; and the pelvic cavity, housing the sexual organs, organs of elimination, and related structures.

The abdomen is, for the most part, contained within a membrane called the peritoneum. The stomach lies immediately below the chest cavity and connects directly with the small intestine, a long tube. It fills the bulk of the abdominal cavity, winding around and down to the pelvic bones in the hips. The small intestine then connects to the large intestine, which extends upward and crosses the abdomen just below the stomach and then turns down to connect with the rectum. Other vital organs within the abdominal cavity include the liver, kidneys, spleen, pancreas, and adrenal glands. All these structures are subject to infection by viruses, bacteria, and other infective agents; to cancer; and to a wide range of conditions specific to individual organs and systems.

Diseases in the abdominal cavity are usually signaled by pain. Identifying the exact cause of abdominal pain is one of the most difficult and important tasks that the physician faces. The familiar stomachache may be simple indigestion, or it may be caused by spoiled, toxic foods, or by infection, inflammation, cancer, obstruction, and tissue erosion, among other causes. It may arise in the stomach, the intestines, or other organs contained within the abdominal cavity. In addition, pain felt in the abdomen may be referred from other sources outside the abdominal cavity. A good example would be a heart attack, which arises in the chest cavity but is often felt by the patient as indigestion. Another example is the abdominal cramping that is often associated with menstruation and premenstrual syndrome (PMS). Because abdominal pain could mean that the patient is in great danger, the physician must decide quickly what is causing the pain and what to do about it.

By far the most common cause of stomach pain is indigestion, but this term is so broad as to be almost meaningless. Indigestion can be brought on by eating too much, eating the wrong foods or tainted foods, alcohol, smoking,

poisons, infection, certain medications such as aspirin, and a host of other causes. It may be merely an annoyance, or it may indicate a more serious condition, such as gastritis, gastroenteritis, ulcer, or cancer.

The stomach contains powerful chemicals to help digest foods. These include hydrochloric acid and chemicals called pepsins (digestive enzymes). In order to protect itself from being digested, the stomach mounts a defense system that allows the chemical modification of foods while keeping acid and pepsin away from the stomach walls. In certain people, however, the defense mechanisms break down and bring the corrosive stomach chemicals into direct contact with the stomach walls. The result can be irritation of the stomach lining, called gastritis. Gastritis may progress to a peptic ulcer, identified as a gastric ulcer if the inflammation occurs in the stomach wall or a duodenal ulcer if it occurs in the wall of the duodenum, the first section of the small intestine. In most cases, the ulcer is limited to the surface of the tissue. In severe cases, the ulcer can perforate the entire wall and can be life-threatening.

A common cause of stomach pain is the medication used to treat arthritis and rheumatism. These drugs include aspirin and a group of related drugs called nonsteroidal anti-inflammatory drugs (NSAIDs). As part of their activity in reducing bone and joint inflammation and pain, they interfere with part of the stomach's network of self-protective devices and allow acids to attack stomach and duodenal walls.

Bacterial and viral infections often result in abdominal distress. Foods that sit too long unrefrigerated can be infected by bacteria, or they can become infected by pathogens on the hands of people who prepare and serve them. The bacteria release toxins into the food. Once eaten, these poisons can cause pain and diarrhea. This can be a mere annoyance, a debilitating illness, or a deadly infection, depending upon the organism involved. Salmonella and staphylococcus are two of the many bacteria that can cause food poisoning. *Clostridium botulinum* is occasionally found in canned or preserved foods. It is probably the most serious infective agent in food; victims often do not recover.

Bacterial and viral infections of the gastrointestinal tract are also common causes of abdominal disease. Viral gastroenteritis is the second most common disease in the United States (after upper-respiratory tract infections) and a leading cause of death in infants and the elderly.

Appendicitis (inflammation of the appendix) is frequently seen. The appendix is a tiny organ at the end of the small intestine. It has no purpose in the physiology of modern humans, but occasionally it becomes infected. If the infection is not treated quickly, the appendix can burst and spread infection throughout the abdominal area, a condition that can be life-threatening.

Diarrhea, with or without accompanying abdominal pain, is a major symptom of gastrointestinal disease. It is com-

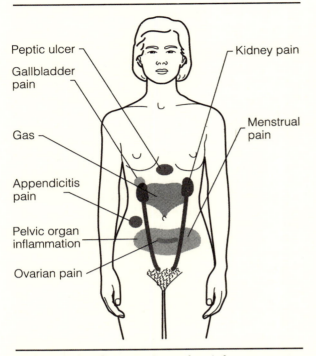

Peptic ulcer

Gallbladder pain

Gas

Appendicitis pain

Pelvic organ inflammation

Ovarian pain

Kidney pain

Menstrual pain

Abdominal disorders are many and varied; some common disorders and their sites are shown here.

monly associated with bacterial or viral infection but may also be attributable to the antibiotics used to treat bacterial infections.

Other gastrointestinal diseases are peritonitis (inflammation of the membrane that covers the abdominal organs), diverticulitis, constipation, Crohn's disease, obstruction, colitis, and the various cancers that can afflict the gastrointestinal system, such as stomach and colon cancers.

The liver is the largest internal organ in the human body and perhaps the most complicated; it is subject to a wide range of disorders. It is the body's main chemical workshop and is responsible for a large number of activities that are vital to body function. The liver absorbs nutrients from the intestinal tract and metabolizes them, that is, modifies them so that they can be used by the cells. The liver introduces nutrients into the bloodstream, supplying it with the glucose, protein, and other substances that the body needs. The liver detoxifies the blood and allows poisons, drugs, and other harmful agents to be eliminated. The liver also manufactures and stores many important substances, such as vitamin A and cholesterol.

Chief among liver disorders are the various forms of hepatitis and cirrhosis. Hepatitis can be caused by a viral infection, related to the use of alcohol or drugs, or the result of poisoning. There are many forms of viral hepatitis; the two most significant are hepatitis A and hepatitis B.

Hepatitis A is the most common form; it is caused by a virus that is transmitted through contaminated food or water. Hepatitis B is a blood-borne disease, that is, the virus is carried in the blood and other body fluids of the victim, such as semen and saliva. It can be transmitted only when infected body fluids are transferred from one person to another. The disease is commonly spread by sexual contact, bites, the use of contaminated needles, and during surgical and dental procedures. Nurses and other staff members in health care facilities are constantly exposed to hepatitis B when taking and handling infected blood samples. Pregnant women who are infected can pass the disease on to their children.

Cirrhosis develops when the liver is damaged by some substance such as alcohol. Liver cells are destroyed, and as the liver attempts to regenerate, scar tissue is formed. The steady flow of blood through the organ is impeded, as are vital functions such as the removal of waste materials from the blood.

The liver is also subject to a number of cancers. Cancer cells can spread to liver tissue from other parts of the body, or they can originate there as a result of hepatitis B or other chronic liver diseases such as cirrhosis.

The gallbladder is a small sac connected to the liver. The liver manufactures bile, a substance that aids in the digestion of fats. Bile is stored in the gallbladder and passes through the bile duct into the small intestine. A common disorder of the gallbladder is the formation of gallstones, crystalline growths that can be as fine as sand or as large as a golf ball. If the stones clog the passage to the bile duct, severe pain may result.

The pancreas, a vital gland situated near the liver, is subject to a number of disorders. The most prominent is diabetes mellitus, a condition in which the pancreas ceases to produce insulin or produces defective insulin. Pancreatitis is a disorder characterized by inflammation of the pancreas.

The other major organ system in the abdomen comprises the kidneys and the urinary tract. The system includes the two kidneys, which sit in the middle of the back on either side of the spine; the two ureters, which transport urine from the kidneys; the bladder, a pouchlike organ that collects the urine; and the urethra, which expels urine from the body. The kidneys and related organs are subject to several disorders, some inborn and some caused by infection, illnesses in other organs and systems, or cancer.

TREATMENT AND THERAPY

Many abdominal disorders are related to the overproduction of stomach acids, which damage the intestinal walls; the treatment of such conditions is often associated with changes in lifestyle. In treating gastrointestinal reflux disease, in which stomach acid backs up into the throat, physicians may suggest that the patient change habits that may be contributing to the condition, such as stopping smoking, reducing the intake of alcohol, losing weight, and avoiding certain foods and medications. Preparations to neutralize stomach acids are used, as well as drugs that reduce the amount of stomach acid produced. Surgery is rarely indicated.

Hiatal hernia, the protrusion of part of the stomach through the diaphragm, usually produces no symptoms. There may be reflux of stomach acids into the esophagus, which can be treated by the same methods used in treating gastrointestinal reflux disease. Surgery is sometimes indicated.

Gastritis is commonly treated with agents that neutralize stomach acid or others that reduce the production of stomach acid. When gastritis appears to be caused by drugs taken for arthritis or rheumatism (for example, aspirin or NSAIDs), the physician may change the drug or the dosage to reduce stomach irritation.

In treating gastric and duodenal ulcers, the physician seeks to heal the ulcer and prevent its recurrence. Acid-neutralizing agents are sometimes helpful, but more often agents that reduce the flow of stomach acids are used. It has been suggested that gastritis and ulcers are associated with certain bacteria. Consequently, some physicians add an antibiotic to the antacid regimen in order to destroy the pathogens. Surgery is sometimes required to heal ulcers.

Bacterial infections in the gastrointestinal tract are, as a rule, self-limiting. They run their course, and the patient recovers. Sometimes, however, appropriate antibiotics are needed. For viral infections, few medications are useful in eradicating the pathogens.

Appendicitis is usually treated surgically. Peritonitis, whether resulting from appendicitis or other gastrointestinal infection, is also treated surgically in order to remove infected tissue. In addition, antibiotic therapy is often used.

For two of the major liver diseases, hepatitis A and hepatitis B, there is no treatment once the person has become infected. For the most part, the diseases resolve without incident. Bed rest, dietary measures, and general support procedures are the only steps that can be taken. In a small percentage of patients, however, hepatitis B can progress to chronic active hepatitis, which may lead to liver failure, cirrhosis, liver cancer, and death. The main defense against hepatitis B is immunization. A vaccine is available and is recommended for all children and all adults who are at high risk. There is no treatment for cirrhosis, although physicians may be able to treat some of its complications.

PERSPECTIVE AND PROSPECTS

Medical science has made great progress in the treatment of disorders arising in the abdominal cavity, but there is much to be done. Most important is the identification of agents to treat or immunize against various viral diseases, particularly those that occur in the gastrointestinal tract and the liver.

A vaccine against hepatitis A is being sought. The vaccine against hepatitis B has been in use for years, but the incidence of the disease has remained relatively constant. In the United States, the practice now is to vaccinate all young children. If this immunization approach is successful, the rate of hepatitis B infection among American children should drop.

New treatment modalities are being developed for many of the diseases that occur in the abdominal cavity. One of the most significant successes has been in the treatment of peptic ulcers. The new drugs being used not only neutralize acid in the stomach but also cut off the secretion of acid into the stomach. One of these agents was the most-prescribed drug in the world for many years, indicating the importance of this therapeutic approach.

Innovations are also occurring in the treatment of diabetes mellitus, the disease caused by malfunction in the pancreas. Medications have been found that promise to treat and prevent some of the potentially fatal diseases that diabetes can cause.

Because the abdominal area contains so many vital organ systems, it is the seat of perhaps the widest range of diseases that afflict the human body—and hence, the target for the greatest amount of research and, potentially, the greatest advances in medicine. —*C. Richard Falcon*

See also Appendicitis; Bacterial infections; Cholecystitis; Cholesterol; Cirrhosis; Colitis; Colon cancer; Constipation; Crohn's disease; Diarrhea and dysentery; Diverticulitis and diverticulosis; Food poisoning; Gallbladder diseases; Gastrointestinal disorders; Heartburn; Hemorrhoids; Hepatitis; Hernia; Indigestion; Intestinal disorders; Jaundice; Liver cancer; Liver disorders; Nausea and vomiting; Obstruction; Pain, types of; Pancreatitis; Peritonitis; Renal failure; Stomach, intestinal, and pancreatic cancers; Ulcers; Viral infections.

FOR FURTHER INFORMATION:

Guillory, Gerard. *IBS: A Doctor's Plan for Chronic Digestive Disorders*. Point Roberts, Wash.: Hartley & Marks, 1991. Guillory includes both preventive and treatment recommendations for people suffering from chronic gastrointestinal problems, often referred to as irritable bowel syndrome (IBS).

Janowitz, Henry D. *Indigestion*. New York: Oxford University Press, 1992. This book covers upper-intestinal problems, such as heartburn, stomach disorders, ulcers, and gallstones. Designed for the lay reader.

Larson, David E., ed. *Mayo Clinic Family Health Book*. New York: William Morrow, 1990. Diseases of the abdominal cavity are discussed in chapters devoted to the individual organs or organ systems involved: "The Digestive System" (which includes liver disorders) and "The Kidneys and the Urinary Tract."

ABSCESSES

SYSTEMS AFFECTED: Skin (commonly), most tissues in the body

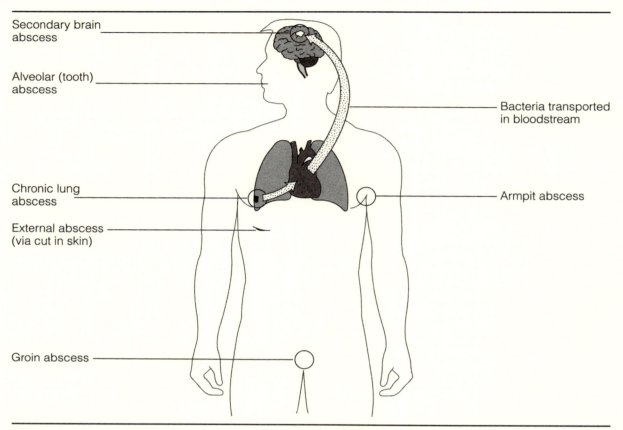

Secondary brain abscess

Alveolar (tooth) abscess

Bacteria transported in bloodstream

Chronic lung abscess

Armpit abscess

External abscess (via cut in skin)

Groin abscess

Abscesses are commonly located in soft tissues and near lymph nodes but may appear in internal organs and may cause other abscesses via bacterial migration.

SPECIALISTS: Dermatologists, family physicians, microbiologists

DEFINITION: An abscess is a localized collection of pus resulting from infection, usually by bacteria such as staphylococci. The pus that fills an abscess contains leukocytes (white blood cells), microorganisms, and cells that have been destroyed by the infection. Abscesses generally form at sites where the immune system fights invading organisms, such as around lymph nodes, but they may develop anywhere in soft tissues or in any organ of the body. Common sites include the breasts, skin, lungs, and gums, but more serious sites can be the brain and liver. Abscesses in the skin may cause only localized swelling, tenderness, redness, and pain, while larger abscesses can cause fever, sweating, and general malaise. An abscess that does not subside on its own may be drained by a physician.

See also Acne; Breast disorders; Cysts and ganglions; Liver disorders; Skin disorders; Staphylococcal infections; Tumors.

ACNE
SYSTEM AFFECTED: Skin

SPECIALISTS: Dermatologists, family physicians, pediatricians

DEFINITION: A group of skin disorders, the most common of which, acne vulgaris, usually affects teenagers; another form, acne rosacea, usually afflicts older people.

KEY TERMS:

acne rosacea: a skin eruption that usually appears between the ages of thirty and fifty; unlike acne vulgaris, it is not characterized by comedones

acne vulgaris: a skin eruption that usually occurs in puberty and is characterized by the development of comedones, which may be inflamed

comedo (pl. comedos, comedones): the major lesion in acne vulgaris; it occurs when a hair follicle fills with keratin, sebum, and other matter, and may become infected

pilosebaceous: referring to hair follicles and the sebaceous glands

sebaceous glands: glands in the skin that usually open into the hair follicles

sebum: a semifluid, fatty substance secreted by the sebaceous glands into the hair follicles

testosterone: the most potent male hormone, which exists in both sexes; it starts the chain of events that leads to acne vulgaris

CAUSES AND SYMPTOMS

Many skin disorders are grouped together as acne. The two most common are *acne vulgaris* and *acne rosacea*. Other acne diseases include *neonatal acne* and *infantile acne*, seen respectively in newborn babies and infants. *Drug acne* is a consequence of the administration of such medications as corticosteroids, iodides, bromides, anticonvulsants, lithium preparations, and oral contraceptives, to name some of the more common agents that are sometimes involved in acne outbreaks. *Pomade acne* and *acne cosmetica* are associated with the use of greasy or sensitizing substances on the skin, such as hair oil, suntan lotions, cosmetics, soap, and shampoo. They may be the sole cause of acne in some individuals or may aggravate existing outbreaks of acne vulgaris. *Occupational acne*, as the name implies, is associated with exposure to skin irritants in the workplace. Chemicals, waxes, greases, and other substances may be involved. *Acné excoriée des jeunes filles*, or acne in young girls, is thought to be associated with emotional distress. In spite of the name, it can occur in boys as well. Two forms of acne are seen in young women. One is *pyoderma faciale*, a skin eruption that always occurs on the face. The other is *perioral dermatitis (peri*, around; *ora*, the mouth), characterized by redness, pimples, and pustules. *Acne conglobata* is a rare but severe skin disorder that is seen in men between the ages of eighteen and thirty.

Acne vulgaris. In acne vulgaris, a disruption occurs in the normal activity of the pilosebaceous units of the dermis, the layer of the skin that contains the blood vessels, nerves and nerve endings, glands, and hair follicles. Ordinarily, the sebaceous glands secrete sebum into the hair follicle, where it travels up the hair shaft and onto the outer surface of the skin, to maintain proper hydration of the hair and skin and prevent loss of moisture. In acne vulgaris, the amount of sebum increases greatly and the hair shaft that allows it to escape becomes plugged, holding in the sebum.

Acne vulgaris usually occurs during puberty and is the result of some of the hormones released at that time to help the child become an adult. One of the major hormones is testosterone, an androgen (*andros*, man or manhood; *gen*, generating or causing), so called because it brings about bodily changes that convert a boy into a man. In boys, testosterone and other male hormones cause sexual organs to mature. Hair begins to grow on the chest and face, in pubic areas and armpits. Musculature is increased, and the larynx (voice box) is enlarged, so the voice deepens. In males, testosterone and other male hormones are produced primarily in the testicles. In girls, estrogens and other female hormones are released during puberty, directing the passage of the child from girlhood to womanhood. Testosterone is also produced, mostly in the ovaries and the adrenal glands.

In both sexes during puberty, testosterone is taken up by the pilosebaceous glands and converted to dihydrotestosterone, a substance that causes an increase in the size of the glands and increased secretion of the fatty substance sebum into hair follicles. At the same time, a process occurs that closes off the hair follicle, allowing sebum, keratin, and other matter to collect. This process is called intrafollicular

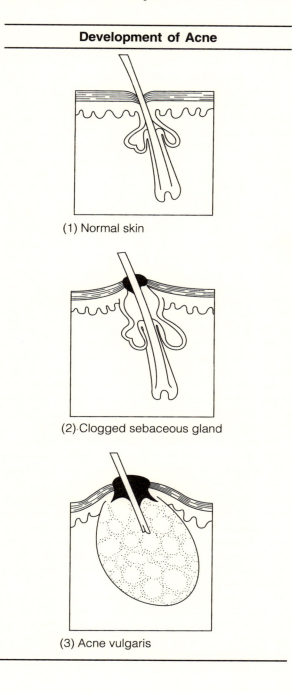

Development of Acne

(1) Normal skin

(2) Clogged sebaceous gland

(3) Acne vulgaris

hyperkeratosis (from *intra*, inside, *follicular*, referring to the follicle, *hyper*, excessive, and *keratosis*, production of keratin). Keratin buildup creates a plug that blocks the follicle opening and permits the accumulation of sebum, causing the formation of a closed comedo. As more and more material collects, the comedo becomes visible as a white-capped pimple, or whitehead. Closed comedones are the precursors of the papules, pustules, nodules, and cysts characteristic of acne vulgaris. *Papula* means "pimple," a pustule is a pimple containing pus, *nodus* means a small knot, and *kystis* means "bladder," or in this case a sac filled with semi-solid material. Sometimes cysts are referred to generically as sebaceous cysts, but the material inside is usually keratin.

Another lesion in acne vulgaris, called an open comedo, occurs when a sac in the outer layer of the skin fills with keratin, sebum, and other matter. Unlike the closed comedo, it is open to the surface of the skin and the material inside appears black—hence the term "blackhead." Blackheads are unsightly, make the skin look dirty, and suggest that they are caused by bad hygienic habits. This is not true, but exactly why the material in the sac turns black is not fully understood. Some believe that the natural skin pigment melanin is involved.

Blackheads are usually easily managed and rarely become inflamed. It is the closed comedo, or whitehead, that causes the disfiguring lesions of acne vulgaris. As the closed comedo fills with keratin and sebum, colonies of bacteria, usually *Propionibacterium acnes*, develop at the site. The bacteria secrete enzymes that break down the sebum, forming free fatty acids that inflame and irritate the follicle wall. With inflammation, white blood cells are drawn to the area to fight off the bacteria.

The comedo enlarges with further accumulation of white blood cells, keratin, and sebum until the follicle wall ruptures, spreading inflammation. If the inflammation is close to the surface of the skin, the lesion will usually be a pustule. If the inflammation is deeper, a larger papule, nodule, or cyst may form.

Clothing, cosmetics, and other factors may exacerbate acne vulgaris. Headbands, chin straps, and other items can cause trauma that ruptures closed comedones and spreads infection. Ingredients in cosmetics, soaps, and other preparations used on the skin can contribute to the formation of comedones in acne vulgaris. Lanolin, petrolatum, laurel alcohol, and oleic acid are among the chemicals commonly found in skin creams, cosmetics, soaps, shampoos, and other preparations applied to the skin. They have been shown to aggravate existing acne in some people and to bring on acne eruptions in others.

It was long thought that fatty foods—such as chocolate, ice cream, desserts, and peanut butter—contributed to acne, perhaps because teenagers eat so much of them. This theory has been largely discarded. Except for specific allergic sensitivities, foods do not appear to cause or in any other way affect the eruptions of acne vulgaris.

Cases of acne vulgaris are classified as mild, moderate, or severe. In mild and moderate acne vulgaris, the number of lesions ranges from a few to many, appearing regularly or sporadically and occurring mostly in the top layer of the skin. Consequently, these cases are sometimes called "superficial acne." In severe cases, the acne lesions are deep, extending down into the skin, and characterized by inflamed papules and pustules.

Superficial acne, or mild-to-moderate acne vulgaris, is easily managed with the therapies available. The teenager goes through a year to two dealing with "zits." The problem may be irritating and may cause inconvenience and discomfort, but it is so common among teenagers that little lasting harm is done. With time and treatment, the skin clears and the problem is over.

With deep or severe acne, however, the condition can be devastating, physically and psychologically. In these cases, the lesions may come in massive eruptions that cover the face and extend to the neck, chest, and back. The lesions can be large and deep, frequently causing disfiguring pits and craters that become lifelong scars. The victims of severe acne can suffer profound psychological damage. The disease strikes at a time when most teenagers are especially concerned with being gregarious, popular, and well liked. The chronic, constant disfigurement effectively isolates the individual, however, often making him or her unwilling to risk social contact.

Acne rosacea. The other common form of acne is acne rosacea, so called because of the "rosy" color that appears on the face. Unlike acne vulgaris, it rarely strikes people under thirty years of age and is not characterized by comedones, although papules and pustules are common. It is predominantly seen in women, although its most serious manifestations are seen in men. The cause of acne rosacea is unknown, but it is more likely to strike people with fair complexions. It is usually limited to the center of the face, but eruptions may occur on other parts of the body.

Acne rosacea is progressive; that is, it gets worse as the patient grows older. It seems to occur most often in people who have a tendency to redden or blush easily. The blushing, whether it is caused by emotional distress, such as shame or embarrassment, or by heat, food, or drink, may be the precursor of acne rosacea. The individual finds that episodes of blushing last longer and longer until, eventually, the redness becomes permanent. Papules and pustules break out, and surface blood vessels become dilated, causing further redness. As the disease progresses, tissue overgrowth may cause the nose to swell and become red and bulbous. Inflammation may develop in and around the eyes and threaten vision. These severe symptoms occur more often in men than in women.

TREATMENT AND THERAPY

The majority of acne patients are treated at home with over-the-counter preparations applied topically (that is, on the skin). For years, many of the agents recommended for acne contained sulfur, and some still do. Sulfur is useful for reducing comedones, but it has been suggested that sulfur by itself may also cause comedones; however, sulfur compounds, such as zinc sulfate, are not suspected of causing comedones. Resorcinol and salicylic acid are commonly included in topical over-the-counter preparations to promote scaling and reduce comedones. Sometimes sulfur, resorcinol, and salicylic acid are used singly, sometimes together, and sometimes combined with topical antiseptics or other agents.

While most patients will be helped by the available over-the-counter agents, many will not respond adequately to such home therapy. These patients must be seen by a doctor, such as a family practitioner or dermatologist. The physician attempts to eliminate existing lesions, prevent the formation of new lesions, destroy microorganisms, relieve inflammation, and prevent the occurrence of cysts, papules, and pustules. If the patient's skin is oily, the physician may advise washing the face and other affected areas several times a day. This has little effect on the development of comedones, but it may improve the patient's appearance and self-esteem. The physician will also use medications that are similar to over-the-counter antiacne agents but more powerful. These include drying agents, topical antibiotic preparations, and agents to abrade the skin, such as exfoliants or desquamating (scale-removing) agents.

Various topical antibiotics have been developed for use in acne vulgaris, such as topical tetracycline, clindamycin, and erythromycin. One that is often used is benzoyl peroxide, a topical antibiotic that can penetrate the skin and reach the sites of infection in the hair follicle. It is also a powerful irritant that increases the growth rate of epithelial cells and promotes sloughing, which helps clear the surface of the skin. It is effective in resolving comedones and seems to suppress the release of sebum. Because it has a high potential for skin irritation, benzoyl peroxide must be used carefully. Physicians generally start with the weaker formulations of the drug and increase the strength as tolerance develops.

Vitamin A has been given orally to patients with acne vulgaris in the hope of preventing the formation of comedones. The effective oral dose of the vitamin for this purpose is so high, however, that it could be toxic. Therefore, a topical form of vitamin A was developed called vitamin A acid, retinoic acid, or tretinoin (marketed as Retin-A). Applied directly to the skin, it has proved highly beneficial in the treatment of acne vulgaris. It clears comedones from the hair follicles and suppresses the formation of new comedones. It reduces inflammation and facilitates the transdermal (through-the-skin) penetration of medications such as benzoyl peroxide and other topical antibiotics. Like benzoyl peroxide, vitamin A acid can be irritating to the skin, so it must be used carefully. When benzoyl peroxide and vitamin A acid are used in combination in the treatment of acne

vulgaris, their therapeutic effectiveness is significantly increased. The physician generally prescribes a morning application of one and an evening application of the other.

When large comedones, pustules, or cysts form, the physician may elect to remove them surgically. The procedure is quite effective in improving appearance, but it does nothing to affect the course of the disease. Furthermore, it demands great skill on the part of the physician to avoid causing damage and irritating the surrounding skin, rupturing the comedo wall, and allowing inflammation to spread. The patient should be advised not to try to duplicate the process at home: Picking at pimples could create open lesions that may take weeks to heal and may produce deep scars. Sometimes, the physician will insert a needle into a deep lesion in order to drain the material from it. Sometimes, the physician tries to avoid surgery by injecting a minute quantity of corticosteroid, such as triamcinolone acetonide, into a deep lesion to reduce its size.

The physician may wish to add the benefits of sunlight to medical therapy. Sunlight helps dry the skin and promotes scaling and clearing of the skin, which is probably why acne improves in summer. The physician may suggest sunbathing, but an overzealous patient could become sunburned or chronically overexposed to the sun, thereby risking skin cancer. The beneficial effects of natural sunlight are not necessarily achievable with a sunlamp and, over a long period of exposure, the ultraviolet light produced by some lamps may actually increase sebum production and promote intrafollicular hyperkeratosis.

About 12 percent of patients with acne vulgaris develop severe or deep acne. In devising a treatment regime for these cases, the physician has many options to help clear the patient's skin, reduce the number and occurrence of lesions, and prevent the scarring that can disfigure the patient for life. Both the topical medications benzoyl peroxide and vitamin A acid are used, singly and in combination, as well as many other topical preparations. Nevertheless, these patients often also require oral antibiotics to fight their infection from within.

It may take weeks for oral antibiotic therapy to achieve results, and it may even be necessary for the patient to continue the therapy for years. Therefore, the physician looks for an antibiotic that is effective and safe for long-term use. Oral tetracycline is often the physician's choice because it has been proven effective against *Propionibacterium acnes*, and it seems to suppress the formation of comedones. Oral tetracycline is usually safe for long-term therapy, and it is economical. Other oral antibiotics used to treat acne vulgaris are erythromycin, clindamycin, and minocycline.

Yet in long-term therapy with any broad-spectrum antibiotic, there is always the possibility that the agent being used will not only kill the offending organism but also destroy "friendly" bacteria that aid in bodily processes and help protect the body from other microorganisms. When this happens, disease-causing pathogens may be allowed to flourish and cause infection. For example, prolonged use of antibiotics in women may allow the growth of a yeastlike fungus, *Candida*, which can cause vaginitis. Prolonged use of clindamycin may allow the proliferation of *Clostridium difficile*, which could result in ulcerative colitis, a severe disorder of the lower gastrointestinal tract.

If, for any reason, the physician believes that oral antibiotics are not working or must be discontinued, there are other therapeutic agents and other procedures that may be helpful in treating severe, deep acne vulgaris. One medication that is highly effective, but also potentially very harmful, is isotretinoin. As the name implies, isotretinoin (meaning "similar to tretinoin") is derived from vitamin A, but it is both more effective and more difficult to use. Unlike the topical vitamin A acid preparations, isotretinoin is taken orally. It is highly effective in inhibiting the function of sebaceous glands and preventing the formation of closed comedones by reducing keratinization, but isotretinoin also produces a wide range of side effects. The majority of these are skin disorders, but the bones and joints, the eyes, and other organs can be affected. Perhaps the most serious adverse effect of isotretinoin is that it can cause severe abnormalities in the fetuses of pregnant women. Therefore, pregnancy is an absolute contraindication for isotretinoin. Before they take this drug, women of childbearing age are checked to ensure that they are not pregnant. They are advised to use strict contraceptive measures one month before therapy, during the entire course of therapy, and for at least one month after therapy has been discontinued.

Estrogens, female hormones, have been used to treat severe acne in women who are more than sixteen years of age. The aim of this therapy is to counteract the sebum-stimulating activity of circulating testosterone and to reduce the formation of comedones by reducing the amount of sebum produced. Estrogens cannot be used in males because the dose required to reduce sebum production could produce feminizing side effects.

Persistent lesions can be treated with cryotherapy. In this procedure, an extremely cold substance such as dry ice or liquid nitrogen is carefully applied to the lesion. This technique is effective in reducing both small pustules and deeper cysts. For patients whose skin has been deeply scarred by acne, a procedure called dermabrasion, in which the top layer of skin is removed, may help improve the appearance.

Although its cause is unknown, acne rosacea can be treated. The topical antiparasitic drug metronidazole, applied in a cream, and oral broad-spectrum antibiotics, such as tetracycline, have been found effective. It may be necessary to continue antibiotic therapy for a long period of time, but the treatment is usually effective. Surgery may be required to correct the bulbous nose that sometimes occurs with this condition.

PERSPECTIVE AND PROSPECTS

Most acne vulgaris (about 60 percent) is treated at home. There has been significant improvement in the treatment of mild-to-moderate acne vulgaris, so for most of these patients, the condition can be limited to an annoyance or an inconvenience of the teen years. Only recalcitrant cases of acne vulgaris are seen by physicians. Of those cases treated by doctors, the majority are seen by family physicians, general practitioners, and other primary care workers. Severe acne is usually referred to the dermatologist, who is skilled in the use of the more serious medications and the more exacting techniques that are required in treatment.

For at least 85 percent of those experiencing puberty, acne vulgaris is a fact of life. It is a natural consequence of the hormonal changes that occur at this time. It is not likely that any drugs or techniques will be found to avoid acne in the teenage years, as this would involve tampering with a fundamental growth process. It can be expected, however, that in this disease condition, as in so many others, progress will continue to be made, and newer, more effective, and safer agents will be developed.

—*C. Richard Falcon*

See also Abscesses; Cysts and ganglions; Keratoses; Pimples; Puberty and adolescence; Rosacea; Skin disorders.

FOR FURTHER INFORMATION:

Dvorine, William. *A Dermatologist's Guide to Home Skin Treatment.* New York: Charles Scribner's Sons, 1983. Offers descriptions of various skin diseases, including acne, and sensible instructions about how to deal with them at home.

Flandermeyer, Kenneth L. *Clear Skin.* Boston: Little, Brown, 1979. Billed as "a step-by-step program to stop pimples, blackheads, acne," a good general text for the layperson that details one dermatologist's views on acne and how to treat it.

Handbook of Nonprescription Drugs. 9th ed. Washington, D.C.: American Pharmaceutical Association, 1990.

Horton, Edward, Felicity Smart, and Trevor Weston, eds. *The Marshall Cavendish Illustrated Encyclopedia of Family Health.* 24 vols. London: Marshall Cavendish, 1984. This multivolume set provides "doctor's answers" to common questions about various diseases. Acne is covered in volume 1.

Larson, David E., ed. *Mayo Clinic Health Book.* New York: William Morrow, 1990. One of the most thorough and accessible medical texts for the layperson.

ACQUIRED IMMUNODEFICIENCY SYNDROME (AIDS)

SYSTEM AFFECTED: Immune

SPECIALISTS: Epidemiologists, family physicians, immunologists, infectious disease physicians, internists

DEFINITION: AIDS arises from chronic infection with the human immunodeficiency virus (HIV) and is characterized by progressive loss of immune function and susceptibility to secondary infections.

KEY TERMS:

CD4: an abbreviation for a protein found on the surface of certain human cells; CD4 is a specific receptor for HIV, and it determines the range of cells that HIV can infect

macrophages: cells involved in the presentation of antigen to the immune system, found in a number of tissues; macrophages, which have CD4 on their surfaces, may be a major reservoir of infection for HIV

opportunistic infections: infections caused by pathogens that take advantage of a dysfunctional immune system; much of the morbidity and mortality of AIDS results from opportunistic infections

retroviruses: the family of ribonucleic acid (RNA) viruses to which HIV belongs, characterized by a multiplication cycle that includes reverse transcription

reverse transcriptase: an enzyme, encoded by an HIV gene, that causes a deoxyribonucleic acid (DNA) copy of the HIV genes to be inserted into the chromosomes of the target cell; drugs directed against HIV target reverse transcriptase

T helper cells: CD4-expressing cells involved in immune recognition and the coordination of immune responses; the destruction of T helpers by HIV multiplication contributes to AIDS immunodeficiency

zidovudine: a drug, also known as azidothymidine (or AZT), used to treat HIV infection; it interferes with the functioning of the virus' reverse transcriptase enzyme

CAUSES AND SYMPTOMS

Acquired immunodeficiency syndrome (AIDS) is a condition that occurs in persons infected with the human immunodeficiency virus (HIV). The morbidity and mortality attributed to AIDS result primarily from opportunistic viral and protozoal infections arising from a generalized failure in cell-mediated immunity caused by HIV infection, or from certain characteristic malignancies of uncertain etiology. There may also be tissue damage, especially in the central nervous system, that can be attributed directly to the destruction of HIV-infected cells. From a clinical standpoint, AIDS can be considered as a terminal manifestation of HIV infection, and there is no single diagnostic criterion to distinguish it from other disease states associated with HIV. AIDS is most widespread in central Africa and southern Asia, but it occurs with some degree of prevalence in most parts of the world.

HIV is a member of the Retroviridae, a family of enveloped viruses whose life cycles are characterized by the phenomenon of reverse transcription, by which the nucleotide sequence of the virus' ribonucleic acid (RNA) genome is used to synthesize deoxyribonucleic acid (DNA) that is subsequently incorporated into an infected cell's chromosomes; this is the reverse of the normal flow of genetic information in cells and is catalyzed by a unique viral enzyme, reverse transcriptase. Another retrovirus causing disease in humans is the human T-cell lymphotropic virus type I (HTLV-I), which may be associated with adult T-cell leukemias. There are two genetically distinct forms of HIV, HIV-1 and HIV-2, with HIV-1 being dominant worldwide.

HIV has evolved for transmission during sexual intercourse. HIV-susceptible cells are found in association with the epithelia of the vagina, rectum, and urethra. In HIV-infected persons, both HIV-infected cells and free virus particles (virions) may be found at these sites, as well as in seminal fluid and in vaginal secretions. There is evidence that the rate of HIV transmission (the proportion of sexual contacts between an infected and a susceptible individual that result in transmission of the virus), which is normally very low, may be increased by the presence of other sexually transmitted infections; presumably, the inflammation associated with these infections causes an increase in the number of HIV-infected and HIV-susceptible cell populations. Because HIV-infected cells and HIV virions are found in the blood of an infected person, HIV can be transmitted through accidental transfer of blood, as may occur in needle sharing by intravenous drug users, needle-stick injuries to health care workers, and the administration of blood products. Infection by vertical transmission to a developing fetus occurs in approximately one-third of children born to HIV-infected mothers. There is no evidence that HIV can be spread by airborne transmission, by indirect or direct nonsexual contact, or by arthropod vectors, such as mosquitoes.

The major cellular targets for the multiplication of HIV are macrophages and T-helper lymphocytes. Both of these cell populations display a surface protein designated as CD4, to which HIV can attach through interaction with proteins (gp120 and gp41) found on the surface of the virion. This interaction leads to entry of the virus into the cell, probably involving fusion of the cell membrane and the viral envelope. After the nucleoprotein core (the HIV genome and associated proteins) migrates to the cell's nucleus, reverse transcriptase uses the viral RNA as a template for producing a DNA copy that is inserted into the chromosomal DNA of the cell.

At this point, the virus exists in the infected cell as a collection of genes. Conceivably, these genes could remain unexpressed, the virus persisting in this state without affecting the cell or giving evidence to the immune system of its presence; this condition of biological latency can be shown in cultured cells, though its significance in an infected person is unknown. For production of progeny virus particles (virions), HIV genes are expressed, leading to the synthesis of viral proteins and full-length RNA genomes. After assembly, the virions leave the cell by a process of budding through the cell membrane. The entire reproductive cycle is regulated by viral gene products and is influenced by the metabolic state of the cell. In culture, macrophages can continue releasing virions over a long period of time, while HIV infection of T helpers often leads to their rapid destruction. In an infected person, multiplication of HIV occurs primarily in lymphoid tissues, including lymph nodes and the spleen, where HIV-susceptible macrophages and lymphocytes are abundant.

HIV strains isolated from different persons, or even from the same person at different times in the course of an infection, may display genetic variability, especially in the genes encoding the virion surface proteins. Apparently, reproduction of HIV is associated with a high rate of spontaneous mutation, which may help the virus to evade an effective immune response. Such mutation places a significant restraint on development of an HIV vaccine.

The earliest stages of HIV infection may be unapparent or may be expressed in symptoms similar to those of many other viral infections, including mild fever, malaise, and swollen lymph nodes. Antibodies to HIV proteins are usually produced within twelve weeks of exposure, although they do not contain the infection.

Primary infection is followed by a period of clinical latency, during which signs and symptoms of HIV infection are absent or subtle. The length of this period varies and may exceed fifteen years. It is important to distinguish this state of clinical latency from biological latency of the virus. During clinical latency, HIV may continue to multiply, and the infected person continues to serve as a potential reservoir of infection, transmitting the virus to new hosts.

In virtually all HIV infections, continued multiplication of the virus eventually leads to a state of impaired cellular immunity. The mechanisms whereby this characteristic immunodeficiency of AIDS develops are complex. Both macrophages and T helpers are critical players in the immune response, and their destruction by HIV may be responsible in part for dysfunctional immunity. The immunodeficiency is not, however, entirely attributable to the depletion of HIV-susceptible cells, since cells not infected by HIV also show aberrant behavior in infected persons; these include the cytolytic T lymphocytes that are essential to the defense against intracellular parasites and antibody-producing B lymphocytes. These indirect effects may arise from shifts in relative amounts of cytokines—small proteins produced by cells that influence the activity of surrounding cells—produced by HIV-infected cells.

Later stages of HIV infection, leading to AIDS, are distinguished by a measurable drop in absolute numbers of peripheral T helpers and weak delayed hypersensitivity responses. At this point the HIV-infected person becomes susceptible to a variety of opportunistic infections—infections caused by pathogens that are normally incapable of infecting humans but that can invade the tissues of a person whose immune response is impaired. Some of the opportunistic infections that afflict HIV-infected persons are also seen in other immunodeficiency states, such as those that occur in transplant patients receiving immunosuppressive drugs, while others are especially prominent in persons with AIDS.

The most common opportunistic infection accompanying advanced HIV infection, and one of the most commonly documented causes of death from AIDS, is pneumonia resulting from invasion by the eukaryotic parasite *Pneumocystis carinii*. *P. carinii* pneumonia can be treated with drugs, but unfortunately reinfection is common. Other fungal and parasitic infections common among persons with AIDS are oropharyngeal candidiasis, cryptococcal meningitis, and toxoplasmosis. Among bacterial pathogens, mycobacteria are especially important, including *Mycobacterium intracellulare* and *Mycobacterium tuberculosis*; persistence of *M. tuberculosis* in the United States is attributed in part to its association with AIDS. Herpesvirus infections, which are very common in the general population but are usually held in a state of biological latency by the immune system, may become reactivated in persons with AIDS, leading to systemic tissue damage.

Characteristic malignancies may also accompany advanced HIV infection, including Kaposi's sarcoma and non-Hodgkin's lymphomas. Kaposi's sarcoma is diagnosed primarily in the Western Hemisphere among homosexual and bisexual males; the significance of this unusual pattern of incidence is unclear.

Although opportunistic infections remain the major cause of death from AIDS, advanced HIV infections may also be accompanied by disease states more directly attributable to the viral infection. These include a wasting syndrome characterized by chronic or recurrent diarrhea and a pattern of neurological damage known as AIDS dementia.

Diagnosis. The early stages of HIV infection are most commonly diagnosed by the identification of antibodies in patient serum that are specific for viral antigens, using an enzyme immunoassay (EIA). Test serum is incubated with a solid matrix coated with material containing HIV proteins; if the serum contains HIV-specific antibodies, these will bind to the matrix with high affinity. After the matrix is washed to remove nonspecific antibodies, it is incubated with a solution of secondary antibodies that are specific for human immunoglobulin; these will attach to any HIV-specific patient antibodies that are bound to the matrix. The secondary antibodies are covalently linked to an enzyme that catalyzes the formation of a detectable product, signaling the presence of the secondary antibodies and thus of HIV-specific antibodies in the test serum. While this test is very sensitive for the detection of HIV-specific antibodies, false-positive results may arise from the presence of antibodies in the test serum that bind to non-HIV proteins on the matrix.

Sera that test positive in the EIA test are therefore subjected to Western blot tests, which also detect antibodies in the serum but which allow greater discrimination of antibodies specific for HIV proteins. In terms of number of tests performed, the most significant application of the EIA and Western blot tests is in screening donor blood to prevent transfusion-associated HIV transmission. Immunoassays have also been developed to allow detection of HIV proteins in serum; these may have the advantage of allowing HIV infection to be diagnosed prior to the production of antibodies by the infected person. Methods for the detection of HIV that have been limited to the research setting include direct assay of viral activity in cell culture and amplification of the viral genome by polymerase chain reaction (PCR). PCR amplification of HIV nucleic acids was used to demonstrate the importance of lymphoid tissues as sites for HIV multiplication.

The course of HIV infection is commonly monitored by measuring the concentration, in cells per cubic millimeter, of peripheral blood lymphocytes displaying the CD4 protein, which is the major receptor for HIV. A drop in this CD4+ T-cell count below 500 may be an indicator of progression of HIV infection beyond the clinically latent phase, and CD4+ T-cell counts are one piece of information used to determine appropriate therapies, including the initiation of antiviral drug treatment and secondary infection prophylaxis. CD4+ T-cell counts can be obtained by a variation of flow cytometry known as fluorescence-activated cell sorting, or FACS. In FACS, leukocytes in a blood sample are incubated with antibodies specific for cell surface proteins such as CD4; the antibodies have fluorescent chemical groups attached to allow their detection by fluorometry. The antibody-labeled cells are subsequently channeled into a stream that carries them, one at a time, past a detector that measures the fluorescent intensity of each cell. FACS detectors can simultaneously distinguish fluorescent groups attached to different antibodies, and consequently different cell surface proteins. This allows the counting of several cell populations in the same sample. For example, the ratio of lymphocytes displaying CD4 to those displaying CD8 (another cell surface protein) may be significant in monitoring HIV infection.

TREATMENT AND THERAPY

By the early 1990's, the only available therapeutic agents for treating HIV infection directly were nucleoside analogues, the most widely used being zidovudine (formerly azidothymidine, or AZT). Nucleoside analogues such as zidovudine are phosphorylated in HIV-infected cells, where they interfere with the functioning of the virus' reverse transcriptase enzyme. This interference may block the production of a DNA copy of the virus' RNA genome, an essential step in HIV multiplication. Other nucleoside analogues used in HIV infection are deoxycytidine (ddC) and deoxyinosine (ddI).

Zidovudine produces measurable improvement in survival, immune reactivity, and quality of life in persons with AIDS; the benefit is significant enough that the earliest clinical trials were abandoned at six months so that placebo

subjects could be offered the drug. Unfortunately, when given early in HIV infection, zidovudine has not been shown to lengthen the period of clinical latency significantly, and if given immediately after HIV exposure (as may be done in the case of needle stick injury to health care workers), may not block the establishment of HIV infection. Zidovudine therapy is usually initiated when CD4+ T-cell counts drop below 500.

Adverse reactions to zidovudine are common, the most important being suppression of blood cell formation in bone marrow, leading to leukopenia (a reduction in leukocytes) and anemia. Dosage adjustment may help, as may the co-administration of cytokines that promote granulocyte and erythrocyte formation. With severe anemia, administration of zidovudine may be temporarily withdrawn, or zidovudine may be replaced with another nucleoside analogue.

Continued administration of zidovudine can result in the selection of HIV strains that are resistant to the action of the drug, as a result of mutations in the gene for reverse transcriptase. The effect of this resistance on the clinical course of HIV infection is unknown. Concern with drug resistance and a desire to limit adverse reactions, however, has led to recommendations for multidrug therapies, in which different nucleoside analogues are administered either together or during alternate periods.

In addition to reverse transcription, potential targets for drug development include the process by which HIV attaches to host cells and the protein factors that regulate the expression of HIV genes.

Because opportunistic pathogens play such an important role in the pathology of AIDS, the control of opportunistic infections is central to the medical treatment of AIDS. Treatment of opportunistic infections is complicated by the fact that many of the relevant microorganisms are eukaryotic parasites, mycobacteria, or viruses, for which effective agents are often highly toxic and require long-term administration. Additionally, successful treatment with antimicrobials typically relies on immune responses that may not be effective in patients with AIDS. Nevertheless, early diagnosis and treatment of opportunistic infections can significantly improve the health and extend the life of persons infected with HIV. For example, treatment of *P. carinii* pneumonia with available antimicrobials, combined with the prophylactic administration of pentamidine, can dramatically limit episodes of this often-fatal opportunistic infection.

PERSPECTIVE AND PROSPECTS

There can be little doubt that the epidemiologic concentration of early Western AIDS patients among marginalized groups—homosexual men and intravenous drug users—contributed to a response that was tragically inadequate in terms of policy and resource allocation. Public concern became apparent only in the early 1980's, when the possibility of transmission by blood transfusion was revealed. This, in turn, led to a degree of irrational fear of casual transmission, contributing further to discrimination against persons infected with HIV. At one point, there was serious discussion of universal EIA testing of health care personnel, without regard to the tremendous cost of such an enterprise or the absence of evidence that health care workers could accidentally transmit HIV to their patients.

The HIV epidemic has dramatically influenced the health care system in the United States. In larger metropolitan areas, the presence of large numbers of young adults with a terminal infectious disease has contributed to a reassessment of health care objectives, with greater emphasis on patient care and health maintenance. Thanks in part to the efforts of patient advocacy groups, many HIV-infected persons are exceptionally well informed as to their medical options, leading physicians to recognize the importance of patient contribution to therapeutic decision making. One area of public health policy arising from the HIV epidemic that has affected large numbers of people is the implementation of workplace policies for preventing transmission of blood-borne pathogens. Along with minimizing exposure to HIV, such practices are likely to lead to reduced prevalence of infection with hepatitis B virus, which is far more readily transmitted.

The devastating manner in which AIDS progressively degrades the health of an HIV-infected person, along with its usually fatal outcome, tends to promote an aura of despair surrounding discussion of the disease. Certainly, AIDS has resisted many efforts at control, casting doubt on the traditional faith in biomedical solutions. It is important, however, to recognize that HIV is not a supernatural agent of evil. HIV is a virus and, from long experience, medical researchers know that viruses always possess points of vulnerability. One of these—the reverse transcriptase enzyme, which can be targeted by nucleoside analogues—has already been identified, as will others. With due recognition of predictable setbacks, there is every reason to expect continued progress in the effort to extend the lives and improve the health of persons infected with HIV.

—*Kenneth A. Pidcock*

See also Human immunodeficiency virus (HIV); Immunodeficiency disorders.

FOR FURTHER INFORMATION:

Corey, Lawrence, ed. *AIDS: Problems and Prospects*. New York: W. W. Norton, 1993. A compiled collection of review articles first published in *Hospital Practice*. Some familiarity with medical terminology and concepts is helpful, though the authors have been careful to limit

AIDS-Related Deaths in the United States Since 1982

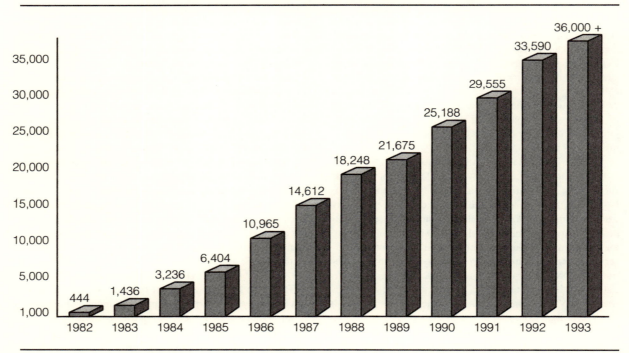

Note: Statistics for 1993 are projected based on 33,260 deaths for the first eleven months of that year. Data are from the U.S. Centers for Disease Control, National Center for Health Statistics, Atlanta, Georgia.

technical discussions. Outstanding illustrations and bibliographies are included.

Fan, Hung, Ross F. Connor, and Luis P. Villareal. *The Biology of AIDS*. 2d ed. Boston: Jones and Bartlett, 1991. A highly readable, concise account of the HIV epidemic considered from the perspectives of virology, immunology, and epidemiology. The authors succeed in providing a comprehensive account that is easy to read. A limited number of illustrations are provided.

Global AIDS Policy Coalition. *AIDS in the World*. Cambridge, Mass.: Harvard University Press, 1992. Considers the impact of AIDS as a global pandemic, looking at worldwide patterns of infection along with economic and political impacts. A useful source of information that is extensively documented with numerous graphs and tables.

Levy, Jay A. "Pathogenesis of Human Immunodeficiency Virus Infection." *Microbiological Reviews* 57 (March, 1993): 183-289. From a leader in AIDS research, a detailed overview of all aspects of HIV biology, including molecular events involved in its reproduction and its interaction with various host cells. Very difficult for the nonspecialist to read, but its depth makes it worth knowing about, and it should be available in almost all college libraries. Heavily referenced.

Shilts, Randy. *And the Band Played On*. New York: St. Martin's Press, 1987. A thorough journalistic account of the United States' tragically limited response to AIDS through 1985 and the parts played by the biomedical community, politicians, journalists, and gay activists. Although the author is meticulous in placing blame, the book is admirably lacking in malice.

Sontag, Susan. *AIDS and Its Metaphors*. New York: Farrar, Straus & Giroux, 1989. An extended essay on themes the author developed in her 1978 book *Illness as Metaphor*, applied to the AIDS epidemic. Sontag's dense writing style may not appeal to all readers, but her reflections on what AIDS is and is not contribute to rational discourse.

Stine, Gerald J. *Acquired Immune Deficiency Syndrome: Biological, Medical, Social, and Legal Issues*. Englewood Cliffs, N.J.: Prentice Hall, 1993. Successfully covers a wide variety of topics, from the biology of HIV to legal barriers faced by HIV-infected persons. While the presentation is somewhat choppy—with tables of information competing for page space with article reprints—this is an excellent single-volume reference work on AIDS and HIV.

ADDICTION

SYSTEMS AFFECTED: Psychic-emotional, brain, nervous
SPECIALISTS: Psychiatrists, psychologists
DEFINITION: A psychological and sometimes physiological process whereby an organism comes to depend on a substance; addiction is defined by a persistent need to use the substance and to increase the dosage used as a result of tolerance, as well as the experience of withdrawal symptoms when the substance is withheld or use is reduced.

KEY TERMS:

abstinence: complete, voluntary refrainment from the use of a substance of abuse

compulsion: a persistent, irresistible urge to perform a stereotyped behavior or irrational act, often accompanied by repetitious thoughts (obsessions) about the behavior

pharmacodynamics: changes in tissue sensitivity or physiologic systems in response to pharmacological substances

pharmacokinetics: the action of pharmacological substances within a biological system; pharmacologic substance absorption, distribution, metabolism, and elimination by an organism

physiological dependence: a state of tissue adaptation to a substance of abuse marked by tolerance and withdrawal

positive reinforcement: a process that increases the frequency or probability of a response and increases the strength of a learning process

psychological dependence: habitual substance use across various situations, or a persistent need for a substance for the sense of well-being provided by its reinforcing properties

substance abuse: the continued use of a psychoactive substance for at least one month despite impairment of psychological, social, occupational, or physical functioning

tolerance: a condition in which the same dose achieves a lesser effect, or in which successively greater doses of an abusable substance are required to achieve the same desired effect

withdrawal: a physical and mental condition following decreased intake of an abusable substance, with symptoms ranging from anxiety to convulsions

CAUSES AND SYMPTOMS

Addiction is a disorder that can affect any animal and may result from the use of a variety of psychoactive substances. Typically, it involves both psychological and physiological dependence. Psychological dependence is marked by compulsions to use a substance of abuse because of its positively reinforcing qualities. Physiological dependence results when the body responds to the presence of the addictive substance. Both tolerance and withdrawal characterize physiological dependence.

Tolerance involves pharmacokinetics, pharmacodynamics, and environmental or behavioral conditioning. Pharmacokinetics refers to the way in which a biological system, such as a human body, processes a drug. Substances are subject to absorption into the bloodstream, distribution to different organs (such as the brain and liver), metabolization by these organs, and then elimination. Over time, the processes of distribution and metabolism may change, such that the body eliminates the substance more efficiently. Thus, the substance has less opportunity to affect the system than it did initially, reducing any desired effects. As a result, dose increases are needed to achieve the initial or desired effect.

Pharmacodynamics refers to changes in the body as a result of a pharmacologic agent being present. Tissue within the body responds differently to the substance at the primary sites of action. For example, changes in sensitivity may occur at specific sites within the brain, directly or indirectly impacting the primary action site. Direct changes at the primary sites of action denote tissue sensitivity. An example might be an increase in the number of receptors in the brain for that particular substance. Indirect changes in tissue remote from the primary action sites denote tissue tolerance, or functional tolerance. In functional tolerance, physiologic systems that oppose the action of the drug compensate by increasing their effect. Once either type of tolerance develops, the only way for the desired effect to be achieved is for the dose of the substance to be increased.

Finally, environmental or behavioral conditioning is involved in the development of tolerance. Organisms associate the reinforcing properties of substances with the contexts in which the drugs are experienced. Such contexts may be physical environments, such as places, or emotional contexts, such as when the individual is depressed. Over the course of repeated administrations in the same context, the tolerance that develops is associated with that specific context. Thus, an organism may experience tolerance to a drug in one situation, but not another. Greater doses of the reinforcing substance would be needed to achieve the same effect in the former situation, but not in the latter.

Tolerance develops differently depending on the type of substance taken, the dose ingested, and the routes of administration used. Larger doses may contribute to quicker development of tolerance. Similarly, routes of administration that produce more rapid and efficient absorption of a substance into the bloodstream tend to increase the likelihood of an escalating pattern of substance abuse leading to dependence. For many drugs, injection and inhalation are two of the fastest routes of administration, while oral ingestion is one of the slowest. Other routes include intranasal, transdermal, rectal, sublingual, and intraocular administration.

For some substances, the development of tolerance also depends on the pattern of substance use. For example, even though two individuals might use the same amount of alcohol, it is possible for tolerance to develop more quickly in one person than in the other. Two individuals might each drink fourteen drinks per week, but they would develop tolerance at different rates if one consumes two drinks each of seven nights and the other consumes seven drinks each of two nights in a week. Because of their patterns of use, the first drinker would develop tolerance much more slowly than the second, all other things being equal.

Withdrawal occurs when use of the substance significantly decreases. Withdrawal varies by the substance of abuse and ranges from being minor or nonexistent with some drugs (such as hallucinogens) to quite pronounced with other drugs (such as alcohol). Mild symptoms include anxiety, tension, restlessness, insomnia, impaired attention, and irritability. Severe symptoms include convulsions, perceptual distortions, irregular tremors, high blood pressure, and rapid heartbeat. Typically, withdrawal symptoms can be alleviated or extinguished by readministration of the substance of abuse. Thus, a compounding problem is that the addicted individual often learns to resume drug use in order to avoid the withdrawal symptoms.

Addiction occurs with both legal and illegal drugs. Alcohol and nicotine are two of the most widely used legal addictive drugs. Over-the-counter drugs, such as sleeping aids, and prescription drugs, such as tranquilizers (for example, sedative-hypnotics) and antianxiety agents, also have addiction potential. Common illegal addictive drugs include cocaine, marijuana, hallucinogens, heroin, and methamphetamine.

Not everyone who uses these substances will automatically become addicted (although addiction is nearly assured with the repeated use of potent substances such as cocaine and heroin). In the United States, for example, surveys have shown that approximately 65 percent of adults drink alcohol each year. In contrast, less than 13 percent of the population goes on to develop alcohol problems serious enough to warrant a medical diagnosis of alcohol abuse or dependence. Similarly, despite the fact that large numbers of individuals are prescribed opiates or sedative-hypnotics for pain while hospitalized, roughly 0.7 percent of the adult population is addicted to opiates and 1.1 percent is addicted to sedative-hypnotics or antianxiety drugs. Thus, the development of addiction often requires repeated substance administration, as well as other biological and environmental factors.

When addiction is present, the consequences are multiple and complex. While substance abuse involves deteriorated functioning in psychological, social, occupational, or physical functioning, substance dependence usually involves each of these areas for significantly longer amounts of time. Psychologically, problems with depression, anxiety, the ability to think clearly or remember information, motivation, judgment, and one's sense of self may result. Socially, one can become isolated from friends and family, or even unable to deal with the stresses and demands of normal, everyday relationships. Finally, occupational disruptions can result from the inability to plan, to manage one's feelings and thoughts, and to deal with social interactions.

In terms of health, there are many acute and chronic effects of addiction. With cocaine, for example, acute cardiac functioning may be affected, such that the risk of heart attacks is increased. Similarly, individuals addicted to opiates, alcohol, and sedative-hypnotics must contend with such risks as falling into a coma or experiencing depressed respiratory functioning. Finally, the acute effects of any of these drugs can impair judgments and contribute to careless behavior. As a result, accidents, severe trauma, and habitually dangerous behavior, such as risky sexual behavior, may be associated with addiction.

Chronic health consequences are common. Smoking is associated with cancers of the mouth, throat, and lungs, as well as premature deterioration of the skin. Alcohol is associated with cancers of the mouth, throat, and stomach, as well as ulcers and liver problems. General malnutrition is a risk for heroin and alcohol users, since they often fail to eat properly. Injected drugs such as heroin and cocaine are associated with problems such as hepatitis and acquired immunodeficiency syndrome (AIDS), since shared needles may transmit blood-borne diseases. Finally, addiction contributes to health problems in the unborn children of addicted individuals. Problems such as low birth weight in the children of smokers, fetal alcohol syndrome in the children of female drinkers, and withdrawal difficulties in the children born to other types of addicts are well documented.

TREATMENT AND THERAPY

Because of the combination of psychological and physiological dependence, addiction is a disorder that often demands both psychological and pharmacological treatments. Typically, interventions focus on reestablishing normal psychological, social, occupational, and physical functioning in the addicted individual. Though the length and type of treatments may vary with the particular addictive drug and the duration of the addiction problem, similar principles are involved in the treatment of all addictions.

Psychological treatments focus primarily on extinguishing psychological dependence, as well as on facilitating more effective functioning by the addicted individual in other areas of life. Attempts to change the behavior and thinking of the addicted individual usually involve some combination of individual, group, and family therapy. Adjunctive training in new occupational skills and healthier lifestyle habits are also common.

In general, treatment focuses on understanding how the addictive behavior developed, how it was maintained, and how it can be removed from the person's daily life. Assessments of the situations in which the drug was used, the needs for which the drug was used, and alternative means of addressing those needs are primary to this understanding. Once these issues are identified, a therapist then works with the client to break habitual behavior patterns that were contributing to the addiction (for example, driving through neighborhoods where drugs might be sold, going to business meetings at restaurants that serve alcohol, or maintaining relationships with drug-using friends). Concurrently, the therapist helps the client design new behavior patterns that will decrease the odds of continued problems with addiction. Problems related to the drug use would then be addressed in some combination of individual, family, or group therapy.

The therapy or therapies selected depend on the problems related to drug use. For example, family therapy might be more appropriate in cases in which family conflicts are related to drug use. In contrast, individual therapy might be more appropriate for someone whose drug use is linked to thinking distortions or mood problems. Similarly, group therapy might be most appropriate for individuals lacking social support to deal with stress, or whose social interactions are contributing to their drug use. Regardless of the type of therapy, however, the basic goal remains: facilitating the client's solving of his or her specific problems. Additionally, the development of new ways of coping with intractable problems, rather than relying on drug use as a means of coping, would be critical.

Cognitive and behavioral therapies have been quite useful for breaking the conditioned effects of addiction. Some psychological dependence, for example, is placed on placebo effects. A placebo effect occurs as a result of what people believe a drug is doing for them, rather than from anything that the drug actually has the power to accomplish. In addition, the practice of using addictive drugs within certain contexts is associated with drug tolerance, such that certain situations trigger compulsions leading to drug use. In this way, cognitive therapy can be used to challenge any faulty thinking associations that individuals have made about what the drugs do for them in different situations. This may involve increasing patients' awareness of the negative consequences of their drug use and challenging what they perceive to be its positive consequences. As a complement, such therapies correct distorted thinking that is related to coping with stressful situations or situations in which drug use might be especially tempting. In such situations, individuals might actually have the skill to handle the stress or temptation without using drugs. Without the confidence that they can successfully manage these situations, however, they may not even try, instead reverting to drug use. As such, therapy facilitating realistic thinking about stress and coping abilities can be quite beneficial.

Similarly, behavioral therapies are used to break down conditioned associations between situations and drug use. For example, smokers are sometimes made to smoke not in accordance with their desire to smoke, but according to a schedule over which they have no control. As a result, they are made to smoke at times or in situations where it is inconvenient, leading to an association between unpleasant feelings and smoking. While such assigned drug use would not be used with illegal drugs, the basic principles of increasing negative or unpleasant feelings with drug use in specific situations can be used. Rewarding abstinence has also been a successful approach to treatment. In this way, positive reinforcement is associated with abstinence and may contribute to behaviors related to abstinence being more common than behaviors related to drug use.

Pharmacological treatments concentrate on decreasing physical dependence on the substance of abuse. They rely on behavioral principles and on five primary strategies. The first strategy, based on positive reinforcement, is pharmacological replacement. Prescribed drugs with similar effects at the sites of action as the addictive drug are used. These prescribed drugs, however, usually fail to have reinforcing properties as powerful as the addictive drug and focus mainly on preventing the occurrence of withdrawal symptoms. Nicotine patches for smokers and methadone for heroin users are examples of replacement therapies.

A second strategy involves the use of both reinforcement and extinction, the behavioral process of decreasing and eventually extinguishing the drug-taking behavior. Partially reinforcing and partially antagonistic drugs are prescribed. The net effect is that the prescribed drug staves off withdrawal symptoms, but yields less reinforcement than drug replacement therapy, serving to facilitate the process of extinction for the drug taking.

Antagonists, or drugs that completely block the receptors responsible for the reinforcing effects of the drug action, are prescribed alone as a third strategy. With this strategy, extinction is the primary behavioral principle in effect. The prescribed drug blocks the primary receptor sites and does not yield positively reinforcing drug effects. Even if the addictive drug is taken in addition to the antagonist, no positively reinforcing effects are experienced. Thus, without reinforcement, drug-taking behavior should eventually cease. Naltrexone, typically used for opiate addiction, is a good example of this strategy.

Punishment is another behavioral principle used in pharmacological therapy. Metabolic inhibitors, or drugs that make the effects of the addictive substance more toxic, are often used to discourage drug use. Antabuse, a drug often given for problems with alcohol, is such a substance. When metabolic inhibitors are prescribed, individuals using these drugs in combination with their substance of abuse experience toxic and unpleasant effects. Thus, they begin to associate use of the addictive substance with very noxious results and are discouraged from continuing their drug use.

Symptomatic treatment of withdrawal effects is used as a fifth strategy. Based on reinforcement, this strategy simply encourages the use of drugs likely to reduce withdrawal effects. Unfortunately, these drugs may also have abuse potential. For example, when benzodiazepines are given to individuals with alcohol or opiate dependence, one dependency may be traded for another. As such, symptomatic treatment is helpful but is not a treatment of choice by itself. In fact, none of these pharmacological treatments is recommended for use in isolation; they are recommended for use with complementary psychological treatments.

PERSPECTIVE AND PROSPECTS

The use of substances to alter the mind or bodily experiences is a practice that has been a part of human cultures for centuries. Time and again, even through legislated acts such as Prohibition, drug and alcohol use have persisted. The continued use of drugs for recreational and medicinal practices seems virtually inevitable, and it is unlikely that substance abuse and dependence will disappear from the world's societies. Consequently, an understanding of substance use, how it leads to addiction, ways to minimize the development of addiction problems, and strategies for improving addiction treatments will be critical.

At different times in history, addiction has been viewed as strictly a moral, medical, spiritual, or behavioral problem. As the science of understanding and treating addiction has progressed, the variety of ways in which these aspects of addiction combine has been noted. Modern treatments and theories no longer view addiction from one strict point of view, but instead recognize the heterogeneity of paths leading to addiction. Such an approach has been helpful not only in treating addiction but also in preventing it. Efforts to curb the biological, social, and environmental forces contributing to addiction have become increasingly important.

Addiction remains a disorder with no completely effective treatment. Of individuals seeking treatment across all addictive disorders, fewer than 20 percent succeed the first time that they attempt to achieve long-term abstinence. As a result, individuals suffering from addiction often undergo multiple treatments over several occasions, with some individuals experiencing significant problems throughout their lives. Even though treatments for physiological and psychological dependence offer some improvement, much work remains to be done. In this context, the challenge ahead is not to prevent all substance use, but rather to decrease the odds that a person will become addicted. Improving the pharmacological and psychological treatments currently available will be important. Discoveries of new ways of tailoring treatment for addiction to the needs and backgrounds of the different individuals affected will be one critical task for health professionals. Continued exploration of new pharmacological treatments to combat withdrawal and facilitate abstinence is necessary.

—*Nancy A. Piotrowski*

See also Alcoholism; Eating disorders; Obsessive-compulsive disorder; Stress.

FOR FURTHER INFORMATION:

American Psychiatric Association. *Diagnostic and Statistical Manual of Mental Disorders.* Rev. 3d ed. Washington, D.C.: Author, 1987. This manual provides detailed descriptions of the behaviors and types of symptoms used to describe and diagnose different addictive disorders. It is written by mental health professionals from psychiatric, psychological, and social work backgrounds.

Brickman, Philip, et al. "Models of Helping and Coping." *American Psychologist* 37 (April, 1982): 368-384. This article describes a four-model perspective on helping and coping with problems related to addiction. A classic in the addiction field, providing a good review of historical factors influencing different treatment models.

Julien, Robert M. *A Primer of Drug Action.* 5th ed. New York: W. H. Freeman, 1988. A nontechnical guide to drugs written by a medical professional. Describes the different classes of drugs, their actions in the body, their uses, and their side effects. Basic pharmacologic principles, classifications, and terms are defined and discussed.

Miller, William R., and Nick Heather, eds. *Treating Addictive Behaviors: Processes of Change.* New York: Plenum Press, 1986. This book, written by medical and psychological scientists, is an overview of treatment strategies for problems ranging from nicotine to opiate addiction. Psychological, behavioral, interpersonal, familial, and medical approaches are outlined and discussed.

Schlaadt, Richard G., and Peter T. Shannon. *Drugs of Choice: Current Perspectives on Drug Use.* Englewood Cliffs, N.J.: Prentice Hall, 1982. A good introduction to the complex issues surrounding addiction and drug use. Describes different drugs of abuse, individual differences in drug use, legal and social issues, and continuing controversies. Also included is an overview of the differences between illegal and legal drugs, as well as drug myths and facts.

Weil, Andrew, and Winifred Rosen. *From Chocolate to Morphine: Everything You Need to Know About Mind-Altering Drugs.* Rev. ed. Boston: Houghton Mifflin, 1993. This book on psychoactive substances provides basic information to the general reader. Psychoactive substances are identified and defined. Also outlines the relationships between different types of drugs, the motivations to use drugs, and associated problems. As the title suggests, the discussion ranges from legal, caffeinated substances to illegal and prescription drugs.

ADDISON'S DISEASE

SYSTEM AFFECTED: Endocrine

SPECIALISTS: Endocrinologists, internists

DEFINITION: Addison's disease, also known as adrenal insufficiency or adrenal hypofunction, is a chronic condition in which the adrenal glands do not produce adequate amounts of corticosteroid hormones. Symptoms include fatigue, dizziness, nausea, diarrhea, weight loss, a weak and irregular pulse, and a general darkening of the skin and mucous membranes. These symptoms are easily managed with corticosteroid drugs over the patient's lifetime, but with injury, surgery, or stress—when the body's immune system is compromised—acute episodes of the disease can occur. These Addisonian crises, or adrenal crises, require hospitalization. The disease was fatal before hormone-replacement therapy was developed, but proper long-term care and prompt treatment when crises occur can allow patients to live with the disease.

See also Endocrine disorders.

ADOLESCENCE. *See* PUBERTY AND ADOLESCENCE.

ADRENAL DISORDERS. *See* ADDISON'S DISEASE; CUSHING'S SYNDROME.

AGING

SYSTEMS AFFECTED: Psychic-emotional, all bodily systems

SPECIALISTS: Audiologists, cardiologists, emergency physicians, general surgeons, geneticists, geriatric specialists, neurologists, oncologists, psychiatrists, psychologists

DEFINITION: The process of growing old, regardless of one's chronological age; with the number of old persons dramatically increasing, medical researchers are striving to understand the causes and effects of the aging process.

KEY TERMS:

Alzheimer's disease: a disorder characterized by progressive deterioration of intellectual capacity with memory loss, impaired judgment, and personality change

arthritis: inflammation or degenerative joint change often marked by stiffness, swelling, and pain

atherosclerosis: a condition of an artery characterized by lipid deposits and a thickening of the inner wall

free radical theory: the idea that aging may be brought about by the production within the body of very reactive chemicals (free radicals) that damage chromosomes and other cell parts

geriatrics: the branch of medicine that treats the conditions and diseases associated with aging and old age

hypertension: a condition characterized by higher-than-normal blood pressure in the blood vessels

immunocompetence: the ability of the body to produce a proper immune response to infectious organisms

osteoporosis: a progressive loss of density in new bone as it replaces old bone

transient ischemic attack (TIA): a brief period of insufficient circulation to the brain

PROCESS AND EFFECTS

Aging is an ongoing process begun at conception and eventually leading to death. The effects of aging, however, tend to be more observable after the age of forty. These age-related changes occur in every organ and system of the body.

Most changes that occur in the skin do not directly affect a person's physical health, but they may greatly affect one's self-concept and general attitude. Age spots form because pigment cells tend to clump together. Wrinkles become common when elastic fibers become less resilient and the fat layer below the skin is greatly reduced. The loss of many oil glands leaves skin dry and scaly. Hair gradually loses pigment and may become thin and fragile.

The chief age-related skeletal system change is a loss of calcium from bone. This loss begins at a younger age and progresses more rapidly in women than in men. Accompanied by a loss of protein fibers in the bone, this calcium depletion leaves bones frail, brittle, and prone to break easily.

The cartilage in aging joints becomes thin and erodes away, causing discomfort and restricting movement. Cartilage between the ribs and breastbone hardens, becomes less flexible, and makes breathing more difficult. Progressive degeneration of cartilage discs between vertebrae leads to painful compression of the spine, especially in the neck and lower back.

A gradual reduction in strength, endurance, and coordination results from changes in aging muscle. As old muscle fibers are lost, new ones are not produced; instead, they are replaced by pockets of fat and of stringy connective

Aging and the Body

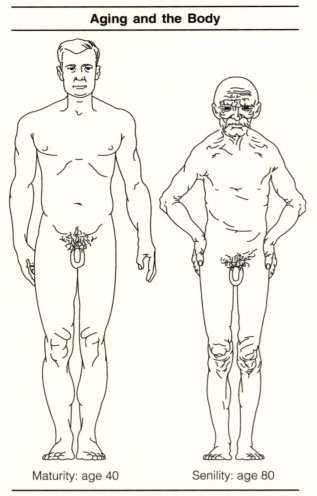

Maturity: age 40   Senility: age 80

Among the most obvious effects of aging are reduced body mass, a "shrinking" of height with loss of bone mass, sagging and wrinkling skin, and graying or loss of hair.

tissue. In addition, the nerves that cause muscle contraction degenerate and lose their ability to bring about smooth, swift movement.

Because the nervous system directs and coordinates all other parts of the body, its age-related changes are of particular concern. Because nerve cells lose some ability to produce and receive neurotransmitters (chemicals that move impulses from one nerve cell to another), impulses move more slowly in the elderly.

As nerve cells die, they are not replaced. This loss of neurons, especially in the brain, is believed to cause a decline in intelligence and in the capacity to learn new skills. It also triggers memory loss, especially of more recent memories. The loss of about 25 percent of the cells in the cerebellum of the brain adversely affects balance and the coordination of fine movements. Those exhibiting the most mental disabilities have a significant number of defects called neurofibrillary tangles within their nerve cells and neuritic plaques or debris between their nerve cells.

Age-related changes in the inner ear affect both hearing and balance. The spiral-organ cells in the cochlea, which enable sound to be perceived, die off as blood capillaries thicken and prevent nutrients from reaching the cochlea. The death of nerve cells in the semicircular canals greatly reduces the ability of the elderly to maintain equilibrium and to coordinate movements.

It is not unusual for an eighty-five-year-old to have lost 80 percent of his or her ability to see clearly. This dramatic difference in vision is caused by many cumulative changes. The cornea in front of the eye loses its ability to bend light correctly, while the lens becomes harder, thicker, less elastic, and unable to change shape as needed. The aqueous humor or fluid that cleanses and nourishes the lens and cornea becomes insufficient to do so in many older people, leaving the eye dry and irritated. In addition, the vitreous humor that gives shape to the eyeball may shrink and become opaque. This allows little light to reach the retina and images are, therefore, poorly received.

Elderly persons often fail to eat properly because food does not taste or smell appealing. A loss of taste stems from a decrease in the amount of saliva secreted, from changes in the taste-processing centers in the brain, and possibly from a decline in the number of taste buds. The loss of neurons involved in smell causes that sense to begin to decline in most people by middle age.

Structural changes occur in all parts of the digestive system with aging. There is a tendency to develop gum disease and to lose one's teeth. The degeneration of digestive glands leaves the mouth, stomach, and small intestine with less of their digestive juices. In spite of these changes, digestion and absorption are not appreciably interfered with in otherwise healthy older persons.

Aging brings a major reduction in the elasticity of arteries and a narrowing of their diameter as a result of an ac-

Aging and the Brain

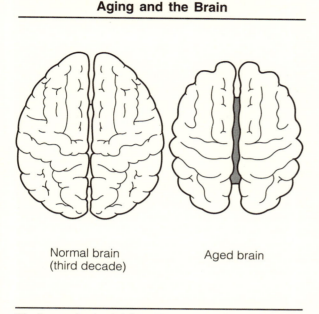

Normal brain
(third decade)

Aged brain

The human brain shrinks with age as nerve cells are lost and brain tissue atrophies.

cumulation of fats (lipids) in arterial walls. Blood pumped by the heart thus encounters more resistance to its easy movement through the vessels. The result is some degree of high blood pressure, or hypertension, in all the elderly. The heart of an older person is often enlarged and pumps less blood with less force than that of a young adult. Fat deposits gather on its surface, and valves may become less flexible. The heart, working much harder yet achieving increasingly less, is unable to supply adequate oxygen for all the body's needs.

The amount of red bone marrow also diminishes with age. Although sufficient marrow remains to form new blood cells under ordinary circumstances, it is not sufficient to form them rapidly should the elderly person bleed extensively for any reason.

Those who are aging experience a decreased ability of the respiratory organs to acquire and deliver the oxygen needed for normal physical activity. Hardening of the trachea and bronchi hampers the movement of air into the lungs, which themselves become inelastic. The walls of the alveoli, or lung air sacs, become increasingly unable to allow oxygen through them and into the blood.

In an aging woman, the degeneration of follicle cells in the ovary results in lowered secretion of estrogens and progesterone. These declining hormone levels cause changes in the uterus and the cessation of menstrual cycles known as the menopause. Some women experience hot flashes and irritability at this time. The diminished hormonal levels also cause fat to accumulate below the waist area, breast tissue to sag, and the vagina to become dry and thin.

In the older man, changes within the testes cause less testosterone to be produced, reducing muscle strength and resulting in a general wasting appearance. Sperm production is greatly decreased, although there may still be an adequate number to bring about fertilization at an advanced age. The penis tends to become smaller, and its erectile tissue becomes somewhat rigid; this inability to expand makes the attainment of an erection very difficult for many older men. Meanwhile, hard masses appear in the prostate, and the whole gland may double in weight. Its enlargement often constricts the urethra and makes urination difficult.

In both sexes, large numbers of glomeruli, the filters that make up the kidneys, are lost as one ages, as is an efficient blood supply to these vital organs. Consequently, the kidneys lose much ability to form urine and purify the blood correctly. By the age of seventy-five, the kidneys are usually only half as efficient as they are in a young adult.

COMPLICATIONS AND DISORDERS

An accumulation of age-related changes can cause a serious dysfunction or disease to develop. Two major dysfunctions that medical science must treat in the skeletal system are arthritis and osteoporosis.

Arthritis is a general term used to describe the various kinds of degenerative changes or inflammation that occur in joints. These changes are seen in the membranes surrounding the joints, in the protective, cushioning cartilage at the ends of bones, and in the bones themselves. The most common form of arthritis, called osteoarthritis, is a chronic and debilitating degeneration of that protective, or articular, cartilage. The pain in stiff, swollen joints is caused by the wearing away of the smooth cartilage and the rubbing together of the rough, exposed bones. Bony growths or spurs may appear, causing the characteristic joint enlargement.

Osteoarthritis causes misshaped, painful fingers. More important, it affects the lower limbs and the vertebrae of the spine. It thus severely hampers posture and limits normal walking, while producing constant leg pain and backaches. No single cause of osteoarthritis has been discovered. It seems to result from a combination of the stress on joints and changes in the collagen and elastic fibers within the bones and cartilage. An additional cause may be the decreased blood supply to the joints found in most older people. It is thought that heredity also influences the degree to which cartilage thins, as well as the rate.

Osteoporosis ("porous bone") is a common dysfunction in elderly persons but especially in postmenopausal women. It is a progressive reduction in the density of the new bone that is replacing old bone. Osteoporosis can cause curvature of the spine, backache, diminished height, and brittle bones that are easily broken. From middle adulthood, everyone's bones begin a gradual decline in mass and strength. If bone volume reaches a level that is low enough, osteoporosis results. The cause of this disease is unclear, but contributing factors in both sexes include a deficiency of vitamin D and calcium in the diet over many years. Women may lose 50 percent of their bone mass by the age of seventy; their hormonal deficiencies after the menopause are believed to be the major factor in such extensive osteoporosis.

Two fairly common dysfunctions of the aging central nervous system are Parkinson's disease and Alzheimer's disease. The former is a chronic and slowly progressive condition which generally develops after the age of fifty. More common in men than in women, Parkinson's disease involves useless contractions of skeletal muscles, a rhythmic tremor, and muscle rigidity. It becomes difficult for the patient to begin movement or to walk without a characteristic shuffling gait. Drooling from the mouth, slow and monotonous speech, and a loss of facial expression accompany this disease.

Parkinsonism results from changes in the part of the brain called the basal ganglia when cells there lose the ability to produce and use properly the neurotransmitter called dopamine. There is a direct relationship between the degree of dopamine deficiency and the severity of symptoms. Some degree of memory loss or decreased ability to comprehend new concepts afflicts patients with Parkinson's disease.

Alzheimer's disease is also progressive but has three recognizable stages. Impairment of recent memories, a lessening of spontaneous emotions, and confusion about one's surroundings are among the earliest symptoms seen. In the second stage, the ability to read, write, calculate, and think clearly are lost; the patient even becomes unable to recognize a spouse or other family members. Finally, the patient becomes unable to speak and begins to have seizures.

These symptoms may result from a deficiency of the neurotransmitter called acetylcholine. This lack is caused by the death of many neurons which had previously produced acetylcholine in the correct amount for normal brain functioning. The brains of Alzheimer's patients have a large number of neurofibrillary tangles and neuritic plaques. In addition, their brains tend to contain accumulations of metals such as aluminum. It has yet to be proven whether the tangles, the plaques, or the metal deposits are the causes or effects of this disease.

Dysfunctions of the circulatory system, all of which are potential causes of death, are more common in older people. Though patients who suffer from one often suffer from other, related conditions, the dysfunctions can be categorized by their primary symptoms as ischemic heart disease, myocardial infarction, cardiac arrhythmias, congestive heart failure, atherosclerosis and arteriosclerosis, and hypertension.

Coronary artery disease is an ischemic (anemic) condition in which the heart tissue does not receive an adequate supply of blood. The reduced blood flow is caused by a narrowing of the coronary arteries. Most sixty-year-olds are believed to have only one-third the blood flow through the

heart's vessels when compared to a young adult. The most frequent cause of the constriction is a plaque which partially or completely blocks the vessel. If the plaque protrudes into the artery, its rough edges can cause a thrombus, or stationary blood clot, to block that vessel. If the thrombus detaches, it is called an embolus; it will then cause a blockage when it enters a smaller vessel.

A myocardial infarction, or heart attack, results when the muscle cells deprived of blood and oxygen are damaged and die. A heart thus damaged has much less, if any, ability to pump blood to the whole body.

When the heart does not contract in the regular manner with a predictable sequence of heartbeats, the condition is called cardiac arrhythmia. It may result from too few heartbeats or from many extra contractions per minute. The latter is more dangerous because it does not allow the heart chambers to fill properly and move the blood efficiently through the heart. An extremely rapid and irregular beat, known as fibrillation, puts great strain upon the heart.

Congestive heart failure may result from a heart attack, from valve damage, or from prolonged high blood pressure. It is also called cardiac insufficiency because the heart is not able to pump enough blood to meet the needs of the body. The insufficiency to the kidney causes less urine to be produced and blood volume to increase; the heart must work even harder to pump this greater blood volume and, in time, may fail.

Atherosclerosis and arteriosclerosis are very closely related conditions. Atherosclerosis is the presence in an artery wall of plaques composed of lipids, connective tissue, and abnormal smooth muscle cells. Plaques can cause ischemic heart disease directly by constricting a coronary artery or indirectly by causing a blood clot to form. Often, atherosclerotic plaques become hardened by the accumulation of calcium, producing arteriosclerosis, or "hardening of the arteries." These inelastic walls are one cause of hypertension, or high blood pressure. The excessive blood pressure creates kidney damage and thus more strain upon the heart.

A malfunctioning cardiovascular system has great potential to damage the delicate nervous system. A transient ischemic attack (TIA) can result if the atherosclerosis prevents sufficient blood from reaching the brain for a very brief period. TIAs often serve as a prediction that a stroke will soon occur. A stroke or cardiovascular accident (CVA) involves either a blood clot or a rupture of a weakened blood vessel in the brain. A CVA is always accompanied by some destruction of fragile nervous tissue, and the severity of its effects depends on the size and location of the brain subdivision in which it occur.

PERSPECTIVE AND PROSPECTS

The understanding of the aging process holds a key position in modern medical science. Although people have observed and described many age-related changes for centuries, it was only in the twentieth century that scientists began to comprehend why the elderly suffer from so many diseases and dysfunctions. This understanding marked the birth of the science of geriatrics. In the 1980's, using the tools of biochemistry, microbiology, and genetics, gerontologists began to accumulate meaningful data to answer the ultimate question: What actually causes aging? If the underlying cause could be determined, it might be possible to interfere with the process and increase the human life span.

It seems most likely that there is no single cause of aging but rather a complex combination of causes. Many tentative theories have been advanced, including aging by program, gene-caused, gene mutation, cross-linkage, free radical, cellular garbage, and the wear-and-tear theories. The causes of aging seem closely interwoven with the role of the endocrine glands and the immune system.

There are strong arguments supporting the idea that aging is somehow programmed into all species. Some scientists believe the hypothalamus, located at the base of the brain, may be the timekeeper of life because of its key role in normal hormone production; others think the thymus gland might control life span because of its work in immunity. Still others assume that an individual organ is not responsible and that each cell has its own internal "life clock."

The gene-caused theory suggests that aging is programmed by harmful genes that only become active late in life or useful genes that are altered and become harmful over the years.

The gene mutation theory postulates that an accumulation of mistakes in deoxyribonucleic acid (DNA) production with the passage of time results in large numbers of altered, malfunctioning cells. This theory further assumes that the many methods of gene repair that are possessed by young cells become ineffective over the years.

The cross-linkage theory proposes that, with age, abnormal bonds form within numerous proteins, altering their structure and therefore the functioning of the organs in which they are found. These proteins include the thousands of enzymes responsible for body processes, and especially the collagen that makes up 30 percent of the protein found in organs.

The free radical theory postulates that highly reactive chemicals are formed in the course of normal living and combine with cell membranes and chromosomes, thus damaging and altering them. The number of free radicals can be suppressed by substances such as vitamins C and E, called antioxidants. If this theory is correct, there is hope that these vitamins could be used to increase life span.

The cellular garbage theory suggests that the accumulation over the years of large amounts of chemical waste products can interfere with normal cell activities and bring about the aging of all organs. The wear-and-tear theory includes the concept of cellular garbage and a possible accumulation of improperly produced proteins. It further focuses on the supposition that each animal has a specific amount of metabolic energy available to it; the length of life is determined by the rate at which that energy is used up.

The immune system seems to have a central role in aging for two reasons. First, autoimmune conditions, in which the person's immune system mistakenly attacks and destroys body parts, are very prevalent in the elderly. Second, the aging immune system's ability to recognize and destroy foreign invading organisms, its immunocompetence, becomes extremely reduced. —*Grace D. Matzen*

See also Alzheimer's disease; Amnesia and memory loss; Death and dying; Dementia; Depression; Diabetes mellitus; Growth; Hearing loss; Heart disease; Menopause; Midlife crisis; Osteoporosis; Parkinsonism; Stress; Strokes and TIAs.

FOR FURTHER INFORMATION:

Bonner, Joseph, and William Harris. *Healthy Aging: New Directions in Health, Biology, and Medicine*. Claremont, Calif.: Hunter House, 1988. A brief but highly readable and informative book. Contains both theories of aging and practical applications. A useful glossary and an extensive bibliography are included.

Fries, James F. *Aging Well*. Reading, Mass.: Addison-Wesley, 1989. Offers precise explanations of all age-related changes and ways to prevent or cope with them. The format of the book makes information very easy to locate.

Kahn, Carol. *Beyond the Helix: DNA and the Quest for Longevity*. New York: Times Books, 1985. The story of the scientists working at laboratories throughout the United States to discover why organisms age and whether one can retard the aging process. Explains highly technical material in an exciting, comprehensible manner for the layperson.

Kart, Cary S., Eileen K. Metress, and Seamus P. Metress. *Aging, Health, and Society*. Boston: Jones and Bartlett, 1988. An introduction to the basic health concerns of older people. Includes some social and psychological aspects of aging. Each chapter contains a lengthy bibliography.

Rossman, Isadore. *Looking Forward: The Complete Medical Guide to Successful Aging*. New York: E. P. Dutton, 1989. Offers sound medical advice on the prevention of most of the ills that can afflict the elderly. Contains reprints of innumerable, pertinent magazine and journal articles. Written in a warm, direct, personal style.

Rusting, Ricki L. "Why Do We Age?" *Scientific American* 267 (December, 1992): 130. An excellent summary of significant experiments in the 1980's and projected research in the 1990's on the genetic and biochemical causes of aging.

Spence, Alexander P. *Biology of Human Aging*. Englewood Cliffs, N.J.: Prentice-Hall, 1989. A general overview of the aging process. Spence makes a clear distinction between normal age-related changes and possible age-related dysfunctions. Contains a very thorough bibliography.

Weiss, Robert, and Genell J. Subak-Sharpe, eds. *Complete Guide to Health and Well-Being After Fifty*. New York: Times Books, 1988. An excellent volume sponsored by the Columbia University School of Public Health. Contains a clear, complete explanation of the aging process and what one can do to remain healthier to a more advanced age. Each chapter includes extensive lists of further resources.

AIDS. *See* ACQUIRED IMMUNODEFICIENCY SYNDROME (AIDS).

ALBINISM

SYSTEMS AFFECTED: Skin, visual

SPECIALISTS: Dermatologists, geneticists, ophthalmologists

DEFINITION: An inherited defect in the production of melanin, albinism is a rare condition characterized by a lack of pigmentation. Oculocutaneous albinism, the more common type, affects the skin and the eyes. Whites affected with albinism have extremely pale skin and white or yellow hair, and blacks with the defect have very light brown skin and hair that is white, slightly yellow, or yellowish brown. Albinos with a less severe form of the disorder may experience some darkening of the skin and hair with age. Albinism causes such eye problems as myopia (nearsightedness), squinting, and photophobia (dislike of bright light), but its main danger is to the skin: Albinos have no melanin to protect them from the sun's harmful radiation and often develop skin cancers. *See also* Skin cancer; Skin disorders.

ALCOHOLISM

SYSTEMS AFFECTED: Psychic-emotional, liver, brain, nervous

SPECIALISTS: Family physicians, internists, psychiatrists, psychologists

DEFINITION: The compulsive drinking of and dependency on alcoholic beverages; viewed as psychological in origin, it can be arrested but not cured.

KEY TERMS:

cerebral cortex: the outer part of the cerebrum, responsible for higher nervous functions

cirrhosis: chronic liver disease; its symptoms include nonfunctional tissue, blocked blood circulation, liver failure, and death

delirium tremens: severe alcohol withdrawal syndrome, with symptoms including confusion, delirium, terrifying hallucinations, and severe tremors

distillation: the use of heat to separate mixtures of liquid chemicals that boil at different temperatures by vaporization and cooling back into the liquid state

Korsakoff's psychosis: brain damage that may require hospitalization because of disorientation and impaired or false memory

manic-depressive syndrome: a psychosis involving rapid alternations between extreme elation and depression

metabolism: the chemical and physical processes involved in the interconversion of foods and the maintenance of life

proof: a designation of beverage alcohol content; divided by two, it approximates the percentage of alcohol present

psychosis: a severe mental disorder characterized by loss of normal intellectual and social function and withdrawal from reality

substance abuse: the overuse of a controlled substance that causes physical dependence and psychological abnormality

CAUSES AND SYMPTOMS

The basis for alcoholism is compulsive abuse of alcoholic beverages. It probably began in antiquity after prehistoric humans discovered that fruit or grain, mashed and suspended in water, fermented into beverages that produced euphoria in users. The first recorded production of fermented beverages was of beer and wine in ancient Babylon and Egypt, respectively.

The active ingredient in fermented beverages is ethyl alcohol (alcohol), a colorless, mild-smelling liquid that boils at 79 degrees Celsius. Alcohol content in such beverages is indicated as "proof." If divided by two, the proof number indicates the approximate percentage of alcohol present. For example, 20-proof wine contains about 10 percent alcohol. In contrast, 80-proof brandy and vodka—"hard liquors"—contain about 40 percent alcohol, because such hard liquors have been "fortified" by adding pure alcohol prepared via distillation.

Substance abuse of alcoholic beverages first became epidemic during the Middle Ages, when development of widespread alcohol distillation produced hard liquors and made it easy to attain alcoholic euphoria and stupor. In 1992, it was estimated that nearly 70 percent of Americans used alcoholic beverages, that more than ten million such people were involved in the severe substance abuse of alcohol, and that about 250,000 alcohol-related deaths occur each year.

Some deaths attributable to alcohol occur as a result of its excessive consumption in a short time period. The drug depresses the action of the central nervous system, creating the desired euphoric effects of alcohol consumption. Given a drink or two, a drinker becomes relaxed and uninhibited. A few more drinks, however, further depress the central nervous system, causing lack of coordination, slurred speech, and stuporous sleep. If just a little more alcohol is imbibed before stupor occurs, further depression of the central nervous system stops breathing and kills.

People engaged in substance abuse of alcohol, alcoholics, carry out repeated, compulsive abuse that may make them unable to retain their jobs, to obtain an education, or to engage in responsible societal roles. Eventually, alcoholics damage their brains and other body tissues irreversibly.

Often, they die of these afflictions or by suicide triggered by depression or terrifying hallucinations. They also engage in crimes that range from driving under the influence to armed robbery and murder. It is estimated that more than half of all motor vehicle accidents are caused by drunk drivers.

Unlike nonalcoholics, once an alcoholic takes a single drink, all self-control vanishes and a drinking spree begins that ends only in stupor, when intoxication is complete. Chronic alcoholism damages many body organs. Best known is brain damage: Mental disorders caused by injury to the cerebral hemispheres may include delirium tremens (the D.T.'s) and Korsakoff's psychosis. Both the D.T.'s, characterized by hallucination and other psychotic symptoms, and Korsakoff's psychosis, which is accompanied by huge memory loss and the lies manufactured to cover this loss, may be accompanied by severe physical debility requiring hospitalization.

In addition, alcoholism damages the liver (causing potentially fatal cirrhosis), the kidneys, the heart, and the pancreas. In fact, a large number of instances of diseases of these other organs are thought to arise from alcohol abuse. Also, much evidence suggests that alcoholism, which impairs the immune system, greatly enhances the incidence of mouth and throat cancer resulting from smoking tobacco.

Severe effects in the liver occur because most ingested alcohol is metabolized there. In the presence of alcohol, most other substances normally metabolized by the liver—the factory bloc of the body—are not changed into the useful and essential forms made in nonalcoholics. One example has to do with fat, a major dietary source of energy. Decreased fat metabolism in the livers of alcoholics results in the fat accumulation—a fatty liver—that precedes cirrhosis of the liver. Cirrhosis results in the replacement of liver cells with nonfunctional fibrous tissue.

Another problem that results from excessive alcohol metabolism is that the liver no longer destroys the many other toxic chemicals that are eaten. This defect adds to problems seen in cirrhosis and leads to dissemination of such chemicals through the body, where they can damage other body parts. In addition, resistance to the flow of blood through the alcoholic liver develops, which can burst blood vessels and cause dangerous internal bleeding. As a consequence of these problems, alcoholic liver disease, or cirrhosis, has become a major, worldwide cause of death from disease.

There is no clear physical explanation for the development of alcoholism. Most often, it is viewed as the result of social problems and psychological stresses, especially in those socioeconomic groups in which consumption of alcoholic beverages is equated with manliness or sophistication. Other proposed causes of behaviors that lead to alcoholism include domineering parents, adolescent peer pressure, personal feelings of inadequacy, loneliness, job pressures, and marital discord.

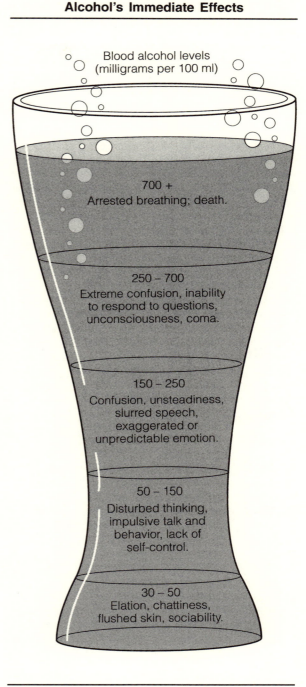

Alcohol's Immediate Effects

Blood alcohol levels
(milligrams per 100 ml)

700 +
Arrested breathing; death.

250 – 700
Extreme confusion, inability
to respond to questions,
unconsciousness, coma.

150 – 250
Confusion, unsteadiness,
slurred speech,
exaggerated or
unpredictable emotion.

50 – 150
Disturbed thinking,
impulsive talk and
behavior, lack of
self-control.

30 – 50
Elation, chattiness,
flushed skin, sociability.

The presence of 30-50 milligrams of alcohol per every 100 milliliters of blood, which represents the effects of an average drink (a glass of beer, wine, or an ounce of hard liquor), has immediate effects; as the amount increases, effects progress toward death.

The fact that 20 percent of children of alcoholics tend to develop the disease, compared to 4 percent of the children of nonalcoholics, has led to investigations of the genetic proclivity for alcoholism. The fact that 80 percent of the progeny of alcoholic parents escape alcoholism, however, diminishes support for such theories. On the other hand, there are clearer indications that genetic factors are important to distaste for alcohol, precluding the development of alcoholism in some ethnic and national groups.

Another disease attributable to alcoholism is fetal alcohol syndrome, which occurs in many children of mothers who drank heavily during pregnancy. Such children may be hyperactive, mentally retarded, and facially disfigured, and they may exhibit marked growth retardation. Fetal alcohol syndrome is becoming more frequent as alcohol consumption increases worldwide.

Commonly observed symptoms of alcoholism are physical dependence on alcohol consumption shown by tremor, shakes, other physical discomfort, and excitability reversed only by alcohol intake; blackout and accompanying memory loss; diminished cognitive ability, exhibited as an inability to understand verbal instructions or to memorize simple series of numbers; and relaxed social inhibitions. These symptoms are attributable to the destruction of tissues of the central nervous system. Diminished sexual activity and sexual desire, especially in men, may also result

from excessive alcohol consumption. A high level of alcohol appears to trigger a significant decrease in the production of the male hormone testosterone, causing diminished libido and impotence. In addition, alcohol may even increase the rate of destruction of existing testosterone in the body. In some cases, the combined effect of lowered testosterone production and the increased destruction of this hormone is feminization of appearance in male alcoholics.

TREATMENT AND THERAPY

There is no known cure for alcoholism. As noted by Diane M. Riley and her coauthors in their article "Behavioral Treatment of Alcohol Problems: A Review and Comparison of Behavioral and Nonbehavioral Studies," in *The Treatment and Prevention of Alcohol Problems* (1987),

> treatments for alcohol problems with demonstrated enduring effectiveness do not exist, regardless of treatment orientations or goals. It is a disease that can be handled only by total abstinence from alcoholic beverages, all medications that contain alcohol, and any other potential sources of alcohol in the diet.

A single contact with alcohol derived from any source usually leads to relapse.

The recognition of alcoholism as a medical problem has led to the establishment of alcoholic rehabilitation centers, where combined psychiatric treatment, medication, and

Alcohol's Long-Term Effects

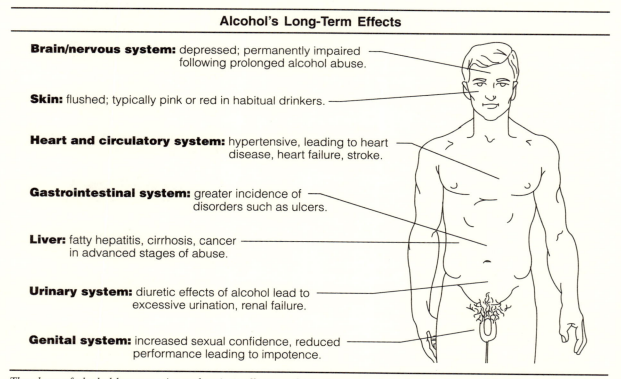

Brain/nervous system: depressed; permanently impaired following prolonged alcohol abuse.

Skin: flushed; typically pink or red in habitual drinkers.

Heart and circulatory system: hypertensive, leading to heart disease, heart failure, stroke.

Gastrointestinal system: greater incidence of disorders such as ulcers.

Liver: fatty hepatitis, cirrhosis, cancer in advanced stages of abuse.

Urinary system: diuretic effects of alcohol lead to excessive urination, renal failure.

Genital system: increased sexual confidence, reduced performance leading to impotence.

The abuse of alcohol has extensive and serious effects on the body; unarrested, alcohol abuse will lead inevitably to death.

physical therapy are used in widely different combinations. The psychosocial programs of the organization Alcoholics Anonymous are also viewed as effective deterrents to a return to alcohol abuse.

In the mid-1930's, alcoholism, previously viewed as criminal behavior, was first conceived to be a disease. The resulting study of alcoholism has made it clear that complete abstinence from alcohol is the only hope for most alcoholics. There are three main means for accomplishing this goal: the use of chemicals that make drinking very unpleasant or facilitate withdrawal from alcohol abuse; membership in an organization such as Alcoholics Anonymous; and enrollment at an alcohol rehabilitation center.

Two well-known medical treatments for enforcing sobriety are the drugs disulfiram (Antabuse) and citrated calcium carbonate (Abstem). These drugs are given to alcoholics who wish to avoid all use of alcoholic beverages and who require a deterrent to drinking to achieve this goal. Neither drug should ever be given secretly by well-meaning family or friends because of the serious dangers that Antabuse and Abstem pose if an alcoholic backslides and drinks alcohol.

These dangers are the result of the biochemistry of alcohol utilization via the two enzymes (biological protein catalysts) alcohol dehydrogenase and aldehyde dehydrogenase. Normally, alcohol dehydrogenase converts alcohol to the toxic chemical acetaldehyde, and aldehyde dehydrogenase quickly converts the acetaldehyde to acetic acid, the main biological fuel on which the body runs. Either Abstem or Antabuse will turn off aldehyde dehydrogenase and cause acetaldehyde levels to build up in the body when alcohol is consumed. The presence of acetaldehyde in the body then quickly leads to violent headache, great dizziness, heart palpitation, nausea, and vertigo. When the amount of alcohol found in a drink or two (or even the amount taken in cough medicine) is consumed in the presence of either drug, these symptoms can escalate to the extent that they become fatal.

An interesting sidelight is the view of many researchers that abstinence from alcohol may be genetically related to the presence of too much alcohol dehydrogenase and/or too little aldehyde dehydrogenase in the body. Either of these unbalanced conditions is thought to produce enough acetaldehyde from a small amount of any alcohol source to cause aversion to all alcohol consumption. This is viewed as particularly relevant in Japan, where about 50 percent of the population lacks aldehyde dehydrogenase, and this lack correlates well with the low predisposition of many Japanese to become alcoholics.

Other therapeutic drugs utilized to treat alcoholics are lithium (more often given to the manic-depressive psychiatric patient), tranquilizers, and sedative hypnotics. The function of these psychoactive drugs is to diminish the discomfort of alcohol withdrawal. Lithium treatment, which must be done with great care because it can become very toxic, appears to be effective only in the alcoholics who drink because of depression or manic-depressive psychosis.

The use of tranquilizers and the related sedative hypnotics must also be done with great care, under close supervision of a physician. Many such drugs are addictive, and their abuse will often substitute another drug for alcohol. In addition, some of these psychoactive drugs have strong synergistic (additive) effects when mixed with alcohol, and such synergism can be fatal if alcoholics backslide during therapy. Detailed information on the uses and dangers of these therapeutic drugs in the treatment of alcoholism can be found in *The Merck Manual of Diagnosis and Therapy* (1987), edited by Robert Berkow and Andrew J. Fletcher.

It is believed that the advent of Alcoholics Anonymous in the 1930's has been crucial to the successful treatment of alcoholism. This organization operates on the premise that abstinence is the best course of treatment for alcoholism—an incurable disease that can, however, be arrested by the cessation of all alcohol intake. The methodology of the organization is psychosocial. First, alcoholics are brought to the realization that they can never use alcoholic beverages without succumbing to alcoholism. Then, the need for help from a "higher power" is identified as crucial to abstinence. In addition, the organization develops a support group of people in the same situation. As stated by Andrew M. Mecca in *Alcoholism in America* (1980), "Alcoholics Anonymous never pronounces the disease as cured. . . . [I]t is arrested." More detailed information on Alcoholics Anonymous is found in most of the bibliography citations for this article.

Estimates of the membership of Alcoholics Anonymous in 1992 ranged between 1.5 and 4 million, meaning up to one-third of American alcoholics were affected by its tenets. These people, ranging widely in age, achieve results varying from periods of sobriety (lasting longer and longer as membership in the organization continues) to lifelong sobriety. A deficit of the sole utilization of Alcoholics Anonymous for alcoholism treatment—in the opinion of some experts—is lack of medical, psychiatric, and trained sociological counseling. The results of the operation, however, are viewed by most as extremely beneficial to all parties who seek help from the organization.

Alcohol rehabilitation centers apply varied combinations of drug therapy, psychiatric counseling, and social counseling, depending on the treatment approach for the individual center. The great value of the psychiatrist in alcoholism therapy can be identified from various sources, including David H. Knott's *Alcohol Problems: Diagnosis and Treatment* (1986). Knott points out that, while psychotherapists cannot perform miracles, psychotherapy can be very valuable in helping the alcoholic patient. It can identify the factors leading to "destructive use of alcohol," explore and help to rectify the problems associated with inability to abstain from alcohol abuse, provide emotional support that helps patients to rebuild their lives, and refer patients to Alcoholics Anonymous and other long-term support efforts. The psychotherapist also has experience with psychoactive drugs, understands behavioral modification techniques, and can determine whether an individual requires institutionalization.

Knott and others also point out the importance of behavior modification as a cornerstone of alcoholism psychotherapy and make it clear that many choices are available to all alcoholics desiring psychosocial help. An interesting point made by several sources is that autopsy and a variety of other sophisticated medical techniques, including CT (computed tomography) and PET (positron emission tomography) scans, identify the atrophy of the cerebral cortex of the brain in many alcoholics. This damage—and cortical damage that is not extensive enough to see with existing technology—is viewed as participating in the inability of alcoholics to stop drinking, their loss of both cognitive and motor skills, and the eventual development of serious conditions such as Korsakoff's psychosis and the D.T.'s.

PERSPECTIVE AND PROSPECTS

Modern efforts to deal with alcoholism are often considered to have begun in the early twentieth century, with the activities of the American temperance movement and the Anti-saloon League. These activities culminated in the period called Prohibition after Congress passed the 1919 Volstead Act, proposed by Minnesota congressman Andrew J. Volstead. The idea behind the act was that making intoxicating beverages impossible to obtain would force sobriety on Americans. Prohibition turned out to be self-defeating, however, and several sources point out that it increased the incidence of alcoholism. Subsequently, the act was repealed in 1933, ending Prohibition.

The next, and much more useful, effort to combat alcoholism was the psychosocial Alcoholics Anonymous organization, started in 1935 by William Griffith Wilson and Robert Holbrook Smith. Because that organization does not reach the majority of alcoholics, other efforts have evolved as treatment methodologies. Among these have been psychiatric counseling, alcohol rehabilitation centers, family counseling, and alcohol management programs in the workplace. These endeavors, funded by the federal government and private industry, reached workable levels in the last quarter of the twentieth century.

Alcoholics Anonymous and all the other options for treating alcoholism, alone or in various combinations, have had considerable success in reaching alcoholics, and combined alcoholism therapy seems to work best. It has not yet been possible to cure the disease, however, partly because there is no clear understanding of the cause of alcoholism. It is obvious that solving the riddle of alcoholism is essential because of its epidemic proportions. Frightening observations of the late twentieth century were estimates that up to 25 percent of American teenagers got drunk weekly and that 50 percent of alcoholics were children of alcoholic par-

ents. The main hope for curing alcoholism is ongoing basic research in the areas of biochemistry, pharmacology, and physiology. —*Sanford S. Singer*

See also Addiction; Cirrhosis; Dementia; Fetal alcohol syndrome; Intoxication; Jaundice; Liver disorders; Manic-depressive disorder; Psychosis.

FOR FURTHER INFORMATION:

Becker, Charles E. "Pharmacotherapy in the Treatment of Alcoholism." In *The Diagnosis and Treatment of Alcoholism*, edited by J. H. Mendelson and N. K. Mello. New York: McGraw-Hill, 1979. This article describes the uses and pitfalls of therapeutic drugs. Topical coverage includes managing intoxication, alcohol withdrawal syndrome, and related problems; chronic assistance; and handling depression in patients.

Bennett, Abram E. *Alcoholism and the Brain*. New York: Stratton International Medical Book, 1977. The relationships between brain function and alcoholism as a brain disease are considered. Coverage includes alcohol action in the brain; tests for alcoholism-related brain disease; constructive relationships between psychiatry and other alcoholism treatments; and rehabilitation methodology.

Berkow, Robert, and Andrew J. Fletcher, eds. *The Merck Manual of Diagnosis and Therapy*. 13th ed. Rahway, N.J.: Merck Sharp & Dohme Research Labs, 1977. This book contains a compendium of data on the etiology, diagnosis, and treatment of alcoholism. Contains good cross-references to the psychopathology related to the disease, drug rehabilitation, and Alcoholics Anonymous. Designed for physicians, it is also valuable to less specialized readers.

Collins, R. Lorraine, Kenneth E. Leonard, and John R. Searles, eds. *Alcohol and the Family*. New York: Guilford Press, 1990. This book is divided into genetics, family processes, and family-oriented treatment. Genetic testing and markers are well covered, and adolescent drinking, children of alcoholics, and alcoholism's effect on a marriage are also discussed. Evaluates the ability of the family to cope with stresses of alcoholism and its treatment.

Cox, W. Miles, ed. *The Treatment and Prevention of Alcohol Problems: A Resource Manual*. Orlando, Fla.: Academic Press, 1987. This work contains much information on the psychiatric and behavioral aspects of alcoholism. It is also widely useful in many other related issues, including Alcoholics Anonymous, marital and family therapy, and alcoholism prevention.

Eskelson, Cleamond D. "Hereditary Predisposition for Alcoholism." In *Diagnosis of Alcohol Abuse*, edited by Ronald R. Watson. Boca Raton, Fla.: CRC Press, 1989. This article provides useful data on the genetic aspects of alcoholism, concentrating on metabolism, animal and human studies, teetotalism, familial alcoholism, and genetic markers. Sixty-five references are included.

Knott, David H. *Alcohol Problems: Diagnosis and Treatment*. New York: Pergamon Press, 1986. This book provides physicians with useful information. Topics include alcohol use and abuse; biochemical factors; epidemiology, diagnosis, and treatment; information on special populations affected by the disease; and perspectives on control and prevention.

Mecca, Andrew M. *Alcoholism in America: A Modern Perspective*. Belvedere, Calif.: California Health Research Foundation, 1980. Entertaining reading about the history of alcoholic beverages, the nature of alcoholism, its effects on the body, its treatment, community alcoholism prevention, and future perspectives. Includes a useful glossary.

Riley, Diane M., Linda C. Sobell, Gloria I. Leo, Mark B. Sobell, and Felix Klajner. "Behavioral Treatment of Alcohol Problems: A Review and a Comparison of Behavioral and Nonbehavioral Studies." In *The Treatment and Prevention of Alcohol Problems: A Resource Manual*, edited by W. Miles Cox. Orlando, Fla.: Academic Press, 1987. State-of-the-art behavioral treatment of alcoholism and the efficacy of existent and future treatments are evaluated. Included are sections on behavioral treatment, relaxation training, skills training, marital and family training, contingency management, self-management, nonbehavioral treatment, and future prospects. More than two hundred references are given.

Rix, Keith J. B., and Elizabeth Lumsden Rix. *Alcohol Problems: A Guide for Nurses and Other Health Professionals*. Bristol, England: John Wright and Sons, 1983. This book, with more than two hundred references, provides nurses with "information that will contribute to . . . improved education." Contains information on the causes of alcoholism, its epidemiology, characteristics of alcohol intoxication and withdrawal, medical treatment, psychosocial aspects, and intervention models.

Watson, Ronald R., ed. *Diagnosis of Alcohol Abuse*. Boca Raton, Fla.: CRC Press, 1989. This work contains chapters on various aspects of alcoholism research. They include basic science issues in biochemistry, genetics, enzymology, and nutrition. Other topics covered are the diagnosis of alcoholic liver disease, the identification of problem drinkers, and alcohol testing and screening.

ALLERGIES

SYSTEM AFFECTED: Immune

SPECIALISTS: Allergists, family physicians, immunologists, internists

DEFINITION: Hyperimmune reactions to materials that are intrinsically harmless; the body's release of pharmacologically active chemicals during allergic reactions may result in discomfort, tissue damage, or, in severe responses, death.

KEY TERMS:

allergen: any substance that induces an allergic reaction

anaphylaxis: an immediate immune reaction, triggered by mediators that cause vasodilation and the contraction of smooth muscle

basophil: a type of white blood cell which contains mediators associated with allergic reactions; represents approximately 1 percent of total white cells

histamine: a compound released during allergic reactions which causes many of the symptoms of allergies

IgE: a type of antibody associated with the release of granules from basophils and mast cells

mast cell: a tissue cell with granules containing vasoactive mediators such as histamine, serotonin, and bradykinin; the tissue equivalent of basophil

CAUSES AND SYMPTOMS

Allergies represent inappropriate immune responses to intrinsically harmless materials, or antigens. Most allergens are common environmental antigens. Approximately one in every six Americans is allergic to material such as dust, cigarette smoke, animal dander, or pollen. The effects range from a mere nuisance, such as the rhinitis associated with hay fever allergies or the itching of poison ivy, to the life-threatening anaphylactic shock that may follow a bee sting. Allergies are most often found in children, but they may affect any age group.

Allergies are generally classified according to the types of effector molecules that mediate their symptoms and according to the time delay that follows exposure to the allergen. P. G. H. Gell and Robin Coombs defined four types of hypersensitivities. Three of these, Types I through III, follow minutes to hours after the exposure to an allergen. Type IV, or delayed-type hypersensitivity (DTH), may occur anywhere from twenty-four to seventy-two hours after exposure. People are most familiar with two of these forms of allergies: Type I, or immediate hypersensitivity, commonly seen as hay fever or asthma; and Type IV, most often following an encounter with poison ivy or poison oak.

Type I hypersensitivities have much in common with any normal immune response. A foreign material, an allergen, comes in contact with the host's immune system, and an antibody response is the result. The response differs according to the type of molecule produced. A special class of antibody, IgE, is secreted by the B lymphocytes. IgE, when complexed with the specific allergen, is capable of binding to any of several types of mediator cells, mainly basophils and mast cells.

Mast cells are found throughout skin and tissue. The mucous membranes of the respiratory and gastrointestinal tract in particular have high concentrations of these cells, as many as ten thousand cells per cubic millimeter. Basophils, the blood cell equivalents of the mast cells, represent 1 percent of the total white-cell count. Though the cells are not identical, they do possess features related to the role that they play in an allergic response. Both basophils and mast cells contain large numbers of granules composed of pharmacologically active chemicals. Both also contain surface re-

The Body's Response to Allergens

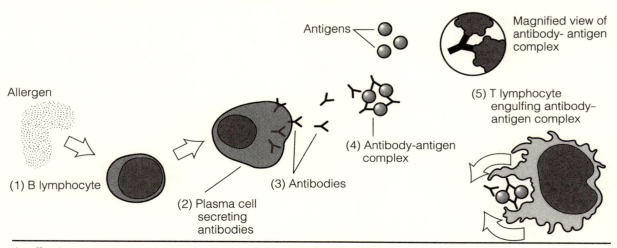

An allergic reaction is caused when foreign material, or antigens, enter the immune system, which produces (1) B lymphocytes that (2) cause blood plasma cells to secrete antibodies. The (3) antibodies link with antigens to form (4) antigen-
antibody complexes, which then are engulfed and destroyed by (5) a T lymphocyte.

ceptors for IgE molecules. The binding of IgE/allergen complexes to these cells triggers the release of the granules.

A large number of common antigens can be associated with allergies. These include plant pollens (as are found in rye grass or ragweed), foods such as nuts or eggs, bee or wasp venom, mold, or animal dander. A square mile of ragweed may produce as much as 16 tons of pollen in a single season. In fact, almost any food or environmental substance could serve as an allergen. The most important defining factor as to whether an individual is allergic to any particular substance is the extent and type of IgE production against that substance.

Type I allergic reactions begin as soon as the person is exposed to the allergen. In the case of hay fever, this results when the person inhales the pollen particle. The shell of the particle is enzymatically dissolved, and the specific allergens are released in the vicinity of the mucous membranes in the respiratory system. If the person has had prior sensitization to the materials, IgE molecules secreted by localized lymphocytes bind to the allergens, forming an antibody/antigen complex.

Events commonly associated with allergies to pollen—a runny nose and itchy, watery eyes—result from the formation of such complexes. A sequence of events is set in place when the immune complexes bind to the surface of the mast cell or basophil. The reactions begin with a cross-linking of the IgE receptors on the cell. Such cross-linking is necessary because, in its absence, no release of granules occurs. On the other hand, artificial cross-linking of the receptors in laboratory experiments, even in the absence of IgE, results in the release of vasoactive granules.

Following the activation of the cell surface, a series of biochemical events occurs, the key being an influx of calcium into the cell. Two events rapidly follow: The cell begins production of prostaglandins and leukotrienes, two mediators that play key roles in allergic reactions, and preexisting granules begin moving toward the cell surface. When they reach the cell surface, the granules fuse with the cell membrane, releasing their contents into the tissue.

The contents of the granules mediate the clinical manifestations of allergies. These mediators can be classified as either primary or secondary. Primary mediators are those found in preexisting granules and that are released initially following the activities at the cell surface. They include substances such as histamine and serotonin, associated with increased vascular permeability and smooth muscle contraction. Histamine itself may constitute 10 percent of the weight of the granules in these cells. The result is the runny nose, irritated eyes, and bronchial congestion with which so many are familiar. Secondary mediators are synthesized following the binding of the immune complexes to the cell surface. These substances include the leukotrienes (also called slow reactive substances of anaphylaxis, or SRS-A) and prostaglandins. Pharmacological effects from these chemicals include vasodilation, increased capillary permeability, and contraction of smooth muscles in the bronchioles.

Foods to which one is allergic may trigger similar reactions in the gut. Mast cells in the gastrointestinal tract also contain receptors for IgE, and contact with food allergens results in the release of mediators similar to those in the respiratory passages. The result may be vomiting or diarrhea. The allergen may also pass from the gut into the circulation or other tissues, triggering asthmatic attacks or ur-ticaria (hives).

In severe allergic reactions, the response may be swift and deadly. The venom released during a bee sting may trigger a systemic response from circulating basophils or mast cells, resulting in the contraction of pulmonary mus-cles and rapid suffocation, a condition known as anaphy-lactic shock. The leukotrienes and prostaglandins play key roles in these reactions.

Delayed-type hypersensitivities, also known as contact dermatitis reactions, are most commonly manifested follow-ing the presentation of a topical allergen. These may include the catechol-containing oils of poison oak, the constituents of hair dyes or cosmetics, environmental contaminants such as nickel or turpentine, or any of a wide variety of environ-mental agents. Rather than being mediated by antibodies, as are the other types of hypersensitivities, DTH is medi-ated through a specific cellular response. These cells appear to be a special class of T (for thymus-derived) lymphocytes.

DTH reactions are initiated following the exposure to the appropriate antigen. Antigen-presenting cells in the skin bind and "present" the allergen to the specific T lymphocytes. This results in the secretion by these T cells of a variety of chemicals mediating inflammation. These mediators, or cy-tokines, include gamma interferon, interleukin-2, and tumor necrosis factor. The result, developing over a period of twenty four to seventy-two hours, is a significant inflamma-tory response with subsequent localized damage to tissue.

The other classes of hypersensitivity reactions, Types II and III, are less commonly associated with what most peo-ple consider to be allergies. Yet they do have much in com-mon with Type I, immediate hypersensitivity. Type II reac-tions are mediated by a type of antibody called IgG. Clinical manifestations result from the antibody-mediated destruction of target cells, rather than through the release of mediators. One of the most common forms of reaction is blood transfusion reactions, either against the A, B, or O antigen blood groups or as a result of an Rh incompati-bility. For example, if a person with type O blood is acci-dentally transfused with type A, an immune reaction will occur. The eventual result is destruction of the incompatible blood. Rh incompatibilities are most commonly associated with a pregnant woman who is lacking the Rh protein on her blood (that is, Rh negative) carrying a child who is Rh positive (a blood type obtained from the father's genes). The production of IgG directed against the Rh protein on the child's blood can set in motion events that result in the destruction of the baby's blood, a condition known as erythroblastosis fetalis.

Type III reactions are known as immune complex dis-eases. In this case, sensitivity to antigens results in forma-tion of IgG/antigen complexes, which can lodge in the kid-ney or other sites in the body. The complexes activate what is known as the complement system, a series of proteins which include vasoactive chemicals and lipolytic com-pounds. The result can be significant inflammation or kid-ney damage. Type III reactions can include autoimmune diseases such as arthritis or lupus, or drug reactions such as penicillin allergies.

It should be kept in mind, however, that none of these reactions is inherently abnormal. Under normal circum-stances, these same reactions mediate an inflammatory de-fense against foreign pathogens. For example, the normal role of IgE appears to be associated with the destruction of parasites such as are found in helminthic infections (such as parasitic worms). The release of mediators under these conditions is important as a defensive reaction leading to the destruction of such agents. It is only when these same mediators are released inappropriately that one observes the symptoms of allergies.

Most individuals are familiar with immediate hypersen-sitivities as reactions involving a localized area. The most common form of allergy is rhinitis, known as hay fever, which affects approximately 10 percent of the population. When a person inhales an environmental allergen such as ragweed pollen, the result is a release of pharmacologically active mediators from mast cells located in the upper res-piratory tract. If the release occurs in the lower respiratory tract, the condition is known as asthma. In both instances, the eyes and nose are subject to inflammation and the re-lease of water. In mild cases, the person suffers from watery discharges, coughing, and sneezing. In more severe asthma attacks, the bronchioles may become constricted and ob-struct the air passages.

TREATMENT AND THERAPY

There exist three methods for dealing with allergies: avoidance of the allergen, palliative treatments, and desen-sitization. Ideally, one can attempt to avoid the allergen. For example, cow's milk, a common allergen, should not be given to a child at too young an age, and one can stay away from patches of poison ivy or avoid eating strawber-ries if one is allergic to them.

Yet avoidance is not always possible or desirable, as the problem may be the fur from the family cat. In any event, it is sometimes difficult to identify the specific substance causing the symptoms. This is particularly true when dealing with foods. Various procedures exist to identify the irritating substance, skin testing being the most common. In this pro-cedure, the patient's skin is exposed to small amounts of suspected allergens. A positive test is indicated by hives or reddening within about twenty to thirty minutes. If the per-son is hypersensitive to a suspected allergen, the Prausnitz-Kustner, or P-K, test may be substituted. In addition to run-ning a battery of tests, a patient's allergy history (including family history, since allergies are in part genetic) or envi-ronment may give clues as to the identity of the culprit.

The most commonly used method of dealing with aller-gies is a palliative treatment—that is, treatment of the symptoms. Antihistamines act by binding to histamine receptors on target cells, interfering with the binding of histamine. There exist two types of histamine receptors: H-1 and H-2. Histamine binding to H-1 receptors results in contractions of smooth muscles and increased mucous secretion. Binding to H-2 receptors results in increased vasopermeability and swelling. Antihistamines that act at the level of the H-1 receptor include alkylamines and ethanolamines and are effective in treating symptoms of acute allergies such as hay fever. The H-2 blockers such as cimetidine are a newer class of antihistamines and are effective in the symptomatic treatment of duodenal ulcers through the control of gastric secretions.

Many antihistamines can be obtained without a prescription. If they are not used properly, however, the side effects can be serious. Overuse may result in toxicity, particularly in children; overdoses in children can be fatal. Because antihistamines can depress the central nervous system, side effects include drowsiness, nausea, constipation, and drying of the throat or respiratory passage. This is particularly true of H-1 blockers.

Other symptomatic treatments include the use of cromolyn sodium, which blocks the influx of calcium into the mast cell, and of theophylline and adrenaline, both of which act to block steps leading to degranulation and the release of mediators. In more severe cases, the administration of steroids (cortisone) may prove useful in limiting symptoms of allergies.

Anaphylaxis is the most severe form of immediate hypersensitivity, and unless treated promptly, it may be fatal. It is often triggered in susceptible persons by common environmental substances: bee or wasp venom, drugs such as penicillin, or foods such as peanut oil or seafood. Symptoms include labored breathing, rapid loss of blood pressure, itching, hives, and/or loss of bladder control. The symptoms are triggered by the release of mast cell or basophil mediators such as histamine, leukotrienes, or prostaglandin derivatives. Treatment consists of the immediate injection of epinephrine and the maintenance of an open air passage into the lungs. If cardiac arrest occurs, cardiopulmonary resuscitation must be undertaken. Persons in known danger of encountering such a triggering allergen often carry with them an emergency kit containing epinephrine and antihistamines.

Contact dermatitis is a form of delayed-type hypersensitivity, developing several days after exposure to the sensitizing allergen. Rather than resulting from the presence of IgE antibody, the symptoms of contact dermatitis result from a series of chemicals released by sensitized T lymphocytes in the area of the skin on which the allergen (often poison ivy or poison oak) is found. Treatments generally involve the application of topical corticosteroids and soothing or drying agents. In more severe cases, systemic use of corticosteroids may be necessary.

In some persons, the relief of allergy symptoms may be achieved through desensitization. This form of immunotherapy involves the repeated subcutaneous injection of increasing doses of the allergen. In a significant number of persons, such therapy leads to an improvement in symptoms. The idea behind such therapy is that repeated exposure to the allergen may lead to production of another class of antibody, either localized IgA (or secretory antibody) or the more systemic IgG. These molecules can serve as blocking antibodies, competing with IgE in binding to the allergen. Because IgA/allergen or IgG/allergen complexes can be phagocytosed (destroyed by phagocytes) and do not bind receptors on mast cells or basophils, they should not trigger the symptoms of allergies. Unfortunately, for reasons that remain unclear, not all persons or all allergies respond to such therapy.

Immediate hypersensitivity reactions commonly run in families, a fact that is not surprising if one realizes that the level and type of IgE trigger such reactions. These factors, particularly the regulation of IgE production, are genetically determined. Thus, if both parents have allergies, there is little chance that their offspring will escape the problem. On the other hand, if one or both parents are allergy-free, the odds are at least even that the offspring will also be free from such reactions.

PERSPECTIVE AND PROSPECTS

Though allergies in humans have probably existed since humans first evolved from ancestral primates, it was only in the nineteenth century that an understanding of the process began to develop. Type I hypersensitivity reactions were first described in 1839, when dogs repeatedly injected with egg albumin suffered immediate fatal shock. The term "anaphylaxis" was coined for this phenomenon in 1902, when Paul Portier and Charles Richet observed that dogs repeatedly immunized with extracts of sea anemone tentacles suffered a similar fate. Richet was awarded the 1913 Nobel Prize in Physiology or Medicine for his work on anaphylaxis.

In the 1920's, Sir Henry Dale established that at least some of the phenomena associated with immediate hypersensitivity were caused by the chemical histamine. Dale sensitized guinea pigs against various antigens. He then observed that, when the muscles from the uterus were removed and exposed to the same antigen, histamine was released and the muscles underwent contraction (known as the Schultz-Dale reaction).

The existence of a component in human serum which mediates hypersensitive reactions was demonstrated by Otto Prausnitz, a Polish bacteriologist, and Heinz Kustner, a Polish gynecologist, in 1921. Kustner had a strong allergy to fish. Prausnitz removed a sample of serum from his colleague and injected it under his own skin. The next day, Prausnitz injected fish extract in that same region. Hives immediately appeared, indicating that the serum contained components that mediated the allergy. The P-K test has remained a means of testing for allergens under circumstances in which a person cannot be tested directly for sensitivity. In this test, a serum sample from the test subject is injected under the skin of a surrogate (usually a relative) and later followed with test allergens. The presence of a wheal and flare reaction (hives) indicates sensitivity to the allergen. The serum component responsible for this sensitivity was identified as the antibody IgE by K. and T. Ishizaka in 1967. The target cells to which the IgE bound were later identified as mast cells and basophils.

Once the components of the immune system associated with the symptoms of allergies were identified, it became possible to study the reactions at the molecular level. At the very least, by understanding the sequence of events that followed exposure to the allergen, it was feasible to develop therapies that were able to act at various steps along the pathway. Thus, newer and better drugs for intervention were produced.

The eventual goal of the research was to understand the molecular defects that result in allergies and ultimately to find a means to eliminate the problem, rather than simply offer palliative measures. For example, the Ishizakas determined that levels of IgE are in part determined by factors secreted by T lymphocytes. These factors can either raise IgE levels or lower them. By exploring the means of such regulation, it may become possible to inhibit IgE production in allergic persons selectively and without affecting the desired functions of the immune response. —*Richard Adler*

See also Asthma; Dermatitis; Food poisoning.

FOR FURTHER INFORMATION:

Joneja, Janice M. V., and Leonard Bielory. *Understanding Allergy, Sensitivity, and Immunity*. New Brunswick, N.J.: Rutgers University Press, 1990. The authors provide extensive discussion on allergies and the roles played by the immune system. They describe the means by which one can learn to cope with allergies and discuss various testing methods for the identification of allergens. Written for the nonscientist.

Kuby, Janis. *Immunology*. New York: W. H. Freeman, 1992. The section on hypersensitivity in this immunology textbook is well written and includes a mixture of detail and overview of the subject. Particularly useful are discussions of the various types of hypersensitivity reactions. Some knowledge of biology is useful.

Norback, Craig T., ed. *The Allergy Encyclopedia*. New York: Penguin Books, 1981. A concise discussion of allergies and their causes. Much of the book is in the form of questions or terms related to the subject. Describes the symptoms associated with various types of allergies, as well as the role of psychosomatic disorders. Written for the nonscientist.

Roitt, Ivan. *Essential Immunology*. 7th ed. Boston: Blackwell Scientific Publications, 1991. Written by a leading author in the field, the text provides a fine description of immunology. The section on hypersensitivity is clearly presented and profusely illustrated. Though too detailed in places, most of the material can be understood by individuals who have taken high school-level biology. The first choice as a reference for the subject.

Young, Stuart, Bruce Dobozin, and Margaret Miner. *Allergies*. Yonkers, N.Y.: Consumer Reports Books, 1991. An excellent review of the subject from Consumer Reports. In addition to discussing the diagnosis and treatment of allergies, the authors evaluate the various remedies on the market at the time of publication. Also useful are lists of organizations to contact for further information and various clinics that specialize in the treatment of allergies.

ALTITUDE SICKNESS

SYSTEMS AFFECTED: Brain, nervous, respiratory, visual

SPECIALISTS: Aerospace physicians, emergency physicians, neurologists, occupational medicine physicians

DEFINITION: A condition resulting from altitude-related hypoxia (low oxygen levels).

CAUSES AND SYMPTOMS

There are four types of altitude sickness: acute mountain sickness, high-altitude pulmonary edema (HAPE), high-altitude cerebral edema (HACE), and high-altitude retinopathy (HAR). Though most patients have mild symptoms, death is not uncommon in severe cases. Illness is associated with rapid ascent to mountain areas by tourists, skiers, and mountaineers. Residents of mountainous regions are less susceptible because their bodies have adapted to lower oxygen levels. It is estimated that up to one-quarter of tourists skiing in the mountains of the western United States have experienced some manifestations, although mild ones, of altitude sickness.

Acute mountain sickness is characterized by headache, decreased appetite, insomnia, fatigue, nausea, and onset at altitudes above 1,980 meters (6,500 feet). The risk of becoming affected increases with young age, quick ascent, and a past history of acute mountain sickness. Symptoms usually last for a few days. Between 5 and 10 percent of patients with acute mountain sickness progress to HAPE, which occurs when the small pulmonary blood vessels leak, allowing fluid accumulation in the lungs. Mortality from HAPE ranges from 11 to 44 percent. The related condition HACE occurs when fluid accumulation in the brain causes increased pressure within the skull. Neurologic signs such as confusion and coma may be noted.

TREATMENT AND THERAPY

Prevention is crucial to the reduction of morbidity and mortality from altitude sickness. Ascents should be slow, especially when involving physical exertion. Sedatives and salt should be avoided. Most people adapt to altitude changes within three days. Returning to lower altitudes at night is advised. Premedication with acetazolamide, a prescription drug, will hasten adaptation and reduce symptoms. In serious cases, descent to lower altitudes is vital. Corticosteroids, oxygen, and hyperbaric treatments may be used. Chronically ill persons should check with their doctors before attempting strenuous activity at high altitudes.

—Louis B. Jacques

See also Asphyxiation.

FOR FURTHER INFORMATION:

Auerbach, Paul S. *Medicine for the Outdoors.* Boston: Little, Brown, 1986.

Rennie, D. "The Great Breathlessness Mountains." *JAMA* 256 (July 4, 1986): 81-82.

Wilkerson, James A., ed. *Medicine for Mountaineering & Other Wilderness Activities.* 4th ed. Seattle: Mountaineers, 1992.

ALZHEIMER'S DISEASE

SYSTEMS AFFECTED: Brain, nervous

SPECIALISTS: Family physicians, geneticists, geriatric specialists, internists, neurologists, psychiatrists

DEFINITION: The most common cause of dementia in old age, affecting between 3 and 11 percent of those over sixty-five.

KEY TERMS:

agnosia: an inability to recognize persons or various objects even though the patient sees them clearly

anomia: an inability to remember the names of persons or objects even though the patient sees and recognizes the persons or objects

aphasia: difficulty in understanding and talking to other people in the absence of hearing impairment

apraxia: difficulty in carrying out coordinated voluntary activities (such as dressing, undressing, or brushing one's teeth) in the absence of any muscular weakness

benign senescent forgetfulness: a common source of frustration in old age, associated with memory impairment; unlike dementia, it does not interfere with the individual's social and professional activities

brain imaging techniques: tests performed to examine brain anatomy and functioning; these include computed tomography (CT) scans, magnetic resonance imaging (MRI), and single photon emission computed tomography (SPECT)

cognitive deficit: an impairment in mental functions, including anomia, agnosia, aphasia, and apraxia; it is usually associated with an impairment in the ability to make rational decisions

dementia: also called dementing illness; a disease characterized by memory impairment of sufficient severity to interfere with the individual's daily social and professional activities

neuropsychological testing: a series of tests administered by a neuropsychologist to examine the efficiency of various parts of the brain

neurotransmitters: chemical substances inside the brain that allow the flow of electrical impulses from one part of the brain to another; at least five neurotransmitters are absent with Alzheimer's disease

CAUSES AND SYMPTOMS

Alzheimer's disease is the most common dementing illness in old age. In the United States, it is estimated that its prevalence increases from 3 percent in those aged sixty-five to seventy-four years, to 18.7 percent in those seventy-five to eighty-four years of age, to as much as 47.2 percent of those over the age of eighty-five. While both sexes are about equally affected, there are more women than men with Alzheimer's disease because women tend to live longer. As with other dementing illnesses, the characteristic memory impairment initially affects the recent, rather than the remote, memory and interferes with the patient's daily social and professional activities; the patient's attention span is also significantly reduced.

The disease typically has a slow, insidious onset, and a very slow, gradual progress. Caregivers observing this decline are often unable to agree about when the symptoms began to manifest themselves. The memory deficit is usually accompanied by an impaired ability to make good, rational decisions. One of the most common and earliest problems is an inability to take care of one's financial affairs. In addition to being unable to balance a checkbook, the patient may attempt to pay the same bill several times, while disregarding other financial obligations. Similarly, the patient may be overly generous at times and extremely mean on other occasions.

In Alzheimer's disease, the dementing process is also associated with other evidence of cognitive deficit. When anomia is present, patients often use paraphrases to describe various objects because they have difficulty finding the correct words. For example, they may say "milk pourer" instead of "milk jug." This condition is usually present very early in the disease process, but it is often so slight that it may only be detected by neuropsychological testing. Agnosia develops later and can be quite hazardous. For example, a patient may confuse a knife with a comb. As the disease progresses, a patient may develop aphasia and find it difficult to communicate with other people. Finally, the patient develops apraxia, experiencing difficulty carrying out coordinated activities such as dressing or undressing, even though there is no loss of muscular power. The apraxia may also be responsible for unsteadiness, and the patient may fall repeatedly and may become chairbound or bedfast. Anomia, agnosia, aphasia, and apraxia are sometimes referred to as the "four A's" that accompany the memory deficit seen in Alzheimer's disease.

Alzheimer's disease is progressive, and there is much individual variability in the rate of progress. A number of staging classifications, most of them arbitrary, are available. One of the most practical is the three-stage classification.

In stage 1, the memory impairment and degree of cognitive deficit are so slight that patients may still be able to function socially and even professionally, although family members and close associates may have observed strange behavioral patterns. Superficially, the patients may appear "normal," although somewhat eccentric. Although the memory deficit and impaired mental functions are present, patients may use various tricks to mask this deficit. They may ask a partner to keep score of a game they are playing because they have "left their reading glasses at home" or may decline invitations to play card games or socialize altogether. Patients with this disease may also stop engaging in their favorite hobbies and activities. Patients at this stage usually have difficulties balancing their checkbooks. Errors of judgment are not infrequent, although they are initially often attributed by family and friends to age, to eccentricity, or to the patient's having too many things on his or her mind. Patients may buy large quantities of the same item and start hoarding various articles. As time progresses, they may lose their way, and their errors in judgment while driving may result in traffic accidents. One of the main problems in this stage is the inability to learn and retain new information. This mental deficit becomes particularly problematic if the patient's work is being reorganized or if the patient relocates. Agitation, irritability, and anxiety are not uncommon in this stage and probably represent the patient's inability to cope with a loss of control over the environment and a declining mental ability.

In stage 2, the memory impairment, cognitive deficit, and degree of impaired judgment are so great that even a stranger who has never met the patient cannot help but conclude that there is something wrong with the patient's mental functions. In this stage, patients frequently become lost, even in very familiar surroundings, such as in their own houses. They may no longer be able to find their way to the toilet, they may no longer recognize people they know well, and they are unable to take care of their own hygienic needs. They tend to walk aimlessly and wander constantly and are likely to become agitated, irritable, and even aggressive. These symptoms are often pronounced late in the afternoon or early evening and are often referred to as "sundowning syndrome."

In stage 3, in addition to their mental impairment, patients become unsteady on their feet and may sustain repeated falls. Because they have become physically frail, they tend to wander much less and to spend most of their time confined to a chair or bed. They are completely dependent on their caregivers for most activities. Swallowing is often difficult, and feeding through a small tube inserted in the nose (a nasogastric tube) may be required. Patients are at risk of becoming dehydrated and malnourished, and urinary and even fecal incontinence are not uncommon. Mutism gradually sets in, and communication with the patient becomes difficult. Flexion (bending) contractures

gradually develop, and the patient slowly adopts the fetal position, with the arms and knees bent. The development of pressure ulcers, or bedsores, is likely. The common cause of death is septicemia (blood poisoning) resulting from a respiratory tract infection, a urinary tract infection, or an infected pressure ulcer.

Alzheimer's disease is characterized by a loss of brain cells, affecting in particular the cerebral cortex. The brain appears smaller in size and atrophic, with the gyri (grooves) much less prominent and the ventricles (cavities inside the brain) enlarged. Multiple deficiencies in the neurotransmitters, chemical substances inside the brain that carry impulses from one cell to another, have been identified with this disease.

Diagnosis. At present, there are no positive tests available to make a definitive diagnosis of Alzheimer's disease without examining brain tissue under the microscope. Before such a diagnosis can be considered, several factors should be present. First, the memory impairment should be of sufficient magnitude and consistency to interfere with one's social and professional activities, and it should be accompanied by evidence of cognitive deficit and impaired judgment. These are the main differentiating features between Alzheimer's disease and benign senescent forgetfulness, which is also very common in old age. Although the latter can be quite irritating, it does not significantly interfere with the person's professional and social activities and tends to be selective, with one's forgetting only unimportant and relatively trivial matters. The forgetfulness seen in

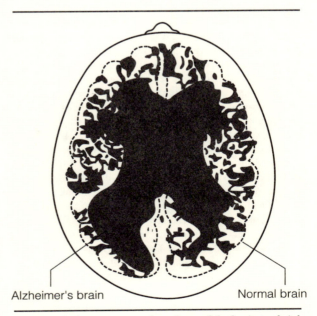

Alzheimer's brain   Normal brain

Alzheimer's disease causes the volume of the brain to shrink substantially.

Alzheimer's disease, on the other hand, is global and does not distinguish between trivial and important matters.

Second, in Alzheimer's disease, the onset of memory impairment is insidious, and the progress is slow. This differentiates it from multiple infarct dementia, which is caused by multiple strokes and which has an abrupt onset and progress marked by bouts of deterioration. Whenever a stroke develops, the patient's condition deteriorates and then stabilizes until the next stroke occurs.

Third, the patient must be alert, not drowsy—one of the main distinctions between Alzheimer's disease and delirium. The latter, in addition to having a sudden onset, is associated with clouding of consciousness, a rambling and incoherent speech, disorganized thinking, hallucinations, and sensory misperceptions.

Finally, as the diagnosis of Alzheimer's disease is still based on a process of exclusion, all other possible causes of impaired mental functions must be ruled out. These causes are numerous and can be conveniently remembered by the mnemonic device DEMENTIA.

The *D* stands for drugs. Older patients are particularly susceptible to the effects of many medications that may impair mental functions. These indications include not only those acting specifically on the brain, such as the sedatives and hypnotics, but also other medications such as those that lower blood pressure. Finally, alcohol is often abused by older people and may significantly interfere with the older person's mental abilities.

The *E* stands for emotional disorders. Depression is very common in old age and may manifest itself with cognitive impairment. Unlike patients with Alzheimer's disease, who except in the very early stages of the disease are not aware of their deficit, those with depression are acutely aware of their problem and often exaggerate it. Often, patients with depression also have a long list of complaints. They lack animation, their appetite is reduced, and they take a diminished interest in their environment and pleasure in their daily activities. Sleep disturbances, in the form of insomnia or increased sleepiness, are common. Although most cases of depression are easily recognized, some may be difficult to diagnose and therefore may require neuropsychological testing to differentiate them from Alzheimer's disease. This differentiation is important, because unlike Alzheimer's disease, depression can be treated, and the outlook is good. Additionally, it is important to emphasize that about 20 percent of patients with Alzheimer's disease have a coexistent depression that often responds to appropriate therapy.

The *M* stands for metabolic disorders. In old age, both overactivity and underactivity of the thyroid gland may be responsible for mental impairment without a patient's exhibiting any of the characteristic clinical features. Dehydration is a common cause of confusion in older patients because their sense of thirst is often reduced. Liver and kidney diseases also may be responsible for impaired mental func-

tions. Similarly, patients with diabetes mellitus are susceptible to a number of metabolic disorders, including an increased or decreased blood sugar level, both of which may cause cognitive impairment. Serum electrolyte disorders also may result in confusional states and can be precipitated by severe vomiting, diarrhea, or the intake of medication. Finally, vitamin B_{12} deficiency may be responsible for impaired mental functions, occasionally without there being any other clinical evidence of this deficiency. Patients who have had a gastrectomy (surgical removal of their stomach) and no vitamin B_{12} replacement are likely to develop B_{12} deficiency a few years after surgery. By this time, however, the patient may have relocated, changed physicians, and probably "forgotten" about the surgery.

The *E* stands for both eyes and ears. For individuals to interact appropriately with others and the environment, they must be aware of the various circumstances surrounding them. If an individual cannot hear properly and guesses at the questions asked, he or she often will not give an appropriate answer and may give the impression of being confused. Hearing impairment is very common among the older population, and often older people choose not to wear a hearing aid because of difficulties manipulating the controls or because of embarrassment. Visual impairment may also interfere with an individual's appropriate interaction with the environment and give the impression of dementia. There are many causes of visual impairment in old age, including glaucoma, cataracts, and macular degeneration (a progressive disorder of the retina).

The *N* stands for neurological disorders; these include other dementias such as multi-infarct dementia and hydrocephalus (increased fluid in the brain).

The *T* stands for both tumors and trauma. A subdural hematoma (a collection of blood inside the skull) may be precipitated by trauma that is usually trivial. The symptoms do not become apparent until a few days or even weeks after the trauma, by which time the patient and caregivers may have forgotten about the physical trauma. Brain tumors may also manifest themselves with impaired mental functions. The computed tomography (CT) scan and magnetic resonance imaging (MRI) are useful tools in diagnosing these conditions.

The *I* stands for infections. Infections, regardless of their location but especially those of the respiratory and urinary tracts, may be associated with confusional states in older people. Unlike younger people, they often do not exhibit a rise in body temperature, thus making the diagnosis of infection difficult. Acquired immunodeficiency syndrome (AIDS) is another cause of dementia that is related to infection; this condition must be suspected when mental functions deteriorate rapidly, especially if the patient has risk factors for AIDS.

The *A* stands for atherosclerosis and includes arteriosclerotic cardiovascular diseases. Older patients who experience myocardial infarction (a "heart attack" caused by a sudden reduction of blood flow to the heart muscle) may not experience any chest pain but may nevertheless develop an acute confusional state. Generalized arteriosclerosis also might be responsible for multiple, small, repeated strokes that can eventually interfere with the patient's cognitive functions.

The accuracy of the clinical diagnosis of Alzheimer's disease can be increased to about 90 percent if a few investigations are conducted. These include a complete blood count, Chem-18 (a series of blood tests to check on the blood levels of many substances and the functioning of the kidneys and liver), thyroid function tests, serum B_{12} measurement, electrocardiogram, and brain imaging tests. Single photon emission computed tomography (SPECT) seems to be a promising test in the diagnosis of Alzheimer's disease and may represent the first step toward being able to make a diagnosis without examining brain tissue microscopically.

TREATMENT AND THERAPY

Although the understanding of the pathophysiology of Alzheimer's disease has increased tremendously since it was first described by Alois Alzheimer in the early years of the twentieth century, this understanding has not been translated into effective therapeutic opportunities. A large number of compounds have been and are being tried for the treatment of Alzheimer's disease but, unfortunately, without any significant degree of success. At present, therefore, it is essentially a disease without a cure.

Nevertheless, many things can be done to aid a patient with Alzheimer's disease. It is important to detect the presence of any other disease that may worsen the patient's condition, and unnecessary medications must be avoided for the same reason. Medication may nevertheless be required to control agitation and the sundowning syndrome. Physicians will generally start with the smallest possible dose of medication and then gradually increase it according to the patient's symptoms.

The patient's environment and daily routine should be left as constant as possible, as any change may precipitate or worsen the symptoms and degree of confusion. The patient should be spared the task of having to choose an option among several ones (such as which dress to wear) and to make decisions (such as which activity in which to become involved). Instead, the daily routine should be as structured as possible and yet retain enough flexibility for the patient to withdraw from any activity that is disliked and to join any that is enjoyed.

The patient with Alzheimer's disease should be treated not in isolation but by caregivers and family members, who will also need support and help if they are to cope effectively with their loved one's illness. Social workers and various community agencies, such as the Area Agency on Aging, can help develop a management program tailored to the individual patient's needs and those of his or her caregivers. A number of community programs are available, and the Alzheimer's Association and support groups are very useful resources. Caregivers and family members should also be given advice concerning financial, legal, and ethical issues, such as obtaining a durable power of attorney and finding out the patient's wishes concerning advance directives prior to incapacitation.

PERSPECTIVE AND PROSPECTS

It is hoped that effective and safe medication to treat Alzheimer's disease specifically will soon become available. An analogy can be made between Alzheimer's disease and Parkinson's disease. Although their signs and symptoms are different, both are associated with a reduction of neurotransmitters in the brain. Scientists have found effective drugs to treat Parkinson's disease, and it is believed it is only a matter of time before a drug will be found to treat Alzheimer's disease as well. —*Ronald C. Hamdy, Louis A. Cancellaro, and Larry Hudgins*

See also Aging; Amnesia and memory loss; Brain disorders; Dementia.

FOR FURTHER INFORMATION:

Coons, Dorothy H., ed. *Specialized Dementia Care Units.* Baltimore: The Johns Hopkins University Press, 1991. Contains articles that assess the treatment of dementia patients in care units designed to address their special needs. The advantages of such specialized care are weighed against the problems that these units encounter.

Cummings, Jeffrey L., and Bruce L. Miller, eds. *Alzheimer's Disease.* New York: Marcel Dekker, 1990. Explores the available therapies for Alzheimer's disease patients, including the management of behavioral symptoms and the need to provide long-term care. The various authors of this edited text also speculate on future treatments for this disease.

Hamdy, Ronald C., J. M. Turnbull, L. D. Norman, and M. M. Lancaster, eds. *Alzheimer's Disease: A Handbook for Caregivers.* St. Louis: C. V. Mosby, 1990. Offers practical advice for researchers and caregivers about how to deal with the patient with Alzheimer's disease or another type of dementia. Presents a thorough discussion of the symptoms of these disorders, as compared to normal brain structure and function and the natural effects of aging.

Howe, M. L., M. J. Stones, and C. J. Brainerd, eds. *Cognitive and Behavioral Performance Factors in Atypical Aging.* New York: Springer-Verlag, 1990. Using younger patients as a point of reference, this work addresses the factors that control brain function and behavior in older individuals.

Terry, Robert D., ed. *Aging and the Brain.* New York: Raven Press, 1988. The structure and function of the brains of both normal elderly people and those with various types of dementias (including Alzheimer's disease) are compared. Reviews the neurobiological and technological concepts developed in the 1980's in this field of study.

U.S. Congress. Office of Technology Assessment. *Confused Minds, Burdened Families: Finding Help for People with Alzheimer's and Other Dementias.* Washington, D.C.: Government Printing Office, 1990. This official government report describes the current system of services in the United States set up to care for those with Alzheimer's disease and other dementias. Details its many inadequacies and presents an alternative vision of a more efficient system, including recommendations for congressional policy options to make it a reality.

U.S. Congress. Office of Technology Assessment. *Losing a Million Minds: Confronting the Tragedy of Alzheimer's Disease and Other Dementias.* Washington, D.C.: Government Printing Office, 1987. Offers a comprehensive assessment of the impact of Alzheimer's disease on the United States, including the psychoeconomic effects of this disease on patients and caregivers, personnel training and quality assurance in public and private programs that serve patients with dementia, and future governmental policies regarding these issues.

West, Robin L., and Jan D. Sinnott, eds. *Everyday Memory and Aging.* New York: Springer-Verlag, 1992. This work discusses the methodology of research into the human memory. Focuses on the changes in memory that occur naturally with age, as well as those that are brought about by various forms of dementia in the older individual.

AMENORRHEA

SYSTEM AFFECTED: Reproductive (female)

SPECIALISTS: Gynecologists

DEFINITION: In girls or women suffering from amenorrhea, menstruation has not occurred or is abnormally suppressed. Primary amenorrhea is diagnosed if a young woman has not experienced menarche (the first menstruation) by the age of eighteen; it may be caused by a hormone imbalance, a tumor in the pituitary or adrenal glands, or an underactive thyroid. Secondary amenorrhea is defined as the cessation of menstruation for at least three months in a woman who has menstruated previously; in addition to the above causes, it may be attributable to rapid weight loss or gain, overly strenuous exercise, prolonged use of oral contraceptives, or emotional trauma. Treatment depends on the cause of the amenorrhea, such as hormone therapy for imbalances, surgery for tumors, or psychiatric counseling for self-destructive behaviors.

See also Menstruation.

AMNESIA AND MEMORY LOSS

SYSTEMS AFFECTED: Brain, psychic-emotional

SPECIALISTS: Geriatric specialists, neurologists, psychiatrists, psychologists

DEFINITION: An impairment of memory which may be total or limited, sudden or gradual.

CAUSES AND SYMPTOMS

Memory impairment is a common problem, especially among older people. It occurs in various degrees and may be associated with other evidence of brain dysfunction. Amnesia is complete memory loss.

Benign forgetfulness. In this condition, the memory deficit affects mostly recent events, and although a source of frustration, it seldom interferes with the individual's professional activities or social life. An important feature of benign forgetfulness is that it is selective and affects only trivial, unimportant facts. For example, one may misplace the car keys or forget to return an unwanted phone call, respond to a letter, or pay a bill. Cashing a check or telephoning someone with whom one is particularly keen to talk, however, will not be forgotten. The person is aware of the memory deficit, and written notes often are used as reminders. Patients with benign forgetfulness have no other evidence of brain dysfunction and maintain their ability to make valid judgments.

Dementia. In dementia, the memory impairment is global, does not discriminate between important and trivial facts, and interferes with the person's ability to pursue professional or social activities. Patients with dementia find it difficult to adapt to changes in the workplace, such as the introduction of computers. They also find it difficult to continue with their hobbies and interests.

The hallmark of dementia is no awareness of the memory deficit, except in the very early stages of the disease. This is an important difference between dementia and benign forgetfulness. Although patients with early dementia may write themselves notes, they usually forget to check these reminders or may misinterpret them. For example, a man with dementia who is invited for dinner at a friend's house may write a note to that effect and leave it in a prominent place. He may then go to his host's home several evenings in succession because he has forgotten that he already has fulfilled this social engagement. As the disease progresses, patients are no longer aware of their memory deficit.

In dementia, the memory deficit does not occur in isolation but is accompanied by other evidence of brain dysfunction, which in very early stages can be detected only by specialized neuropsychological tests. As the condition progresses, these deficits become readily apparent. The patient is often disoriented regarding time and may telephone relatives or friends very late at night. As the disease progresses, the disorientation affects the patient's environment: A woman with dementia may wander outside her house and be unable to find her way back, or she may repeatedly ask to be taken back home when she is already there. In later stages, patients may not be able to recognize people whom they should know: A man may think that his son is his father or that his wife is his mother. This stage is particularly distressing to the caregivers. Patients with dementia may often exhibit impaired judgment. They may go outside the house inappropriately dressed or at inappropriate times, or they may purchase the same item repeatedly or make donations that are disproportional to their funds. Alzheimer's disease is one of the most common causes of dementia in older people.

Multiple infarct dementia. Multiple infarct dementia is caused by the destruction of brain cells by repeated strokes. Sometimes these strokes are so small that neither the patient nor the relatives are aware of their occurrence. When many strokes occur and significant brain tissue is destroyed, the patient may exhibit symptoms of dementia. Usually, however, most of these strokes are quite obvious because they are associated with weakness or paralysis in a part of the body. One of the characteristic features of multiple infarct dementia is that its onset is sudden and its progression is by steps. Every time a stroke occurs, the patient's condition deteriorates. This is followed by a period during which little or no deterioration develops until another stroke occurs, at which time the patient's condition deteriorates further. Very rarely, the stroke affects only the memory center, in which case the patient's sole problem is amnesia. Multiple infarct dementia and dementia resulting from Alzheimer's disease should be differentiated from other treatable conditions which also may cause memory impairment, disorientation, and poor judgment.

Depression. Depression, particularly in older patients, may cause memory impairment. This condition is quite common and at times is so difficult to differentiate from dementia that the term "pseudo-dementia" is used to describe it. One of the main differences between depression that presents the symptoms of dementia and dementia itself is insight into the memory deficit. Whereas patients with dementia are usually oblivious of their deficit and not distressed (except those in the early stages), those with depression are nearly always aware of their deficit and are quite distressed. Patients with depression tend to be withdrawn and apathetic, given a marked disturbance of affect, whereas those with dementia demonstrate emotional blandness and some degree of lability. One of the problems characteristic of depressed patients is their difficulty in concentrating. This is typified by poor cooperation and effort in carrying out tasks with a variable degree of achievement, coupled with considerable anxiety.

Head trauma. Amnesia is sometimes seen in patients who have sustained a head injury. The extent of the amnesia is usually proportional to the severity of the injury. In most cases, the complete recovery of the patient's memory occurs, except for the events just preceding and following the injury.

PERSPECTIVE AND PROSPECTS

Memory impairment is a serious condition which can interfere with one's ability to function independently. Every attempt should be made to identify the underlying condition because, in some cases, a treatable cause can be found and the memory loss reversed. Furthermore, it may soon be possible to arrest the progress of amnesia and memory loss and even to treat the dementias which now are considered as irreversible, such as Alzheimer's disease and multiple infarct dementia.

—*Ronald C. Hamdy and Louis A. Cancellaro*

See also Aging; Alzheimer's disease; Dementia; Head and neck disorders.

FOR FURTHER INFORMATION:

Cummings, Jeffrey L., and D. Frank Benson. *Dementia: A Clinical Approach.* Boston: Butterworths, 1983.

Cummings, Jeffrey L., and Bruce L. Miller, eds. *Alzheimer's Disease.* New York: Marcel Dekker, 1990.

Hamdy, Ronald C., et al., eds. *Alzheimer's Disease: A Handbook for Caregivers.* 2d ed. St. Louis: Mosby Year Book, 1994.

Terry, Robert D., ed. *Aging and the Brain.* New York: Raven Press, 1988.

West, Robin L., and Jan D. Sinnott, eds. *Everyday Memory and Aging.* New York: Springer-Verlag, 1992.

ANEMIA

SYSTEM AFFECTED: Blood

SPECIALISTS: Family physicians, hematologists, internists

DEFINITION: A pathological deficiency in the oxygen-carrying material of the blood. Not a disease but a sign of the presence of a variety of diseases, anemia is a frequent and significant worldwide health problem.

KEY TERMS:

aplastic anemia: anemia caused by lack of a functioning bone marrow; also known as bone marrow aplasia

erythrocytes: red blood cells

hemoglobin: the protein whose major function is to transport oxygen throughout the body

hemolytic anemia: anemia resulting from hemolysis, the excessive destruction of red blood cells

hypoxia: a deficiency in the amount of oxygen reaching the body tissues

iron-deficiency anemia: anemia characterized by low serum iron concentration

megaloblastic anemia: anemia caused by the failure of red blood cells to mature; also known as pernicious anemia, Addisonian anemia, or maturation failure anemia

microcytic or hypochromic anemia: anemia that ensues after blood loss

CAUSES AND SYMPTOMS

Hemoglobin, the red blood pigment, is a protein whose major function is to transport oxygen throughout the body. It is contained in the erythrocytes (red blood cells), which are flexible, biconcave disks that can squeeze through capillary blood vessels that are smaller in diameter than they are and ensure the rapid diffusion of oxygen. Anemia is defined as a reduction in either the volume of red blood cells or the concentration of hemoglobin in a sample of venous blood when compared with similar values obtained from a reference population. The anemic condition is considered to exist if hemoglobin levels are below 13 grams per 100 milliliters of blood in males and below 12 grams per 100 milliliters in adult, nonpregnant females.

The initial symptoms of patients with anemia are related to efforts by the body to compensate for the diminished oxygen supply. Later symptoms reflect the failure of these compensatory mechanisms. The viscosity of the blood is dependent almost entirely on the concentration of red blood cells. In severe anemia the blood viscosity may fall to as low as one and a half times that of water, rather than the normal value of around three times the viscosity of water. The greatly decreased viscosity decreases the resistance to blood flow in the blood vessels so that far greater than normal quantities of blood return to the heart. Also, hypoxia caused by the diminished transport of oxygen by the blood causes the tissue vessels to dilate, increasing the return of blood to the heart. As a result, the cardiac output can increase to as much as two to three times its normal value.

The increased cardiac output in anemia offsets many of its symptoms: Even though each unit quantity of blood carries only small quantities of oxygen, the rate of blood flow may be increased so much that normal quantities of oxygen are delivered to the tissues. As long as an anemic person's rate of activity is low, he or she can live without fatal hypoxia of the tissues, even when his or her concentration of red blood cells may be reduced to a quarter of the normal quantity. When the patient begins to exercise, the heart is not capable of pumping much greater quantities of blood than it is already pumping. Therefore, during exercise, which increases tissue demand for oxygen, extreme tissue hypoxia results and acute cardiac failure can ensue.

Anemia is a process that evolves within a clinical context produced by any condition that causes the quantity of oxygen transported to the tissues to decrease. Some of the most important types of anemia are microcytic or hypochromic anemia, iron-deficiency anemia, aplastic anemia, megaloblastic anemia, and hemolytic anemia.

Microcytic or hypochromic anemia is the type of anemia that ensues after blood loss. In the case of rapid hemorrhage, the body normally replaces plasma within one to two days, but this leaves a low concentration of red blood cells, creating the anemia condition. If another hemorrhage does not occur, the red blood cell count goes back to normal within three to four weeks. In the case of chronic blood loss, the person cannot absorb enough iron through the intestines to form hemoglobin as fast as it is lost. Therefore, red blood cells are produced in too few numbers and with too little hemoglobin in them, again creating the anemic condition. The symptoms of microcytic anemia depend on whether the anemia is sudden in onset, as in severe hemorrhage, or

gradual. In all cases, it is frequently manifested by pallor of the skin and mucous membranes, shortness of breath, palpitations of the heart, soft systolic murmurs in the heartbeat, lethargy and fatigability, and low blood pressure.

Iron-deficiency anemia is characterized by low serum iron concentration. There are two possible causes of this type of anemia. One is a condition in which the storage sites in macrophages are depleted of iron and cannot supply it to the plasma. The other possibility is a chronic disorder, in which the macrophage iron level is normal or increased but iron flow to the plasma appears to be partially blocked. Both abnormalities are among the most common causes of anemia. Iron deficiency in macrophages predominates in children and young women, while chronic disorders are the most common cause of this type of anemia among elderly individuals.

Aplastic anemia is serious and usually lethal. It is caused by an inability of the bone marrow to function properly, a condition also known as bone marrow aplasia. Red blood cell numbers are greatly reduced, and the bone marrow does not regenerate them. Examples of patients with this type of anemia are persons exposed to gamma radiation, excessive X-ray treatments, certain industrial chemicals, and even drugs. Symptoms include paleness and a tendency to suffer hemorrhages under the skin and mucous membranes.

Megaloblastic anemia—also known as pernicious anemia, maturation failure anemia, or Addisonian anemia—occurs when red blood cells fail to mature. In pernicious anemia, there is atrophy of the stomach mucosa, or loss of the stomach lining. Patients with intestinal sprue, in which folic acid and other vitamin B compounds are poorly absorbed, also experience maturation failure. The bone marrow cannot proliferate rapidly enough to form normal numbers of red blood cells, and the cells that are formed are oversized and have bizarre shapes and fragile membranes. These cells rupture easily, leaving the patient in dire need of an adequate number of red blood cells. This is commonly a disease of the middle aged, rarely occurring before the age of forty. It affects both men and women, and because its onset is insidious, it is usually well developed before medical help is sought. Patients have a lemon yellow complexion, and their tongue is sore and appears thinner and redder than normal. Other symptoms include soreness of and cracks in the skin at the corners of the mouth, slight enlargement of the spleen, and a complete absence of free hydrochloric acid in the stomach. One of the most serious complications of this anemia is a degenerative condition of the spinal cord (subacute combined degeneration) that can be cured by treating the anemia. The adult form of pernicious anemia is particularly common among individuals of Scandinavian, English, and Irish ancestry and is most common in late adult life.

Vitamin B_{12} is required for nuclear maturation and division. Since tissues that produce red blood cells are among

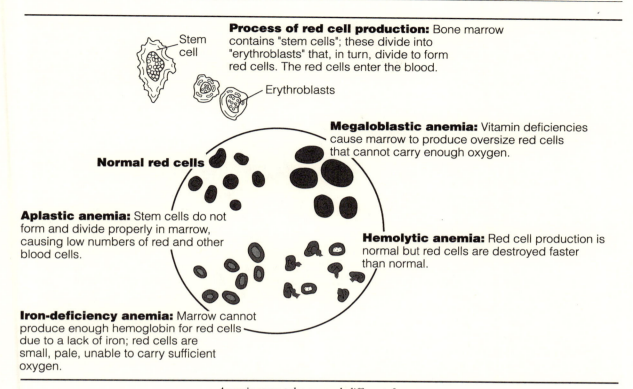

Process of red cell production: Bone marrow contains "stem cells"; these divide into "erythroblasts" that, in turn, divide to form red cells. The red cells enter the blood.

Stem cell

Erythroblasts

Megaloblastic anemia: Vitamin deficiencies cause marrow to produce oversize red cells that cannot carry enough oxygen.

Normal red cells

Aplastic anemia: Stem cells do not form and divide properly in marrow, causing low numbers of red and other blood cells.

Hemolytic anemia: Red cell production is normal but red cells are destroyed faster than normal.

Iron-deficiency anemia: Marrow cannot produce enough hemoglobin for red cells due to a lack of iron; red cells are small, pale, unable to carry sufficient oxygen.

Anemia may take several different forms.

the most rapidly growing and proliferating of all the body's tissues, lack of vitamin B_{12} especially inhibits the rate of red blood cell production. Therefore, it is said that deficiency of vitamin B_{12} causes maturation failure. In the mucus secreted by the stomach is a mucopolysaccharide or mucopolypeptide called intrinsic factor which combines with the vitamin B_{12} of the food and makes it available for absorption by the gut. The intrinsic factor binds tightly with the vitamin, and in this bound state the vitamin is protected from digestion by the gastrointestinal enzymes. Still in the bound state, the B_{12} and intrinsic factor attach to the membranes of the small intestine. The combination is then transported into the cells and, about four hours later, free vitamin B_{12} is released into the blood. Lack of intrinsic factor causes loss of much of the vitamin and also results in failure of absorption. Therefore, either a lack of the intrinsic factor in gastric secretions or a lack of the vitamin will produce this type of anemia. Once the vitamin has been absorbed from the gastrointestinal tract, it is stored in large quantities in the liver and then released slowly as needed. Consequently, there is normally a long period of defective B_{12} absorption before anemia results.

Hemolytic anemia results from hemolysis, the excessive destruction of red blood cells. Different abnormalities of the red blood cells, most of which are hereditary, make the cells very fragile so that they rupture easily as they go

through the capillaries, especially through the spleen. Therefore, even when the number of red blood cells produced is normal, the cell life span is so short that serious anemia results. Acquired hemolytic anemia can also result from transfusion reactions, malaria, reactions to certain drugs such as penicillin, sulfonamides, and burns or as an autoimmune process. Some of these types of anemia are hereditary spherocytosis, sickle-cell anemia, thalassemia, and erythroblastosis fetalis.

In hereditary spherocytosis, the red cells are very small in size and spherical in shape rather than biconcave disks. They cannot be compressed because they do not have the normal loose, baglike cell membrane structure of the disks. Therefore, they are easily ruptured by even slight compression when they pass through capillaries.

With sickle-cell anemia, the red cells contain an abnormal type of hemoglobin called hemoglobin S, caused by abnormal composition of the globin portion of the hemoglobin. When this type of hemoglobin is exposed to small amounts of oxygen, it precipitates into long crystals inside the red blood cell. The crystals elongate the cell and give it the appearance of a sickle instead of a biconcave disk. The precipitated hemoglobin also damages the cell membranes so that the cells are highly fragile, leading to anemia. Patients sometimes enter a cycle in which low oxygen tension in tissues causes sickling, impeding the blood flow through the tissue and causing a further decrease in oxygen tension. Once this process starts, it progresses rapidly, leading to a serious decrease in red blood cell mass in a few hours. These episodes or crises are characterized by severe pain because of microvascular occlusions. The sickle-cell trait and disease occur mainly in persons of equatorial African descent.

Thalassemia is also called Cooley's anemia or Mediterranean anemia. In this type of hemolytic anemia, the red cells are small and have fragile membranes and are therefore easily ruptured. This type of anemia is common in people from Mediterranean regions and areas of Asia where malaria is prevalent. The disease is characterized by a reduction in the rate of synthesis of the beta chain of hemoglobin, and severely affected individuals do not survive childhood.

In erythroblastosis fetalis, Rh-positive red blood cells in the fetus are attacked by antibodies from an Rh-negative mother. The antibodies make the red cells fragile, and the child is born with serious anemia.

TREATMENT AND THERAPY

Fundamentally, anemia is attributable to loss of blood, excessive destruction of red blood cells, or impaired red cell production. The optimal treatment of anemia requires eradication of its cause or, if that is not possible, at least modification of the underlying disorder.

Anemia is usually insidious in its onset and in some cases has no specific symptoms to alert the physician to its presence. Unusual fatigue is the earliest and most common complaint, but other, more subtle changes such as loss of libido or alterations in mood or sleep patterns may be elicited. The level of anemia at which symptoms occur is highly variable among individuals. Since oxygen transport is much more compromised by impaired circulation than by diminished oxygen-carrying capacity per se, patients with vascular or cardiac disease may show stronger symptoms with milder degrees of anemia.

The first step in the treatment of the anemic patient is evaluation. First, the physician should make sure that the symptoms are not caused by other diseases. If the condition is proven to be anemia, it must be determined whether it is inherited or acquired. Evidence of blood loss is sought, such as pregnancy, ulcers, cancers, anomalous vessels, or parasites. Hemolytic anemias are considerably less common than the anemias of iron deficiency or chronic disease and may be more difficult to recognize, since inherited disorders show a wide spectrum of severity. Therefore, the practitioner would ask the patient about jaundice, dark urine, gallbladder disease, or other conditions. It should also be determined if there has been exposure to medication or toxins that can result in anemia; drug-induced anemias may be associated with marrow aplasia, maturational effects, and hemolysis by both direct or immune-mediated mechanisms. Lastly, the physician should determine if there is a systematic illness or nonhematologic organ dysfunction. The anemia of chronic disease is present in most patients with active inflammatory disease or advanced malignant disease. Chronic infections such as subacute bacterial endocarditis and active inflammatory processes such as rheumatoid arthritis and inflammatory bowel syndrome are almost always associated with it. Patients with diminished renal, hepatic, or endocrine function are often anemic. In each case, a significant degree of organ failure must be present to result in anemia, so these conditions are easily excluded by measuring renal, hepatic, thyroid, or pituitary function. Red blood cell production and destruction are intimately modulated by the immune system, so immune dysfunction is commonly complicated by anemia.

Therapy for anemia may be specific, as in the replacement of deficient iron, vitamin B_{12}, or folate; diagnostic, as in the therapeutic trial; or symptomatic, as in the administration of blood transfusions. Specific therapy requires a definitive diagnosis. The duration of treatment must be correlated with response and based on a thorough understanding of the requirements and body stores to avoid harm to patients. For megaloblastic anemia, administration of vitamin B_{12} by injection for the rest of the patient's life is the normal treatment. For microcytic or hypochromic anemia, treatment consists primarily of giving sufficient iron by mouth to restore and then maintain a normal blood picture. The main iron preparation is ferrous sulfate. Iron can also be given intravenously, but only when rapid results are needed. If there is hemorrhage, however, this process must be arrested, and if the loss of blood is severe, a blood transfusion may be necessary. In the case of aplastic anemia, the treatment consists primarily of regular blood transfusion. The disease is often fatal, but 25 percent of the patients recover when adequately treated and others survive several years. Promising results are reported with the use of bone marrow transplantation.

PERSPECTIVE AND PROSPECTS

The study of the blood has a long history, since it is likely that even primitive humans realized that loss of blood, if sufficiently great, is associated with death. The therapeutic use of iron was mentioned in Greek mythology in the story of Iphiclus, who was cured of impotence by drinking iron rust dissolved in wine. Iron was used to treat a variety of ailments in ancient Egypt and the Roman Empire, but the specific use of iron salts was not reported until the 1700's. In the 1830's, anemia, hypochromia, and lack of iron in the blood were detected.

Credit for reporting the first case of pernicious (megaloblastic) anemia is generally given to George Combe in 1822, while Thomas Addison is given credit for recognizing the condition as a clinical entity in 1855. As early as 1860, Austin Flint expressed the view that the anemia resulted from deficient gastric secretions and consequent inadequate assimilation of food. The relation of the gastric defect to the cause of pernicious anemia was demonstrated by William Castle and coworkers in 1929. In 1926, two Americans, G. R. Minot and W. P. Murphy, reported that pernicious anemia responded to treatment with liver. Vitamin B$_{12}$ is needed for the formation of normal red blood cells. The efficient absorption of this vitamin into the body is dependent on the presence of the intrinsic factor that is produced normally by the mucous lining of the stomach. It is the inability of the patient to produce the intrinsic factor that leads to the onset of pernicious anemia. The use of whole liver by mouth led to the development of liver extracts of increasing potency that could be administered parenterally. The search for the active principle of liver extract culminated in the discovery of vitamin B$_{12}$ in 1948.

In 1945, Linus Pauling correctly hypothesized that sickle-cell anemia is the result of the presence of a mutant hemoglobin. He and his coworkers demonstrated an ionic difference between normal human hemoglobin (HbA) and sickle-cell hemoglobin (HbS). In 1956, Vernon Ingram developed the technique of peptide mapping in order to pinpoint the difference between HbA and HbS—one peptide in the beta subunits. This discovery marked the first time that an inherited disease was shown to arise from a specific amino acid change in a protein. Some individuals are homozygous (cells have two copies of the gene for sickle-cell anemia) or heterozygous (one copy of the gene). Heterozygous individuals, who are said to have sickle-cell trait, can live normally even though their erythrocytes have a shortened life span. *—Maria Pacheco*

See also Sickle-cell anemia; Thalassemia; Vitamin and mineral deficiencies.

FOR FURTHER INFORMATION:

Guyton, Arthur C. *Textbook of Medical Physiology.* 5th ed. Philadelphia: W. B. Saunders, 1976. An in-depth presentation of various medical subjects. Several chapters deal with the different types of anemias, their diagnosis and treatment.

Landau, Sidney I., ed. *International Dictionary of Medicine and Biology.* Vol. 1. New York: John Wiley & Sons, 1986. Offers an accessible and concise presentation of various medical terms and subjects.

Leavell, Byrd S., and Oscar A. Thorup, Jr. *Fundamentals of Clinical Hematology.* 4th ed. Philadelphia: W. B. Saunders, 1976. A comprehensive presentation of the fundamentals of hematology. Relatively easy to read, although it uses a large number of medical terms. A good science background is recommended for those who use this reference.

Lee, G. Richard, et al. *Wintrobe's Clinical Hematology.* 9th ed. Vol. 1. Philadelphia: Lea & Febiger, 1993. An extensive treatise on blood and its diseases. Includes excellent, very detailed coverage of the different types of anemia, their discovery, symptoms, and treatment. A good back-

ground in chemistry and biology is recommended for use of this reference.

Stedman, Thomas L. *Stedman's Medical Dictionary.* 25th ed. Baltimore: Williams & Wilkins, 1990. A presentation of the basic of medical subjects and terms that is easy to use and understand.

ANEURYSMS

SYSTEM AFFECTED: Circulatory

SPECIALISTS: Cardiologists, emergency physicians, thoracic surgeons, vascular surgeons

DEFINITION: A localized dilatation of a blood vessel, particularly an artery, that results from a focal weakness and distension of the arterial wall.

CAUSES AND SYMPTOMS

The arterial distension associated with aneurysms will take one of several forms. For example, fusiform aneurysms create a uniform bulge around an artery, while those of the saccular variety distend on one side of the blood vessel. Some saccular aneurysms found in the brain are called berry aneurysms for their protruding shapes.

Hypertension and arteriosclerosis commonly produce dilatation of the thoracic aorta. Very large aneurysms of the abdominal aorta (possibly the most common type) are usually caused by advanced atherosclerosis. The pathologic processes associated with the production of aortic aneurysms are varied, but certain factors are common to all. The media (middle arterial layer) of the normal aorta must remain intact in order for the aorta to withstand the systolic blood pressure. When the media is damaged, there is progressive dilation of the weakened area and an aneurysm develops. An aortic aneurysm is a serious disease with poor prognosis. Many such aneurysms rupture and cause death before surgical intervention can take place.

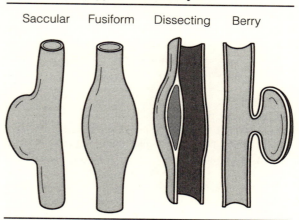

Types of Aneurysm

| Saccular | Fusiform | Dissecting | Berry |

Aneurysms may cause a variety of different shapes of distension of the affected blood vessel.

There are several types of aneurysms. Dissecting aneurysms are actually hematomas. Blood enters the wall of the aorta and splits the media of the vessel. The dissection of the media usually begins as a transverse tear in the region above the aortic valve. Some believe that hypertension promotes the tear by increasing the tension on the aorta. Traumatic aneurysm is usually caused by penetrating wounds or by blunt trauma; the most common cause of such injuries is automobile accidents. Mycotic aneurysms of the aorta may be associated with bacterial endocarditis and sometimes with organisms such as salmonella. Aneurysms of the sinuses of Valsalva may be attributable to syphilitic aortitis, bacterial endocarditis, or congenital defect.

TREATMENT AND THERAPY

Surgical therapy for thoracic aortic aneurysms varies with the type and location of the lesion. Aneurysms involving the aortic arch are often surgically corrected by employing a bypass technique. One method sutures a large prosthetic graft between the ascending and descending aortas, thus bypassing the diseased area. Surgical techniques sometimes offer the only hope for the survival of a patient with aneurysm. —*Jane A. Slezak*

See also Hypertension.

FOR FURTHER INFORMATION:

Beeson, Paul B., Walsh McDermott, and James B. Wyngaarden, eds. *Textbook of Medicine*. 15th ed. Philadelphia: W. B. Saunders, 1979. A comprehensive text which provides a valuable reference for all diseases, disorders of the nervous and neuromuscular systems, and environmental and physical factors in disease.

Burch, George E. *A Primer of Cardiology*. 3d ed. Philadelphia: Lea & Febiger, 1963. A text covering fundamental clinical cardiology and basic hemodynamic phenomena in healthy individuals and those with cardiac disease.

Kernicki, Jeanette, Barbara Bullock, and Joan Matthews. *Cardiovascular Nursing*. New York: G. P. Putnam's Sons, 1970. A book covering the clinical aspects of dealing with cardiac patients. Includes chapters on the anatomy and physiology of the cardiovascular system, problems of fluid and electrolyte disturbances, congestive heart failure, and cardiac arrhythmias.

ANGINA

SYSTEM AFFECTED: Heart

SPECIALISTS: Cardiologists, family physicians, internists

DEFINITION: Chest pain ranging from mild indigestion to a severe crushing, squeezing, or choking sensation.

CAUSES AND SYMPTOMS

Usually located below the sternum, angina may radiate down the left arm and/or left jaw, or down both arms and jaws. It is ischemic in nature, meaning that the pain is produced by a variety of conditions that result in insufficient supply of oxygen-rich blood to the heart. Some examples include arteriosclerosis (hardening of the arteries), atherosclerosis (arteries clogged with deposits of fat, cholesterol, and other substances), coronary artery spasms, low blood pressure, low blood volume, vasoconstriction (a narrowing of the arteries), anemia, and chronic lung disease.

Precipitating factors for angina include physical exertion, strong emotions, consumption of a heavy meal, temperature extremes, cigarette smoking, and sexual activity. These factors can cause angina because they may increase heart rate, cause vasoconstriction, or divert blood from the heart to other areas, such as the gastrointestinal system. Angina usually lasts from three to five minutes and commonly subsides when the precipitating factors are relieved. Typically, it should not last more than twenty minutes after rest or treatment.

Diagnosis consists of a physical examination which includes a chest X ray to determine any cardiac abnormalities; blood tests to screen risk factors such as lipids or to detect enzymes that can indicate if a heart attack has occurred; electrocardiography (ECG, or EKG); nuclear studies such as Thallium stress tests, which measure myocardial perfusion; coronary angiography to evaluate the anatomy of the coronary arteries and to note the location and nature of artery narrowing or constriction; cardiac catheterization to measure cardiac output; and Holter monitor studies to evaluate chest pain during the performance of daily activities for a twenty-four-hour period.

Treatment depends on the specific cause of the angina. Three types of drugs are the most common form of treatment: nitrates, to increase the supply of oxygen to the heart by dilating the coronary arteries; beta blockers, to lower oxygen demand during exercise and improve oxygen supply and demand; and calcium blockers, to decrease the work of the heart by decreasing cardiac contractility. —*John A. Bavaro*

See also Atherosclerotic disease; Heart attack; Heart disease; Hyperlipidemia; Hypertension; Ischemia; Thrombosis and thrombus.

ANOREXIA NERVOSA

SYSTEMS AFFECTED: Psychic-emotional, many other systems

SPECIALISTS: Endocrinologists, gynecologists, internists, psychiatrists, psychologists, registered dietitians

DEFINITION: Anorexia nervosa is an eating disorder characterized by a compulsive aversion to food. The anorectic (usually a young woman) fears obesity and creates a false body image; as a result, she intentionally starves herself. The extreme weight loss that often results can cause such medical problems as skeletal muscle atrophy, dental caries, constipation, hypotension, hair loss, amenorrhea (cessation of menstruation), and electrolyte imbalance. Cardiac arrest or circulatory collapse can occur and may prove fatal. Intensive psychiatric counseling and perhaps

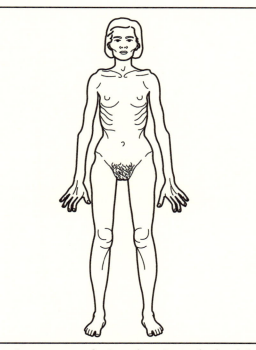

Anorexia nervosa results in undereating and other behaviors that lead to emaciation and, if unchecked, death; most often seen in women, its incidence among men is on the rise.

hospitalization to correct the symptoms of severe malnutrition are required.

See also Addiction; Anxiety; Depression; Eating disorders; Malnutrition; Obsessive-compulsive disorder; Stress; Vitamin and mineral deficiencies; Weight loss and gain.

ANXIETY

SYSTEMS AFFECTED: Psychic-emotional, heart, nervous, skin

SPECIALISTS: Cardiologists, internists, psychiatrists, psychologists

DEFINITION: Heightened fear or tension that causes psychological and physical distress; the American Psychiatric Association recognizes six types of anxiety disorders, which can be treated with medications or through counseling.

KEY TERMS:

anxiety: abnormal fear or tension, which may occur without any obvious trigger

brain imaging: any of several techniques used to visualize anatomic regions of the brain, including X rays, magnetic resonance imaging, and positron emission tomography

compulsion: a repetitive, stereotyped behavior performed to ward off anxious feelings

GABA/benzodiazepine receptor: an area on a nerve cell to which gamma aminobutyric acid (GABA) attaches and

that causes inhibition (quieting) of the nerve; benzodiazepine drugs enhance the attachment of GABA to the receptor

obsession: a recurrent, unwelcome, and intrusive thought

panic: a sudden episode of intense fearfulness

CAUSES AND SYMPTOMS

Anxiety is a subjective state of fear, apprehension, or tension. In the face of a naturally fearful situation, anxiety is a normal and understandable condition. When anxiety occurs without obvious provocation or is excessive, however, anxiety may be said to be abnormal or pathological (existing in a disease state). Normal anxiety is useful because it provides an alerting signal and improves physical and mental performance. Excessive anxiety results in a deterioration in performance and in emotional and physical discomfort.

There are several forms of pathological anxiety, known collectively as the anxiety disorders. As a group, they constitute the fifth most common medical or psychiatric disorder. In the United States, 14.6 percent of the population will experience anxiety at some point in their lives. More women suffer from anxiety disorders than do men, by a 2:1 ratio.

The anxiety disorders are distinguished from one another by characteristic clusters of symptoms. These disorders include generalized anxiety disorder, panic disorder, obsessive-compulsive disorder, phobias, adjustment disorder with anxious mood, and post-traumatic stress disorder. The first three disorders are characterized by anxious feelings that may occur without any obvious precipitant, while the latter three are closely associated with anxiety-producing events in a person's life.

Generalized anxiety disorder is thought to be a biological form of anxiety disorder in which the individual inherits a habitually high level of tension or anxiety that may occur even when no threatening circumstances are present. Generally, these periods of anxiety occur in cycles which may last weeks to years. The prevalence is unknown, but this disorder is not uncommon. The male-to-female ratio is nearly equal.

Evidence suggests that generalized anxiety disorder is related to an abnormality in a common neurotransmitter receptor complex found in many brain neurons. These complexes, the GABA/benzodiazepine receptors, decrease the likelihood that a neuron will transmit an electrochemical signal, resulting in a calming effect on the portion of the brain in which they are found. These receptors exist in large numbers in the cerebral cortex (the outer layer of the brain), the hippocampus (the sea horse-shaped structure inside the temporal lobe), and the amygdala (the almond-shaped gray matter inside the temporal lobe). The hippocampus and amygdala are important parts of the limbic system, which is significantly involved in emotions. Benzodiazepine drugs enhance the efficiency of these receptors and have a calming effect. In contrast, if these receptors are inhibited, feelings of impending doom result.

Panic disorder is found in 1.5 percent of the United States population, and the female-to-male ratio is 2:1. This disorder usually begins during the young adult years. Panic disorder is characterized by recurrent and unexpected attacks of intense fear or panic. Each discrete episode lasts about five to twenty minutes. These episodes are intensely frightening to the individual, who is usually convinced he or she is dying. Because people who suffer from panic attacks are often anxious about having another one (so-called secondary anxiety), they may avoid situations in which they fear an attack may occur, in which help would be unavailable, or in which they would be embarrassed if an attack occurred. This avoidance behavior may cause restricted activity and can lead to agoraphobia, the fear of leaving a safe zone in or around the home. Thus, agoraphobia (literally, "fear of the marketplace") is often secondary to panic disorder.

Panic disorder appears to have a biological basis. In those people with panic disorder, panic attacks can often be induced by sodium lactate infusions, hyperventilation, exercise, or hypocalcemia (low blood calcium). Normal people do not experience panic attacks when these triggers are present. Highly sophisticated scans show abnormal metabolic activity in the right parahippocampal region of the brain of individuals with panic disorder. The parahippocampal region, the area surrounding the hippocampus, is involved in emotions and is connected by fiber tracts to the locus ceruleus, a blue spot in the pons portion of the brain stem that is involved in arousal.

In addition to known biological triggers for panic attacks, emotional or psychological events may also cause an attack. To be diagnosed as having panic disorder, however, a person must experience attacks that arise without any apparent cause. The secondary anxiety and avoidance behavior often seen in these individuals result in difficulties in normal functioning. There is an increased incidence of suicide attempts in people with panic disorder; up to one in five have reported a suicide attempt at some time. The childhoods of people with panic disorder are characterized by an increased incidence of pathological separation anxiety and/or school phobia.

Obsessive-compulsive disorder (OCD) is an uncommon anxiety disorder with an equal male-to-female ratio. It is characterized by obsessions (intrusive, unwelcome thoughts) and compulsions (repetitive, often stereotyped behaviors that are performed to ward off anxiety). The obsessions in OCD are often horrifying to the afflicted person. Common themes concern sex, food, aggression, suicide, bathroom functions, and religion. Compulsive behavior may include checking (such as repeatedly checking to see if the stove is off or the door is locked), cleaning (such as repetitive handwashing or the wearing of gloves to turn a doorknob), or stereotyped behavior (such as dressing by using an exact series of steps that cannot be altered). Frequently, the compulsive behaviors must be repeated many times. Sometimes, there is an exact, almost magical number of times the behavior must be done in order to ward off anxiety. Although people with OCD have some conscious control over their compulsions, they are driven to perform them because intense anxiety results if they fail to do so.

The most common psychological theory for OCD was proposed by Sigmund Freud, who believed that OCD symptoms were a defense against unacceptable unconscious wishes. Genetic and brain imaging studies, however, suggest a biological basis for this disorder. Special brain scans have shown increased metabolism in the front portion of the brain in these patients, and it has been theorized that OCD results from an abnormality in a circuit within the brain (the cortical-striatal-thalamic-cortical circuit). Moreover, OCD is associated with a variety of known neurological diseases, including epilepsy, brain trauma, and certain movement disorders.

Phobias are the most common anxiety disorders. A phobia is an abnormal fear of a particular object or situation. Simple phobias are fears of specific, identifiable triggers such as heights, snakes, flying in an airplane, elevators, or the number thirteen. Social phobia is an exaggerated fear of being in social settings where the phobic person fears he or she will be open to scrutiny by others. This fear may result in phobic avoidance of eating in public, attending church, joining a social club, or participating in other social events. Phobias are more common in men than in women, and they often begin in late childhood or early adolescence.

In classic psychoanalytic theory, phobias were thought to be fears displaced from one object or situation to another. For example, fear of snakes may be a displaced fear of sex because the snake is a phallic symbol. It was thought that this process of displacement took place unconsciously. Many psychologists now believe that phobias are either exaggerations of normal fears or that they develop accidentally, without any symbolic meaning. For example, fear of elephants may arise if a young boy at a zoo is accidentally separated from his parents. At the same time that he realizes he is alone, he notices the elephants. He may then associate elephants with separation from his parents and fear elephants thereafter.

Adjustment disorder with anxious mood is an excessive or maladaptive response to a life event in which the individual experiences anxiety. For example, an individual may become so anxious after losing a job that he or she is unable to eat, sleep, or function and begins to entertain the prospect of suicide. While anxiety is to be expected, this person has excessive anxiety (the inability to eat, sleep, or function) and a maladaptive response (the thought of suicide). The exaggerated response may be attributable to the personality traits of the individual. In this example, a dependent person will be more likely to experience an adjustment disorder than a less dependent person.

Adjustment disorders are very common. In addition to adjustment disorders with anxious mood, people may experience adjustment disorders with depressed mood, mixed emotional features, disturbance of conduct, physical complaints, withdrawal, or inhibition in school or at work. These disorders are considered to be primarily psychological.

Post-traumatic stress disorder (PTSD) is similar to adjustment disorder because it represents a psychological reaction to a significant life event. PTSD only occurs, however, when the precipitating event would be seriously emotionally traumatic to a normal person, such as war, rape, natural disasters such as major earthquakes, or airplane crashes. In PTSD, the individual suffers from flashbacks to the precipitating event and "relives" the experience. These episodes are not simply vivid remembrances of what happened but a transient sensation of actually being in that circumstance. For example, a Vietnam War veteran may literally jump behind bushes when a car backfires.

People who suffer from PTSD usually are anxious and startle easily. They may be depressed and have disturbed sleep and eating patterns. They often lose normal interest in sex, and nightmares are common. These individuals usually try to avoid situations that remind them of their trauma. Relationships with others are often strained, and the patient is generally pessimistic about the future.

In addition to the anxiety disorders described, abnormal anxiety may be caused by a variety of drugs and medical illnesses. Common drug offenders include caffeine, alcohol, stimulants in cold preparations, nicotine, and many illicit drugs, including cocaine and amphetamines. Medical illnesses that may cause anxiety include thyroid disease, heart failure, cardiac arrhythmias, and schizophrenia.

TREATMENT AND THERAPY

When an individual has difficulty with anxiety and seeks professional help, the cause of the anxiety must be determined. Before the etiology can be determined, however, the professional must first realize that the patient has an anxiety disorder. People with anxiety disorders often complain primarily of physical symptoms that result from the anxiety. These symptoms may include motor tension (muscle tension, trembling, and fatigue) and autonomic hyperactivity (shortness of breath, palpitations, cold hands, dizziness, gastrointestinal upset, chills, and frequent urination).

When an anxiety disorder is suspected, effective treatment often depends on an accurate diagnosis of the type of anxiety disorder present. A variety of medications can be prescribed for the anxiety disorder. In addition, several types of psychotherapy can be used. For example, patients with panic disorder can be educated about the nature of their illness, reassured that they will not die from it, and taught to ride out a panic attack. This process avoids the

development of secondary anxiety, which complicates the panic attack. Phobic patients can be treated with systematic desensitization, in which they are taught relaxation techniques and are given graded exposure to the feared situation so that their fear lessens or disappears.

The origin, diagnosis, and treatment of anxiety disorders can best be portrayed through case examples. Three fictional cases are described below to illustrate typical anxiety disorder patients.

Hypothetical case examples. Ms. Smith is a twenty-four-year-old married mother of two young children. She works part-time as a bookkeeper for a construction company. Her health had been good until a month ago, when she began to experience spells of intense fearfulness, a racing heart, tremors of her hands, a dry mouth, and dizziness. The spells would come on suddenly and would last between ten and fifteen minutes. She was convinced that heart disease was causing these episodes and was worried about having a heart attack. As a result, she consulted her family physician.

Physical examination, electrocardiogram, and laboratory studies were all normal. Her physician had initially considered cardiac arrhythmia (abnormal rhythm of the heartbeat) as a cause but diagnosed panic disorder on the basis of Ms. Smith's history and the outcome of the tests. Treatment consisted of medication and comforting explanations of the nonfatal nature of the disorder. Within three weeks, the panic attacks stopped altogether.

This case illustrates many common features of panic disorder. The patient is a young adult female with classic panic attacks striking "out of the blue." Most patients fear that they are having a heart attack or a stroke or that they are going insane. Typically, they present their symptoms to general medical physicians rather than to psychiatrists. Treatment with medication and simple counseling techniques are usually successful.

Mr. Jones is a thirty-five-year-old single man who works as an accountant. He has always been shy and has adopted leisure activities that he can do alone, such as reading, gardening, and coin collecting. As a child, he was bright but withdrawn. His mother described him as "highstrung," "a worrier," and "easily moved to tears." Recently, he has been bothered by muscle achiness, frequent urination, and diarrhea alternating with constipation. He thinks constantly about his health and worries that he has cancer.

Mr. Jones makes frequent visits to his doctor, but no illness is found. His doctor tells him that he worries too much. The patient admits to himself that he is a worrier and has been his whole life. He ruminates about the details of his job, his health, his lack of friends, the state of the economy, and a host of other concerns. His worries make it hard for him to fall asleep at night. Once asleep, however, he sleeps soundly. Finally, Mr. Jones is given a tranquilizer by his physician. He finds that he feels calm, no longer broods over everything, falls asleep easily, and has relief from his physical symptoms. To improve his social functioning, he sees a psychiatrist, who diagnoses a generalized anxiety disorder and an avoidant (shy) personality disorder.

This case illustrates many features of patients with generalized anxiety disorder. These individuals have near-continuous anxiety for weeks or months that is not clearly related to a single life event. In this case, some of the physical manifestations of anxiety are prominent (muscle tension, frequent urination, and diarrhea). Difficulty falling asleep is also common with anxiety. In contrast, patients who are depressed will often have early morning wakening. In this case example, the patient also has a concomitant shy personality that aggravates his condition. Such a patient usually benefits from treatment. Medication may be required for many years, although it may be needed only during active cycles of anxiety. Because some patients attempt to medicate themselves with alcohol, secondary alcoholism is a potential complication.

Ms. Johnson is a forty-two-year-old married homemaker and mother of four children. She works part-time in a fabric store as a salesclerk. She is friendly and outgoing. She has also been very close with her family, especially her mother. Ms. Johnson comes to her family physician because her mother has just had a stroke. Because her mother lives on the other side of the country, Ms. Johnson needs to take an airplane if she is to get to her mother's bedside quickly. Unfortunately, Ms. Johnson has a long-standing fear of flying; even the thought of getting into an airplane terrifies her. She has not personally had a bad experience with flying but remembers reading about a plane crash when she was a teenager. She denies any other unusual fears and otherwise functions well.

Her family physician refers her to a psychologist for systematic desensitization to relieve her phobia for future situations. As a stop-gap measure for the present, however, she is taught a deep-muscle relaxation technique, is shown videotapes designed to reduce fear of flying, and is prescribed a tranquilizer and another drug to reduce the physical manifestations of anxiety (a beta-blocker). This combination of treatments allows her to visit her mother immediately and, eventually, to be able to fly without needing medication.

This case illustrates a typical patient with an isolated phobia. Phobias are probably the most common anxiety disorders. Treatments such as those described above are usually quite helpful.

PERSPECTIVE AND PROSPECTS

Anxiety has been recognized since antiquity and was often attributed to magical or spiritual causes, such as demonic possession. Ancient myths provided explanations for fearful events in people's lives. Pan, a mythological god of mischief, was thought to cause frightening noises in forests, especially at night; the term "panic" is derived from his name. An understanding of the causes of panic and other anxiety disorders has evolved over the years.

Sigmund Freud (1856-1939) distinguished anxiety from fear. He considered fear to be an expected response to a specific, identifiable trigger, whereas anxiety was a similar emotional state without an identifiable trigger. He postulated that anxiety resulted from unconscious, forbidden wishes that conflicted with what the person believed was acceptable. The anxiety that resulted from this mental conflict was called an "anxiety neurosis" and was thought to result in a variety of psychological and physical symptoms. Psychoanalysis was developed to uncover these hidden conflicts and to allow the anxiety to be released.

Freud's theories about anxiety are no longer universally accepted. Many psychiatrists now believe that several anxiety disorders have a biological cause and that they are more neurological diseases than psychological ones. This is primarily true of generalized anxiety disorder, panic disorder, and obsessive-compulsive disorder. It is recognized that anxiety can also be triggered by drugs (legal and illicit) and a variety of medical illnesses.

Psychological causes of anxiety are also recognized. Adjustment disorder with anxious mood, phobias, and post-traumatic stress disorder are all thought to be primarily psychological disorders. Unlike with Freud's conflict theory of anxiety, most modern psychiatrists consider personality factors, life experiences, and views of the world to be the relevant psychological factors in such anxiety disorders. Nonpharmacological therapies are no longer designed to uncover hidden mental conflicts; they provide instead support. Specific therapies include flooding (massive exposure to the feared situation), systematic desensitization (graded exposure), and relaxation techniques.

—Peter M. Hartmann

See also Death and dying; Depression; Grief and guilt; Hypochondriasis; Manic-depressive disorder; Midlife crisis; Neurosis; Obsessive-compulsive disorder; Panic attacks; Paranoia; Phobias; Postpartum depression; Psychiatric disorders; Psychosomatic disorders; Sexual dysfunction; Stress; Suicide.

FOR FURTHER INFORMATION:

American Psychiatric Association. *Diagnostic and Statistical Manual of Mental Disorders*. Rev. 3d ed. Washington, D.C.: Author, 1987. This textbook contains the official diagnostic criteria and classification for all the anxiety disorders. Provides useful descriptions, definitions, and prevalence data.

Greist, John H., James W. Jefferson, and Isaac M. Marks. *Anxiety and Its Treatment*. Washington, D.C.: American Psychiatric Press, 1986. A short book written by three psychiatrists with a special interest in the anxiety disorders. Intended for a lay audience, it describes the nature of the anxiety disorders and their treatment.

Kleinknecht, Ronald A. *Mastering Anxiety: The Nature and Treatment of Anxious Conditions*. New York: Plenum Press, 1991. This book provides a good overview, with statistics and good explanations of the different types of anxiety disorder.

Leaman, Thomas L. *Healing the Anxiety Diseases*. New York: Plenum Press, 1992. A helpful text written by a family physician with an interest in anxiety disorders. Provides a good overview to the subject in nontechnical terms, and contains practical advice on dealing with anxiety.

Sheehan, David V. *The Anxiety Disease*. New York: Bantam Books, 1983. A classic book written for the layperson that explains the nature of anxiety, the different types of anxiety disorder, and treatment approaches.

Weekes, Claire. *Hope and Help for Your Nerves*. New York: Hawthorne Books, 1969. A classic text describing the nature of panic disorder. Weekes describes her pioneering approach to the nonpharmacological management of this disorder.

APHASIA AND DYSPHASIA

SYSTEM AFFECTED: Brain

SPECIALISTS: Neurologists, speech pathologists

DEFINITION: Dysphasia is a disturbance of such language skills as speaking, reading, writing, and comprehension, while aphasia is the total absence of these skills. Both conditions occur with damage to areas of the brain that are important to language, usually as a result of a head injury or stroke. Damage to Broca's area causes slow, labored speech. When there is damage to Wernicke's area, comprehension of speech becomes difficult (that of others as well as of the patient's own speech), resulting in grammar and word selection errors. Nominal aphasia refers to a difficulty in naming objects, while widespread brain damage can cause global aphasia, the complete inability to speak, write, or understand words.

See also Speech disorders; Strokes and TIAs.

APNEA

SYSTEMS AFFECTED: Nervous, respiratory

SPECIALISTS: Neurologists, sleep specialists

DEFINITION: Apnea is the temporary cessation of breathing; sleep apnea, the most common type, occurs during the night and causes frequent waking. This condition can be physical, caused by obstruction of the upper airway, or neurological, caused by a failure of the respiratory center to stimulate adequate breathing. The occurrence of sleep apnea is linked to stress, strokes, senility, obesity, smoking, excess alcohol consumption, and the use of mind-altering drugs. As an extreme, chronic condition, sleep apnea can result in sleep deprivation, permanent brain damage, and cardiac arrhythmias leading to heart failure. In babies, it is sometimes associated with sudden infant death syndrome (SIDS). Sleep apnea can usually be avoided by sleeping on one's side, rather than on the back.

See also Abdominal disorders; Gastrointestinal disorders; Intestinal disorders; Peritonitis.

APPENDICITIS

SYSTEM AFFECTED: Gastrointestinal

SPECIALISTS: Emergency physicians, gastroenterologists, general surgeons

DEFINITION: Inflammation of the human vermiform appendix.

CAUSES AND SYMPTOMS

Appendicitis may be acute or chronic. The inflammation characteristic of the condition may be associated with infection or the causes may be various or even unknown.

In the human digestive system, the small intestine empties into the large intestine, or colon, in the lower right abdomen. Movement of waste from that point is generally upward through the ascending colon, but the colon begins with a downward-projecting blind end called the cecum, to which is attached the vermiform ("wormlike") appendix. The appendix is 7.5 to 15 centimeters long and less than 2.5 centimeters in diameter, and it has no known function. Occasionally, its opening into the cecum becomes obstructed, and inflammation, swelling, and pain follow. Sometimes the cause of the obstruction is identifiable, such as pinworms or other parasites, or hardened fecal material; more often, it is not. Symptoms, including pain that is general at the outset but localizes in the lower right abdomen, can include nausea, fever, and an elevated white blood cell count. If the swollen appendix bursts, peritonitis—infection and poisoning of the abdominal cavity—can result. Peritonitis is usually signaled to the patient by an abrupt cessation of pain, when the swelling is relieved, but is followed by serious and life-threatening complications.

TREATMENT AND THERAPY

The treatment of choice is almost invariably surgical removal of the inflamed appendix, an operation that is no longer considered major surgery. The patient is usually out of bed in a day or two and fully recovered in a few weeks. Peritonitis, however, calls for emergency surgery to remove the toxic material released by the ruptured appendix, as well as the appendix itself. Because a greater or lesser portion of the abdominal cavity must be cleansed with saline solution and treated with antibiotics, this surgery can become a major procedure. —*Robert M. Hawthorne, Jr.*

See also Abdominal disorders; Gastrointestinal disorders; Intestinal disorders; Peritonitis.

FOR FURTHER INFORMATION:

Clayman, Charles B., ed. *The American Medical Association Encyclopedia of Medicine*. New York: Random House, 1989.

Larson, David E., ed. *Mayo Clinic Family Health Book*. New York: William Morrow, 1990.

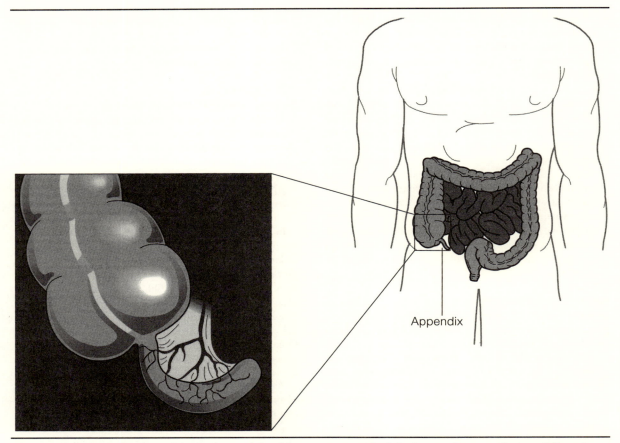

The vermiform appendix, located in the lower-right abdomen at one end of the large colon, may become inflamed as a result of obstruction; surgery is nearly always required to avoid bursting and the release of deadly toxins into the body.

Wagman, Richard J., ed. *New Complete Medical and Health Encyclopedia.* 4 vols. Chicago: J. C. Ferguson, 1992-1993.

ARRHYTHMIAS

SYSTEM AFFECTED: Heart

SPECIALISTS: Cardiologists, internists

DEFINITION: An arrhythmia is an irregularity in the heartbeat, in rhythm or rate. The heartbeat is an electrical impulse that normally originates in the sinoatrial node (S-A node) and then travels to the atrioventricular node (A-V node). A disturbance in either node can cause such cardiac abnormalities as sinus tachycardia (a regular, rapid beat), ventricular tachycardia (an irregular, rapid beat originating in the ventricles), supraventricular tachycardia (a regular, very rapid beat originating in the tissue above the ventricles), sinus bradycardia (a regular, slow beat), atrial fibrillation (a very irregular, rapid beat), and heart block (alternating tachycardia and bradycardia). Arrhythmias are usually caused by coronary heart disease, especially after a myocardial infarction (heart attack) occurs. In the case of heart block, the implantation of an artificial pacemaker may be required.

See also Atherosclerotic disease; Heart attack; Heart disease; Hypertension; Ischemia; Palpitations; Panic attacks.

ARTHRITIS

SYSTEMS AFFECTED: Immune, joints, skeletal

SPECIALISTS: Internists, orthopedic surgeons, physical therapists, rheumatologists

DEFINITION: A group of more than one hundred inflammatory diseases that damage joints and their surrounding structures, resulting in symptomatic pain, disability, and systemwide inflammation.

KEY TERMS:

anti-inflammatory drugs: drugs to counter the effects of inflammation locally or throughout the body; these drugs can be applied locally or introduced by electric currents (in a process called ionthophoresis), by injections into the joint or into the muscles, or by mouth; the three classes of these drugs are steroidal, immunosuppressant, and nonsteroidal

cartilage: material covering the ends of bones; it does not have a blood supply or nerve supply but may swell or break down

inflammation: the body's defensive and protective responses to trauma or foreign substances by dilution, cellular efforts at destruction, and the walling-off of irritants; characterized by pain, heat, redness, swelling, and loss of function mediated through a chemical breakdown

physical modalities: the physical means of addressing a disease, which include heat, cold, electricity, exercises, braces, assistive devices, and biofeedback

rehabilitation: a physician-led program to evaluate, treat, and educate patients and their families about the sequelae of birth defects, trauma, disease, and degenerative conditions, with the goals of alleviating pain, preventing complications, correcting deformities, improving function, and reintegrating individuals into the family and society

synovium: the cellular lining of a joint, having a blood supply and a nerve supply; the synovium secretes fluid for lubrication and protects against injury and injurious agents

Causes and Symptoms

Approximately one in six people (more than 15 percent) suffers from one of approximately one hundred varieties of arthritis, and 2.6 percent of the population suffer from arthritis that limits their activities. Although 12.6 percent of those over seventy-five years of age experience arthritis, the disease can occur in the young as a result of infections, rheumatic conditions, or birth defects. Young and middle-aged adults experience the disease as a result of trauma, infections, and rheumatic or immune reactions. Arthritis may be located in joints, joint capsules, the surrounding muscles, or diffusely throughout the body. Inflammation of the joint lining (synovium) can similarly afflict the linings of other organs: the skin, colon, eyes, heart, and urinary passage. Those suffering from the disease may therefore suffer from psoriasis and rashes, spastic colitis and diarrhea, dryness of the eyes, inflammations of the conjunctiva or iris, frequent urination, discharge and burning upon urination, and other symptoms.

The collagen-type arthritic diseases involve the binding materials in the body or connective tissues and may be rheumatologic, generally more diffuse and in the distal joints (as in juvenile rheumatoid arthritis and rheumatic fever), or located in the skin and muscles (dermatomyositis). Psoriatic arthritis causes severe punched-out defects in the joints. Reiter's and Sjögren's syndromes involve the eyes and the joints. Genetic conditions, such as Gaucher's disease, frequently run in families. Metabolic disturbances, such as gout, can leave uric acid deposits in the skin and in the joints. Gout sufferers experience very painful, hot, tender, and swollen joints—often in the large toe. Immunologically mediated arthritides may be associated with infections, liver diseases, bowel disturbances, and immune deficiencies. Localized infections may be bacterial, viral, or fungal. "Miscellaneous disorders," a basket category, include conditions that do not fit into any of the aforementioned categories: Psychogenic disorders and arthritis associated with cystic disorders are examples. Arthritis may also be associated with tumors that grow from cartilage cells, blood vessels, synovial tissue, and nerve tissue. Blood abnormalities may give rise to hemorrhages into joints (a side effect of sickle-cell anemia and hemophilia) and can be disabling and very painful, sometimes requiring surgery. Traumatic and mechanical derangements—sports and occupational injuries, leg-length disparity, and obesity—may elicit acute synovial inflammation with subsequent degenerative arthritis. Finally, wear-and-tear degeneration can occur in joints after years of trauma, repetitive use, and (especially in the obese) weight-bearing. The most common arthritic entities are rheumatoid arthritis (also called atrophic or proliferative arthritis), osteoarthritis, hypertrophic arthritis, and degenerative arthritis.

The inflammatory reactions in response to injury or disease consist of fluid changes—the dilation of blood vessels accompanied by an increase in the permeability of the blood-vessel walls and consequent outflow of fluids and proteins. Injurious substances are immobilized with immune reactions and removed by the cellular responses of

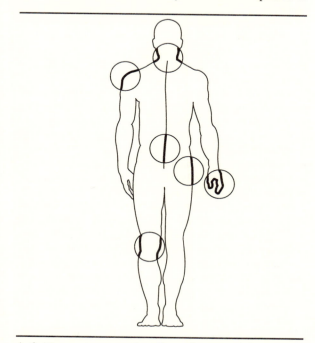

Arthritis most commonly affects the joints of the neck, shoulders, hands, lower back, hips, and knees.

Osteoarthritis

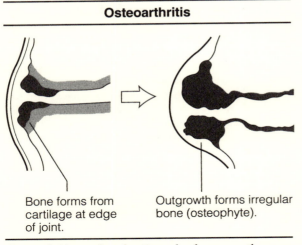

Bone forms from cartilage at edge of joint.

Outgrowth forms irregular bone (osteophyte).

Osteoarthritis results when irregular bone growth occurs at the edge of a joint, causing impaired movement of the joint and pressure on nerves in the area.

phagocytosis and digestion of foreign materials, resulting in the proliferation of fibrous cells to wall off the injurious substances and in turn leading to scar formation and deformities. The chemical reactions to injury commence with a degradation of phospholipids when enzymes are released by injured tissue. Phospholipids—fatty material that is normally present—break down into arachidonic acid, which is further broken down by other enzymes, lipoxygenase and cycloxygenase, resulting in prostaglandins and eicosanoid acids. Most anti-inflammatory medications attempt to interfere with the enzymatic degradation process of phospholipids and could be damaging to the liver and kidneys and to the body's blood-clotting ability.

The physician bases the diagnosis of arthritic disease on the patient's medical history and a physical examination. Specific procedures such as joint aspiration, laboratory studies, and X-ray or magnetic resonance imaging may help to establish the diagnosis and the treatment. The history will elicit the onset of pain and its relation to time of day and difficulties performing the activities of daily living. A functional classification has evolved that is similar to the cardiac functional classification: Class 1 patients perform all usual activities without a handicap; class 2 patients perform normal activities adequately with occasional symptoms and signs in one or more joints but still do not need to limit their activities; class 3 patients find that they must limit some activities and may require assistive devices; and class 4 patients are unable to perform activities, are largely or wholly incapacitated, and are bedridden or confined to a wheelchair, requiring assistance in self-care.

A person's medical history or surgical conditions and the medications that he or she is taking can influence the physician's diagnosis and prescription for treatment. Patients may present a gross picture of the body to the physician showing the joints involved in their symmetry (whether distal or proximal, and whether weight-bearing or post-traumatic in distribution). Physicians may ask (verbally or by questionnaire) for a history of other system complaints, which can then be checked more thoroughly. During a physical examination, the physician will check the joints, skin, eyes, abdomen, heart, and urinary tract. The neuro-muscular evaluation may reveal localized tenderness of the joints or muscles, swelling, wasting, weakness, and abnormal motions. Joints may have weakened ligamentous, muscle, and tendon supports that could give rise to instability or grinding of joints, with subsequent roughening of cartilage surfaces. The arthritides are frequently associated with muscular pains, called fibrositis and myofascial pain syndromes.

Fibrositis is a diffuse muscular pain syndrome with tenderness in the muscles, no muscle spasm, and no limitations in motion; all laboratory tests are within normal limits. It is frequent in postmenopausal women who have a history of migraines, cold extremities, spastic colitis, softening of the bone matrix accompanied by loss of minerals, and irritability. Myofascial trigger points can be found in both men and women, at all ages, with acutely tender nodules or cords felt in muscles. The pain of these trigger points is referred to more distal areas of the muscles that may not be tender to touch. Physicians may frequently miss the acutely tender trigger points. Tests will show whether pain is elicited when muscles are contracted with motion, when muscles are contracted without motion, or when motion is carried out passively by the examiner without muscular effort by the patient.

Joint pathology is generally associated with some limitation in the range of motion. Sensation testing, muscle strength, and reflex changes may also indicate nerve tissue damage. Nerves occasionally pass close to joints and may be pinched when the joint swelling encroaches upon the passage opening. This condition may result in carpal tunnel syndrome, in which the median nerve at the wrist becomes pinched, causing pain, numbness, and weakness in the hand. Pinched nerves may also be associated with tarsal tunnel syndrome, in which the nerve at the inner side of the ankle joint may be compressed and cause similar complaints in the feet. Other nerves may be constricted in exiting from the spine and when passing through muscles in spasm.

The medications used to treat arthritis can involve the nervous system. An evaluation and estimation of the severity of the disease can be obtained by electrical testing, as in electroneuromyography. The nerves are stimulated and their rate of transmitting the stimulus is measured. The normal transmission rate for nerves is 45 meters per second. Delays at areas of impingement can be determined by measuring the transmission rate of a stimulus from different points along the nerve paths. Abnormal or damaged muscles will cause muscle fibers to contract spontaneously, or "fibrillate." Chest expansion during inspiration and after expiration may be limited because of arthritis at the spine or because of lung pathology. Involvement of the spine can also be measured by the posture, the ability to move the neck, and the ability to move the lower back.

Arthritis of the spine leads to progressive loss in motion. The amount lost can be measured by comparing the normal motion with the restricted motion of the patient. The neck may be limited in all directions, rotation of the head to the sides can restrict the driving view, and the head may gradually tilt forward. The lower back may also exhibit restriction in all directions; for example, it may be limited in forward bending because of spasms in the muscles in the back. Tilting backward of the trunk may be limited and painful when the vertebral body overgrowth of osteoarthritis or degenerative arthritis restricts the space for the spinal cord. The nerves pinched in their passage from the vertebrae may thus cause radiculitis, irritation of the nerves as they exit from the spine that leads to pain and muscle involvement. Circumferential measurements of the involved joints and the structures above and below can confirm swelling, atrophy from disuse or inaction, or atrophy from a damaged nerve supply. When measurements are repeated, they can indicate improvement or deterioration.

Testing of blood for cells, chemicals, or enzymes is helpful. The simplest test—the sedimentation (or "sed") test—measures the rate at which blood cells settle out of the plasma. Normally, women have a more rapid rate of sedimentation than men. When this rate exceeds the normal range, active inflammation in the body is indicated. Comparisons of sed tests performed at different stages can reveal the disease's rate of progression or improvement. The chemicals tested may include uric acid for gout and sugar for diabetes. Blood tests for immune substances and antibodies are also possible. The joint fluid can be aspirated and analyzed, particularly for appearance, density, number of blood cells, and levels of sugar. Cloudy fluid, the tendency to form clots, a high cell count, and lower-than-normal levels of sugar in the joint fluid (compared to the overall blood sugar level) indicate abnormalities. With inflammatory arthritides, the X rays will show the results of synovial fluid and cellular overabundance. Clumps of pannus break off and may destroy the cartilage and bone. Bones about these joints, because of increased vascularity and blood flow, have less minerals and will appear less dense, a condition known as osteoporosis.

Deformities in inflammatory arthritis may be the result of unequal muscle pulls or the destruction or scarring of tissues; such deformities can occasionally be prevented by the use of resting splints, which is most important for the hands.

Degenerative and post-traumatic arthritis show joint narrowing, thinning of the cartilage layer, hardening of the underlying bone (called eburnation), and marginal overgrowth of the underlying bone (called osteophytes), resulting in osteoarthritis. Osteophytes, or marginal lipping in the

Rheumatoid Arthritis

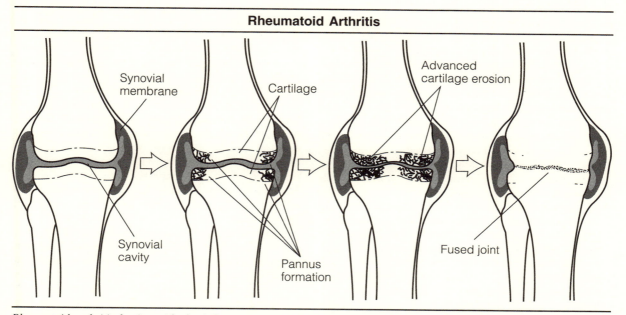

Rheumatoid arthritis begins with the inflammation of the synovial membrane and progresses to pannus formation and erosion of cartilage; eventually, the joint cavity is destroyed and the bones (here, the knee bones) become fused.

back, may enhance symptoms of lower back pain. The cushions between the vertebrae, called discs, are more than 80 percent water, a figure which diminishes with aging, bringing the joints in the back (the facets) closer together and compressing the facet joints between the vertebrae. Irritation and arthritis of these joints are the result. Other organ structures may be involved as well.

A diagnosis of rheumatoid arthritis should include two to four of the following criteria: morning stiffness, three or more joints involved symmetrically (especially the hands), six weeks or longer in duration, rheumatoid nodules that can be felt under the skin, blood tests showing a serum rheumatoid factor, and the radiographic evidence described above.

TREATMENT AND THERAPY

Treatment of arthritis may vary from home treatment to outpatient treatment to hospitalization for acute, surgical, and/or rehabilitative care. Educating patients as to their condition, the prognosis, the treatment goals, and the methods of treatment is necessary. Patients must be made aware of warning signs of progression, drug effects, local and systemic side effects of drug therapy, and diet associated with relieving pain, stiffness, and inflammation. If surgery is contemplated for joint replacement or other reasons, patients should be fully informed as to expectations and rate of functional activities. Postoperative restrictions in the range of motion must be given; in hip replacement, for example, hip bending should not exceed 90 degrees. The rotation and overlapping of legs must be limited initially after surgery.

Some physicians provide a questionnaire that outlines the activities of daily living and recommends how a patient should perform such activities and how much time should be spent at rest. The goals generally are to maintain function, to alleviate pain, to limit the progression of deformities, to prevent complications, and to treat associated and secondary disease states. In patients with degenerative arthritis—most often the elderly, who are at risk for other organ failures—arthritides associated with systemic diseases and other organ involvements may require care. Patients with rheumatoid arthritis, for example, frequently are anemic. Anti-inflammatory drugs, normally used to treat the arthritis, may cause blood loss through the gastrointestinal tract and even ulcerations. The physician may therefore prescribe alternative therapies.

Other therapies can include assistive devices, counseling patients and their families regarding home management, medicinal regimen and compliance, behavior modification, sexual advice, and biofeedback. The aim is to reduce the need for and frequency of medical care, through a balance between rest and activity and between effective drug dose, toxicity, and physical modalities. To protect joints and allow function, various braces and assistive devices may be needed. Scarring of a wrist joint can be alleviated by avoid-

ing positions that inhibit function. Shoulders should not be left with arms close to the body, since frozen shoulders aggravate neck and arm problems.

Physicians may offer physical therapy, occupational therapy, assistive devices for self-care, ambulation, or home and automobile modifications. Assistive devices may include reachers, an elongated shoe-horn handle, thickened handles for utensils, walkers, canes, crutches, and wheelchairs. Homes may require ramps for easier access, widened doors to allow wheelchair passage, grab bars in bathtubs, or raised toilet seats for easier transference from a wheelchair.

Heat therapy may reduce the pain, loosening and liquefying tightened tissues. Somewhat like gelatin, tissue liquifies when heated and solidifies when cooled. Patients frequently will be stiffer after protracted rest periods (for example, on waking) and feel better after some activity and exercise. Heated pools offer an excellent heating and exercise modality. The type of heat modality used will depend upon the depth of heating desired. Hot packs and infrared lamps will heat predominantly the skin surface areas and some underlying muscles. Diathermy units heat the muscular layers, and ultrasound treatments heat the deepest bony layers. Ultrasound (but no diathermy) can even be used in patients who have metallic implants such as joint replacements.

Transcutaneous electrical nerve stimulation can be used to alleviate pain. The units can regulate the frequency of electrical impulses. The usual starting rate is 100 cycles, which can alleviate pain in a few minutes; this rate is later changed to 4 cycles, which will give hours of relief even when discontinued. The intensity can also be varied. The sensation desired is a slight tingle. The effect described induces an increase in the release of beta endorphin, a substance naturally produced by the body with effects similar to those of morphine. Endorphin is produced by other physical therapy procedures as well: hypnosis, acupuncture, suggestion, and stress, among others.

Patients in chronic pain may show a reduced level of the beta endorphins and an increase in a substance P, and they may find no relief of pain with physical therapy. The P chemical increases the nerves' sensitivity to stimuli, producing greater pain. Patients with chronic pain may show depression, hysteria, and hypochondriasis on the Minnesota Multiphasic Personality Inventory test and may require antidepressants. Exercise programs can help to increase endorphin levels. These exercises may range from simple movements performed by a therapist (the patient remaining passive) to active exertion against loads for strength. Stretching or gentle, intermittent traction may gradually decrease contractures, but neck traction should not be used in patients with rheumatoid arthritis of the neck.

Surgery may occasionally be necessary to alleviate pain, to replace joints, or to alleviate contactures. Isometric or static exercises can mobilize muscles without joint movement and maintain muscle viability during joint pain. Individuals can, however, be trained to perform activities more efficiently and effectively, thus saving energy. Posture training may alleviate postural muscle fatigue. In acute stages of inflammation, the treatment choices are rest, ice, compression, and proper positioning and medicinals for pain and inflammation. The stepped-up medicinal approach utilizes nonsteroidal anti-inflammatory drugs (NSAIDS), adding other drugs as necessary, including antimalarials and gold, immune suppressants, and systemic corticosteroids. Irradiation of lymphoid tissues may also be used at the acute stages. Heat modalities should not be used in acute cases, since the speed of chemical reactions increases on heating; the chemical enzyme activity of collagenase that destroys cartilage could increase the rate and extent of damage. The simplest way to prepare cold applications is to fill a plastic container with water and refrigerate it. Physicians may also use fluoromethane or other refrigerant sprays. The hot packs sold in pharmacies can similarly be soaked in water and placed in the refrigerator to create an ice pack.

PERSPECTIVE AND PROSPECTS

Historically, arthritis was treated with electric eels (as the source of electric shocks) and warm baths or sands. Some experimental treatments presently being tried include electric current to joints to bring about reductions in intra-articular pressures and in the fluid and cellular content in joints. Acupuncture has been shown to bring an increase in the beta endorphin levels and consequent relief of pain. Topical use of capsaicin, an extract from peppers, is reported to counteract substance P. One group is attempting the experimental procedure of washing out inflamed joints with a saline-type solution. Exercises continue to maintain and improve strength, dexterity, the range of motion, and endurance. Good health habits—including adequate rest, good nutrition, and nutritional supplements—can be beneficial. —*Eugene J. Rogers*

See also Bursitis; Gout; Inflammation; Muscle sprains, spasms, and disorders; Osteoarthritis; Rheumatoid arthritis; Tendon disorders.

FOR FURTHER INFORMATION:

Dachman, Ken, and John Lyons. *You Can Relieve Pain.* New York: HarperCollins, 1990. This book approaches pain from a psychological point of view. Discusses methods for behavior modification, relaxation techniques, and mental imagery. Lists the names and addresses of various support groups and offers a suggested reading list for pain management.

Dong, Collin, and Jane Banks. *New Hope for the Arthritic.* New York: Ballantine Books, 1990. The emphasis in this book is predominantly on nutrition. The authors believe that food allergies and chemical additives in foods contribute to arthritis. They outline exercise programs to benefit arthritic patients.

Fries, James F. *Arthritis: A Comprehensive Guide to Understanding Your Arthritis.* 3d ed. Reading, Mass.: Addison-Wesley, 1990. This book is recommended by the Arthritis Foundation. The fifteen chapters discuss the major categories of arthritis, as well as pathology, quackery, surgery, employment, prevention, home treatment, and the effects of medications.

Gach, Michael R. *Acupressure's Potent Points: A Guide to Self-Care for Common Ailments.* New York: Bantam Books, 1990. Outlines the various acupressure points for treatment of various pain sites. The instructions for self-administration of acupressure techniques are specific and outlined in a steplike manner. The author also includes tips on proper eating and lifestyles.

Gordon, Neil F. *Arthritis: Your Complete Exercise Guide.* Champaign, Ill.: Human Kinetics, 1993. The author is eminently qualified to discuss and illustrate the various types of exercise modalities; he suggests a schedule of frequencies and durations for each. The illustrations are easily understood and followed.

Lorig, Kate, and James F. Fries, eds. *The Arthritis Handbook: A Tested Self-Management Program for Coping with Your Arthritis.* 3d ed. Reading, Mass.: Addison-Wesley, 1990. This book states that it is recommended by the Arthritis Foundation. The contributors, who include allied health professionals from the fields of physical therapy, occupational therapy, and public health, address pain management principles, body mechanics, and exercises.

MacLean, Helene. *Relief from Chronic Arthritis Pain.* New York: Dell Medical Library, 1990. This small book describes how to make a diagnosis of arthritis, stresses the importance of making the right diagnosis, and discusses treatments from aspirin to gold. Also includes chapters on alternative treatments, exercises, and vitamins and minerals. The glossary and index are helpful.

Pisetsky, David S., and Susan Trien Flamholtz. *The Duke University Medical Center Book of Arthritis.* New York: Fawcett Columbine Press, 1992. Discusses some of the major types of arthritis in three sections. The first discusses the major facts about arthritis, including its effects and some of the tests for the disease. The second portion delves into the major forms of arthritis. The third section goes into detail about the Duke University Basic Treatments, including physical therapy, diet, rest, exercises, and early medical interventions.

Yates, George, and Michael Shermer. *Meeting the Challenges of Arthritis: Motivational Program to Help You Live a Better Life.* Los Angeles: Lowell House, 1990. The book describes the personal struggle in overcoming marked disability from arthritis. Discusses the mental and physical effort expended and the techniques used to overcome the hardship of arthritic disabilities experienced by a young adult.

ARTHROPOD-BORNE DISEASES

SYSTEMS AFFECTED: Gastrointestinal, nervous, skin, blood

SPECIALISTS: Epidemiologists, infectious disease physicians, public health specialists, tropical medicine specialists

DEFINITION: Diseases that employ arthropods as vectors to animal or human hosts.

KEY TERMS:

arbovirus: an abbreviation for "arthropod-borne virus"

enzootic: referring to a disease that maintains itself in an animal reservoir

filariasis: infection with filaria, very slender parasitic worms mostly found in the tropics

helminthic: worm-related

host: the organism that harbors a disease agent, usually providing habitat and nourishment and often suffering harm from the infection or infestation

pathogen: a disease-causing agent (usually a virus, bacterium, protozoan, or parasitic worm)

vector: the agent that transfers a disease organism from host to host; may also be an intermediate site of propagation of the disease agent

zoonosis: a disease continuously transmitted in an animal population and for which humans are a side infection

CAUSES AND SYMPTOMS

From the perspective of a disease agent (virus, bacteria, protozoan, or parasitic worm) there are two major problems: adjusting to live in the host organism and avoid its defenses, and moving to new victims when the host eventually dies. Arthropods—the very successful group of small animals that includes mites, ticks, insects, and related organisms—are major vectors that shuttle many diseases to new hosts.

Size is a major factor in the success of arthropods. To both the massive blue whale and the microscopic bacterium, food items and natural media appear fairly uniform. It is at the size of insects and other arthropods that the world is most varied, and their one-million-plus known species outnumber all other animals and plants together. Because different arthropods live on roots and stems or infest the specific parts of all animals, disease agents that evolved an ability to live in ticks, fleas, or mosquitoes have shared the success of the arthropods. The control of these diseases requires a knowledge of the biology of insects and their relatives in order to interrupt this route of transmission.

Yet disease agents are not simply ingested and expelled by roving mosquitoes. Disease organisms must be finely adapted to survive the harsh gut environment of an insect or be able to migrate across insect membranes, migrate to salivary ducts, or proliferate wildly in the arthropod's own body fluids. Many disease agents simply cannot cross these barriers and are therefore not arthropod-borne. The range of disease agents includes viruses, protozoa, bacteria, and parasitic worms. That such a wide range of organisms have succeeded in using this route of transmission indicates that the strategy of using arthropod vectors has evolved many times.

Arthropod-Borne Viral Diseases

Disease	Principal Vectors
Colorado tick fever	Tick: *Dermacentor andersoni*
Encephalitis, California	Mosquitoes: *Culex tarsalis, Aedes* species
Encephalitis, Eastern equine	Mosquitoes: *Aedes sollicitans, Culiseta melanura*
Encephalitis, Far East Russian	Tick: *Ixodes persulcatus*
Encephalitis, St. Louis	Mosquitoes: *Culex pipiens pipiens, C. p. quinquefasciatus, C. tarsalis*
Encephalitis, Venezuelan	Mosquitoes: *Aedes serratus, Ae. scapularis, Ae. taeniorhynchus, Anopheles aquasalis, Culex vomifer, C. taeniopus, Haemogogus* species, *Mansonia titillans, Psorophora confinnis, P. ferox*
Encephalitis, Western equine	Mosquitoes: *Culex tarsalis* and others
Louping ill	Tick: *Isodes ricinus*
Pappataci or sandfly fever	Sandfly: *Phlebotomus papatasii*
Rift Valley fever	Mosquitoes: *Eretmapodites chrysogaster, Aedes caballus, Ae. deboeri, Ae. circumluteolus, Ae. tarsalis, Culex theileri*
Yellow fever	Mosquitoes: *Aedes aegypti* (urban and jungle strains), *Ae. africanus, Ae. simpsoni, Ae. leucocelaenus, Sabethes chloroterus,* and others

Arthropod-Borne Bacterial and Rickettsial Diseases

Disease	Disease Agent	Principal Vectors
Anthrax	*Bacillus anthracis*	Various horse flies by mechanical transmission
Boutonneuse fever	*Rickettsia conori*	Ticks: *Rhipicephalus sanguineus, R. secundus*, and species of *Haemaphysalis, Hyalomma, Amblyomma, Boophilis, Dermacentor*, and *Ixodes*
Carrion's disease	*Bartonella bacilliformis*	*Phlebotomus* sandflies
Food poisoning	*Shigella* and *Salmonella*	Various flies by mechanical transmission
Plague	*Yersinia pestis*	*Xenopsylla cheopis* and some other fleas
Q fever	*Coxiella burneti*	Ixodid ticks
Relapsing fever	*Borrelia*	*Ornithodoros* ticks
Rickettsialpox	*Rickettsia akari*	Mite: *Liponyssoides sanguineus*
Rocky Mountain spotted fever	*Rickettsia rickettsi*	Ticks: *Dermacentor andersoni, D. variabilis, Amblyomma americanus, Haemaphysalis leporispalustris* (rabbit-to-rabbit transmission)
Trench fever	*Rickettsia quintana*	Human body louse *Pediculus humanus humanus*
Tularemia	*Francisella tularensis*	Deer flies and ticks
Typhus, louse-borne	*Rickettsia prowazekii*	Human body louse *Pediculus humanus humanus*
Typhus, murine	*Rickettsia mooseri*	Rat flea *Xenopsylla cheopis*; the rat louse *Polyplax spinulosa* and the tropical rat mite *Ornthonssus bacoti* are zoonotic vectors
Typhus, scrub	*Rickettsia tsutsugamushi*	Mites: *Leptotrombidium akamushi* and *L. deliensis*
Yaws	*Treponema pertenue*	*Hippelates* gnats

In a strict sense, viruses are not living entities that can metabolize or move on their own. Merely elegant chunks of hereditary material protected by protein, viruses resemble living agents and are infectious only when they are taken in and reproduced by host cells. Plant bugs transmit many serious plant virus diseases; likewise a limited number of human viruses are transmitted by arthropods.

Some species of bacteria have adapted to transmission through arthropods. In some cases, they serve as simple mechanical carriers; other insects and ticks serve as true vectors by providing the pathogen with a medium in which to propagate and then actively injecting the bacteria into a new host. Rickettsias are smaller relatives of the bacteria that are particularly adapted for arthropod transmission. Rickettsias develop only inside the cells of susceptible hosts and vectors.

Protozoa are cellular organisms that are more complex than bacteria. Amebic dysentery caused by *Entamoeba histolytica* may occasionally be transmitted mechanically by cockroaches and flies. Yet some of the most serious tropical human afflictions—malaria, sleeping sickness, and leishmaniasis (kala-azar)—are also caused by protozoans. The trypanosomes and *Leishmania* are flagellates that belong to the subphylum Mastigophora; the malaria organisms are part of the Apicomplexa, a group of protozoa specialized for parasitism.

The last group of organisms that are transmitted with the help of arthropods is the parasitic worms. "Worms" is a nonscientific term that includes the flatworms (Trematoda), spiny-headed worms (Acanthocephalans), tapeworms (Cestoda), and roundworms (Nematoda). Many are quite large in size, but those that utilize arthropod vectors have microscopic stages. While most of the nematode parasites need to enter the bloodstream and are vectored by various blood-sucking flies, the other worms—those that mostly target the digestive system—are contracted when people ingest the arthropod host.

The involvement of arthropods in carrying diseases varies greatly. House flies and horseflies may merely pick up bacteria and mechanically transmit it to food or a wound.

Arthropod-Borne Protozoan Diseases

Disease	Disease Agent	Principal Vectors
Chagas disease	Trypanosoma cruzi	Assassin bugs: Panstrongylus megistus and many species of Triatoma
Kala-azar	Leishmania donovani	Sandflies: Phlebotomus chinensis, P. major, P. argentipes, P. perniciosus
Leishmaniasis, American mucocutaneous	Leishmania braziliensis	Sandflies: Phlebotomus intermedius, P. longipalpus, P. pessoai
Leishmaniasis, Mexican	Leishmania mexicana	Sandfly: Phlebotomus flaviscutellatus
Malaria, benign tertian	Plasmodium vivax	Mosquitoes: species of Anopheles
Malaria, malignant tertian	Plasmodium falciparum	Mosquitoes: Anopheles stephensi, A. labranchiae
Malaria, ovale tertian	Plasmodium ovale	Mosquitoes: Anopheles gambiae, A. funestus
Malaria, quartan	Plasmodium malariae	Mosquitoes: many species of Anopheles
Nagana (cattle, etc.)	Trypanosoma brucei	Tsetse fly: Glossina morsitans
Oriental sore	Leishmania tropica	Sandflies: Phlebotomus papatasii and P. sergenti
Sleeping sickness, East African	Trypanosoma rhodesiense	Tsetse flies: Glossina morsitans and G. swynnertoni
Sleeping sickness, West African	Trypanosoma gambiense	Tsetse flies: Glossina tachinoides and G. palpalis
Surra (camels, etc.)	Trypanosoma evansi	Horse flies in the family Tabanidae
Texas cattle fever	Babesia bigemina	Ticks: Boophilus annulatus, B. microplus, B. decoloratus, Haemaphysalus punctata, and species of Rhipicephalus

In such cases, it is difficult to determine accurately the extent to which such casual transmission is involved in diseases. Other arthropods are actually required by the disease agent for the completion of their developmental stages; without some time in the insect's gut, for example, a pathogen may be unable to infect another host. Finally, some arthropods are critical because they seek out and target the host with accuracy.

Treatment and Therapy

Unlike some viral and bacterial infections that have been thoroughly controlled or even eliminated, most arthropod-borne diseases remain serious health threats, especially in tropical areas. For example, smallpox (which is not insect-borne) was easier to control and eliminate because it only occurred in humans; it was transferred directly from human to human; a survivor or inoculated person had lifetime immunity from further infection; inoculation was cheap and provided long-term protection; and smallpox was easy to diagnose (few other diseases could be mistaken for it).

In contrast, arthropod-borne diseases generally reside in an animal reservoir. This animal reservoir may provide the natural cycle for the parasite or disease agent; this is known from cases in which the disease agent is mild in its natural animal host, indicating that the organism and the disease have evolved together over a long time. For both parasites and disease agents, mild strains that preserve the host are selected over time, and virulent strains that rapidly kill the host have less chance of surviving themselves. Therefore, when a new arthropod-borne disease appears that is extremely virulent, it is an indication that humans are a new host with little adaptation to the parasite.

Arthropod-borne diseases may be unusually resistant to the human immune system, which usually eliminates invaders in a short time. Some organisms such as malaria Plasmodium are constantly changing the stage that they present to the immune system. Parasitic worms, on the other hand, may seal themselves up in cysts or inside protective cuticles and live protected lives. Because one often cannot reach the infective agent in the human body, attempts to control arthropod-borne diseases have centered heavily on interrupting the transmission by the vectors.

Because humans do not form immunity to worms and some other disease agents, an individual can be infected repeatedly. Moreover, the symptoms of many of these diseases are fevers easily confused with other ailments. Thus, in many tropical regions it is the norm for people to have

Arthropod-Borne Worm (Helminthic) Diseases:
Diseases Contracted Through Ingesting Arthropod Host

Disease	Parasite	Arthropod Host
Broad tapeworm	*Dibothriocephalus latus*	Crustaceans eaten by fish that in turn are eaten by humans
Dog tapeworm	*Dipylidium caninum*	Dog flea *Pulex irritans* and lice
Dracunculosus or guinea worm	*Dracunculus medinensis*	Copepod crustaceans: *Cyclops* species
Oriental lung fluke	*Paragonimus westermani*	Snails via crabs and crayfish
Rodent tapeworm	*Hymenolepis diminuta*	Fleas including *Xenopsylla cheopis*; also roaches, moth and beetle larvae
Spiney-headed worm	*Macracanthorhynchus hirudinaceus*	Beetle larvae

a parasite load. Since the disease agents are generally protected inside the relatively uniform environment of the body of host animals and humans, the fact that many of these diseases do not extend to the temperate areas of the world indicates that harsh winters are important in controlling the range of insect vectors. This fact also explains why tropical diseases do not spread in a temperate country when immigrants bring them: The arthropod vector is absent.

PERSPECTIVE AND PROSPECTS

Following the work of Louis Pasteur and Robert Koch and their students, the late 1800's saw a shift away from a belief in night air miasmas ("malaria" means "bad air") toward germ theory—that disease agents are at the cause of all ailments. Indeed, nutritional deficiencies such as pellagra were even suspected to be caused by some disease agent. Therefore, in 1878 when Patrick Manson observed the development of *Wuchereria bancrofti* in the bodies of *Culex*

mosquitoes, it did not take long for him and other workers to prove that this insect was the intermediate host and vector for this medically important worm infection. The discovery of vector-borne diseases gave birth to the field of medical entomology, and a sequence of important discoveries followed: malaria parasites in the blood of humans; tsetse fly transmission of nagana, cattle sleeping sickness, and human sleeping sickness; malaria parasites in mosquitoes; mosquito transmission of yellow fever; transmission of the plague organism through sick rats by fleas; and the role of the body louse in carrying typhus fever (1909).

Whenever science becomes aware of a new infectious disease—as in the cases of Lyme disease, Legionnaires' disease, AIDS, or Hantavirus—the possibility that the disease is arthropod-borne is an early concern. (Of these new diseases, only Lyme disease involves an arthropod vector.) In addition to working out the etiology—the mechanisms by

Arthropod-Borne Worm (Helminthic) Diseases:
Diseases Contracted from Blood-Sucking Flies

Disease	Parasite	Principal Vectors
Acanthocheilonemasis	*Acanthocheilonema perstans*	Biting midges: *Culicoides austeni* and *C. grahami*
Bancroft's filariasis	*Wuchereria bancrofti*	Mosquitoes: *Culex pipiens quinquefasciatus* and other *Culex*, *Aedes*, *Anopheles*, and *Mansonia* species
Brug's filariasis	*Brugia malayi*	Mosquitoes: *Mansonia*, *Anopheles*, *Aedes*, and *Armigeres* species
Dog heartworm	*Dirofilaria immitis*	Mosquitoes: *Culex pipiens*, *Aedes aegypti*, and others
Loiasis or African eyeworm	*Loa loa*	Mango flies: *Chrysops dimidiatus* and *C. silaceus*
Onchocerciasis	*Onchocerca volvulus*	Black flies: *Simulium damnosum*, *S. neavei*, *S. ochraceum*, and others
Ozzard's filariasis	*Mansonella ozzardi*	Biting midge *Culicoides furens*

Mosquito-Borne Diseases

Mosquito	Habits	Features	Diseases
Aedes	Day biter, urban or rural	Head bent, body parallel to surface, black and white in color	Dengue, yellow fever, viral encephalitis
Anopheles	Night biter, mainly rural	Head and body in line, at angle to surface	Malaria, filariasis
Culex	Day biter, urban or rural	Shaped like *Aedes* but brown; whines in flight	Viral encephalitis, filariasis

which the disease agent actually causes the illness—it is important to confirm if an insect or mite is spreading the disease in order to put effective control measures into place.

Clues that a new disease may be arthropod-borne could include epidemiological evidence, such as a pattern of disease occurrence that matches the range of a mosquito or the common report of insect bites by all patients. Eventually, confirmation of the role of an arthropod as a vector for the disease will come after extensive clinical work proves the identity of the disease agent and additional laboratory work shows this disease agent to be present in natural populations of the vector. This knowledge proves beneficial when control of arthropod populations results in dramatic improvements in the health of human populations.

—*John Richard Schrock*

See also Bites and stings; Lice, mites, and ticks; Parasitic diseases; Zoonoses; *specific diseases.*

FOR FURTHER INFORMATION:

Busvine, J. R. *Insects, Hygiene, and History.* London: Athlone Press, 1976. An accurate summary of human rela-

tionships with ectoparasites, primarily insects and mites. With abundant illustrations and further references to classics in parasite biology.

Desowitz, Robert S. *The Malaria Capers: More Tales of Parasites and People, Research, and Reality.* New York: W. W. Norton, 1991. The best modern overview of how social and political factors are involved in the science of public health medicine is this set of two stories on kala-azar and malaria. Honest false leads in early research contrast with modern research fraud impeding the effort to hold the line against these two major world diseases.

James, Maurice T., and Robert F. Harwood. *Herm's Medical Entomology.* 6th ed. New York: Macmillan, 1969. Entomologists, scientists who study insects, are also called upon to identify noninsect arthropods involved in bites, stings, and vector-transmitted diseases. An authoritative text for training medical entomologists and a standard reference.

Learmonth, Andrew. *Disease Ecology: An Introduction to Ecological Medical Geography.* Oxford, England: Basil Blackwell, 1988. Important chapters on the history of diseases, tropical diseases, mosquito-borne diseases, and onchocerciasis place arthropod-borne diseases in a wider perspective.

McKelvey, John J., Jr., Bruce F. Eldridge, and Karl Maramorosch. *Vectors of Disease Agents: Interactions with Plants, Animals and Man.* New York: Praeger, 1981. Authorities in the biology of vectored diseases explain the problems encountered by disease agents and by humans trying to control their transmission.

Snow, Keith R. *Insects and Disease.* New York: John Wiley & Sons, 1974. A clear and simple explanation of the biology of both insects and pathogens.

ASPHYXIATION

SYSTEMS AFFECTED: Circulatory, respiratory

SPECIALISTS: Emergency physicians, occupational medicine physicians

DEFINITION: The state of unconsciousness or death resulting from oxygen deprivation.

The phenomenon whereby the body experiences a decrease in oxygen below normal levels is called hypoxia; extreme cases of hypoxia lead to anoxia, a complete lack of oxygen. The difference between anoxia and asphyxia is that in asphyxia an accumulation of excess carbon dioxide (hypercapnia) takes place, as the normal exchange of oxygen and carbon dioxide in the lungs is obstructed.

Respiration is regulated in the medulla, while chemoreceptors present in the aortic arch and the carotid sinus respond to levels of oxygen, carbon dioxide, and the pH in blood and the cerebrospinal fluid. The concentration of carbon dioxide pressure in the plasma is proportional to the oxygen pressure. Generally, oxygen deprivation may be the consequence of one or more of several conditions. In all cases, damage results that leads first to hypoxia and eventually to death.

Types of oxygen deprivation. In the first condition, respiration may be slowed or stopped by injury or foreign material blocking the air passage. The most common example of this case is asphyxia that results from the inhalation of water by exhausted swimmers or persons who cannot swim. Large quantities of water fill the lung and cut off the oxygen supply. Other examples include the entrapment of food or liquid in the respiratory tract, strangulation, and residence in high altitude. In these cases, the carbon dioxide pressure is drastically increased. Artificial respiration may save the victim's life; it should be performed as soon as possible and after the removal of the inhaled foreign substance via vomiting. Strangulation provides the more serious problem of capillary rupturing and internal bleeding.

A second condition, hypoxic anoxia, is caused by an inadequate concentration of oxygen in the atmosphere, which occurs in poorly ventilated enclosed spaces such as in mine tunnels, sewers, or industrial areas. Odorless gases such as methane (which is produced in decomposing sewage) or nitrogen may be dangerous because they generally go undetected. A former way of detecting such gases involved taking along a bird in a cage and monitoring its well-being during the exploration of unknown caves or ancient tombs.

In anemic anoxia, respiration may not be effective because of the reduced capacity of the blood to become oxygenated; as a result, less oxygen is transferred to the tissues. Carbon monoxide behaves differently than methane or nitrogen, since it binds much more strongly to hemoglobin than oxygen does. Thus the hemoglobin, which is the oxygen-carrying component of blood, does not transfer oxygen to the tissues, which are starved of it. The passage of oxygen from the lung alveoli to the adjacent blood capillaries may also be affected, such as with chronic lung disease, infections, or developmental effects.

A fourth category is stagnant anoxia, whereby a reduced flow of blood through the blood tissues takes place. This may be a generalized condition, attributable to heart disease, or localized, which may take place in a pilot during aerial maneuvers. The blackout of the aviator is a result of the heart's inability to pump enough blood to these regions against the high centrifugal force. In some cases, the carbon dioxide pressure cannot be removed in the usual manner by the lung. Any lung disease will decrease the effective removal of carbon dioxide and therefore result in elevated levels of it in the blood. Thus in emphysema, a disease in which the alveoli increase in size and which leads to a reduction of the surface area available for gas exchange, carbon dioxide will be retained in the blood. In bronchopneumonia, the alveoli contain secretions, white cells, bacteria, and fibrin, which prevent an efficient gas exchange.

In histotoxic anoxia, the failure of cellular respiration is observed. The body's cells are unable to utilize oxygen as a result of poisoning, as from cyanide. The supply of oxygen is normal, but the cells are unable to metabolize the oxygen that is delivered to them.

Symptoms. All cases of anoxia may lead to oxygen deprivation in the brain, which may be fatal if it lasts more than a few minutes. Nerve cell degeneration may start and continue, despite the fact that the original cause of anoxia is removed and normal breathing is resumed. Many health conditions may interfere with the blood transport of oxygen, which is accomplished via the red blood cells. Such diseases include cases of anemia, trauma, hemorrhage, and circulatory disease.

The body responds toward oxygen deprivation with an increase in the rate of depth of breathing. The normal, sea-level oxygen pressure of the air is approximately 160 millimeters (6.2 inches) of mercury. When the oxygen pressure is reduced to 110 millimeters (4.2 inches) of mercury at an altitude of about 3,000 meters (10,000 feet), the pulse rate increases and the volume of blood pumped from the heart also increases. Although prolonged exposure to low oxygen pressure may bring the pulse rate back to normal, the output of the heart remains elevated. Despite the lack of oxygen, both the heart and the brain function because of the dilation of their blood cells and the increased oxygen extraction from the blood. Anoxia leads to vision problems first, while hearing is generally the last sense to go. It is not unusual for a person who is suffering from anoxia to be incapable of moving but able to hear. —*Soraya Ghayourmanesh*

See also Altitude sickness; Unconsciousness.

ASTHMA

SYSTEM AFFECTED: Respiratory

SPECIALISTS: Allergists, immunologists, pulmonologists

DEFINITION: A chronic obstructive pulmonary disease that obstructs the airways to the lungs and makes it difficult or, in severe attacks, nearly impossible to breathe.

KEY TERMS:

allergen: any substance that causes an overreaction of the immune system; also called an antigen

allergic reaction: the presence of adverse symptoms that are part of the body's overreaction to an antigen

allergy: an overreaction of the immune system to a substance that does not affect the general population; the tendency to be allergic is inherited

beta-stimulators: chemicals that attach to the beta-receptors on cells; often used in inhalers, they cause the bronchioles to dilate, or open

bronchioles: small air tubes leading to the air sacs of the lungs; the functional units of the airway that are involved in asthma

mast cells: cells in connective tissue capable of releasing chemicals that cause allergic reactions

trigger: the substance or event that sets off an asthma attack; triggers may be allergens or some other type of stimulus

CAUSES AND SYMPTOMS

Asthma is a Greek word meaning "grasping" or "panting." It is a chronic obstructive pulmonary (lung) disease that involves repeated attacks in which the airways in the lungs are suddenly blocked. The disease is not completely understood, but asthma attacks cause the person to experience tightening of the chest, sudden breathlessness, wheezing, and coughing. Death by asphyxiation is rare but possible. Fortunately, the effects can be reversed with proper medication. The severity of symptoms and attacks varies greatly among individuals, and sufferers can be located on a continuum running from mild to severe. Mild asthmatics have fewer than six minimal attacks per year, with no symptoms between attacks, and they require no hospitalizations and little or no medication between attacks. Severe asthmatics have more than six serious attacks each year, have symptoms between attacks, lose more than ten school days or workdays, and require two or more hospitalizations per year. Attacks are typically spaced with symptom-free intervals but may also occur continuously. Rather than focusing only on the specific attacks, one should view and treat asthma as a chronic disease, a nagging, continuing condition that persists over a long period of time.

A review of the path of air into the body during normal breathing helps in understanding asthma. During inhalation, air travels into the nose and mouth and then into the trachea (windpipe); it then divides into the two tubes called bronchi and enters the lungs. Inside each lung, the tubes become smaller and continue to divide. The air finally moves into the smallest tubes, called bronchioles, and then flows into the millions of small, thin-walled sacs called alveoli. Vital gas exchange occurs in the alveoli.

This gas exchange involves two gases in particular, oxygen and carbon dioxide. Oxygen must cross the membrane of the alveoli into the blood and then travel to all the cells of the body. Within the cells, it is used in chemical reactions that produce energy. These same reactions produce carbon dioxide as a by-product, which is returned by the blood to the alveoli. This gas is removed from the body through the same pathway that brought oxygen into the lungs.

The parts of this airway that are involved in asthma are the bronchioles. These tubes are wrapped with smooth, involuntary muscles that adjust the amount of air that enters. The lining of the bronchioles also contains many cells that secrete a substance called mucus. Mucus is a thick, clear, slimy fluid produced in many parts of the body. Normal production of mucus in the lungs catches foreign material and lubricates the pathway to allow smooth airflow. People suffering from asthma have very sensitive bronchioles.

Three mechanisms in the bronchioles contribute to an asthma attack. One is an abnormal sensitivity and constriction of the involuntary muscles surrounding the airways, which narrows the diameter of the airway. Another is an inflammation and swelling of the tissues that make up the

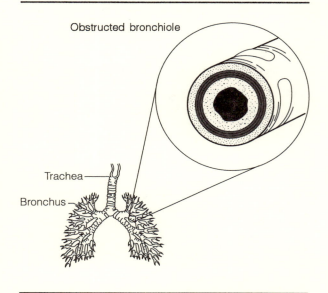

During an asthma attack, obstructed bronchioles limit or halt airflow, resulting in severely restricted breathing.

bronchioles themselves. The third is an increased production of mucus, which then blocks the airways. These three mechanisms may work in combination. The result can be extreme difficulty in taking air into the lungs until the attack subsides. The characteristic "wheeze" of asthma is caused by efforts to exhale, which is more difficult than inhaling. In the most serious attacks, the airways may close down to the point of suffocating the patient if medical help is not given.

Attacks can vary in severity at different times because of variations in tension within the bronchiole muscles. Although there is still debate about the general function of these muscles, they probably help to distribute the air entering the alveoli evenly. Control of the tension in these smooth muscles is involuntary and follows a circadian (twenty-four-hour) rhythm. Accordingly, for most people this cycle causes maximum constriction to occur at about 6:00 A.M. and maximum relaxation to occur at about 6:00 P.M. Hence, asthma attacks tend to be more severe in the late night and early morning.

Following a given asthma attack, patients are sometimes susceptible to additional, more severe attacks. This period of high risk, called a late-phase response, occurs five or six hours after the initial symptoms pass and may last as long as a day. Some researchers believe that the increase in deaths from asthma in the United States may be tied to this danger, which often goes unrecognized.

The initial cause and mechanism of an asthma attack can vary from person to person. Accordingly, asthma is usually divided into two types. One type is extrinsic, that is, caused by external triggers that bring about an allergic response. Allergic reactions involve the immune system. Normal functioning of the immune system guards the body against harmful substances. With an allergy, the body incorrectly identifies a harmless substance as harmful and reacts against it. This substance is then called an allergen. If the symptoms of this reaction occur in the lungs, the person has extrinsic or allergic asthma. Pollens, dust, animal dander, molds, and feathers are common allergens.

When allergens enter the body, the white blood cells make specific IgE antibodies that can bond with the invaders. Next, the IgE antibodies attach to the surfaces of mast cells; these cells are found all over the body and are numerous in the lungs. The allergens attach to the IgE antibodies located on the mast cells, and the mast cells are stimulated to produce and release chemicals called mediators, such as histamine, prostaglandin D_2, and leukotrienes. These mediators cause sneezing, tighten the muscles in the bronchioles, swell the surrounding tissues, and increase mucus production.

The second type of asthma is intrinsic and does not involve allergies. People who suffer from intrinsic asthma have hyperactive or twitchy airways that overreact to irritating factors. The mechanism for this form is not always understood, but no IgE antibodies for the irritant are placed on the mast cells. Examples of such nonallergic stimuli are cigarette smoke, house dust, artificial coloring, aspirin, ozone, or cold air. Odors from insecticides, cleaning fluids, cooking foods, and perfume can also trigger attacks. Also included in this category are attacks that are caused by viral infections (including colds and flu), stress, and exercise. Asthma can be triggered by many different substances and events in different people. While the symptoms are the same whether the asthma is intrinsic or extrinsic, asthmatics need to identify what substances or events trigger their attacks in order to gain control of the disease.

Why people develop asthma is not well understood. Asthma can begin at any age, but it is more likely to arise in childhood. While it is known that heredity predisposes an individual to asthma, the pattern of inheritance is not a simple one. Most geneticists now regard allergies as polygenic, which means that more than one pair of genes is involved. Height, skin color, and intelligence are other examples of polygenic traits. Exposure to particular external conditions may also be important. The children who develop asthma are more likely to be boys, while girls are more likely to show signs of the disease at puberty (about age twelve). Childhood asthma is also most likely to disappear or to be "outgrown" at puberty; about half of the cases of childhood asthma eventually disappear.

Early exposures to some triggers may be a key in the development of asthma. Smoking by mothers can cause children with a genetic disposition to develop asthma. Apparently, the early exposure to secondhand smoke develops an allergy. Early studies in this area were confusing until

the data were sorted by level of education. Lung specialist Fernando Martinez of the University of Arizona believes that less-educated women who smoke are more likely to cause this effect because their homes are likely to be smaller and therefore expose the children to more smoke. Another study, this one in Great Britain, indicated that more frequent and thorough housecleaning might keep children from developing asthma. Early exposure by genetically susceptible children to dust and the mites that thrive in dust may also cause some to develop asthma.

Asthma is a major health problem in the United States. As many as 20 million Americans may have the disease, and the number has been mysteriously increasing since 1970. While attacks can cause complications, there is no permanent damage to the lungs themselves, as there is in emphysema. Complications include possible lung collapse, infections, chronic dilation, rib fracture, a permanently enlarged chest cavity, and respiratory failure. Furthermore, millions of days of work and school are lost as victims recuperate; asthma is the leading cause of missed school days. Even though attacks can be controlled by medication, occasionally fatalities do occur. The death rate in the United States reached 4,600 in 1987.

TREATMENT AND THERAPY

The key to gaining control of asthma is discovering the particular factors that act as triggers for an attack in a given individual. These factors vary and at times can be surprising; for example, one person found that a mint flavoring in a particular toothpaste was a trigger for his asthma. Nevertheless, most common triggers fall in the following groups: allergies; irritants, including dust, fumes, odors, and vapors; air pollution, temperature, and dryness; colds and flu; and stress. Even types of food may be important. Diets low in vitamin C, fish, or a zinc-to-copper ratio, as well as diets with a high sodium-to-potassium ratio, seem to increase the risk of asthma attacks and bronchitis. There have also been correlations between low niacin levels in the diet and tight airways and wheezing.

Various medications are available to keep the airways open and to lower their sensitivity. In an emergency, drugs may be injected, but medications are usually either inhaled or taken orally as pills. Because inhaling transports the medication directly to the lungs, lower doses can be used. Many asthmatics carry inhalers, which allow them to breathe in the medication during an attack. Because this action requires a person to coordinate inhaling with the release of the spray, young children are sometimes better off with a device that requires them to wear a mask. The choice and dosage of medicine vary with the patient, and physicians need to determine what is safest and most effective for each individual. Self-treatment with nonprescription drugs should be avoided.

Some of the most commonly prescribed drugs are bronchodilators, inflammation reducers, and trigger-sensitivity reducers. The bronchodilators include albuterol, metaproterenol, and terbutaline. They are beta-stimulators that mimic the way in which the body's nervous system relaxes or dilates the airways. (Any drug that functions as a beta-blocker should be avoided by asthmatics because of its opposite effects.) Another bronchodilator is adrenaline (or epinephrine), but it is a less specific drug that also affects the heart and pulse rate. Theophylline, a stimulant chemically related to caffeine, relaxes the airways and also helps clear mucus. The use of corticosteroids (or steroids) for asthma has been increasing because they reduce inflammation and relax airways. Initially, corticosteroids were used if other drugs were ineffective, but in 1991 they were strongly recommended for long-term preventive use. As another way of addressing asthma as a long-term problem, cromolyn sodium is sometimes inhaled on a daily basis to prevent attacks by decreasing sensitivity to triggers.

The concern for safety with these medications increases when asthmatics use high doses (more than two hundred inhalations monthly) of beta-stimulator inhalers. A higher risk of fatal or near-fatal attacks has been found with a high usage of fenoterol, a beta-stimulator that is not used in the United States. Paul Scanlon, a chest physician at the Mayo Clinic, warns that individuals should not exceed their prescribed dosage when using an inhaler. An individual who feels the need to use an inhaler more often to obtain adequate relief should see a doctor. The increased need is a sign of worsening asthma, and a doctor needs to investigate and perhaps change the treatment.

Some doctors have improved their diagnosis of asthma with a tool called the peak flow meter. The meter can also be used by patients at home to predict impending attacks. This inexpensive device measures how fast air can be moved out of the lungs. Therefore, it can be discovered that airways are beginning to tighten before other symptoms occur. The early warning allows time to adjust medications to head off attacks. This tool can help asthmatics take charge of their disease.

Research is continuing with a new family of drugs that interfere with the chemical moderators, such as leukotriene, released by mast cells. Two drugs, zileuton and MK-571, have shown promise. Zileuton interferes with leukotriene production in the mast cells. MK-571 does not affect production but blocks the receptor sites for leukotriene on the smooth muscle. Zileuton reduced the feeling of congestion in volunteers in one experiment and allowed another group to withstand much more cold air before having an attack. MK-571 reduced airway constriction by about 70 percent during a stationary bicycle test. This line of research represents a hopeful new direction for asthma sufferers.

Over-the-counter drugs are often used by asthmatics to treat their symptoms. These drugs often use ephedrine, metaraminol, phenylephrine, methoxamine, or similar chemicals. All these drugs are structurally related to amphetamine or adrenaline. Unfortunately, some people may be getting relief without discovering the cause of their asthma. The National Asthma Education Panel (NAEP) maintains that self-treatment without a doctor's guidance is risky.

That asthmatics should generally avoid exercise is a myth. With a doctor's approval, regular sports and exercise may be pursued. Furthermore, exercise may be helpful in reducing the frequency and severity of attacks. Many athletes compete at high levels in spite of their asthma. An outstanding example is Olympic gold medalist Jackie Joyner-Kersee, who is asthmatic and who was named the best all-around woman athlete in the world in 1988. Another is Jeanette Bolden, who had been especially affected as a child but sprinted to an Olympic gold medal in 1984. Sports that do not require continuous activity or exposure to cold, dry air are preferred. Swimming is considered ideal. Doctors can help the athlete with a pre-exercise medication plan and a backup plan if symptoms occur during or after the exercise.

Another damaging belief about asthma needs comment. Early Freudian psychology held that asthma could be caused by a mother who failed to answer her baby's crying. Accordingly, the onset of asthma, with its gasping for air, was seen as a continuation of that crying. This sad hypothesis is false: Asthma is not connected to any abnormal relationships between mother and child, and it is not caused by early or deep psychological problems.

Researchers continue to search for new ways to reduce the frequency and the effects of asthmatic attacks. The National Heart, Lung, and Blood Institute in Bethesda, Maryland, found that caffeine in coffee seems to help. The study showed that asthmatics who are regular coffee drinkers suffer one-third fewer symptoms (particularly, less wheezing) than those who do not drink coffee. The most promise, however, seems to be in developing a new line of drugs that will prevent the mast cells from releasing their chemicals. Such a medication could stop inflammation before it takes hold, either by curbing the production of leukotrienes or by preventing these chemicals from acting on the airways.

PERSPECTIVE AND PROSPECTS

Asthma was recognized in ancient times in both the East and the West. The Chinese people have a rich collection of traditional remedies going back more than five thousand years that includes the use of *ma huang*, an Asiatic species of the genus *Ephedra*, for asthma and other lung conditions. *Ma huang* is a vinelike, shrubby, almost leafless gymnosperm. In 1887, the alkaloid ephedrine was isolated from *Ephedra* as the active ingredient in the plant; the drug is similar in effect to adrenaline. Alkaloids are bitter in taste and often affect the nervous system. Scientists used the ending *-ine* to identify alkaloids, many of which have strong physiological effects on humans (such as caffeine, morphine, nicotine, and cocaine). *Ma huang* was used in both ancient China and India.

Pliny the Elder (A.D. 23-79) believed that everything had been created for the sake of humans and therefore that nature was a complete storehouse of natural remedies. His encyclopedia *Historia Naturalis* recommended ephedron, a source of ephedrine, for asthma, coughing, and hemorrhages. Some believe that Pliny may have suffered from asthma. He died from the fumes of Mount Vesuvius while investigating the volcano and trying to help refugees.

In the eighteenth century, the discovery of oxygen, nitrous oxide, and other gases led to serious efforts to determine medical uses for these gases. Inhalation allowed a gaseous medication to be removed as soon as the effect was achieved; precise dosage did not have to be calculated. There were legitimate efforts to find painkillers for surgery and dentistry. Soon charlatans falsely claimed, however, to be able to use the new gases to cure asthma and other diseases. Anesthetics such as ether, nitrous oxide, and chloroform were used by doctors in the 1850's to treat asthma and other conditions.

As early as 1190, Maimonides, the physician to the court of Sladin, the sultan of Egypt, noted that asthma tended to run in families. Unfortunately, Maimonides' thoughts about heredity were forgotten until much later. Early in the twentieth century, researchers did find that 48 percent of the asthmatics surveyed had an immediate family history of allergies.

In 1991, the NAEP, a federal panel of experts brought together by the National Heart, Lung, and Blood Institute, issued the first national guidelines for the diagnosis and treatment of asthma. These guidelines recommended that doctors should not approach asthma as treatment for the attacks alone. Rather, NAEP experts urged a focus on long-term prevention, increasing the use of inhaled steroids especially with severe and moderate asthmatics. The report also urged increased use of the peak flow meter to predict attacks. —*Paul R. Boehlke*

See also Allergies; Environmental diseases; Pulmonary diseases.

FOR FURTHER INFORMATION:

Haas, François, and Sheila Sperber Haas. "Living with Asthma." In *The World Book Medical Encyclopedia*. Chicago: World Book, 1988. This special report carefully explains the disease and encourages asthmatics to take control of their lives. A chart details how a house can be asthma-proofed. Side effects and drawbacks of various drugs are charted.

Krementz, Jill. *How It Feels to Fight for Your Life*. Boston: Little, Brown, 1989. A collection of fourteen case studies of children who have serious chronic diseases. In one chapter, Anton Broekman, a ten-year-old, describes what living with asthma is like.

Ostrow, Williams, and Vivian Ostrow. *All About Asthma.*

Morton Grove, Ill.: Albert Whitmany, 1989. A children's book written to inform and encourage. The writers, a boy and his mother, tell about his experience with asthma. He explains causes, symptoms, and ways to lead a normal life. A must for children with asthma.

Paul, Glennon H., and Barbara A. Fafoglia. *All About Asthma and How to Live with It*. New York: Sterling, 1988. A valuable book with tips for coping with asthma at home, in school, and in the workplace. The chapter on drugs is very helpful, pointing out both benefits and risks.

Weinstein, Allan M. *Asthma: The Complete Guide to Self-Management of Asthma and Allergies for Patients and Their Families*. New York: Fawcett Crest, 1987. An excellent guide to asthma which contains an extensive section on the identification of triggers that may be causing an individual's attacks.

ASTIGMATISM

SYSTEM AFFECTED: Visual

SPECIALISTS: Ophthalmologists

DEFINITION: An astigmatism is a relatively common condition in which either the cornea of the eye or the lens is not symmetrical, being flatter or more curved in some places. The vision is blurred because the image that reaches the retina is distorted or out of focus. Astigmatism may occur in combination with myopia (nearsightedness) or hyperopia (farsightedness). The condition can be corrected by placing a cylindrical lens (such as an eyeglass or contact lens) in front of the eye in order to focus the image on the retina.

See also Visual disorders.

ATAXIA

SYSTEMS AFFECTED: Muscular, nervous

SPECIALISTS: Neurologists

DEFINITION: Ataxia is characterized by an inability to coordinate the muscles in voluntary movement. The sufferer may have an awkward, unsteady gait with little balance, jerky movement of the limbs, and slurred speech. It may have many causes, ranging from brain damage from a stroke or tumor to a disorder of the inner ear to excessive alcohol consumption. The symptoms are much more severe and longer lasting, if not permanent, when the cause is neurological, as with brain disorders or multiple sclerosis.

See also Alcoholism; Brain disorders; Multiple sclerosis; Strokes and TIAs.

ATHEROSCLEROTIC DISEASE

SYSTEMS AFFECTED: Heart, circulatory

SPECIALISTS: Cardiologists, internists, vascular surgeons

DEFINITION: Also called arteriosclerosis or "hardening of the arteries," a generalized disease that causes narrowing of the arteries because of deposits on the arterial walls and leading to a multitude of serious medical conditions, notably stroke and heart attack.

KEY TERMS:

angina: chest, jaw, or shoulder pain with exercise or stress—a symptom of atherosclerotic heart disease

embolus: a small piece of atherosclerotic plaque, thrombus, or other debris that breaks off and lodges in a blood vessel

infarct: tissue death resulting from lack of blood flow

intermittent claudication: a symptom of lower-extremity arteriosclerosis manifested by pain or cramping in the leg while walking, relieved by rest; from the Latin word *claudicatio*, "to limp"

ischemia: lack of blood in a particular tissue

rest pain: pain noted in the most distal portion of the extremity at rest, relieved by analgesics

revascularization: procedures to reestablish the circulation to a diseased portion of the body

thrombosis: aggregation of platelets and other blood cells to form a clot

CAUSES AND SYMPTOMS

The human body's arterial system is designed to carry oxygen, hormones, various types of blood cells (such as red and white blood cells), and other nutrients in the blood from the heart to the periphery and all organ structures of the body. The arteries are composed of three separate layers: adventia (the outer layer), media (the middle layer), and intima (the inner layer). Atherosclerosis or arteriosclerosis, derived from the Greek words that mean "hardening of the arteries," refers to the different diseases that compromise one or more of the layers of the large- or medium-sized arteries or smaller arterioles. Most commonly, fat, cholesterol, and calcium deposits are laid down along the intima and inner portion of the media. These components build up, forming plaques, which then may produce stenosis (narrowing) or occlusion (closure) of the arterial lumen. Accumulation of platelets and other blood cells can form a thrombus along with plaque buildup, which also obstructs the arteries. Pieces of plaque or thrombotic material can break off, causing emboli to lodge in the vessels acutely.

Depending on the arterial segment in the body that is affected, various diseases and symptoms may occur. As the blood vessels become diseased with plaque buildup, the body will try to compensate by the development of collaterals, small vessels that bypass the diseased artery. Collateral vessels are smaller than the native arteries and cannot accommodate the same amount of blood. Normally, during exercise, there is an increased demand for additional blood flow to the muscles; flow will increase and the arteries will dilate. With atherosclerosis, since the arteries are blocked and collaterals cannot accommodate the additional blood volume, waste products in the muscles build up, causing

pain. In the heart, this process affects the flow in the coronary arteries, and angina (chest pain) may occur. In lower-extremity arteriosclerosis, stenosis or occlusions of the aorta, iliac, femoral, popliteal, or tibial arteries may occur, producing intermittent claudication.

As the disease progresses, more blood vessels become stenosed or occluded and collateral formation will maximize, but the circulation is severely limited and ischemia may result. In atherosclerotic heart disease, significant ischemia may then result in a myocardial infarct, or heart attack. In the lower extremities, patients may develop rest pain. The most severe symptoms of lower-extremity arteriosclerosis are the development of nonhealing ulcers and gangrene (tissue death) in the lower portion of the foot, similar to a heart attack. When the disease process has become this severe, there are multisegmental areas of arterial occlusions and no further compensatory mechanisms.

Acute arterial ischemia is a sudden onset of ischemia as opposed to the more common chronic processes described above. The usual cause of acute arterial ischemia is an embolus (portion of a clot) that lodges in the arteries. The most common source of embolization is the heart; embolization from the heart occurs in patients who have recently had a heart attack, who have mitral valvular disease, or who have atrial fibrillation (irregular heartbeats). Another cause of acute arterial ischemia is thrombosis of, or embolization from, an aneurysm. In such cases, since no significant collaterals have developed in the area of the acute

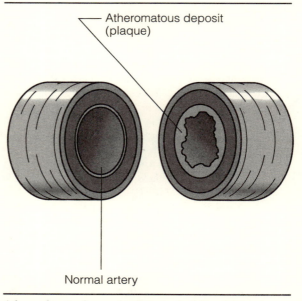

Atheromatous deposit (plaque)

Normal artery

Atherosclerotic disease leads to the buildup of fatty plaques on the walls of arteries, which inhibits blood flow and may lead to obstructions resulting in stroke, heart attack, and other life-threatening events.

blockage, immediate revascularization is mandatory to prevent significant tissue death.

Aneurysms—another disease entity that may be associated with the atherosclerotic disease process—produce a weakening of the adventia and a "ballooning" of the arteries with a thrombus (clot). Rupture or thrombosis (clotting off) may be a consequence of aneurysmal disease.

In cerebrovascular disease, atherosclerosis affects the arteries supplying the circulation to the brain (the carotid and vertebral-basilar system). The most common symptoms noted are transient ischemic attacks (TIAs), also referred to as ministrokes. TIAs usually last less than twenty-four hours. Most TIAs are produced by embolization, in which pieces of plaque in the major arteries break off and temporarily block the blood flow to certain areas of the brain. Once the symptoms last more than twenty-four hours, a cerebrovascular accident (CVA), cerebral infarct, or stroke has occurred. Atherosclerosis in the cerebrovascular system will behave in a manner similar to that previously described, with increasing stenosis and eventual occlusion. Collateral development seems to be especially prominent in the cerebrovascular system, since the brain is a greedy organ needing blood at all times. The majority of CVAs are caused by occlusion or thrombosis of a major vessel, producing significant ischemia in a portion of the brain.

Other sources of CVAs are hemorrhaging (bleeding) from ruptured cerebral aneurysms or from uncontrolled hypertension. This significant bleeding can cause spasm of the arteries in the brain and eventual ischemia. Monckeberg's sclerosis, not usually thought of as a true form of atherosclerosis, refers to the disease in which calcification of the tibial arteries is noted, often in diabetic patients.

Contributing or significant risk factors in the development of atherosclerosis include hypertension (high blood pressure), hyperlipidemia (high cholesterol), smoking, diabetes mellitus, and family history. Also, depending on the significance and the location of atherosclerosis, a variety of symptoms and conditions can result. In atherosclerotic heart disease, the first symptom is angina. As in intermittent claudication, chest, shoulder, or upper back pain may occur during exercise or stress as a result of the decreased blood supply to the tissues of the end-organ, the myocardium (heart muscle). As the disease progresses, the angina will become more unstable and patients will become progressively limited in minor activities. Symptoms of a heart attack may include severe, crushing chest pain, shortness of breath, pain in the left arm, and tingling of the fingers. Cessation of breathing and cardiac arrest indicate a significant heart attack. Immediate medical attention during the severe symptomatic phase or with cardiac arrest will aid in reducing further damage to the heart muscle and may prevent death. Many heart attacks are "silent" in that, although portions of the cardiac muscle are "dead," symptoms will have been negligible or minor, because of sufficient collateralization.

In lower-extremity atherosclerosis, patients with intermittent claudication will complain of pain or cramping in their calves, thighs, or buttocks while walking or exercising; symptoms will be relieved by rest. Claudication is usually described by distances, such as "one block" claudication or "half a mile" claudication. Rest pain occurs mostly at night at the most distal portion of the extremity, usually the toes and forefoot. Often patients will sleep in chairs or with their legs hanging off the bed to relieve the pain. On physical examination, the foot is usually cool to the touch, with a slightly bluish discoloration. There is hardening of the nails, dryness of the skin, and loss of hair in the lower portion of the leg. Pulses are absent or diminished. Often, when the leg is in a dependent position, *dependent rubor*, a purplish discoloration of the leg is seen, produced by dilation of the small blood vessels in the skin to provide the maximum amount of blood. Elevating the leg will produce a cadaverous white pallor. Because of the limited blood supply, ulcers will not heal and gangrene can develop. Patients with symptoms of severe claudication, rest pain, or neuropathic diabetes should be evaluated prior to undergoing any podiatry procedures because their compromised circulation will result in poor healing. Patients with acute arterial ischemia of the lower extremity will complain of the "five P's": pain, pallor, pulselessness, parathesias (loss of feeling), and paralysis. As previously described, emergent revascularization of the acutely ischemic limb is necessary to prevent limb loss or amputation.

Although aneurysmal disease is a separate entity, it may be associated with atherosclerotic disease in certain cases. Most aneurysms produce no symptoms. Detection of aneurysms is usually incidental; during a physical examination, for example, a physician may note a pulsatile mass in the abdomen (aorta, iliac), in the groin (femoral), or behind the knee (popliteal). Incidental diagnosis of aneurysms may also occur during routine chest X rays; the X ray may reveal a calcium rim around the body of the aneurysm. As aneurysms increase in size, the probability of rupture increases; therefore, elective surgery is usually recommended once certain sizes are achieved: more than 6 centimeters for an abdominal aneurysm and more than 2 centimeters for femoral and popliteal aneurysms. Symptoms of a rupturing abdominal aneurysm include severe lower back pain and a decrease in blood pressure, whereas thrombosis of a popliteal or femoral aneurysm will cause an acutely ischemic leg. Symptomatic aneurysms are considered medical emergencies, since ruptures may result in death and thrombosis in limb loss.

Symptoms of TIAs in the carotid arteries, which supply the front of the brain, include hemiparesis (numbness) or hemiplegia (weakness) of an arm and/or leg, affecting the carotid artery on the side opposite the symptom; aphasia (speech disorder), usually affecting the left carotid artery; or amaurosis fugax (blindness in one eye, similar to the sensation of a shade over the eye), which is from the carotid artery on the same side as the blindness. Other symptoms include dizziness, vertigo, imbalance, and other visual disturbances. These more generalized symptoms are referable to the vertebral-basilar circulation, which supplies the back portions of the brain, or are a result of multisegmental cerebrovascular disease in which a low-flow state can affect multiple areas of the brain and produce diverse symptoms. A stroke is an event whose symptoms will last more than twenty-four hours. Often these are permanent deficits, affecting the patient for the rest of his or her life.

Many patients will be asymptomatic (have no symptoms) and not develop TIAs but will have a stroke, which may result from eventual occlusion or thrombosis of the cerebral vessels and infarcts in a particular section of the brain. Asymptomatic cerebrovascular disease is often detected by the presence of a bruit (French for "noise"). Stenosis in arteries resembles rapids in a river: Flow will go very fast through the blockage and then be turbulent. The turbulence will produce a bruit which can be detected with a stethoscope. Turbulence from stenoses ranging from 20 to 80 percent can cause a bruit. The absence of a bruit does not mean that the arteries are disease-free. Once the stenosis reaches critical proportions, the flow is diminished and turbulence may be negligible. An occluded artery will also have no bruit, since there is no flow. Once the narrowing has reached 60 to 80 percent, many doctors will recommend elective surgery to reestablish flow and prevent eventual occlusion and possible stroke. About 75 percent of strokes are ischemic, resulting from this process. Bruits may be appreciable in other parts of the body and can also indicate the presence of atherosclerosis in those areas.

Atherosclerosis of the renal arteries, which supply the kidneys, may cause a condition known as renovascular hypertension. This type of high blood pressure is often difficult to control with medication, and continued high blood pressure will contribute to progression of the atherosclerotic process elsewhere in the body.

Another condition that results from atherosclerosis is chronic mesenteric ischemia. Here the blood vessels supplying the intestines, stomach, and many of the organs associated with the digestive process are affected. Patients may experience pain with eating and significant weight loss. This condition is often missed until an extensive workup for cancer or other chronic diseases yields negative results. In acute mesenteric ischemia, by contrast, thrombosis of the superior mesenteric artery occurs. As with other acute arterial conditions, emergent revascularization is necessary to prevent gangrene of the intestines.

TREATMENT AND THERAPY

A complete history and physical examination are usually the first methods of diagnosing atherosclerosis. Eliciting symptoms, noting significant risk factors and physical findings, will aid the physician in determining areas at risk.

In lower-extremity atherosclerosis, a common noninvasive method utilizes Doppler ultrasound. A series of blood-pressure cuffs are attached to the extremity, and segmental blood pressure and plethysmographic (a technique which measures a change in volume) waveforms are measured. A drop of more than 20 millimeters of mercury (mm Hg) of pressure between segments or extremities is indicative of a significant stenosis at that level. Exercise testing will demonstrate whether there are significant drops in pressure, confirming the diagnosis and severity of claudication. A similar method, ocular pneumoplethysmography (OPG), developed by William Gee, utilizes eye cups placed in the eye to measure the ocular pressure. A vacuum is applied to the eyes, effectively occluding the ophthalmic arteries, the first major branch of the internal carotid artery. As the vacuum is released, the blood flow is reestablished and the appearance of arterial pulsations is noted on a strip chart, denoting the systolic ophthalmic pressures. A difference of 5 mm Hg is consistent with significant (greater than 50 to 70 percent) carotid disease.

Duplex ultrasound machines utilize B-mode (brightness-mode) ultrasound to visualize the vessels and type of plaque, while Doppler ultrasound can audibly evaluate the blood flow in the vessels. Using real-time spectrum analyzers, the Doppler signals are then analyzed in terms of velocities and waveform characteristics. The greater the velocities, the greater the amount of stenosis. Absence of blood flow will denote occlusions. The use of color duplex ultrasound, in which the Doppler signals are color-coded in terms of flow direction and speed to denote the various flow patterns in normal and diseased vessels, has enhanced the diagnostic accuracies in the examinations. The use of color Doppler in many of the ultrasound machines is aiding in more rapid detection of arterial lesions in the heart, cerebrovascular, and lower-extremity arterial circulation.

Arteriography or angiography is an invasive procedure. The delineation of the blockages and collateral pathways detected through this method—in which the patient is hospitalized and a catheter is used to inject dye containing iodine into the arteries—is then used to plan a revascularization procedure.

Ultrasound is the primary diagnostic tool for detecting and measuring the size of aneurysms. Computed tomography (CT) scanning is an alternative radiological modality to visualize aneurysms.

The majority of patients with mild to moderate intermittent claudication can be treated conservatively. Cessation of smoking, alterations to diet, and a carefully controlled exercise plan will alleviate or decrease the progression of symptoms. Less than 5 percent of patients with intermittent claudication will develop gangrene sufficient to warrant a major amputation within a five-year period.

Some medications available work by decreasing the stickiness of the platelets in the blood; these are often prescribed for patients with claudication. Aspirin is often prescribed to alleviate symptoms of TIAs and to protect patients from strokes or heart attacks. Although it is a powerful drug in decreasing the incidence of embolization, a national study has demonstrated that patients with TIAs and severe stenosis of the carotid arteries should undergo surgical revascularization to protect against major strokes.

Severe disabling claudication, rest pain, ulceration or gangrene of the lower extremity, and unstable angina and heart attacks require some sort of surgical intervention. Usually bypass surgery is planned to revascularize the ischemic portion of the extremity or myocardial tissue to prevent limb loss or further cardiac events. The arteriogram will illustrate the areas of blockage, and, depending on the results of this test, various types of bypasses can be performed. Inflow procedures refer to bypasses performed above the groin: Aorto-iliac or aorto-femoral are the most common types performed, usually utilizing a prosthetic (plastic) material. Outflow procedures are those performed below the groin: femoral-popliteal or femoral-tibial bypasses. Prosthetics are sometimes used, but the best bypass material in terms of durability is the patient's own vein, either removed and reversed, or in situ (in place). Depending on the type of bypass procedure performed, the five-year patency rates (number of bypasses open at five years) exceeds 85 percent for aorto-iliac/aorto-femoral bypasses and 75 percent for lower-extremity reconstructions. Coronary artery bypass grafts (CABGs) typically employ the saphenous veins of the legs or the mammary artery of the chest wall to bypass the diseased segments in the heart vessels.

Endarterectomy, a surgical technique in which the intima and part of the media are excised, effectively "scrapes out" atherosclerotic plaques. Although used in other arterial segments, endarterectomy is the most common surgical procedure used to revascularize the carotid arteries.

Other interventional modalities have been developed. Percutaneous balloon angioplasty involves placing a balloon catheter in the diseased segment during an angiogram and opening up the area of stenosis or small segmental occlusion. This method has been employed in the coronary arteries as well as in the vessels of the aorta, iliacs, and lower extremities.

New lytic drugs, which "dissolve" clots, are sometimes employed alone, or in combination with balloon angioplasties or surgery, especially in the more acute cases of lower-extremity arterial ischemia and myocardial infarctions.

PERSPECTIVE AND PROSPECTS

Atherosclerosis of the coronary and cerebrovascular system is a major cause of annual deaths. Heart attacks are the primary cause of death in the United States, with approximately 650,000 people dying annually. Half of those deaths are sudden, with no prior significant symptoms.

Stroke is the third leading cause of death in the United States, with approximately 155,000 deaths annually. There are 400,000 strokes annually, and about one-fourth of all nursing-home patients are permanently impaired from strokes. These statistics have a great impact on the amounts of health care monies spent annually to care for victims of heart disease and strokes.

Since the 1960's, the rates of death from both heart attacks and strokes in the United States have decreased significantly. Control of blood pressure and diet, the development of new drugs and diagnostic techniques, and the advent of cardiovascular surgery in the early 1950's have aided in this decrement. Unfortunately, atherosclerotic diseases are still prevalent. Autopsies of Korean and Vietnam War American soldiers demonstrated that atherosclerotic plaque was evident even at an early age. This was attributed to the high-fat diet of most Americans. It is recognized that this disease is more prevalent in young males and that females are more protected until the onset of menopause; then the death rates tend to equalize. High-salt diets, which may increase the incidence of hypertension, also contribute to the development and progression of atherosclerosis. Since the 1960's, extensive education of the American public regarding dietary control has had a favorable impact. More recently, the benefits of exercise have helped to stem the atherosclerotic process.

The 1950's saw the development of cardiovascular surgery. The first bypass (arterial autograft) probably occurred during the Korean War. Coronary artery bypass surgery and carotid endarterectomies are the most common surgical procedures performed today. Recognition of and prompt treatment of symptomatic cardiac and cerebrovascular symptoms remain the key to better survival rates. With development of newer bypass materials for lower-extremity bypass surgery in the 1970's, as well as better surgical techniques for utilization of the saphenous veins, the amputation rate has significantly decreased. Research into graft materials that better mimic the native arteries and veins continues. The use of lasers to obliterate atherosclerotic plaque, popular in the 1980's and early 1990's, is being discontinued, since the results are not as favorable. Atheroscopy devices, which suction out the diseased segments, are being investigated in some centers.

Since the 1950's, a number of noninvasive and invasive procedures have been developed to diagnose atherosclerotic disease. The development of ultrasound devices in the 1950's initiated the research into using these noninvasive devices to diagnose atherosclerotic disease. The duplex devices, introduced commercially in the late 1970's and early 1980's, opened a new diagnostic field for detection of atherosclerotic disease. These devices allow for visualization of plaque morphology (composition of the plaque such as thrombus, calcium, and hemorrhage) and the blood-flow characteristics for a better understanding of the atherosclerotic process. Future developments in the field of ultrasound include holographic imaging for three-dimensional visualization of plaques. These noninvasive technologies will also allow physicians to monitor the effects of new drugs and techniques in the treatment of atherosclerosis. Advances in digital subtraction and computer enhancement of angiographic techniques, along with new contrast media, are making arteriograms safer and more accurate.

Technologies being developed for future diagnostic use include magnetic resonance imaging (MRI), a nonradiological modality for visualizing structures in the brain and other portions of the body. MRI is being expanded with the aid of computerization to do MR angiography. Magnetic resonance is also being utilized to measure, noninvasively, actual flow in individual arterial segments of the body in terms of cubic centimeters per minute. —*Silvia M. Berry*

See also Angina; Cholesterol; Claudication; Edema; Embolism; Heart attack; Heart disease; Heart failure; Hyperlipidemia; Hypertension; Ischemia; Phlebitis; Strokes and TIAs; Thrombosis and thrombus; Venous insufficiency.

FOR FURTHER INFORMATION:

American Heart Association. *AHA Focus Series: Arteriosclerosis*. Washington, D.C.: Author, 1988. This pamphlet helps educate patients on the causes and symptoms of arteriosclerosis.

Good Housekeeping Family Health and Medical Guide. New York: Hearst Books, 1981. A general reference guide on medical problems and the subspecialties associated with medical care.

Rutherford, Robert B., ed. *Vascular Surgery.* 2d ed. Philadelphia: W. B. Saunders, 1984. The definitive textbook for the understanding, diagnosis, and treatment of vascular disorders.

ATHLETE'S FOOT

SYSTEM AFFECTED: Skin

SPECIALISTS: Dermatologists, family physicians, podiatrists, sports medicine physicians

DEFINITION: Athlete's foot is a contagious fungal infection of the skin on the feet. It usually affects the soles of the feet and can be identified by moist, grayish or red scales, especially between the toes. Sometimes, small blisters may form. It is common for itching to occur in inflamed areas. Athlete's foot is caused by infection by a trichophyton fungus, which can occur with poor hygiene and/or hot or humid weather. Symptoms can be treated by keeping the affected areas cool and dry. Additionally, nonprescription medication may be applied after cleansing.

See also Foot disorders; Fungal infections.

AUTISM

SYSTEMS AFFECTED: Nervous, psychic-emotional

SPECIALISTS: Child psychiatrists, speech pathologists

DEFINITION: An emotional disturbance found in children in which communication, social interactions, and language skills are severely impaired.

CAUSES AND SYMPTOMS

Autism was first delineated in 1943 by Dr. Leo Kanner, who observed that some children seemed unable to relate properly to people. Later, those who worked with autistic children became convinced that the disorder was caused by cold, distant parents. Intensive treatment designed to break through this problem was unsuccessful, and parents were no longer seen as causing the disorder. Investigators now believe autism is the result of brain damage caused by any of several factors, including genetic errors, infectious diseases, metabolic disturbances, and neurological disorders. Autism does not progress, but it has no cure and is a lifelong disability. While some people with autism have normal or better intelligence, most are mentally retarded.

Autistic children demonstrate delays in speech, deficits in interpersonal skills, hearing or sight impairment, severe problems in eating and sleeping, attachments to unusual objects, persistent attention to spinning objects, and endlessly repeated behaviors such as hand flapping. Autism is a relatively rare disorder, occurring in fewer than 15 of every 10,000 children. People with autism may also suffer from other sensory deficits, hyperactivity, obsessive-compulsive disorder, depression, or Tourette's syndrome.

TREATMENT AND THERAPY

Children diagnosed with autism need psychological testing so that the child's deficits and strengths are well understood. A few autistic children are gifted in a specialized

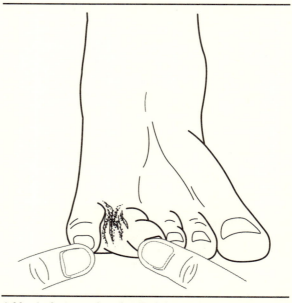

Athlete's foot can be identified by the itchy scaling that appears between the toes.

area, such as puzzle-solving. Proper plans of treatment draw upon the person's strengths to compensate for deficits and are individualized, community-based, family-focused, and well structured. Treatment should emphasize developing the person's social and communication skills. Family members need special training and support to cope with the needs of the autistic person. Psychoactive medication is used increasingly when treating the autistic person. People with autism can have normal life spans, and, with treatment, can live successfully in a community.   —*Russell Williams*

See also Learning disabilities.

FOR FURTHER INFORMATION:

Batshaw, Mark L., ed. *The Child with Developmental Disabilities*. Philadelphia: W. B. Saunders, 1993.

Dulcan, Mina K., and Charles W. Popper. *Concise Guide to Child and Adolescent Psychiatry*. Washington, D.C.: American Psychiatric Press, 1991.

Gillberg, Christopher, ed. *Diagnosis and Treatment of Autism*. New York: Plenum Press, 1989.

AUTOIMMUNE DISORDERS

SYSTEMS AFFECTED: Immune, all physical systems

SPECIALISTS: Immunologists, internists, rheumatologists

DEFINITION: Disorders in which the immune system attacks an individual's own body.

KEY TERMS:

antibodies: proteins of the immune system formed by lymphocytes in response to a specific antigen

antigen: a molecule, usually a foreign invader to the body, which induces the production of antibodies which will bind to it in a highly specific manner

inflammation: a by-product of the attack upon an antigen by antibodies and other cells of the immune system; the aggregation of these cells causes swelling and pain, and increased blood flow to the area results in redness and a sensation of heat

lymphocyte: the major cells of the immune system; one type of lymphocyte produces antibodies

CAUSES AND SYMPTOMS

The body's immune system is a complex, highly coordinated defense system against foreign invaders. Phagocytes digest microorganisms, dust particles, allergens, pollutants, and other cellular debris that does not belong in the body. Macrophages, a type of phagocyte, act in concert with other cell types such as T lymphocytes to destroy invading viruses. B lymphocytes are responsible for the production of antibodies, which in turn are designed to react with and destroy an invader which displays a particular antigen on its surface. Suppressor T cells call off the immune response once the foreign bodies have been eradicated. A low level of antibodies will remain circulating in the bloodstream, poised to eliminate a recurring invasion swiftly.

During fetal development, the cells of the immune system learn to recognize the markers on the cells and tissues of the body as "self" and are programmed to ignore all such components. Occasionally, the immune system is somehow disrupted and components of the body are mistakenly identified as foreign invaders. In this case, antibodies against body components are formed and attack these self cells and tissues. The attack of the body by its own immune system is the basis of autoimmune diseases.

Systemic lupus erythematosus, often simply called lupus, is a chronic disease characterized by inflammation that can affect the skin, blood, kidneys, and joints. Symptoms include a butterfly-shaped rash across the face, fatigue, shortness of breath and/or chest pains caused by inflamed lung or heart lining, sensitivity to light, arthritis, anemia, and oral or nasal lesions. Normally, the immune system will eliminate the body cells that die naturally. In lupus, antibodies are made against these dead self cells. They attach to the debris and form large complexes that cannot be eliminated from the body. These complexes may lodge in the small blood vessels of any body tissue, causing an inflammatory response. Other damage is caused by the direct attack of body cells by these misguided antibodies, as in the destruction of red blood cells. The cause of lupus is unknown.

Multiple sclerosis and diabetes mellitus are two relatively common disorders of an autoimmune nature. In multiple sclerosis, the immune system attacks the insulation along the outside of nerve fibers, called myelin. The holes are replaced with scar tissue that cannot conduct nerve impulses, resulting in symptoms such as blurred vision, muscular weakness, and loss of coordination. In diabetes, the cells of the pancreas that produce insulin are targeted and gradually destroyed by the immune system. Lack of insulin prevents the proper regulation of the uptake of glucose by the brain and other body cells, resulting in severe complications and possible death. The cause of these disorders is unknown, but evidence suggests that an infection of viruses harboring antigens similar in structure to myelin or pancreatic cells may be involved in their onset.

In rheumatoid arthritis, the body manufactures antibodies which attack the membranes that cover the joints. Pain, fatigue, and inflammation in the fingers, knees, hips, and back are common symptoms. In severe cases, the heart, lungs, and kidneys can be affected, as well as the cartilage and tendons, leading to joint degeneration. Myasthenia gravis is a serious disorder in which the immune system attacks and destroys the muscle cell receptors for the neurotransmitter acetylcholine. Thus the muscles are prevented from responding to signals from the brain, and the result is severe muscle weakness.

Pernicious anemia is a potentially fatal disorder in which immune cells attack the intestinal cells that absorb vitamin B_{12}, thus denying the body this vitamin. B_{12} is necessary for the production of red blood cells and for a healthy nervous system; therefore, lack of it produces severe consequences. In a disorder called Hashimoto's thyroiditis, a protein called thyroglobulin which is normally sequestered inside the thyroid cells accidentally leaks into the bloodstream, forming antibodies that destroy the thyroid gland.

Fibromyalgia is characterized by pain and stiffness of the muscles and is often accompanied by sleep disturbances, fatigue, headaches, numbness, and tingling. No cause is known, but it may be associated with damage to the muscle cell membranes. In Sjögren's syndrome, the immune cells attack the body's salivary and tear glands, resulting in a host of mouth and eye disorders as well as fatigue and central nervous system disturbances. Sjögren's syndrome can mimic and coexist with other autoimmune disorders. Scleroderma is an autoimmune disorder which damages the blood vessels and causes thickening and scarring of the skin and malfunction of internal organs. The symptoms can be limited to a small area or can spread throughout the body.

Chronic fatigue syndrome, formerly known as chronic Epstein-Barr virus, is a debilitating disorder characterized by extremely severe fatigue that may last months or years. While the cause is unknown, it is believed that the overproduction of some of the chemicals involved in the immune response are the causative agents. Abnormalities in the levels of specific immune cells are also implicated.

Rheumatic fever is the result of cross-reaction of antibodies produced in response to the bacterium that causes strep throat. These antibodies also recognize the heart valves, attacking them and causing inflammation and damage. Other autoimmune diseases include those targeted against a man's sperm, resulting in severe inflammation of the reproductive tract (orchitis, epididymitis); destruction of the eye (sympathetic ophthalmia); destruction of platelets within the blood (thrombocytopenia); and inflammation of the arteries (periarteritis). Leakage of the silicone from breast implants has been associated with the development of scleroderma and lupus.

TREATMENT AND THERAPY

While for many types of autoimmune disorders there are theories as to the cause—for example, the involvement of a virus or hereditary factors—the actual cause of any of these diseases is unknown. Because of this lack of fundamental information, no cures for autoimmune diseases are available and treatment is based on alleviating the symptoms of the disorders and strengthening the body when appropriate.

Treatment for systemic lupus erythematosus varies from individual to individual. Rest, proper nutrition, and avoiding the sun, which seems to trigger symptomatic episodes, can help to limit symptoms. Other treatments which are used include anti-inflammatory drugs such as aspirin; antimalarial drugs, which can cause eye problems; and steroids, which have a variety of negative side effects. While not normally fatal, this disease can be extremely debilitating. Kidney involvement can lead to serious consequences, per-

haps necessitating the use of kidney dialysis to remove wastes from the body. Because symptoms are so broad and tend to come and go, physicians frequently misdiagnose lupus as a psychological disorder. Choosing a knowledgeable physician and participating in a support group, such as those provided through the National Lupus Foundation, can be extremely helpful in coping with this disorder.

Multiple sclerosis is generally a manageable disease, treated with a variety of drugs and a therapeutic lifestyle. Steroid hormones are prescribed to alleviate symptoms of a severe attack. These drugs function by suppressing the immune system and reducing inflammation, but prolonged use can have serious side effects. The drug baclofen (Lioresal) is used to help reduce jerkiness and spasticity. Physical therapy is also successful in limiting spasticity, as well as in improving flexibility and range of motion. Mild exercise, rest, proper nutrition, health maintenance, and occupational therapy all contribute to maintaining a high level of daily functioning for multiple sclerosis patients.

Individuals affected by diabetes must monitor the sugar levels in their bodies closely, and in the insulin-dependent form of the disease must administer daily injections of insulin. Failure to do so can result in repeated episodes of coma that may lead to death. All forms of diabetes can be controlled by proper diet, exercise, and weight control. If appropriate, drug therapy may be prescribed. Proper monitoring of this disease is critical since it can lead to such complications as blindness, kidney disease, and neurological disorders.

Exercise, relaxation, and nutrition are all useful in the prevention and treatment of rheumatoid arthritis. Walking, yoga, and swimming are examples of exercise that helps to preserve the joints. A diet low in fat has been shown to reduce pain, swelling, and stiffness. Eliminating foods that trigger attacks is important; some of these foods are alcohol, sugar, chocolate, beef, pork, monosodium glutamate (MSG), and artificial preservatives. Drug therapies include the use of aspirin or ibuprofin for mild arthritis. Severe arthritis can be treated with immunosuppressant drugs, steroids, and anti-inflammatory drugs. Unfortunately, all these medications have dangerous side effects. Surgery to repair damaged joints is sometimes performed on individuals with a crippling form of the disease.

Fibromyalgia is treated with muscle exercises and low-impact aerobic exercise, massage, heat, and stress-reduction techniques. Small doses of antidepressants may be used to improve sleep and reduce pain. No therapy has been shown to be totally effective for long periods of time, so the best approach is for individuals to become familiar with the treatments to which their own disorders respond best and to locate and participate in a support group.

So little is known about scleroderma that no generalized treatment exists; however, therapy is aimed at body organs such as the lungs, heart, and kidneys that may become severely affected by the disorder, frequently to the point of fatality. The treatment for Sjögren's syndrome is based on the severity of the symptoms and is aimed at preventing progression of the disease to a debilitating stage.

Once chronic fatigue syndrome has been diagnosed properly, a variety of therapeutic approaches may be tried. Regular periods of uninterrupted rest are essential, especially during the most acute phase of the disorder. A healthy diet including many vegetables and complex carbohydrates, as well as vitamin supplements, can be helpful. Meditation, acupuncture, and avoidance of stress are some techniques that provide relief in some patients. Low dosages of antidepressants can be helpful in combating insomnia and pain, and certain medications to reinforce the immune system are sometimes prescribed. Emotional support for those suffering from chronic fatigue syndrome is comforting to most people, and in the United States there is an active national organization for sufferers of this disorder which can guide individuals to appropriate resources within their communities.

PERSPECTIVE AND PROSPECTS

Autoimmune disorders are, in general, a group of "modern" diseases. Recorded incidents of few, if any, of these disorders are nonexistent prior to the late nineteenth century. According to historical accounts, multiple sclerosis was unheard of prior to the mid-1800's. Some scientists believe that the disease existed at that time but was not properly diagnosed; however, there are no earlier records of any symptoms resembling those of multiple sclerosis. Other disorders seem to have arisen in the latter half of the twentieth century, such as chronic fatigue syndrome. Some speculate that industrial pollutants and toxins, which are unfortunate by-products of contemporary life, may trigger autoimmune diseases in individuals with susceptible immune systems. No specific chemicals or toxins have yet been shown to be the cause of any of these diseases.

The number of new cases of autoimmune disorders is steadily increasing, in part because of improved diagnostic tests. For years, disorders such as fibromyalgia and chronic fatigue syndrome were misdiagnosed or attributed to a psychological disorder. Many of these disorders seem to have a genetic component, in that individuals directly related to an affected individual may have a slightly higher risk of developing the same autoimmune disorder. This knowledge has permitted closer monitoring of at-risk individuals in an effort to begin treatment at the earliest signs of distress.

Before cures can be developed for autoimmune disorders, the causes must be determined. Therapies targeted against the causative agent may completely alleviate the disease. Improved means of enhancing the immune system through greater knowledge of its mechanics will be a huge step in improved maintenance of affected individuals. While treatment that focuses on symptoms does not cure a disease, improvement in the management of symptoms of autoimmune diseases will allow individuals a greater degree of comfort and an improved ability to conduct a normal life. —*Karen E. Kalumuck*

See also Anemia; Arthritis; Chronic fatigue syndrome; Diabetes mellitus; Immunodeficiency disorders; Lupus erythematosus; Multiple sclerosis; Rheumatoid arthritis.

FOR FURTHER INFORMATION:

Boston Women's Health Book Collective. *The New Our Bodies, Ourselves*. New York: Simon & Schuster, 1992. This comprehensive book on women's health issues provides detailed discussions of the most common autoimmune diseases. Includes a useful list of national support organizations and other resources in the United States.

Carroll, David L., and Jon D. Dorman. *Living Well with MS*. New York: HarperPerennial, 1993. This informative book covers all aspects of multiple sclerosis, including its history and diagnosis, a detailed description of the disease, therapies, and research.

Desowitz, Robert S. *The Thorn in the Starfish*. New York: W. W. Norton, 1987. This very accessible book is written in a narrative style and wonderfully simplifies the story of the immune system and how it works. An excellent source for anyone interested in the history or mechanics of immunity, immune health maintenance, and the future of immune research.

Dwyer, John M. *The Body at War*. Sydney, Australia: Allen & Unwin, 1988. This easy-to-read text is an excellent introduction to the functions of the immune system and such related topics as pregnancy, allergies, immune disorders, and research.

Feiden, Karyn. *Hope and Help for Chronic Fatigue Syndrome*. New York: Prentice Hall, 1990. An invaluable resource for those suffering from chronic fatigue syndrome or for anyone with an interest in the topic. Symptoms, treatments, and support resources are thoroughly covered.

Nilsson, Lennart. *The Body Victorious*. New York: Delacorte Press, 1987. This clearly and concisely written description of the human immune system is fabulously illustrated with photographs of the immune processes in action.

BACK DISORDERS. *See* SPINAL DISORDERS.

BACTERIAL INFECTIONS

SYSTEMS AFFECTED: Circulatory, gastrointestinal, immune, lymphatic, respiratory, all bodily tissues

SPECIALISTS: Epidemiologists, family physicians, immunologists, infectious disease physicians, internists, microbiologists

DEFINITION: Infectious diseases caused by bacteria, of which hundreds exist.

KEY TERMS:

antibiotic: a substance that kills microorganisms, including bacteria; antibiotics are used as a primary therapy in combating bacterial diseases

bacteria: small, single-celled organisms with a very simple structure; they live virtually everywhere and most varieties are harmless, although some types are capable of causing disease

cell: the smallest unit of a living thing; a bacterium consists of one cell, whereas humans are made of billions

immune system: the natural defenses of the body, which kill invading organisms such as harmful bacteria

immunity: resistance to infection by a particular disease-causing microorganism, often acquired by vaccination

infectious disease: diseases that can be passed from person to person through direct of indirect contact; many bacterial diseases are infectious

inflammation: a symptom of the body's immune response to some bacterial infections; may include redness, swelling, heat, and the production of pus

metabolism: the chemical reactions in an organism that sustain life and lead to growth and reproduction

microorganism: any small organism, including bacteria, protozoans, mold, fungi, and viruses; in this context, refers to those which cause disease

vaccination: the process of injecting into an individual a substance that provides immunity to a particular disease

CAUSES AND SYMPTOMS

Bacteria are very small, one-celled organisms (the cell being the smallest unit of a living organism) with an average size of twenty one-thousandths of a millimeter. Based on their relatively simple structure, they are classified as prokaryotic cells. Prokaryotic cells have a rigid outer cell wall, very simply organized hereditary material (deoxyribonucleic acid, or DNA) floating free within the cell, and only a few other structures necessary for their survival, growth, and reproduction. Eukaryotic cells, such as those found in humans, plants, and other animals, have highly organized DNA and many more internal structures. Despite the fact that bacteria are relatively "simple," they are still very complex living organisms.

The many types of bacteria can be divided into three categories based on their shape: coccus (round), bacillus (rod-shaped), or spirillum (spiral). Another major distinction between types of bacteria is based on the sugar and lipid (fat) composition of their cell walls. This difference can be identified by Gram-staining bacteria, the result of the stain determining whether the organism is gram-positive or gram-negative. Various types of bacteria may have additional structures that are useful in their identification. Capsules and slime layers are water-rich sugary materials secreted by the bacteria which cling to their surfaces and form halolike structures. Flagella are long, thin, whiplike structures found in one location on the bacterium or occasionally covering its entire surface. These structures are used to enhance the motility, or movement, of the bacteria.

Some bacteria are normal, harmless inhabitants of human bodies, such as those on the surface of the skin. Others, such as those which live in the human intestinal tract, aid in digestion and are essential for good health. Yet the warm, moist, nutrient-rich human body also provides an excellent breeding ground for numerous harmful bacterial invaders. For bacteria to cause infectious disease, several stages must occur. The bacteria must enter the person; they must survive and multiply on or in the person; they must resist the natural defenses of the human body; and they must damage the infected person. Most bacterial diseases are infectious because of the ease with which they can be transmitted from individual to individual by physical contact with the person, a contaminated object, or bacteria expelled into the air, such as by coughing or sneezing. A few bacterial diseases, such as food poisoning, are not classified as infectious.

Bacterial infections cause disease by a variety of mechanisms. Many of them produce chemical compounds that are toxic to human beings. For example, *Salmonella* and *Staphylococcus aureus* are two types of bacteria that are capable of causing food poisoning. *Clostridium botulinum* produces the deadly botulism toxin. In each case, ingestion of the toxin in contaminated food can lead to serious illness. *Clostridium tetanii* can enter the body through puncture wounds and will multiply rapidly deep in tissue where there is little exposure to the air. The toxin that it produces acts on the central nervous system and causes severe muscle spasms, which can lead to death from respiratory failure. Water that has been contaminated with raw sewage is a potent source of disease-causing bacteria. *Vibrio cholera* produces a potent toxin which causes severe diarrhea leading to death if it is not vigorously treated. Certain varieties of *Escherichia coli* and *Shigella* found in contaminated water can also cause severe intestinal disorders. Toxic shock syndrome is associated with the production of toxins by *Staphylococcus aureus*.

Another common cause of disease from bacterial infections is the result of the physical destruction of tissue by the invading organisms. Leprosy (also called Hansen's disease), caused by *Mycobacterium leprae*, if left untreated can lead to severe deterioration and disfiguration of large areas of a person's body. If a wound interrupts the blood supply to an area of the body such as a hand or foot, the tissues begin to decay, thereby providing nutrients for many bacteria, especially *Clostridium perfringens*. These bacteria can greatly accelerate the destruction of the tissue, which causes the condition known as gas gangrene.

In many cases, disease results when the infecting bacteria are recognized by the body's natural defense system (the immune system) as "nonself," that is, as invaders. Certain cells within the body are designed to attack intruders and eliminate them. During this process, disease symptoms that are consequences of the immune system's response may be

The Body's Response to Bacterial Infection

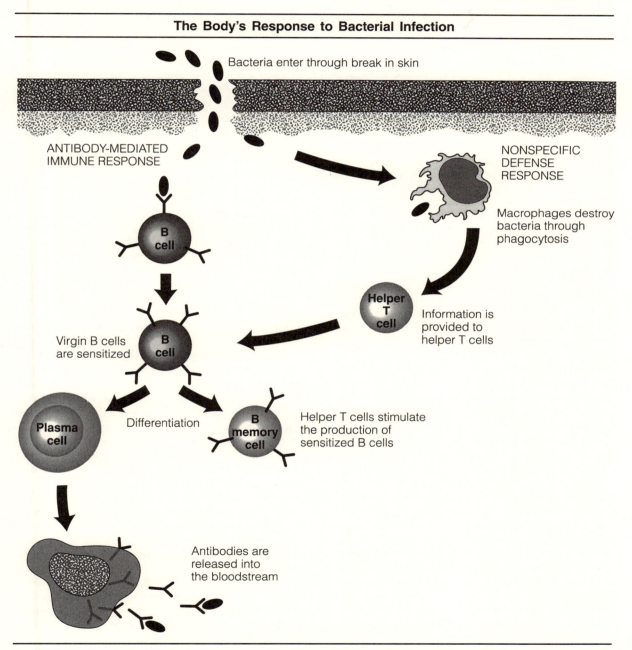

Bacterial infections cause the body to respond with either antibody production or phagocytosis leading to antibody production.

evident: inflammation (redness and swelling), the production of pus, and fever, among other symptoms. In some cases, certain components of the bacteria, such as capsules and slime layers, may protect them from being eliminated by the immune system. The bacteria may also multiply exceedingly rapidly, producing increasing amounts of toxins that overwhelm the capacity of the immune system to eliminate them. In these cases, continued and increasingly elevated disease symptoms such as fever can cause severe, even fatal, damage unless an alternate method for eliminating the infection is found. Failure to eliminate the bacterial invaders can also lead to a long-term, chronic infection that damages body tissues.

Many respiratory diseases are associated with the body's immune response to bacterial invasion. *Streptococcus pyogenes* is the causative agent of strep throat, whose features include severe redness, inflammation, pain, and the production of pus in throat tissue. In a small percentage of cases, strep throat can also lead to an infection of and potential permanent damage to the heart valves in a disease called rheumatic fever. In tuberculosis, *Mycobacterium tuberculosis* enters the lungs through inhalation. The body's defense system walls off the intruders and forms a nodule called a tubercle deep in the lung tissue. Nevertheless, the bacteria continue to multiply in the nodule and can travel to new sites in the lung. Tubercle formation occurs at these new sites. Eventually, this repeated cycle of infection and nodule formation becomes a chronic disease and leads to the destruction of lung tissue. Bacterial pneumonia can be caused by several different organisms, including *Klebsiella pneumoniae* and *Mycobacterium pneumoniae*. A pneumonia-like disease, Legionnaires' disease, was first identified in 1976 after twenty-nine delegates to an American Legion convention died from a mysterious respiratory disorder. The lengthy process of identifying a causative agent led to the discovery of a type of bacteria not previously known, *Legionella pneumophila*.

The human urinary and genital tracts are also potential havens for invading bacteria. Cystitis (bladder infections) are caused by many different types of bacteria. Kidney infections can be acquired as corollaries of urinary tract infections or from contact with infected animals or water. Sexually transmitted diseases (STDs) are contracted through sexual contact with an infected partner, and two common STDs have a bacterial origin. Gonorrhea is caused by *Neisseria gonorrhoeae* and leads to a severe inflammatory response and rapid spread of the organisms throughout the body. If not treated, it can lead to sterility as well as to diseases of the joints, heart, nerve coverings, eyes, and throat. Syphilis, caused by *Treponema pallidum*, can also have serious consequences if left untreated, including dementia and death. In addition, it can be passed to a fetus developing inside an infected mother in a condition known as congenital syphilis.

TREATMENT AND THERAPY

The medical management of the many bacterial infections and the diseases they cause begins with diagnosis. Diagnosis relies on a variety of biochemical tests that are analyzed in conjunction with the symptoms exhibited by the infected individual. Treatment is then designed so that it not only eliminates the disease symptoms but also eradicates all invading bacterial organisms, thereby minimizing the chance of a recurrence of the disease. Prevention involves steps that the individual takes to avoid potential contact with infectious diseases, as well as the use of medical procedures that protect against specific bacterial diseases.

In order to treat a bacterial disease properly, the invading organism must be identified correctly. In some cases, symptomology can be specific enough to identify the offending bacterium, but since there are literally thousands of different types of disease-causing organisms, a systematic approach using a variety of tests is undertaken to make a definitive diagnosis. First, a specimen from the infected person is collected. This may be a blood or urine sample; a swab of the infected area, such as the throat or another skin surface; or a secretion, such as sputum, mucus, or pus. Since human bodies are normally inhabited by a variety of harmless bacteria, the individual types of bacteria are isolated in pure cultures, in which each bacterium present is of the same type. The pure cultures are then tested to determine the identity of the organisms. Staining procedures, such as Gram's stain, and microscopic examination of the stained bacteria to determine the Gram reaction and the shape of the bacteria can narrow down the identity of the organisms considerably.

Based on these results, a standard series of tests is performed, continually narrowing down the possible identities until only one remains. One test measures the organisms' growth requirements. Many identifications are aided by analyzing the types of sugars and proteins that the organisms can use as food sources. The by-products of their metabolism (chemical reactions occurring inside the bacteria), such as acids and gas, are identified. Oxygen requirements, motility, and the presence of a capsule are three other common characteristics that are examined. For cases in which the identification of a particular variety of one type of bacteria is necessary, more complex tests may be undertaken, such as an analysis of the particular sugars and proteins on the surface of the organism or tests for the production of specific toxins. Once the bacterium's identity is confirmed, treatment may begin.

The most common type of treatment for bacterial infection is antibiotic therapy. Antibiotics are chemical compounds that kill bacteria. Originally discovered as antibacterial compounds produced by bacteria, molds, and fungi (such as penicillin from bread mold), many more are synthetically produced. Antibiotics work in a variety of fashions. Some, such as penicillin and the cephalosporins, interfere with the synthesis of cell walls by bacteria, thus preventing the organisms from multiplying. Other commonly used antibiotics prevent the bacteria from synthesizing the proteins that they need to survive and multiply. These includes the tetracyclines (a class of antibiotics which act against a large range of bacteria), erythromycin, and streptomycin. A host of other antibiotics target a variety of bacterial functions, including specific chemical reactions and the propagation of genetic material, and the structural components of the bacteria. Each class of antibiotics works best on certain types of bacteria. For example, penicillin is most efficient in killing cocci (such as *Streptococcus* and *Staphylococcus*) and gram-positive bacilli.

Frequently, the symptoms of a bacterial disease may disappear rapidly after the beginning of antibiotic therapy. This reaction is attributable to the inhibition of bacterial multiplication and the destruction of most of the microorganisms. A small number of the bacteria may not be killed during this initial exposure to antibiotics, however, and if antibiotic therapy is ended before all are killed, a recurrence of the disease is likely. A full prescription of antibiotics should be taken to avoid this situation. For example, effective treatment and eradication of all bacteria in tuberculosis may take six months to a year or more of antibiotic treatment, despite the fact that the symptoms are alleviated in a few weeks.

Upon repeated exposure to a type of antibiotic, some bacteria develop the capacity to degrade or inactivate the antibiotic, thus rendering that drug ineffective against the resistant microorganism. In these cases, other antibiotics and newly developed ones are tested for their effectiveness against the bacteria. Such situations have arisen in the bacteria that cause gonorrhea and tuberculosis.

While antibiotics exist to combat infections of most types of bacteria, in some cases the human immune system is capable of clearing the infection without additional intervention. In these instances, the symptoms of the infection are treated until the body heals itself. This is the common treatment path in mild cases of food poisoning, such as those caused by some *Salmonella* and *Staphylococcus* varieties. Diarrhea and vomiting are treated by replacing water and salts, by drinking large volumes of fluids, and perhaps by using over-the-counter remedies to ease some of the symptoms.

Many bacterial diseases can be easily prevented through good hygiene. Foods that are not thoroughly cooked, such as eggs and meats, may become quickly contaminated by the rapid growth of food-poisoning organisms present on their surfaces. Proper cooking kills these organisms. Similarly, foods that are not properly stored but left out in warm places can also provide a potent breeding ground for toxin-producing bacteria. Picnic food not properly refrigerated is a common source of food poisoning. Similarly, questionable water sources should never be used for drinking or cooking water without proper treatment. Filtering with an ultrafine filter specifically designed to remove bacteria is one safeguard, as is boiling for the required time period based on altitude. Food that may have been washed with contaminated water sources should always be cooked or peeled before consumption.

Many diseases can be prevented with vaccinations. A bacterial vaccine is a mixture of a particular bacterium, its parts, or its inactivated toxins. When this solution is injected into an individual, it provides immunity (resistance to infection) to the particular organism contained in the vaccine. Some vaccines provide lifetime immunity when enhanced with an occasional booster shot, while some are relatively short-acting. Many types of vaccines that are directed against specific diseases are part of standard preventive care given to children. For example, the DPT vaccine confers immunity to diphtheria, pertussis (whooping cough), and tetanus. Some vaccines are useful for individuals who are living, working, or traveling in areas where certain diseases are endemic, or for those who regularly come into contact with infected individuals. Examples of these sorts of vaccines include those for plague (*Yersinia pestis*), typhoid fever (*Salmonella typhi*), cholera, and tuberculosis.

PERSPECTIVE AND PROSPECTS

Bacteria were first described as "animalcules" by the Dutch scientist Antoni van Leeuwenhoek in 1673 after he observed them in water-based mixtures with a crudely designed microscope. In 1860, Louis Pasteur recognized that bacteria could cause the spoiling of wine and beer because of the by-products of their metabolism. Pasteur's solution to this problem was heating the beverages enough to kill the bacteria, but not change the taste of the drink—a process known as pasteurization, which is used today on milk and alcoholic beverages. In addition, Pasteur settled a long-standing debate on the origin of living things that seemed to arise spontaneously in fluids exposed to the air. He demonstrated that these life-forms were seeded by contaminating bacteria and other microorganisms found in the air, in fluids, and on solid surfaces. Pasteur's work led to standard practices in laboratories and food processing plants to prevent unwanted bacterial contamination; these practices are referred to as aseptic techniques.

Prior to the late 1800's, deaths from wounds and simple surgeries were quite common, but the reason for these high mortality rates was unknown. In the 1860's, Joseph Lister, an English surgeon, began soaking surgical dressings in solutions that killed bacteria, and the rate of survival in surgical and wound patients was greatly improved. In 1876, Robert Koch, a German physician, discovered rod-shaped bacteria in the blood of cattle that died from anthrax, a disease which was devastating the sheep and cattle population of Europe. When he injected healthy animals with these bacteria, they contracted anthrax, and samples of their blood showed large numbers of the same bacteria. By these and other experiments, Koch, Lister, and others proved the "germ theory of disease"—that microorganisms cause disease—and appropriate measures were instituted to protect against the transmission of bacteria to humans through medical procedures and food.

A milestone in the prevention of infectious diseases was the development of vaccinations. The first vaccine was developed in 1798, long before the germ theory of disease was proven. The British physician Edward Jenner first used vaccination as a preventive step against the contraction of deadly smallpox, a viral disease. How vaccinations work and their use as a protection against bacterial diseases were discovered around 1880 by Pasteur.

The first antibiotic, penicillin, was discovered by Alexander Fleming in 1928. Since then, scores of others, produced both naturally and synthetically, have been analyzed and used in the treatment of bacterial diseases. All these discoveries have made bacterial disease a much less deadly category of illness than it was in the late 1800's. Yet bacterial diseases are by no means conquered. Overuse of antibiotics in medical practice and in cattle feed results in the appearance of new varieties of bacteria that are resistant to standard antibiotic therapy. Research will continue to develop new means of controlling and destroying such infective organisms. Bacteria also play an important role in synthesizing new antibiotics and other pharmaceuticals in the laboratory through recombinant DNA technology. These organisms will continue to provide challenges and opportunities for human health in the years to come.

—*Karen E. Kalumuck*

See also Arthropod-borne diseases; Botulism; Childhood infectious diseases; Cholecystitis; Cholera; Cystitis; Diphtheria; Endocarditis; Gangrene; Glomerulonephritis; Gonorrhea; Iatrogenic disorders; Infection; Legionnaires' disease; Leprosy; Lyme disease; Mastitis; Parasitic diseases; Pelvic inflammatory disease (PID); Pertussis; Plague; Pneumonia; Salmonella; Scarlet fever; Shigellosis; Staphylococcal infections; Strep throat; Streptococcal infections; Syphilis; Tetanus; Tonsillitis; Toxemia; Tuberculosis; Typhoid fever and typhus; Zoonoses.

FOR FURTHER INFORMATION:

Dixon, Bernard. *Magnificent Microbes*. New York: Atheneum, 1976. This well-written book, written in a narrative style, imparts classic information to those curious about the world of microbes from the perspective of their importance in maintaining health and life. The reader will come away with a true appreciation for the virtues and helpfulness of microbes, including bacteria, to humans—indeed of their necessity for maintaining life.

Finegold, Sydney M., and William J. Martin. *Bailey and Scott's Diagnostic Microbiology*. 6th ed. St. Louis: C. V. Mosby, 1982. A well-organized text that is accessible to the general reader. Describes in detail methods for the isolation and identification of microorganisms, in particu-

lar diagnostic procedures for the identification of bacterial infectious diseases. Includes many illuminating color plates illustrating diagnostic tests.

Gest, Howard. *The World of Microbes*. Menlo Park, Calif.: Benjamin/Cummings, 1987. A very readable, jargon-free book written in an engaging narrative style. Includes a discussion of the history of microbiology, the basic biology and chemistry of microorganisms with an emphasis on bacteria, the roles microorganisms play in the environment and their impact on humans, disease pathology, prevention and cure, and the use of bacteria in biotechnology.

Joklik, Wolfgang K., and Hilda P. Willett, eds. *Zinsser: Microbiology*. 20th ed. East Norwalk, Conn.: Appleton and Lange, 1992. This is the bible of microbiology, with a heavy emphasis on medical microbiology. Features a detailed analysis of the biochemistry of bacteria and other microorganisms. Recommended for its extensive discussions of the many types of diseases and their causative agents.

Pelczar, Michael J., Jr., E. C. S. Chan, and Noel R. Krieg. *Microbiology*. 5th ed. New York: McGraw-Hill, 1986. This general textbook is accessible to the general reader and is a good source of information on bacterial physiology and genetics, diagnostic testing, the prevention and cure of bacterial diseases, and environmental microbiology. Includes many informative photographs and illustrations, as well as an excellent glossary of terms.

Rossmoore, Harold W. *The Microbes, Our Unseen Friends*. Detroit: Wayne State University Press, 1976. An excellent, narrative-style book intended to be read for knowledge and pleasure. In addition to a discussion of bacteria and disease, it includes excellent material on the benefits to human health of microorganisms and their ubiquity and importance in everyday life.

Schlegel, Hans G. *General Microbiology*. 6th ed. Cambridge, England: Cambridge University Press, 1986. This compact version of a classic German textbook provides a concise yet broad account of bacteriology and microbiology for readers with all levels of interest. Topics include cell structure, biochemistry, microbes in the environment, the practical applications of microbes, and the cause, prevention, and cure of diseases.

BALDNESS. *See* HAIR LOSS AND BALDNESS.

BASAL CELL CARCINOMA. *See* SKIN CANCER.

BED-WETTING

SYSTEMS AFFECTED: Muscular, urinary
SPECIALISTS: Family physicians, geriatric specialists, pediatricians, psychiatrists, psychologists, urologists

DEFINITION: A condition characterized by an inability of the bladder to contain the urine during sleep, often a developmental condition in children.

KEY TERMS:

alarm therapy: the practice of utilizing mechanical or electronic devices to detect bed-wetting as it occurs

bed-wetting: the passage of urine during sleep

bladder: a membranous sac in the body that serves as the temporary retention site of urine

diaphragm: a body partition of muscle and connective tissue separating the chest and abdominal cavities

enuresis: an involuntary discharge of urine; incontinence of urine

nervous system: the bodily system that receives and interprets stimuli and transmits impulses to the organs

neurophysiological: pertaining to the nervous system in the human body

phrenic: of or relating to the diaphragm

sphincter: a muscle surrounding and able to contract or close a bodily opening (such as the opening to the bladder)

CAUSES AND SYMPTOMS

Primary enuresis is defined medically as the inability to hold one's urine during sleep. The condition is quite common and occurs most often in children; approximately 20 percent of children under the age of six suffer from the condition. These percentages decrease to about 5 percent at age ten, 2 percent at age fifteen and only about 1 percent of adults. Secondary enuresis is bed-wetting in a child who had previously achieved bladder control. (These terms do not apply, however, to urination problems caused by physical illness, disease, or anatomical defect.) The condition is more common in boys than in girls. Bed-wetting usually occurs during the first third of sleep, although it can occur during all sleep stages and without relation to awakening periods.

It is important to realize that enuresis is considered to be a developmental concern rather than an emotional, behavioral, or physical one. Donald S. Kornfeld and Philip R. Muskin report in *The Columbia University College of Physicians and Surgeons Complete Home Medical Guide* (Rev. ed., 1989) that "enuresis is due to a lag in development of the nervous system's controls on elimination." Many parents fail to understand this neuropsychological element and thus punish the child for a wet bed. Punishing, ridiculing, or shaming the child does not correct the situation; in fact, in many cases, it may prolong the problem as well as cause other unnecessary and undesirable psychological problems. Emotional problems have resulted from enuresis, as the child may be too embarrassed to partake in normal childhood activities such as camping or sleepovers.

TREATMENT AND THERAPY

Techniques for helping the enuretic child achieve dryness range from withholding liquids near bedtime to alarm systems to medical intervention. Generally, restriction of liquid intake after dinner is the first course of action. This treatment method, however, does not have a very high success rate. Should this treatment fail after a trial period of a few weeks, other methods may be employed.

Alarm therapy can help a child achieve control within four months, sometimes in only a few weeks. A beeper- or buzzer-type alarm sounds when moisture touches the bedding or underwear; the desired result is that the child, while sleeping, will eventually recognize the need to urinate and awaken in time to get to the bathroom. Electronic alarms are generally of two types. The first is a wired pad, consisting of two screens, which is placed under the sheets to detect wetness; when the child wets, the moisture activates the battery-operated alarm. The second is a device worn on the body, either in the underpants and connected by a wire to an alarm or a wristwatch-type alarm; the underwear serves as a separating cloth for the contact points. In either case, as wetness occurs, the alarm sounds, thus wakening the child; the child can then be directed to the bathroom to complete urination.

Barry G. Powell and Lynda Muransky cite several case histories in which alarm therapy proved to be effective in stopping enuresis. For example, a six-year-old who never had a dry bed achieved dryness within a week through the use of an alarm. In another case, a fifteen-year-old had been trying to overcome his bed-wetting problem for ten years. Several trips to the doctor showed that he had no physical cause for enuresis. His parents labeled him "lazy, inconsiderate, and difficult." His desire to join his hockey team in overnight travel gave him the impetus to seek help. Powell and Muransky found his problem to be primary enuresis aggravated by family ridiculing. Through the use of his alarm, he achieved dryness within two weeks.

A case involving secondary enuresis is described as well. A child who had suffered through primary enuresis, then achieved dryness, was found to be wetting again. This second bout of bed-wetting seems to have been the result of his parents' marital separation. After a medical examination revealed no physical problems, it appeared the problem was psychological, caused by emotional upset. He resumed dryness in three weeks (although an alarm system on his bed for six months gave him more confidence). It is important to note, however, that alarms can take up to several months' time before a child feels comfortable in stopping its use. Also, parental supervision is imperative in order for this type of therapy to work properly.

Chiropractic spinal manipulation has been found to be effective in the treatment of some cases of enuresis. Some believe that a spinal reflex is involved in bed-wetting. As nighttime breathing slows down (a normal reaction), carbon dioxide builds up in the body. When the carbon dioxide buildup reaches a certain level, a breathing mechanism called the phrenic reflex is triggered. This mechanism normally causes the diaphragm to return breathing to its normal pattern. If the mechanism does not work properly, however, the carbon dioxide continues to increase, resulting in an involuntary relaxation of the sphincter muscle at the opening to the bladder. Fluid (urine) is released and leaks out of the bladder. A child in a deep state of sleep does not recognize that the bed has been wet. Generally, chiropractors believe that the bed-wetting child sleeps in a state of high carbon dioxide intoxication.

While immature development of the phrenic reflex is the most common cause of bed-wetting, in some children a misalignment of the bones in the neck and spine (referred to as "subluxation" by chiropractors) is thought to cause pressure on the nerves that are related to the phrenic reflex. Through chiropractic adjustments, it is argued, the subluxation can be corrected, thus relieving pressure on the nerves. With the spine realigned and bodily functions working normally, enuresis can be eliminated. One child had never had a dry bed in his first ten years of life; after only two spinal adjustments by a licensed chiropractor, the child stopped wetting immediately. Chiropractors usually recommend a series of adjustments in order to realign the spine and nerves and keep them in the proper position.

Drug therapy solely for the treatment of enuresis is controversial. However, when an illness such as diabetes mellitus is the underlying cause of the bed-wetting, the use of drugs may be indicated. The drug imipramine hydrochloride (an antidepressant agent) has been studied to assist in contraction of the sphincter; however, because of the high toxicity and limited effectiveness of such antidepressants, its use is not widespread. Relapse rates are high, and a cure rate of only 25 percent is seen. More success has been achieved with desmopressin acetate, an antidiuretic drug. There is an immediate improvement in 70 percent of treated children. Relapse rates are lower than those associated with imipramine but higher than with the use of bed-wetting alarms, probably because the sphincter muscle is not fully developed in the enuretic child. In general, drug therapy yields a final success rate of 25 percent.

PERSPECTIVE AND PROSPECTS

The history of bed-wetting is probably a lengthy one. The term "enuresis" was first coined around 1800 and has plagued children from every ethnic background and socioeconomic level around the world. It continues to be a problem for many children today and probably will be so in the future as well.

Most enuretics are deep sleepers who are usually quite active during their waking hours. This sleeping pattern, combined with urinary systems that are not yet fully developed, is generally the main cause of bed-wetting. There are some indications that enuresis is hereditary; many children who suffer from the condition have a parent who was enuretic as a child. It is reassuring to know that almost all affected children outgrow the problem by adulthood. While no immediate cure is available, continued experiments with alarm systems and drugs will certainly alleviate the discomfort and embarrassment until the body's lag in development corrects itself. —*Carol A. Holloway*

See also Incontinence; Stress; Urinary disorders.

FOR FURTHER INFORMATION:

"Alarm Bells for Enuresis." *The Lancet* 337 (March 2, 1991): 523. Alarm therapy is discussed as a treatment for enuresis (nocturnal bed-wetting) in children. Attention is given to the importance of parental supervision, family stress, environmental obstacles, and behavioral problems that can contribute to bed-wetting.

"Defining Enuresis." *FDA Consumer* 23 (May, 1989): 10. This article, written for the layperson, is easy to understand and even offers a helpful pronunciation guide for difficult terms. The links between enuresis and sleep patterns, sleepwalking, and nightmares are examined.

Kornfeld, Donald S., and Philip R. Muskin. "Enuresis, or Bed-wetting." In *The Columbia University College of Physicians and Surgeons Complete Home Medical Guide*, edited by Donald Tapley et al. Rev. ed. New York: Crown, 1989. A well-written article explaining the causes, effects, and treatments of bed-wetting in children. Offers the encouraging suggestion that even if all treatments fail, the problem is usually outgrown by adulthood.

Kunz, Jeffrey, ed. *American Medical Association Family Medical Guide*. New York: Random House, 1982. A short, informative article detailing the subject. Medical myths concerning the problem are discussed. Related articles covering such topics as urinary infections in children and nephritis are conveniently located in the same chapter of the book.

Powell, Barry G., and Lynda Muransky. *Bedwetting: Questions and Answers for Parents*. Missasauga, Ontario: Helpful Publications, 1984. This booklet is dedicated to assisting parents in understanding bed-wetting. A strong emphasis on alarm systems is evident, as the writers have also established their own bed-wetting alarm company.

BELL'S PALSY

SYSTEMS AFFECTED: Muscular, nervous

SPECIALISTS: Family physicians, internists, neurologists, physical therapists

DEFINITION: Bell's palsy is a sudden paralysis of one side of the face, including muscles of the eyelid. Pain behind the ear on the affected side, distorted facial expressions, and changes in salivation are common symptoms. The cause is unknown, although reduced blood supply to the facial nerves is believed to trigger most cases. The symptoms of Bell's palsy can be treated by applying heat to painful areas twice a day and by wearing goggles or an eye patch to keep the eye moist and protected. As muscle

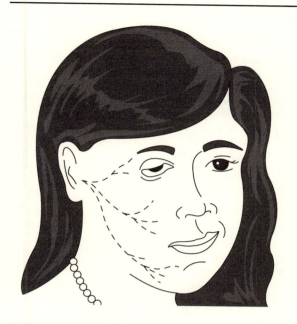

Bell's palsy results in a temporary sagging and paralysis of one side of the face; dashed lines show the main neural pathways affected.

strength returns, facial massage and exercise may be helpful. The mouth should be kept clean with increased brushing and flossing.

See also Palsy.

Beriberi

Systems affected: Heart, muscular, nervous

Specialists: Family physicians, internists, public health specialists, registered dietitians

Definition: Beriberi is a serious vitamin deficiency caused by an inadequate dietary intake of thiamine (B_1). Thiamine, which can be found in green vegetables, whole grains, meat, nuts, and potatoes, is required in order to digest carbohydrates. Its absence in the diet can result in neurological and muscular problems such as numbness and muscle wasting ("dry" beriberi) or heart failure ("wet" beriberi). Except for chronic alcoholics, elderly people who are undernourished, or those in extreme poverty, the disease is rare in developed countries. It is more common, however, in poor countries and is a possibly fatal complication of severe malnutrition. Treatment with thiamine brings about a complete recovery.

See also Vitamin and mineral deficiencies.

Birth. *See* Childbirth; Childbirth, complications of.

Birth defects

Systems affected: All bodily tissues

Specialists: Embryologists, geneticists, obstetricians, pediatricians, perinatologists

Definition: Congenital malformations or structural anomalies and their accompanying functional disorders which originate during embryonic development; they are involved in up to 6 percent of human live births.

Key terms:

deletion: the loss of a portion of a chromosome as a result of induced or accidental breakage

multifactorial inheritance: the interaction of genetic and environmental factors, which leads to certain congenital malformations

mutation: a change in the deoxyribonucleic acid (DNA) which may lead to the occurrence of congenital malformations

nondisjunction: the failure of chromosomes to separate during cell division, resulting in new cells that either lack a chromosome or have an extra chromosome

organogenetic period: the period of embryonic development, from approximately fifteen to sixty days after fertilization, during which most body organs form

spina bifida: a birth defect involving malformation of vertebrae in the lower back, often resulting in paralysis and lower-body organ impairment

teratogen: an environmental factor that can induce the formation of congenital malformations

teratology: the study of congenital malformations

translocation: the structural chromosomal defect that occurs when a piece of one chromosome attaches to another

Causes and Symptoms

As the human embryo develops, it undergoes many formative stages from the simple to the complex, most often culminating in a perfectly formed newborn infant. The formation of the embryo is controlled by both genetic factors and interactions between the various embryonic tissues. Because the genes play a vital role as the blueprint for the developing embryo, they must be accurate and the cellular mechanisms that allow the genes to be expressed must also work correctly. In addition, the chemical and physical communications between cells and tissues in the embryo must be clear and uninterrupted. The development of the human embryo into a newborn infant is infinitely more complex than the design and assembly of the most powerful supercomputer or the largest skyscraper. Because of this complexity and the fact that development progresses without supervision by human eye or hand, there are many opportunities for errors that can lead to malformations.

Errors in development can be caused by both genetic and environmental factors. Genetic factors include chromosomal abnormalities and gene mutations. Both can be inherited from the parents or can occur spontaneously during gamete formation, fertilization, and embryonic development. Environmental factors, called teratogens, include such things as drugs, disease organisms, and radiation.

Chromosomal abnormalities account for about 6 percent of human congenital malformations. They fall into two categories, numerical and structural. Numerical chromosomal abnormalities are most often the result of nondisjunction occurring in the germ cells that form sperm and eggs. During the cell division process in sperm and egg production deoxyribonucleic acid (DNA) is duplicated so that each new cell receives a complete set of chromosomes. Occasionally, two chromosomes fail to separate (nondisjunction), such that one of the new cells receives two copies of that chromosome and the other cell none. Both of the resulting gametes (either sperm or eggs) will have an abnormal number of chromosomes. When a gamete with an abnormal number of chromosomes unites with a normal gamete, the result is an individual with an abnormal chromosome number. The missing or extra chromosome will cause confusion in the developmental process and result in certain structural and functional abnormalities. For example, persons with an extra copy of chromosome number 21 suffer from Down syndrome, which often includes mental deficiency, heart defects, facial deformities, and other symptoms. Abnormal chromosome numbers may also result from an egg's being fertilized by two sperm, failure of cell division during gamete formation, and nondisjunction in one or more cells of the early embryo.

Structural chromosomal abnormalities result from chromosome breaks. Breaks occur in chromosomes during normal exchanges in material between chromosomes (crossing over). They also may occur accidentally at weak points on the chromosomes, called fragile sites, and can be induced by chemicals and radiation. Translocations occur when a broken-off piece of chromosome attaches to another chromosome. For example, an individual who has the two usual copies of chromosome 21 and, as the result of a translocation, carries another partial or complete copy of 21 riding piggyback on another chromosome will have the symptoms of Down syndrome. Deletions occur when a chromosome break causes the loss of part of a chromosome. The cri du chat syndrome is caused by the loss of a portion of chromosome number 5. Infants affected by this disorder have a catlike cry, are mentally retarded, and have cardiovascular defects. Other structural chromosomal abnormalities include inversions (in which segments of chromosomes are attached in reverse order), duplications (in which portions of a chromosome are present in multiple copies), and isochromosomes (in which chromosomes separate improperly to produce the wrong configuration).

Gene mutations (defective genes) are responsible for about 8 percent of birth defects. Mutations in genes occur spontaneously because of copying errors or can be induced by environmental factors such as chemicals and radiation. The mutant genes are passed from parents to offspring; thus certain defects may be present in specific families and geographical locations. Two examples of mutation-caused defects are polydactyly (the presence of extra fingers or toes) and microcephaly (an unusually small cranium and brain). Mutations can be either dominant or recessive. If one of the parents possesses a dominant mutation, there will be a 50 percent chance of this mutant gene being transmitted to the offspring. Brachydactyly, or abnormal shortening of the fingers, is a dominantly inherited trait. Normally, the parent with the dominant gene also has the disorder. Recessive mutations can remain hidden or unexpressed in both parents. When both parents possess the recessive gene, there is a 25 percent chance that any given pregnancy will result in a child with a defect. Examples of recessive defects are the metabolic disorders sickle-cell anemia and hemophilia.

Environmental factors called teratogens are responsible for about 7 percent of congenital malformations. Human embryos are most sensitive to the effects of teratogens during the period when most organs are forming (organogenetic period), that is, from about fifteen to sixty days after fertilization. Teratogens may interfere with development in a number of ways, usually by killing embryonic cells or interrupting their normal function. Cell movement, communication, recognition, differentiation, division, and adhesion are critical to development and can be easily disturbed by teratogens. Teratogens can also cause mutations and chromosomal abnormalities in embryonic cells. Even if the disturbance is only weak and transitory, it can have serious effects because the critical period for development of certain structures is very short and well defined. For example, the critical period for arm development is from twenty-four to forty-four days after fertilization. A chemical that interferes with limb development such as the drug thalidomide, if taken during this period, may cause missing arm parts, shortened arms, or complete absence of arms. Many drugs and chemicals have been identified as teratogenic, including alcohol, aspirin, and certain antibiotics.

Other environmental factors that can cause congenital malformations include infectious organisms, radiation, and mechanical pressures exerted on the fetus within the uterus. Certain infectious agents or their products can pass from the mother through the placenta into the embryo. Infection of the embryo causes disturbances to development similar to those caused by chemical teratogens. For example, German measles (rubella virus) causes cataracts, deafness, and heart defects if the embryo is infected early in development. Exposure to large doses of radiation such as those released by the accident at the Chernobyl nuclear power plant in 1986 or by the atomic bombs dropped on Hiroshima and Nagasaki, Japan, during World War II, can result in death and damage to embryonic cells. There was an increase of about 10 to 15 percent in birth defects in children born to pregnant women exposed to atomic bomb radiation in Japan. Diagnostic X rays are not known to be a cause of birth defects. Some defects such as hip dislocation may be caused by mechanical forces inside the uterus; this could happen if the amnion is damaged or the uterus is malformed, thus restricting the movement of the fetus. About 25 percent of congenital defects are caused by the interaction of genetic and environmental factors (multifactorial), and the causes of more than half (54 percent) of all defects are unknown.

TREATMENT AND THERAPY

Because many birth defects have well-defined genetic and environmental causes, they often can be prevented. Preventive measures need to be implemented if the risk of producing a child with a birth defect is higher than average. Genetic risk factors for such defects include the presence of a genetic defect in one of the parents, a family history of genetic defects, the existence of one or more children with defects, consanguineous (same-family) matings, and advanced maternal age. Prospective parents with one or more of these risk factors should seek genetic counseling in order to assess their potential for producing a baby with such defects. Also, parents exposed to higher-than-normal levels of drugs, alcohol, chemicals, or radiation are at risk of producing gametes that may cause defects, and pregnant women exposed to the same agents place the developing embryo at risk. Again, medical counseling should be sought by such prospective parents. Pregnant women should maintain a well-balanced diet that is about 200 calories higher than normal to provide adequate fetal nutrition. Women who become anemic during pregnancy may need an iron supplement, and the U.S. Public Health Service recommends that all women of childbearing age consume 0.4 milligram of folic acid (one of the B vitamins) per day to reduce the risk of spina bifida and other neural tube defects. Women at high risk for producing genetically defective offspring can undergo a screening technique whereby eggs taken from the ovary are screened in the laboratory prior to in vitro fertilization and then returned to the uterus. Some couples may decide to use artificial insemination by donor if the prospective father is known to carry a defective gene.

The early detection of birth defects is crucial to the health of both the mother and the baby. Physicians commonly use three methods for monitoring fetal growth and development during pregnancy. The most common method is ultrasound scanning. High-frequency sound waves are directed at the uterus and then monitored for waves that bounce back from the fetus. The return waves allow a picture of the fetus to be formed on a television monitor, which can be used to detect defects and evaluate the growth of the fetus. In amniocentesis, the doctor withdraws a small amount of amniotic fluid containing fetal cells; both the fluid and the cells can be tested for evidence of congenital defects. Amniocentesis generally cannot be performed until the sixteenth week of pregnancy. Another method of obtaining embryonic cells is called chorionic villus sampling

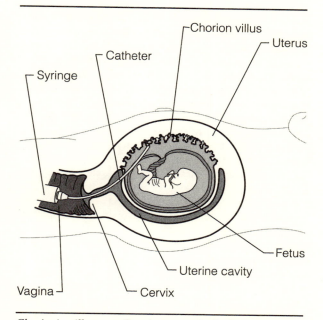

Chorionic villus sampling is one method of obtaining embryonic cells from a pregnant woman; examination of these cells helps physicians determine fetal irregularities or defects, which allows time to assess the problem and make recommendations for treatment.

and can be done as early as the fifth week of pregnancy. A tube is inserted into the uterus in order to retrieve a small sample of placental chorionic villus cells, identical genetically to the embryo. Again, these cells can be tested for evidence of congenital defects. The early discovery of fetal defects and other fetal-maternal irregularities allows the physician time to assess the problem and make recommendations to the parents regarding treatment. Many problems can be solved with therapy, medications, and even prenatal surgery. If severe defects are detected, the physician may recommend termination of the pregnancy.

Children born with defects often require highly specialized and intense medical treatment. For example, a child born with spina bifida may have lower-body paralysis, clubfoot, hip dislocation, and gastrointestinal and genitourinary problems in addition to the spinal column deformity. Spina bifida occurs when the embryonic neural tube and vertebral column fail to close properly in the lower back, often resulting in a protruding sac containing parts of the spinal meninges and spinal cord. The malformation and displacement of these structures result in nerve damage to the lower body, causing paralysis and the loss of some neural function in the organs of this area. Diagnostic procedures including X rays, computed tomography (CT) scans, and urinalysis are carried out to determine the extent of the disorder. If the sac is damaged and begins to leak cerebrospinal fluid, it needs to be closed immediately to reduce the risk of meningitis. In any case, surgery is done to close the opening in the lower spine, but it is not possible to correct the damage done to the nerves. Urgent attention must also be given to the urinary system. The paralysis often causes loss of sphincter muscle control in the urinary bladder and rectum. With respect to the urinary system, this lack of control can lead to serious urinary tract infections and the loss of kidney function. Both infections and obstructions must be treated promptly to avoid serious complication. Orthopedic care needs to begin early to treat clubfoot, hip dislocation, scoliosis, muscle weakness, spasms, and other side effects of this disorder.

The medical treatment of birth defects requires a carefully orchestrated team approach involving physicians and specialists from various medical fields. When the abnormality is discovered (before birth, at birth, or after birth), the primary physician will gather as much information as possible from the family history, the medical history of the patient, a physical examination, and other diagnostic tests. This information is interpreted in consultation with other physicians in order to classify the disorder properly and to determine its possible origin and time of occurrence. This approach may lead to the discovery of other malformations, which will be classified as primary and secondary. When the physician arrives at a specific overall diagnosis, he or she will counsel the parents about the possible causes and development of the disorder, the recommended treatment and its possible outcomes, and the risk of recurrence in a subsequent pregnancy. Certain acute conditions may require immediate attention in order to save the life of the newborn.

In addition to treating the infant with the defect, the physician needs to counsel the parents in order to answer their questions. The counseling process will help them to understand and accept their child's condition. In order to promote good parent-infant bonding, the parents are encouraged to maintain close contact with the infant and participate in its care. Children born with severe chronic disabilities and their families require special support. When parents are informed that their child has limiting congenital malformations, they may react negatively and express feelings of shock, grief, and guilt. Medical professionals can help the parents deal with their feelings and encourage them to develop a close and supportive relationship with their child. Physicians can provide a factual and honest appraisal of the infant's condition and discuss treatments, possible outcomes, and the potential for the child to live a happy and fulfilling life. Parents are encouraged to learn more about their child's disorder and to seek the guidance and help of professionals, support groups, family, and friends. With the proper care and home environment, the child can develop into an individual who is able to interact positively with family and community.

PERSPECTIVE AND PROSPECTS

Birth defects have been recognized and recorded throughout human history. The writer of the Old Testament book of 2 Samuel (21:20) describes the defeat of a giant with six fingers and six toes. Defects were recorded in prehistoric art, and the cuneiform records of ancient Babylon considered birth defects to be omens of great significance. Aristotle described many common human birth defects such as polydactyly. Superstitions about birth defects abounded during the Middle Ages. People believed that events occurring during pregnancy could influence the form of the newborn; for example, deformed legs could be caused by contact with a cripple. Mothers of deformed children were accused of having sex with animals. In a book written about birth defects in 1573, *Monstres et prodiges*, Ambroise Paré describes many human anomalies and attempts to explain how they occur. Missing body parts such as fingers or toes were attributed to a low sperm count in the father, and certain characteristics such as abnormal skin pigmentation, body hair, or facial features were said to be influenced by the mother's thoughts and visions during and after conception.

With advances in science and medicine these superstitions were swept aside. Surgery for cleft palate was performed as early as 1562 by Jacques Honlier. William Harvey, the seventeenth century English physician, recognized that some birth defects such as cleft lip are normal embryonic features that accidentally persist until the time of birth. The study of embryology, including experiments on bird and amphibian embryos, blossomed as a science during the nineteenth century, leading to a better understanding of how defects arise. At the same time, physicians were developing improved ways to treat birth defects. By 1816, Karl von Graefe had developed the first modern comprehensive surgical method for repairing cleft palate. The modern technique for repairing congenital pyloric stenosis (narrowing of the junction between the stomach and small intestine) was developed by Conrad Ramstedt in 1912. The principles of genetic inheritance developed by Gregor Mendel in the mid-1800's were rediscovered by biologists at the beginning of the twentieth century and soon were applied to the study of human heredity, including the inheritance of birth defects. Geneticists realized that defects such as hemophilia and Down syndrome are inherited diseases. Beginning in the 1930's, other scientists began to show that congenital defects could be induced in experimental animals by such factors as dietary deficiencies, hormone imbalances, chemicals, and radiation. Many tragic accidental human experiments also led to a better understanding of environmentally caused birth defects. The tranquilizer thalidomide caused limb malformations in more than seven thousand children in Europe before it was withdrawn from the market in 1961. Pregnant women treated for cervical cancer in the 1960's with large doses of radiation bore children with defects and mental retardation.

Indeed, much of the medical and environmental health research today centers on the effects of drugs, toxic chemicals, radiation, and other factors on human health and development. Genetic counseling and testing of parents at risk for inherited defects has become an accepted part of medical practice. In addition, there have been many advances in the treatment of congenital defects since the 1950's. Modern orthopedic and plastic surgery is used to correct such problems as clubfoot and cleft palate. Transplants are used to correct deficiencies of the liver, kidneys, and other organs. Biomedical engineers have developed improved prosthetic devices to replace lost limbs and to aid in hearing, speaking, and seeing. An understanding of metabolic disorders such as phenylketonuria (PKU) has led to better treatment that utilizes special diets and medications. Because it is difficult to undo the damage of congenital defects fully, the most promise seems to be in the areas of prevention and protection. Prospective parents and their medical care providers need to be alert to potential hereditary problems, as well as to exposure to hazardous environmental agents. Pregnant women need to maintain a healthy diet and check with their physicians before taking any drugs. With advances in preventive medicine, diagnosis, and treatment, the future is much brighter for reducing the health toll of congenital malformations. —*Rodney C. Mowbray*

See also Cerebral palsy; Childbirth, complications of; Cleft palate; Color blindness; Congenital heart disease; Cystic fibrosis; Diabetes mellitus; Down syndrome; Dwarfism; Fetal alcohol syndrome; Genetic diseases; Gigantism; Hemophilia; Hydrocephalus; Mental retardation; Multiple sclerosis; Muscular dystrophy; Phenylketonuria; Porphyria; Reye's syndrome; Sickle-cell anemia; Spina bifida; Thalassemia.

FOR FURTHER INFORMATION:

Bloom, Beth-Ann, and Edward Seljeskog. *A Parent's Guide to Spina Bifida*. Minneapolis: University of Minnesota Press, 1988. Designed to assist the parents of children with spina bifida. The book includes chapters on the nature of the disorder and how it is treated, the medical problems associated with spina bifida, and how to help the afflicted child while he or she is growing up. Also includes a useful glossary, a list of organizations and support groups, and an extensive bibliography.

Moore, Keith L. *The Developing Human*. 4th ed. Philadelphia: W. B. Saunders, 1988. An outstanding textbook on human embryonic development. Chapter 8 deals specifically with the causes of congenital malformations, and several other chapters include more detailed information about common defects occurring in each of the body's systems. The book is easy to understand and well illustrated.

Nixon, Harold, and Barry O'Donnel. *The Essentials of Pediatric Surgery*. 4th ed. Boston: Butterworth Heinemann, 1992. Describes in laypersons' terms the surgical treatment of many congenital abnormalities, including birth injuries, imperforate anus, spina bifida, hydrocephalus, pyloric stenosis, birthmarks, cleft lip and palate, hernias, urinary and digestive tract deformities, undescended testis, intersex problems, limb malformations, and congenital heart disease. The book is well illustrated with descriptive line diagrams and includes a thorough discussion of each procedure.

Stray-Gundersen, Karen, ed. *Babies with Down Syndrome*. Kensington, Md.: Woodbine House, 1986. A complete guide for parents with a Down syndrome child, written by doctors, nurses, educators, lawyers, and parents. The book includes a complete medical description of the disorder and extensive coverage of care concerns, child development, education, and legal rights. Contains an extensive glossary, reading list, and resource guide.

Warkany, Josef, Ronald J. Lemire, and Michael Cohen. *Mental Retardation and Congenital Malformations of the Central Nervous System*. Chicago: Year Book Medical Publishers, 1981. A medical reference book that gives complete descriptions of congenital malformations of the nervous system and their effects on the eyes, ears, heart, skeleton, and skin. The authors also include a thorough discussion of congenitally caused mental illness. The book is technical in nature but informative and authoritative. Well illustrated; includes extensive listings of technical articles.

BITES AND STINGS

SYSTEMS AFFECTED: Heart, immune

SPECIALISTS: Allergists, emergency physicians, immunologists, toxicologists

DEFINITION: Injuries from animals or insects.

Bites and stings cause four major types of damage to the victim's body: physical damage, the introduction of disease-causing organisms, the introduction of poisons (toxins, venoms), and allergic responses, including anaphylactic shock. Often, more than one form of damage is associated with a bite or sting. Alone or in combination, they can be life-threatening, but usually the damage from a bite or sting is minor. A wide variety of organisms can bite or sting, but the most important among them are mammals, reptiles (snakes and lizards), some fish (sharks, rays, moray eels), arthropods (including insects, centipedes, spiders, mites, ticks, and scorpions), and cnidarians (jellyfish, Portuguese man-of-wars, and their relatives).

Bites causing physical damage. Bites delivered by a mammal (most often a dog or cat) are likely to cause the most extensive physical damage. The specialized teeth of mammals, especially carnivores, in combination with powerful jaw muscles, can produce a serious wound. If wounding is in a vulnerable spot or is very extensive, or if the bleeding is not stopped, the physical damage can be fatal. A bite that causes physical damage is almost certain to introduce bacteria, viruses, or other infectious agents. An important example is the rabies virus, but many kinds of organism are dangerous if introduced into the bloodstream, or into the bone marrow of bones broken by the bite. Most mammalian bites do not introduce toxins into the victim. Some shrews have a venom in their saliva, but their small size and secretive habits minimize their threat to human health. Bites from mammals are also of minimal concern with respect to dangerous allergic responses. Physical damage is also the most serious problem in shark and moray eel bites.

Prevention, by avoiding animals prone to bite, is usually readily accomplished. Treatment involves stopping the bleeding, repairing the damage, and preventing infection.

Bites introducing infectious agents. Bites that cause serious physical damage are not the only ones that can introduce infectious agents. Any bite or sting can introduce infection to the victim because it penetrates the first line of defense, the skin. The arthropods are the most important disease vectors. Malaria is caused by a parasitic protozoan (single-celled, animal-type organism) transferred from one host to another by mosquitoes. Lyme disease is caused by a bacterium and is transported between hosts by ticks. Viruses cause yellow fever, and mosquitoes transport the virus to new hosts. Insects and ticks are vectors for a number of other diseases, most of which are introduced to the victim by a bite (including the stabs of blood-sucking arthropods such as mosquitoes).

Prevention of these diseases involves avoiding and/or eliminating the vectors; neither is always possible. Active immunization (stimulating the host to form antibodies against the disease-causing organism) is also used when available. Treatment involves drugs that destroy the disease organism or the use of passive immunization (the injection of preformed antibodies against the disease organism).

Bites and stings introducing toxins. Toxins or poisons are introduced to the victim most often by arthropods (scorpion stings, spider bites), cnidarians (stings), or reptiles (bites). Some mollusks—the cone shell snails, for example—can also inject toxins into a victim. The chemicals involved include enzymes that destroy tissue, neurotoxins that interfere with appropriate nerve cell responses (blocking or stimulating nerve cell signals), and others that interfere with the normal functions of the victim's body chemistry. Rattlesnakes and their relatives, coral snakes, and the Gila monster (a large lizard) are examples of poisonous reptiles. The brown recluse and black widow spiders are dangerous examples of their group. The sea wasp (a jellyfish) and the Portuguese man-of-war are the best known, but by no means the only, dangerous cnidarians in coastal waters off North America.

Prevention involves avoiding the animals that inject the toxin, which is easily accomplished much, but not all, of the time. Treatment involves injection of antivenin, a solution of antibodies that neutralize a specific toxin. Research on snake antivenin indicates that it might be possible to create a single antivenin which inactivates several snake venoms.

Bites and stings causing allergic reactions. Any bite or sting can cause an allergic response in the victim, because all introduce large foreign molecules, called antigens. These are often proteins, and they stimulate a response in the victim's immune system. If the response is more than that needed to destroy the antigen, it is called an allergic response and the foreign protein is called an allergen. The allergic response may simply be a nuisance causing minor inflammation, but it is exceptionally dangerous if it escalates into anaphylaxis. Anaphylaxis is a hyperreaction to a foreign substance in which the heart rate increases; bronchioles in the lungs constrict, making breathing difficult; and blood pressure drops. If symptoms continue, the victim may go into shock and even die. The toxins introduced by venomous arthropods, reptiles, cnidarians, and mollusks are often allergenic, even causing anaphylaxis, but even nonpoisonous or minimally toxic materials such as the venom introduced in a bee or wasp sting can cause life-threatening anaphylactic shock in sensitive people. A painful sting for people not sensitized to the foreign material becomes a threat to the life of a sensitized, hypersensitive person.

Prevention, by avoiding the allergen, is the preferred defense against allergic reactions. If avoidance is not possible or cannot be assured, the injection of small amounts of the substance to which an individual is hypersensitive, followed by increasingly larger doses, is sometimes effective in desensitizing the individual. Treatment of severe anaphylactic reactions involves the injection of adrenaline. Antihistamines, taken orally or injected, are used in less severe situations. —*Carl W. Hoagstrom*

See also Arthropod-borne diseases; Lice, mites, and ticks; Parasitic diseases; Poisoning; Zoonoses.

FOR FURTHER INFORMATION:

"Bites and Stings: It's That Time of Year." *Patient Care* 26 (May 30, 1992): 79-110.

Caras, Roger A. *Dangerous to Man: The Definitive Story of Wildlife's Reputed Dangers.* Rev. ed. New York: Holt, Rinehart and Winston, 1975.

Halstead, Bruce W., and Paul S. Auerbach. *Dangerous Aquatic Animals of the World: A Color Atlas.* Princeton, N.J.: Darwin Press, 1992.

Harvey, Alan L., ed. *Snake Toxins.* New York: Pergamon Press, 1991.

Tu, Anthony T., ed. *Reptile Venoms and Toxins.* New York: Marcel Dekker, 1991.

BLADDER INFECTIONS. *See* **URINARY DISORDERS.**

BLEEDING

SYSTEMS AFFECTED: Blood, circulatory

SPECIALISTS: Emergency physicians, family physicians, hematologists, internists

Definition: Damage or disruption to hemostasis (the normal absence of bleeding)—the appropriate interactions among blood cells, proteins in the blood, and blood vessels—resulting in loss of blood or abnormal clotting.

Key terms:

coagulation: the sequential process by which multiple, specific factors (predominantly proteins in plasma) interact, ultimately resulting in the formation of an insoluble clot made of fibrin

fibrin: the insoluble protein that forms the essential portion of a blood clot; the soluble protein in plasma converted to fibrin is called fibrinogen

fibrinolysis: the process of dissolving clots; the fibrinolytic system dissolves fibrin through enzymatic action

hemostasis: the arrest of bleeding from injured blood vessels, confining circulating blood to those vessels; blood vessels, platelets, the coagulation system, and the fibrinolytic system contribute to the process of hemostasis

plasma: the fluid portion of blood in which the particulate components are suspended; the majority of coagulation factors are proteins in plasma

platelets: disk-shaped structures in blood that are vital for the maintenance of normal hemostasis

vitamin K: a group of fat-soluble vitamins that play an integral role in the production of multiple, properly functioning coagulation factors by the liver

Causes and Symptoms

Patients with bleeding abnormalities are commonly encountered in medicine. Such patients may be evaluated because of previous bleeding episodes, a family history of bleeding, or sometimes abnormalities detected during preliminary studies before surgery or other invasive procedures. Bleeding episodes are often described as local (the source of bleeding is pinpointed to a specific part of the body) or generalized (abnormal bleeding occurring at multiple, distinct anatomic sites). It is important to distinguish between these two possibilities because treatment may differ markedly. Localized bleeding disorders may be correctable with surgery, while the treatment of generalized bleeding disorders may be more complex and long-term. The evaluation of patients with suspected bleeding disorders includes a detailed medical history, a thorough physical examination, and appropriate screening tests for hemostatic functioning. Subsequently, more specific laboratory tests are usually required to define the nature of a bleeding abnormality. Abnormal bleeding may result from blood vessel abnormalities (vascular defects), low platelet counts (thrombocytopenia), excessively high platelet counts (thrombocytosis), platelet function abnormalities, deficiencies or abnormalities of plasma coagulation factors, excessive breakdown of blood clots (excessive fibrinolysis), or a combination of these abnormalities. Bleeding disorders may be inherited or acquired.

Generalized bleeding abnormalities are suggested by several characteristics. Bleeding from multiple sites, bleeding in the absence of a known causative event (often termed spontaneous bleeding), and bleeding following trauma that is much more severe than expected for the degree of injury are all characteristics of generalized bleeding defects. An unexplained increase in bleeding severity may be a sign of a newly acquired generalized bleeding abnormality.

Inherited disorders. There are numerous inherited disorders of hemostasis. Fortunately, most are quite rare. The two most common inherited bleeding disorders are von Willebrand's disease and hemophilia A. Inherited bleeding disorders usually become evident in infancy or early childhood. There is often a family history of abnormal bleeding, and abnormal bleeding may have been experienced in association with surgery or trauma. Bleeding from the umbilical cord at birth or bleeding following circumcision may provide evidence of inherited hemostatic disorders. In contrast, a lack of abnormal bleeding following surgery such as tonsillectomy or dental procedures such as tooth extraction lowers the likelihood that even a mild inherited hemostatic disorder is present. There are, however, exceptions to such trends. Inherited disorders of hemostasis such as Ehlers-Danlos syndrome or hereditary hemorrhagic telangiectasia may not become evident until later in life. Idiopathic (or immune) thrombocytopenic purpura (ITP) is an acquired hemostatic abnormality which may occur in childhood, usually as a result of an infection. Hemorrhagic disease of the newborn is a short-lived bleeding abnormality caused by a transient deficiency of coagulation factors (known as the vitamin K dependent factors) in the newborn period.

Family history is helpful in the evaluation of hemostatic disorders because a pattern of bleeding among family members may be revealed. If only male members of a family are affected, this suggests an X-linked recessive pattern of inheritance (transmitted by the X sex chromosome). Such diseases are usually transmitted from females who are carriers of the trait. Hemophilia A, hemophilia B, and Wiskott-Aldrich syndrome are transmitted as X-linked recessive traits. Inherited bleeding disorders such as von Willebrand's disease occur in both sexes through non-sex-linked, or autosomal, transmission. Some bleeding disorders occur because of a gene mutation. Some individuals, therefore, are the first members of their family to have an inherited bleeding disorder.

Acquired disorders. These may first become evident in adulthood. A negative family history for bleeding may exist, and diseases may be present that are associated with bleeding abnormalities, such as kidney or liver disease. Liver disease may lead to abnormal bleeding for numerous reasons. Causes of abnormal bleeding include decreases in plasma coagulation factors (most coagulation factors are manufactured by the liver), low platelet counts, platelet function abnormalities, production of abnormal coagulation factors (such as abnormal fibrinogen), vulnerability to a

First Aid for Trauma-Related Bleeding

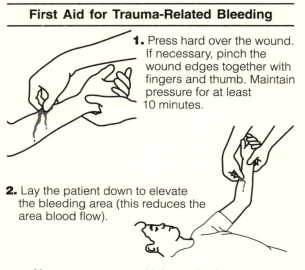

1. Press hard over the wound. If necessary, pinch the wound edges together with fingers and thumb. Maintain pressure for at least 10 minutes.

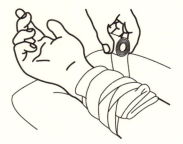

2. Lay the patient down to elevate the bleeding area (this reduces the area blood flow).

Never move a part which may be fractured.

3. Replace the hand pressure with pressure from a pad held firmly in place by a tight bandage or by whatever is at hand: stockings, belts, socks, handkerchiefs, ties.

4. If blood appears to be oozing through, do not investigate by removing the bandage already applied; instead apply additional pressure with more padding and bandage. Continue this procedure until control is achieved.

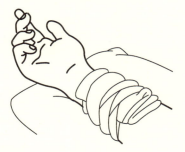

5. Apply antishock measures, as necessary. Get medical aid.

condition called disseminated intravascular coagulation (DIC), and abnormal lysis (breakdown) of blood clots. Platelet function abnormalities are associated with kidney failure and many blood diseases (for example, dysproteinemias, leukemias, and myeloproliferative disorders). Vitamin K is necessary for the production of numerous functional plasma coagulation factors. A deficiency of vitamin K, therefore, may lead to abnormal bleeding. Poor nutrition or antibiotic therapy may lead to vitamin K deficiency, which may also occur in newborns. One source of vitamin K is bacteria located in the gastrointestinal (GI) tract. Because the newborn GI tract is sterile, newborns have no bacterial source of vitamin K. Some medical conditions, such as sprue or biliary obstruction, may lead to inadequate absorption of vitamin K from the GI tract.

Numerous drugs and medications may cause abnormal bleeding. Drugs or medications may cause low platelet counts or platelet dysfunction or may affect coagulation factors. Oral anticoagulant therapy (warfarin therapy), which is used in the treatment of blood clots in the legs, causes a reduction of functional vitamin K dependent coagulation factors and is a common cause of drug-induced bleeding.

Nutritional deficiency, a major problem in many parts of the world, may result in bleeding disorders. One example is severe protein deficiency, a syndrome known as kwashiorkor, which produces severe liver damage. Vitamin C deficiency may cause scurvy, which may result in skin hemorrhages, bleeding gums, and bleeding beneath the lining of the bones (subperiosteal bleeding).

Evaluating hemostatic functioning. Dental extractions are a good measure of hemostatic functioning because bleeding occurs over rigid bone. The bleeding sites, therefore, are not easily compressible. Persistent and excessive bleeding after incisor removal is more significant as a diagnostic indicator than such bleeding following molar removal. (Even patients with normal hemostasis may experience persistent bleeding after molar extractions.) Tonsillectomy is evaluated in a similar manner. Because tonsillectomy may lead to persistent bleeding in the setting of normal hemostasis, the significance of excessive bleeding following tonsillectomy may be difficult to interpret. The lack of bleeding following tonsillectomy, however, implies normal hemostasis.

Investigation of trauma-related bleeding is an important component of hemostatic evaluation. When considering trauma-related bleeding, it is important to determine other details related to the events: Were blood transfusions required? What methods were used to bring bleeding under control? How easily was bleeding brought under control? Was there clearly a local cause of bleeding? Were any medications being taken which could lead to abnormal bleeding? A lack of abnormal bleeding with prior trauma does not absolutely exclude inherited bleeding disorders. Patients with milder forms of hemophilia may only bleed abnormally following severe trauma. Oral contraceptives or pregnancy influence the hemostatic reaction to a degree that may mask von Willebrand's disease in women.

Diagnosis by type of bleeding. In diagnosis, the type of abnormal bleeding may provide important clues. In vascular or platelet abnormalities, bleeding typically occurs in the skin or mucous membranes. Bleeding usually starts within seconds of the time of injury and may continue for hours; however, once the bleeding stops it may not recur. Post-traumatic bleeding in coagulation disorders may be delayed for many hours after a traumatic episode; recurrent episodes of bleeding following trauma are also a characteristic of such disorders.

Petechiae, small, red spots about the size of a pinhead, represent tiny hemorrhages from small blood vessels, such as capillaries. These spots are a sign of platelet or vascular abnormalities. Petechiae caused by vasculitis (the inflammation of blood vessels) are often elevated lesions that are distinct to the touch (palpable) as well as being evident visually. Petechiae associated with low platelet counts or abnormalities of platelet function are not palpable and, while often widespread, may first appear on the lower extremities, such as the ankles, or on mucous membranes, such as in the mouth.

Ecchymoses (bruises) are larger lesions caused by the leakage of blood into tissue of the skin or mucous membranes, usually as the result of trauma. Ecchymoses can be seen with all hemostatic disorders. Spontaneous ecchymoses, bruises appearing in the absence of prior trauma, may be a sign of a hemostatic problem. The location of the ecchymoses may provide diagnostic information. Bruises occurring only on the limbs, which are at greater risk for minor trauma, are less indicative of a possible bleeding abnormality than bruising which occurs on the trunk. Women frequently have one or two bruises, which may be normal. More than a half dozen bruises on a woman, however, warrants further evaluation. Easy bruising in a man also warrants further study.

Hematomas are collections of blood that accumulate in organs, body spaces, or tissues. They produce deformity of the area in which they develop and may be quite painful. Hematomas tend to be associated with abnormalities in the coagulation mechanism, such as hemophilia. Bleeding into joint spaces is known as hemarthrosis. Hemarthroses are characteristic of severe coagulation disorders such as hemophilia. Telangiectases and angiomata, caused by vascular malformations, are red spots or patches caused by the presence of blood in abnormally dilated vessels. Unlike the other lesions previously discussed, these vascular lesions blanch with pressure.

Epistaxis (nose bleeding) is most frequently caused by mild trauma (for example, nose blowing) to dilated vessels of the nose in individuals with normal hemostasis. Epistaxis in the setting of bleeding disorders is often associated with low platelet counts, the vascular abnormality called hereditary hemorrhagic telangiectasia, and von Willebrand's disease. Epistaxis consistently occurring on one side may be the result of a local abnormality, as opposed to a generalized hemostatic defect.

Abnormal bleeding may also be seen in other areas. Gingival bleeding (gum bleeding) may be caused by gum disease; however, it is also seen in association with low platelet counts, platelet dysfunction, scurvy, and in conditions where there are abnormally high levels of proteins in the blood (hyperviscosity syndrome). Hematuria (blood in the urine) may be caused by low platelet counts, platelet dysfunction, coagulation factor abnormalities, and oral anticoagulant therapy. Hematuria is a serious medical symptom that requires medical investigation to determine the cause. Bleeding from the GI tract can be seen with all types of hemostatic disorders. GI bleeding must be completely investigated to determine whether there is local cause for the bleeding or the bleeding is part of a generalized hemostatic defect. Menorrhagia (abnormal bleeding during menstrual periods) is associated with low platelet counts, platelet dysfunction, von Willebrand's disease, and coagulation factor abnormalities. Information such as the number and type of sanitary pads or tampons needed, period duration, the necessity of sanitary pad changes at night, the passage of clots, and the requirement of iron for anemia may be helpful in quantifying menstrual blood loss.

Laboratory tests. Laboratory evaluation of hemostatic functioning consists of screening tests, to aid in the detection of abnormalities, and confirmatory tests, to characterize the disorders. Microscopic examination of a blood smear is a simple screening procedure that may provide valuable information. A disease process associated with abnormal bleeding, such as leukemia, may be detected. Numerous red cell fragments may be present in hemostatic disorders such as DIC or thrombotic thrombocytopenic purpura (TTP). An estimate of the number of platelets and an evaluation of their size and shape can be made. Abnormally low and high platelet counts can lead to abnormal bleeding. Large platelets can be seen in conditions in which they are being destroyed rapidly, such as ITP. Large platelets are also seen in Bernard-Soulier syndrome, an inherited platelet function disorder.

The automated platelet count and bleeding time are screening tests for the evaluation of platelets. A normal interaction between platelets and damaged blood vessels is a necessary first step to control bleeding. This step is often termed primary hemostasis. An adequate number of normally functioning platelets are necessary to provide normal primary hemostasis. A representative normal range for the platelet count is 150,000 to 400,000 platelets per microliter of blood. In the absence of platelet dysfunction, spontaneous bleeding is rare when the platelet count is greater than

20,000 per microliter. The risk of life-threatening hemorrhage does not markedly increase until the platelet count drops below 10,000 per microliter. The bleeding time is primarily used to screen for platelet dysfunction, although it may also indicate some vascular abnormalities. The bleeding time measures the interval required for bleeding to cease following a standard skin incision on the forearm. A blood pressure cuff on the arm is inflated to a pressure of 40 millimeters of mercury during the procedure. A representative normal range for the bleeding time is four to seven minutes. A prolonged bleeding time may be a sign of a platelet or vascular abnormality.

The plasma coagulation system is composed primarily of a set of proteins that interact to produce clotting of blood (fibrin clots). This system is often referred to as secondary hemostasis. Most plasma coagulation factors are identified by a roman numeral (for example coagulation factor VIII). For ease of analysis, the plasma coagulation system has been divided into groups of proteins known as the intrinsic pathway, the extrinsic pathway, and the final common pathway. Screening tests for the plasma coagulation system include the thrombin time (TT), the prothrombin time (PT), and the activated partial thromboplastin time (aPTT). The screening tests detect significant deficiencies or abnormalities of plasma coagulation factors and help localize the defects within the pathways.

Specific, and often more complex, laboratory studies of hemostasis are performed based on information derived from the medical history, physical examination, and screening laboratory tests. The goal of specific tests is to pinpoint the diagnosis of hemostatic abnormalities.

Platelet disorders. Thrombocytopenia, a low platelet count in the blood, has numerous causes. Platelets are produced in the bone marrow and subsequently released into the blood. Bone marrow damage may result in inadequate numbers of platelets. Drugs, toxins, radiation, and infections may damage the bone marrow. Certain diseases, such as leukemia or other cancers, may lead to the replacement of bone marrow cells with abnormal cells or fibrous tissue. Some diseases result in inadequate release of platelets from the bone marrow. Inadequate platelet release may be the result of nutritional deficiencies, such as vitamin B_{12} or folic acid deficiencies, or it can be seen in some rare hereditary disorders, such as May-Hegglin anomaly or Wiscott-Aldrich syndrome. Individuals with an enlarged spleen may develop thrombocytopenia because of the pooling of platelets within the organ. Massive transfusion may result in thrombocytopenia when the blood volume is replaced with transfused solutions that do not contain platelets.

Certain disorders result in the rapid destruction or consumption of platelets. If the production of platelets by the bone marrow does not compensate for the rate of destruction, thrombocytopenia occurs. Platelet consumption with resultant thrombocytopenia is a component of DIC. Thrombocytopenia caused by accelerated destruction may also occur with prosthetic heart valves, blood infections (sepsis), and vascular defects called hemangiomas. The development of antibodies against one's own platelets (such as with ITP) causes platelet consumption. ITP can be a self-limited disorder with a complete return to normal (acute ITP) or a prolonged thrombocytopenic condition (chronic ITP). Acute ITP is seen most frequently in children between two and six years of age. The disease is preceded by a viral infection in about 80 percent of cases. The platelet count returns to normal within six months in more than 80 percent of patients; the usual period of thrombocytopenia is four to six weeks. Mortality from acute ITP occurs in about 1 percent of cases. Chronic ITP typically occurs in young and middle-aged adults, and the disorder is about three times more common in females than in males. As many as 50 percent of children born to mothers with ITP have thrombocytopenia at birth as a result of the transfer of antiplatelet antibodies across the placenta. Isoimmune neonatal thrombocytopenia and post-transfusion purpura are other conditions in which thrombocytopenia is caused by antiplatelet antibodies.

Numerous drugs have been associated with thrombocytopenia. Examples of such drugs include gold salts, quinine, quinidine, sulfonamide drugs, and heparin. Thrombocytopenia may occur within twenty-four hours following exposure to an offending drug. All nonessential medications should be discontinued in patients suspected of having drug-induced thrombocytopenia.

Platelet function defects may be inherited or acquired. They may occur without evidence of an associated disease or be secondary to a recognizable clinical disorder. Platelet function defects are suspected when there is abnormal skin or mucous membrane bleeding, a prolonged bleeding time, and a normal platelet count. Bleeding disorders caused by the inability of platelets to stick to damaged blood vessel walls in a normal manner are called platelet adhesion defects; Bernard-Soulier syndrome and von Willebrand's disease are examples of such defects.

Certain molecules necessary for normal platelet function are contained within platelets (that is, in the storage pool). Deficiencies or defects of these molecules lead to platelet dysfunction and are called storage pool defects. Examples of storage pool defects include gray platelet syndrome and dense granule deficiency. Platelet release defects occur when there is a failure to release storage pool contents normally. Hereditary deficiency of the enzymes cyclooxygenase or thromboxane synthetase causes platelet release defects. Aspirin causes a platelet release defect by inactivating cyclooxygenase.

Disorders that render platelets unable to interact with one another to form large clumps at the site of vascular injury are known as platelet aggregation defects. Ganzmann's thrombasthenia and hereditary afibrinogenemia are examples of such defects.

Platelets also play a key role in secondary hemostasis by providing a surface on which many coagulation factors can interact. A bleeding disorder results if the platelet surface is incapable of supporting secondary hemostasis. Hereditary bleeding disorders caused by this type of platelet defect are quite rare.

Acquired platelet dysfunction is quite common. Renal failure (uremia) may cause acquired platelet dysfunction.

Arterial Pressure Points

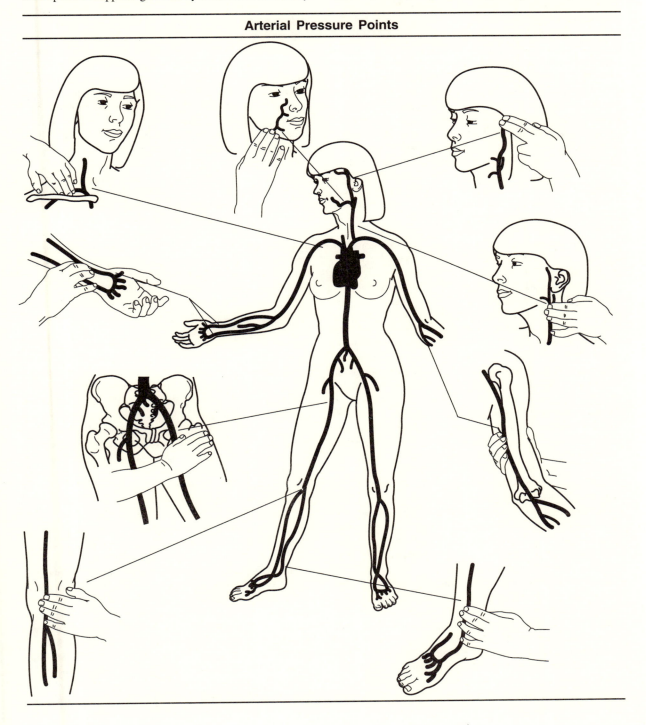

Liver disease can cause multiple bleeding abnormalities, including platelet dysfunction. A vast number of drugs and medications, such as aspirin and penicillin, cause platelet dysfunction. Acquired platelet function defects are seen with cardiopulmonary bypass procedures and in association with numerous blood diseases.

Coagulation disorders. The overall incidence of inherited coagulation factor disorders is about 1 in 10,000. In such conditions, there is either a failure to make a sufficient amount of a coagulation factor (quantitative disorder) or a dysfunctional factor is made (qualitative disorder). An inherited disorder exists for every coagulation factor, although most are quite rare. Symptoms range from serious spontaneous bleeding, which occurs in the severe forms of hemophilia A (factor VIII disorder) or hemophilia B (factor IX disorder), to an absence of abnormal bleeding in other inherited conditions (factors XII, prekallikrein, and high molecular weight kininogen). In general, for disorders which cause bleeding, the more profound the coagulation factor defect, either quantitatively or qualitatively, the more severe the bleeding. Severe disorders are usually easily identified. Moderate or mild disorders are more common and may go undetected until there is a significant hemostatic challenge, such as surgery.

Von Willebrand's disease is probably the most common inherited bleeding disorder. It is caused by deficiencies or defects in a vital group of hemostatic proteins known collectively as von Willebrand factor. Manifestations include epistaxis, menorrhagia, prolonged bleeding after trauma or surgery, frequent ecchymoses, and persistent gum bleeding. Severe episodes of epistaxis may occur during childhood, and such episodes may cease during puberty. In women, epistaxis may recur after the menopause. Important diagnostic clues include a family history of abnormal bleeding, affected members in every generation (males and females), and marked worsening of bleeding following the ingestion of aspirin or other drugs that impair platelet function. Von Willebrand's disease consists of a very diverse spectrum of abnormalities: At least twenty-one distinct subtypes of von Willebrand's disease have been recognized.

Hemophilia A and hemophilia B are clinically indistinguishable; laboratory testing is required for their diagnosis. Hemophilia A is illustrated here. Hemophilia A is an inherited disorder of a portion of coagulation factor VIII. Hemophilia A is typically seen in males, while females are carriers of the abnormal gene and can transmit the disease. Twenty percent of affected individuals have a negative family history and likely developed their disease because of a mutation of the factor VIII gene. Once the abnormal gene is established in a family, the severity of the disease is the same for all affected males. Hemophilia A is divided into severe, moderate, and mild subtypes based on the amount of functional factor VIII present. Bleeding in hemophiliacs may be spontaneous or post-traumatic. Spontaneous bleeding tends to occur only in severe hemophilia. It characteristically affects joints and muscles, and it may lead to crippling injury without prompt and adequate treatment. Post-traumatic bleeding may occur in mild, moderate, or severe hemophilia A. Such episodes are often prolonged and dangerous. Bleeding into the head (intracranial bleeding) remains a common cause of severe disability and death in hemophilia A. Modern treatment, however, has reduced the incidence of this severe complication. Antibodies (inhibitors) directed against factor VIII develop in approximately 12 to 15 percent of patients who require transfusions to provide factor VIII. The development of inhibitors is a serious complication which may compromise the effectiveness of therapy. Factor VIII inhibitors may occur in non-hemophiliacs, leading to serious bleeding in affected males and females.

Acquired coagulation factor disorders may be caused by reduced or absent factor production (for example, in liver disease), the production of defective or inactive factors (such as in liver disease or vitamin K deficiency), factor inhibitors, or accelerated consumption or clearance of factors. Examples in the latter group include DIC (accelerated consumption), kidney disease (factors lost in the urine), and the attachment of factors to abnormal tissue, which occurs in a disease called amyloidosis.

DIC is a hemostatic disorder which arises as part of a disease or medical condition. Examples of associated conditions include obstetrical accidents, abnormal destruction of red blood cells within blood vessels, infections, malignancies, burns, severe injuries, liver disease, and diseases of blood vessels. DIC may be an explosive, life-threatening syndrome (high-grade DIC) or a troublesome, less dramatic feature of a disease (low-grade DIC). Conditions associated with DIC cause abnormal activation of the hemostatic response, resulting in the widespread formation of blood clots in the vascular system. The clots obstruct the blood supply to vital organs (the kidneys, heart, lungs, and brain), leading to impaired organ function. Abnormal bleeding may develop if coagulation factors and platelets become depleted because of their incorporation into widespread blood clots. The breakdown of blood clots may also become inadequately controlled and contribute further to abnormal bleeding.

PERSPECTIVE AND PROSPECTS

The existence of bleeding disorders has been known for many centuries. Abnormal bleeding observed in the males of certain families was described in the Jewish Talmud in the second century. Interest in such disorders increased markedly with the discovery of hemophilia in the royal families of Europe. In 1853, Queen Victoria gave birth to her fifth son, Leopold. She was a carrier of hemophilia, and Leopold had the disease. He died of a brain hemorrhage following a minor blow to the head at the age of thirty-one. Two of Victoria's daughters gave birth to affected sons. Her granddaughter, Alexandra, became the czarina of Russia, and Alexandra's only son, Alexis, suffered from hemophilia.

The transformation of fluid blood to a solid mass has fascinated investigators since ancient times. Aristotle noted that blood contained fibers and, upon cooling, solidified. He also observed that "diseased" blood did not solidify. The realization that blood clotting minimized blood loss from wounds occurred in the early eighteenth century. In the late eighteenth century, William Hewson described the clotting time of whole blood. He found it to be shortened in some diseases and infinite in one woman after delivering a baby. In 1863, work published by Lord Joseph Lister laid the foundation for the discovery of the intrinsic pathway of coagulation. In 1905, Paul Morawitz, aided by the discoveries of such investigators as Alexander Schmidt and Olof Hammarsten, proposed what is now called the classic theory of blood coagulation. This led to the characterization of the extrinsic pathway of coagulation. In 1964, the "cascade" (by Robert Macfarlane) and "waterfall" (by Earl Davie and Oscar Ratnoff) hypotheses of coagulation were proposed. These discoveries paved the way for much of the current understanding of coagulation.

Alfred Donné is credited with the first description of platelets, reported in 1842. In 1881, Giulio Bizzozero became the first author to use the term "blood platelets." Shortly thereafter, discoveries in the late nineteenth century highlighted the importance of platelets in normal hemostasis. In recent times, the study of platelets has intensified. A large volume of information on platelets and platelet function has accumulated since the 1960's.

The study of the cells lining blood vessels (endothelium) and their role in hemostasis is a relatively young discipline. Much has already been learned about these cells, and much more information is anticipated. The future promises great advances in the study of hemostasis and hemostatic disorders. Further definition of the interrelationships of endothelium, platelets, and coagulation factors in normal and abnormal hemostasis is expected. There is hope for a greater understanding of inherited hemostatic disorders. Additional studies on the processes that keep blood from clotting (anticoagulants) and those that break down clots (fibrinolysis) are expected. The effect of diseases such as cancer on hemostasis awaits clarification, as does the effect of hemostasis on other processes, such as the spread of cancer.
—*James R. Stubbs*

See also Hemophilia.

FOR FURTHER INFORMATION:

Colman, Robert W., et al., eds. *Hemostasis and Thrombosis: Basic Principles and Clinical Practice.* 2d ed. Philadelphia: J. B. Lippincott, 1987. This is the bible in the study of hemostasis. An extensive and comprehensive reference textbook that deserves a spot on the bookshelf of all those involved with hemostasis.

Hirsh, Jack, and Elizabeth A. Brain. *Hemostasis and Thrombosis: A Conceptual Approach.* 2d ed. New York: Churchill Livingstone, 1983. A fun book for learning the principles of hemostasis. The text is filled with easy-to-understand illustrations that succeed in making difficult concepts very straightforward.

Owen, Charles A., E. J. Walter, and John H. Thompson. *The Diagnosis of Bleeding Disorders.* 2d ed. Boston: Little, Brown, 1975. A classic in the field of hemostasis. Although this is a somewhat older work, much vital information on hemostasis can still be obtained from the text. The extensive chapter on the history of hemostasis is interesting reading.

Ratnoff, Oscar D., and Charles D. Forbes, eds. *Disorders of Hemostasis.* 2d ed. Philadelphia: W. B. Saunders, 1991. A comprehensive textbook edited by two giants in the field of hemostasis. Although this is a detailed textbook, the authors cover various aspects of hemostasis in an organized and understandable manner.

Thompson, Arthur R., and Laurence A. Harker. *Manual of Hemostasis and Thrombosis.* 3d ed. Philadelphia: F. A. Davis, 1983. This manual provides concise descriptions of the various aspects of hemostasis. It is well written and serves as a valuable "quick source" of information on bleeding disorders.

Triplett, Douglas A. *Hemostasis: A Case Oriented Approach.* New York: Igaku-Shoin, 1985. In a manner similar to the book by Jack Hirsh and Elizabeth A. Brain (above), Triplett has made learning hemostasis quite pleasant. Most of the material in this book is presented in the form of specific patient cases, and it is an effective teaching method.

BLINDNESS

SYSTEM AFFECTED: Visual

SPECIALISTS: Geriatric specialists, ophthalmologists

DEFINITION: The absence of vision, or its extreme impairment to the extent that activity is limited; about 95 percent of all blindness is caused by eye diseases, the rest by injuries.

KEY TERMS:

glaucoma: excessive pressure inside the eye that can damage the optic nerve

laser: an intense light beam used in eye surgery

macular degeneration: a deterioration of vision in the most sensitive, central region of the retina

retina: a paper-thin membrane lining the inside surface of the eyeball, where light is transformed into nerve impulses

trachoma: a contagious eye infection primarily found in Third World countries

CAUSES AND SYMPTOMS

The major cause of blindness among older adults in the Western world is glaucoma. The aqueous fluid produced inside the eye fails to drain properly and causes pressure to build up. In extreme cases, the eyeball becomes hard. Without prompt treatment, the outer layer of the optic nerve starts to deteriorate. The patient can still see straight ahead, but not off to the side. When the cone of forward vision has narrowed to less that 20 degrees (called tunnel vision), the patient is considered legally blind.

Cataracts are another common defect of vision among the elderly. The lens of the eye develops dark spots that interfere with light transmission. Cataracts are not caused by an infection or a tumor but instead are a normal part of the aging process, like gray hair. There is no known treatment to retard or reverse the growth of cataracts.

Macular degeneration and diabetes mellitus can cause blindness as a result of hemorrhages from tiny blood vessels in the retina. The macula is a small region in the middle of the retina where receptor cells are tightly packed together to obtain sharp vision for reading or close work. With aging, blood circulation in the macula gradually deteriorates until the patient develops a black spot in the center of the field of view. Advanced diabetes also causes blood vessel damage in the eye. In serious cases, fluid can leak behind the retina, causing it to become detached. The resulting visual effect resembles a dark curtain that blacks out part of the scene.

Trachoma is a blinding eye disease that afflicts millions of people in poor parts of the world. It is a contagious infection of the eyelid similar to conjunctivitis (commonly known as pinkeye). If untreated, it causes scarring of the cornea and eventual blindness. Trachoma is caused by a virus that is spread by flies, in water, or by direct contact with tears or mucus.

Many kinds of injuries may cause blindness. Car accidents, sports injuries, chemical explosions, battle wounds, or small particles that enter the eye all can result in a serious loss of vision.

TREATMENT AND THERAPY

An indispensable tool in the treatment of serious eye problems is the laser. Its intense light focused into a tiny spot, the laser's heat can burn away a ruptured blood vessel or weld a detached retina back into place. For glaucoma patients, medication to reduce fluid pressure in the eye may be effective for a while. Eventually, a laser can be used to burn a small hole through the iris in order to improve fluid drainage. The laser can only be used to prevent blindness, however, and not to restore sight.

Cataracts formerly were a major cause of blindness among older people. Once the eye lens starts to become cloudy, nothing can be done to clear it. Cataract surgery to remove the defective lens and to insert a permanent, plastic replacement has become common. In the United States, more than a million cataract surgeries are performed annually, with a success rate that is greater than 95 percent.

The infectious eye disease called trachoma has been known for more than two thousand years. Effective modern treatment uses sulfa drugs taken orally, combined with antibiotic eyedrops or ointments. Unfortunately, reinfection is common in rural villages where most people have the disease and sanitation is poor. The World Health Organization has initiated a public health program to teach parents about the importance of cleanliness and frequent eye washing with sterilized water for their children.

PERSPECTIVE AND PROSPECTS

Various techniques have been developed for helping sightless people to live a self-reliant lifestyle. Using a white cane or walking with a trained dog allows a blind person to get around without assistance. Biomedical engineers have designed a miniature sonar device built into a pair of glasses that uses reflected sound waves to warn the wearer about obstacles.

The Braille system of reading, using patterns of raised dots for the alphabet, was invented in 1829 and is still widely used. For blind students, voice recordings of textbooks, magazines, and even whole encyclopedias are available on tape. A recent development is an optical scanner connected to a computer with a voice simulator that can read printed material aloud.

The National Federation of the Blind was founded in 1940. Its goals are to assist the blind to participate fully in society and to overcome the still-prevalent stereotype that the blind are helpless. Blind men and women hold jobs as engineers, teachers, musical performers, ministers, insurance agents, computer programmers, and school counselors. As society becomes more sensitive to all forms of disability, opportunities for blind people continue to expand.

—Hans G. Graetzer

See also Cataracts; Color blindness; Glaucoma; Macular degeneration; Visual disorders.

FOR FURTHER INFORMATION:

Lerman, Sidney. "Glaucoma." *Scientific American*, August, 1959, 110-117. Describes how excess pressure can build up in the eye to cause blindness. Excellent illustrations with clear explanations.

Maurer, Marc. "Reflecting the Flame." *Vital Speeches of the Day* 57 (September 1, 1991): 684-690. A speech by the president of the National Federation of the Blind. He criticizes the media, government agencies, and educators for perpetuating false stereotypes of helplessness. Maurer is a forceful spokesperson for the blind.

Peninsula Center for the Blind. *The First Steps: How to Help People Who Are Losing Their Sight*. Palo Alto, Calif.: Peninsula Center, 1982. A pamphlet designed to help people cope with the emotional trauma of blindness and the process of adjustment. Highly recommended.

Werner, Georges H., Bachisio Latte, and Andrea Contini. "Trachoma." *Scientific American*, January, 1964, 79-86. Describes this infectious eye disease, which is prevalent in poor nations of the world. The efforts to develop effective treatment and a vaccine are reported.

BLOOD POISONING. *See* **SEPTICEMIA.**

BONE CANCER

SYSTEM AFFECTED: Skeletal

SPECIALISTS: Internists, oncologists, orthopedic surgeons

DEFINITION: Cancer of the bone, which may have originated there or have spread from another site in the body.

KEY TERMS:

adjuvant therapy: the use of multiple treatments for cancer, such as chemotherapy following surgery to prevent metastasis

biopsy: the removal of tissue from a suspected cancer site, in order to identify abnormal cells under microscopic examination by a pathologist

bone scan: a diagnostic technique using a radioactive tracer which is strongly absorbed by a tumor, whose location then can be detected by radiation counters

computed tomography (CT) scanning: a method of displaying the outline of a tumor, utilizing a computer to combine information from multiple X-ray beams

magnetic resonance imaging (MRI): a diagnostic technique used to see the outline of an internal organ or a tumor without using X rays

medullary cavity: the interior of a bone, where new blood cells are formed by the bone marrow, surrounded by a hard outer cortex ·

metastasis: the spread of cancer cells from an original tumor site to other parts of the body

palliative treatment: the use of drugs or radiation to suppress a tumor and to provide relief from pain when a cure is not possible

sarcoma: a malignant tumor originating in bone or connective tissue

staging: a numerical classification system used by physicians to describe how far a cancerous growth has advanced

CAUSES AND SYMPTOMS

Out of about one million new cancers that are diagnosed annually in the United States, less than 1 percent are primary bone cancer. Most of these cases arise in children under the age of twenty. If diagnosis is made before the bone cancer has spread to the lungs or other sites in the body, prompt treatment by surgery, radiation, or chemotherapy can provide a good prognosis for recovery.

In older adults, most cases of so-called bone cancer actually are secondary tumors that have spread from other parts of the body, especially from the breast, prostate, thyroid, lung, or kidney. Such metastasized tumors consist of cells that are characteristic of their original, primary site. Secondary bone cancers are far more common than those which start in the bone.

The first symptom of bone cancer in children usually is a localized swelling followed by persistent, dull pain. It is easily mistaken for a sprain or a bruise that might come from a minor injury. Additional symptoms are fatigue, fever, loss of appetite, and other signs of general illness. Unfortunately, early symptoms may be ignored until the disease has already spread to other parts of the body. Before chemotherapy became available in the 1970's, the spread of bone cancer to the lungs occurred within two years for about 80 percent of patients.

A variety of diagnostic techniques are available to the physician if the examination of a patient arouses the suspicion of bone cancer. Blood tests, including a study of liver and kidney functions, have become increasingly useful because of improvements in analytical procedure. X-ray photography and computed tomography (CT) scanning will give pictorial evidence of any lesions or excess bony growth. Magnetic resonance imaging (MRI) provides the best visualization of tumors extending into soft tissue. Finally, the most important diagnostic procedure is biopsy. Usually, the bone is opened surgically and a sample of tissue is taken. Sometimes, a hollow needle inserted through the bone cortex can be used to withdraw a small sample. A pathologist who specializes in oncology examines the tissue under a microscope to confirm if cancer cells are present and to identify their type.

Magnetic resonance imaging as a diagnostic technique was developed in the 1980's, giving remarkable picture clarity for soft tissue. A strong magnetic field and radio waves are used to determine the concentration of hydrogen in a region of the body. Since tissue is mostly water (which contains hydrogen) and bone is dry, the image will show bright areas for tissue or soft organs against a dark background. Also, MRI shows contrast between normal tissue and a denser, tumorous mass.

Another diagnostic technique, the bone scan, is used to investigate whether a tumor has metastasized to other bones in the body. A small amount of radioactive tracer, usually technetium, is injected into the patient. It circulates in the bloodstream and gradually accumulates in the bone marrow. After several hours, radiation counters are used to scan the entire skeleton from head to foot. Regions of rapid cell growth, which may signal a tumorous mass, are indicated by a relatively high counting rate. If secondary tumors are detected by the bone scan, their shape and size can be investigated further using MRI.

Several kinds of bone cancer have been identified. One type is called osteosarcoma. It occurs most frequently during puberty, when a child's bones are growing rapidly. The tumor is likely to develop inside the long bones of the arms, in the legs near the knee, or in the pelvis. As its size increases and the surrounding bone material becomes soft, the bone may fracture because of internal pressure in the bone. Osteosarcomas also may grow on the exterior surface of bones, producing hard spikes that radiate outward. Another type of bone cancer is called Ewing's sarcoma. MRI and CT scans commonly exhibit a "moth-eaten" appearance

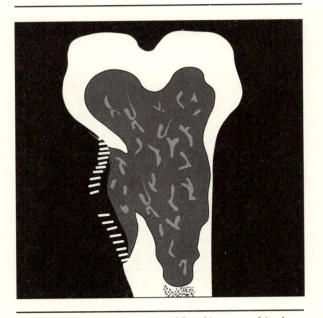

Osteosarcoma in the process of breaking out of its bone compartment.

where bone destruction has taken place. Both the inner (medullary) cavity and the outer cortex of the bone can be affected. Subsequently, a tumorous mass develops within the covering of tissue that surrounds the bone. This abnormal growth tends to form concentric layers, like the skin of an onion. The localized swelling expands in size, causing soreness and eventually impeding motion at the joints.

Bone cancer can take a variety of other forms. For example, a tumor may invade the bone from the outside and then penetrate into the medullary cavity. In order to make an accurate diagnosis and institute the best possible treatment for bone cancer, particularly for children, it is important for patients and their families to find an oncologist and supporting staff with specialized experience in this relatively rare condition. In general, the orthopedic surgeon who does the biopsy should be a specialist who is trained to do the ultimate bone surgery, so that any cancer cell contamination at the site of the biopsy will be completely removed.

TREATMENT AND THERAPY

In order to develop an appropriate treatment plan for a patient with bone cancer, all the relevant diagnostic information must be brought together. A medical team consisting of a radiologist, pathologist, radiation therapist, orthopedic surgeon, and medical oncologist will assess how far the cancer has advanced. This is called staging, that is, classifying its stage of growth.

Three designations commonly are used to characterize a cancer: G for its grade (based on the microscopic tissue analysis), T for tumor size and penetration, and M for evidence of metastasis. For example, (G1) (T2) (M0) would describe a low grade tumor (G1) that has broken out of its bone compartment (T2) but has not metastasized (M0) to the lungs or elsewhere.

Before 1970, treatment of a cancerous bone normally meant amputation. The prognosis for recovery was less than 20 percent, however, because microscopic, invisible metastases to the lungs and other organs usually were already present. The experimental search for drugs that can fight cancer cells started in the 1930's. Dr. Charles B. Huggins discovered that the female sex hormone estrogen could halt the growth of prostate cancer in men. He received the Nobel Prize in Medicine in 1966 for his work. Since that pioneering success, several hundred thousand drugs have been tested, with less than a hundred showing any substantial benefit. The anticancer drugs also can have severe side effects on healthy cells. Fortunately, a rapidly growing tumor has a higher rate of metabolism, so drugs will kill the cancer cells at a lower dose and spare most normal cells.

An effective method of treating bone cancer in children is to use chemotherapy or radiation even before surgery, in order to shrink the size of a tumor. Instead of complete amputation, the surgeon may need to remove only part of a bone, thus saving the limb. Even when a bone joint must be amputated, it may still be possible to salvage the limb by inserting an artificial joint or one from an organ donor.

In older adults, cancer of the bone almost invariably is caused by metastasis from another location in the body. The tumor in the bone may be very painful. Radiation to the affected area can provide palliative treatment, while more aggressive action is taken against the primary cancer site.

A wide range of medications is available to help control pain and to counteract the disagreeable side effects of radiation or chemotherapy. Special attention is given to the diet of cancer patients to prevent weight loss and to maintain body strength. Loss of appetite and digestion problems are common symptoms during therapy. Strong painkilling drugs such as codeine and morphine sometimes are necessary. The dose should be limited, however, so that the patient's ability to interact socially is not completely lost.

Vigorous research to find more effective therapies for cancer is widely supported. The goal is to find procedures that are less mutilating, less expensive, and less painful for the patient. Promising new drugs must be tested to determine how large a dose is needed and how serious the side effects are. Therefore, patients may be asked to become volunteers in clinical trial of an experimental treatment. Although people have a justified sense of reluctance to become "guinea pigs" in an untested therapy, clinical trials with human subjects have been essential in the development of successful medical procedures. Firm guidelines have been established for testing new therapies, such as the requirement to obtain the informed consent of patients and their families. In addition, doctors in the United States are responsible to a medical oversight committee and are obligated to submit their results for professional review. Cancer treatment can make progress through willing participation by patients in the carefully planned clinical trials.

PERSPECTIVE AND PROSPECTS

Bone cancer first came to the attention of the American public in the 1920's through a notorious case of industrial poisoning. A manufacturing company in New Jersey was utilizing radioactive radium to make watch dials that would glow in the dark. The women workers who were hired to apply the luminous paint would twirl the paint brushes between their lips to make a fine tip. The ingested radium, being chemically similar to calcium, became concentrated in bones, especially of the jaw and neck. Eventually, more than forty workers died of bone cancer, including the company's chief chemist.

After this incident, it became clear that radiation has a particularly damaging effect on bone marrow. In fact, any rapidly dividing cells in the body are especially radiosensitive. This would include hair, skin, and the reproductive system. It is unfortunate that it took until the 1950's before X-ray fluoroscopes were removed from shoe stores. Parents were fascinated to see the bones of their child's foot inside a new shoe without realizing that the radiation was harmful.

Until 1970, the outlook for a child who developed bone cancer was very poor. In spite of amputation of the affected limb, 80 percent of the young patients died within two years. In 1972, Norman Jaffe and Emil Frei in Boston made a major breakthrough in therapy by giving their patients large doses of a drug called methotrexate after limb surgery. It was a new approach in chemotherapy to stop the cancer from spreading even though no metastasis was visible yet. The experimental drug was so powerful that other antidote drugs were given to control side effects. The first trial with seventeen children was very successful, with all of them still surviving after twenty-one months.

Yet an article written in 1994 by Tim Beardsley summarizing the status of cancer in the United States came to a rather pessimistic conclusion. The cancer rate was higher and the likelihood of cure had not improved for most types of adult cancer since the "war on cancer" was initiated by President Richard M. Nixon in 1971. The cumulative effects of smoking, poor diet, and continuing exposure to harmful chemicals may help to explain this lack of progress. The good news was that the death rate from childhood cancer fell by almost half in that period. Early diagnosis and improved therapy have helped greatly. The family of a child with cancer can now look forward with substantial hope for a cure without recurrence.

—*Hans G. Graetzer*

See also Cancer; Malignancy and metastasis; Sarcoma; Tumors.

FOR FURTHER INFORMATION:

Beardsley, Tim. "A War Not Won: Trends in Cancer Epidemiology." *Scientific American* 270, no. 1 (January, 1994): 130-138. A summary of factual data about the prevalence of cancer in the United States. In spite of $25 billion spent by the National Cancer Institute, the overall death rate from cancer continues to increase. Critics suggest redirecting funds from expensive cures to prevention.

Brody, Jane E., and Arthur I. Holleb. *You Can Fight Cancer and Win*. New York: Quadrangle-New York Times, 1977. A hopeful and informative book about cancer for the general reader. Symptoms, treatment, possible causes, prevention, and family adjustment to cancer are discussed. Highly recommended.

Cady, Blake, ed. *Cancer Manual*. 7th ed. Boston: American Cancer Society, 1986. A collection of forty essays on various aspects of cancer management, written for health care professionals. The article that discusses sarcomas of the bone requires some knowledge of medical terminology. One interesting chapter deals with worthless cures.

Dollinger, Malin, Ernest H. Rosenbaum, and Greg Cable et al. *Everyone's Guide to Cancer Therapy*. Toronto: Somerville House, 1992. An excellent source of medical information about cancer, written for the general public. Various cancer sites in the body are described, and one essay focuses on sarcomas of the bone. A helpful glossary of medical terminology is provided.

Editors of Time-Life Books. *Fighting Cancer*. Alexandria, Va.: Time-Life Books, 1981. A brief overview of cancer diagnosis and therapy, containing many photographs and color diagrams. How abnormal cancer cells differ from healthy cells can be explained in pictures much more easily than in words. Informative and readable.

Holleb, Arthur I., ed. *The American Cancer Society Cancer Book: Prevention, Detection, Diagnosis, Treatment, Rehabilitation, Cure*. Garden City, N.Y.: Doubleday, 1986. An authoritative reference book on all aspects of cancer, written by forty leading specialists and carefully edited to avoid technical jargon. Contains chapters on chemotherapy, radiation, pain management, and childhood cancer. Clearly written and highly recommended.

Morra, Marion, and Eve Potts. *Choices: Realistic Alternatives in Cancer Treatment*. New York: Avon Books, 1987. A comprehensive reference book written for cancer patients and their families. Uses a question-and-answer format, with explanations given in nontechnical language. Offers good information at an introductory level.

BONE DISORDERS

SYSTEM AFFECTED: Skeletal

SPECIALISTS: Geriatric specialists, oncologists, orthopedic surgeons, rheumatologists

DEFINITION: The various traumatic events that can occur to the bones and the tissues surrounding them, such as fractures, dislocations, degenerative processes, infections, and cancer.

KEY TERMS:

acute: referring to the sudden onset of a disease process

cartilage: connective tissue between bones that forms a pad or cushion to absorb weight and shock

chronic: referring to a lingering disease process

pathogen: any disease-causing microorganism

CAUSES AND SYMPTOMS

Bones are usually studied in combination with their surrounding structures because many of the disorders to which bones can be subjected also involve muscular, cartilaginous, and other tissues to which they are connected. Hence, a common term for this medical category is "musculoskeletal and connective tissue disorders."

There are 206 bones in the human body that serve three functions. Some form protective housing for body organs and structures; these include the skull, which encloses the brain, and the rib cage, which encloses the heart and lungs. Some support the body's posture and weight, including the spine and the bones of the hip and legs. The third function is motion: Most of the bones in the body are involved in movement. These bones include those of the hands, wrists, arms, hips, legs, ankles, and feet.

Bone consists of three sections: an outer layer called the periosteum; the hard bony tissue itself, consisting of mineral compounds that form rigid skeletal structures; and the interior, a spongy mass of cancellous (chambered) tissue, where blood marrow is manufactured and some fat cells are stored. Bone is living tissue. It is a depository for calcium, phosphate, and other minerals that are vital to many body processes. Calcium and phosphate in particular are constantly being deposited in and withdrawn from bone tissue to be used throughout the body.

Bones can be attacked in many ways: They can be broken or dislocated; the processes by which they form, grow, and maintain themselves can be compromised; they can be attacked by pathogens; they can be subject to a series of degenerative diseases that impede function and even destroy bone tissue; and they can become cancerous.

Dislocations take place when the bones of a joint are forced out of alignment. They may occur in the elbows of young children whose arms are forcibly pulled. Fractures are more common. They arise from sports activities, accidents, falls, or hundreds of possible causes, including various disease conditions.

Osteoporosis and other diseases can destroy bone structure to the point where fractures occur with minimal stress. This condition is common in elderly women. The supply of calcium within the bones is gradually drained, leaving the bones porous and brittle. Hip fractures occur often in these people. Also, compression fractures occur in the vertebrae (the bones of the spine), causing the spine to bend forward. A hump develops, and the patient may not be able to raise his or her head.

Osteomalacia is similar to osteoporosis. Called rickets in children, this disease is caused by a deficiency in vitamin D, which impairs the absorption of calcium by the bone. In this condition, bones become soft and pliable. In children, leg bones do not develop correctly and may become bowed. The chest and stomach may protrude.

Bone infection is called osteomyelitis; it occurs most often in children. Infection can be introduced to the bone by fracture or other exposure, or it can be carried to the bone in the blood.

By far the most prevalent long-term bone disorders are those in the general class of diseases called arthritis. Osteoarthritis, a common form, is sometimes called "wear-and-tear arthritis" because it usually surfaces in older people after years of work have constantly challenged certain joints. It occurs often in contact sports such as football, where its progression can be accelerated by years of rough-and-tumble activity. Joints are cushioned by pads of cartilage. Eventually, this cartilage can wear down and become rough. It cannot protect the bones of the joint, and little nodes form at the ends of the bones. Bones of the neck and back are often affected, as are the hips and knees.

Osteoarthritis is painful and debilitating, but it is rarely crippling. More painful and far more serious is rheumatoid arthritis, a progressive disease. It often starts with inflammation in the joints of the hands or feet and is usually bilateral, for example affecting both hands, both feet, or both knees. While rheumatoid arthritis may start with relatively mild inflammation, it can progress to severe deformity and even total destruction of the joint. Fingers and toes can become grossly twisted; the joint can become completely fused and immobile.

There are other relatively common forms of arthritis. People with the skin condition psoriasis can develop psoriatic arthritis. Reiter's syndrome is a form of arthritis that can be transmitted through sexual contact. Ankylosing spondylitis is a form of arthritis that can affect any of the joints in the torso, such as the shoulders and hips, but is most often found in the neck and spine. Patients with inflammatory bowel disease (IBD) may also develop a concomitant arthritis in the joints of the hands or feet.

The bone condition called gout can affect many joints, but it appears most often in the big toe. The body produces a substance called uric acid. If, for any reason, too much is produced, or if it is not properly eliminated, uric acid crystals can form around joints and trigger inflammation. Gout is extremely painful, and an attack may last for weeks.

The spine is subject to a wide range of disorders. One of the most common is the prolapsed (slipped) disk. The individual vertebrae of the spine are separated and cushioned by pads of cartilage called disks. For various reasons, a disk can bulge out and impinge on the nerves of the spinal column. The result can be severe pain, numbness, and loss of movement. In some individuals, the spine fails

Major Bones of the Human Skeleton

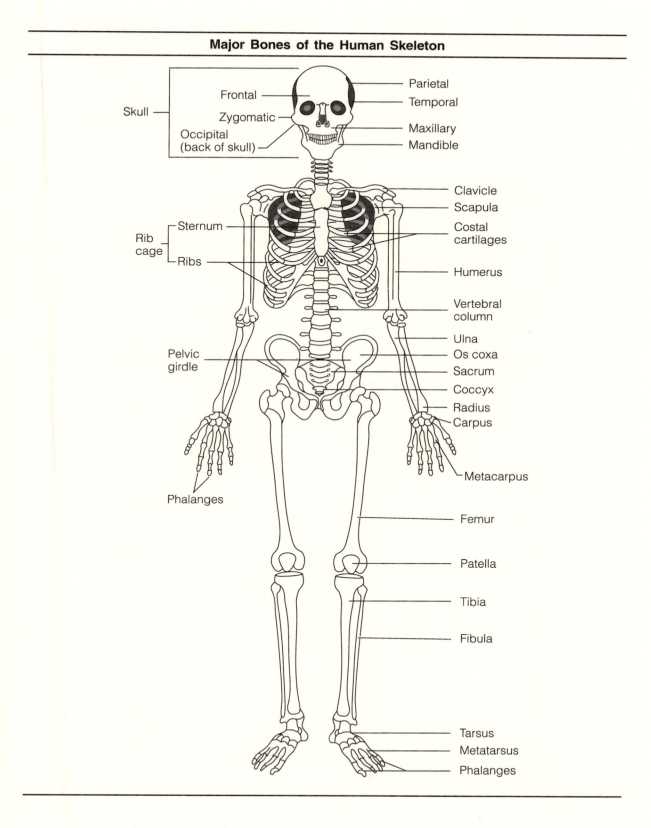

Skull
Frontal
Zygomatic
Occipital (back of skull)
Parietal
Temporal
Maxillary
Mandible

Rib cage
Sternum
Ribs

Clavicle
Scapula
Costal cartilages
Humerus
Vertebral column
Ulna
Os coxa
Sacrum
Coccyx
Radius
Carpus

Pelvic girdle
Phalanges
Metacarpus

Femur
Patella
Tibia
Fibula

Tarsus
Metatarsus
Phalanges

to grow correctly or becomes misaligned, or curved. This condition is called scoliosis. The curvature of the spine can cause the ribs on one side of the body to separate as those on the other side are pushed together. Over time, this separation can cause severe heart and lung problems.

Many cases of joint pain are attributable to inflammation of the tissues surrounding the bony structures. An example is bursitis, in which the bursa, a saclike membrane enclosing many joints, becomes inflamed. Repetitive activities, such as throwing a baseball, hitting a tennis ball, or scrubbing the floor on one's knees, can irritate the membrane and cause inflammation.

Bone cancers or tumors can be benign or malignant. Cancer rarely begins in the bone; it usually spreads there from a tumorous site elsewhere in the body. Of the cancers that arise directly within bone tissue, the most common are multiple myeloma and osteosarcoma.

Treatment and Therapy

In treating a fractured bone, the most important thing is to realign the segments and keep them immobile until they can fuse. Most often, the physician will X-ray the fracture, set the bones correctly, and immobilize the limb in a cast. If injury to the spinal column is suspected, the physician may also order computed tomography (CT) scanning. Surgery is sometimes required in order to set the bones, and the surgeon may join the bone segments together with pins, plates, or screws. In some cases, it is possible to cement bone fragments together with a special glue. Broken arms, legs, fingers, and toes can usually be easily immobilized with appropriate casts or splints. In cases of accidents, falls, or other trauma, if there is any suspicion of injury to the spinal column, it is critical not to move the patient. Movement can worsen the injury and even cause permanent paralysis.

Dislocations, like fractures, should be X-rayed. If the spinal column appears to be involved, CT scanning may be required. The misaligned bones are put back in their proper positions, and the joint is immobilized, often with a splint.

Osteoporosis requires both preventive and therapeutic care. If the physician recognizes that an individual, usually a postmenopausal woman, is at high risk for osteoporosis, supplementary calcium will be prescribed and, in some patients, estrogen replacement therapy. When osteoporosis has begun, supplementary calcium, vitamin D, and hormone therapy may check the progress of the disease.

A patient may suffer from acute back pain because of crushed vertebrae in the spine. Pain relievers such as aspirin may be required, and the patient may need orthopedic support. Gentle exercise is recommended to strengthen back muscles.

In osteomalacia, vitamin D, phosphorus, and calcium supplements are the mainstays of therapy. In osteomyelitis, antibiotics will usually eradicate the infection, but in some cases, surgery is required in order to remove infected tissue.

In other cases, amputation is the only option.

The first line of therapy for osteoarthritis and rheumatoid arthritis is the relief of pain and inflammation. The physician may recommend rest and immobilization of the joint; heating pads and hot baths may give some relief. Exercise can maintain motility in the joints and help the patient avoid stiffness. Most patients are given over-the-counter pain relievers such as aspirin, ibuprofen, or acetaminophen. In a large number of patients, however, these drugs are either not adequate to manage the pain or, as in the case of aspirin, ibuprofen, and others, may be irritating to the gastrointestinal tract. Gastrointestinal disturbances are also common with the drugs proscribed for arthritis. Gastric and duodenal ulcers are often reported and are sometimes so severe that the patient requires surgery. In a small but significant number of patients who develop such ulcers, the outcome is fatal.

Because rheumatoid arthritis is a crippling disease that worsens over the years, the physician has an additional goal: to prevent the progress of the disease, avoiding bone deterioration and degeneration. In these patients, a group of drugs called disease-modifying antirheumatic drugs (DMARDs) may be used in conjunction with pain relievers. Corticosteroids are also used to alleviate acute episodes of pain and inflammation. They can be very effective, but they cannot be used over the long term and may have severe side effects.

Surgery is often required for arthritis patients. Synovectomy is a procedure in which part or all of the synovial membrane that surrounds the diseased joint is removed. It gives temporary relief in inflammation and may help preserve joint function. When a joint has deteriorated severely, the physician may recommend joint replacement therapy. In this procedure, the degenerated bone and joint structures are surgically removed and replaced with an orthopedic device of metal and/or plastic. This procedure is most effective in hip replacement, although it is also used in the knee.

Relief of pain is the main goal of therapy in other arthritic conditions such as psoriatic arthritis and Reiter's syndrome. In ankylosing spondylitis, exercise is also an important facet of treatment, to help avoid stiffening of the spine.

Gout has a tendency to recur. Therefore there are medications for acute episodes, such as pain relievers, and others to control levels of uric acid and prevent attacks.

Benign bone tumors sometimes require surgery. Malignant tumors can be treated surgically and may also require radiation and chemotherapy.

Perspective and Prospects

Radical new therapies for bone disorders are evolving, with exciting possibilities: bone regeneration, bone cements, and glues to knit fractures and replace bone destroyed by disease.

Osteoarthritis, rheumatoid arthritis, and other forms of arthritis continue to afflict vast populations around the world. Current medical treatment is significantly flawed by the incidence of side effects, especially gastrointestinal effects, from the medications used. The search for safer medications is ongoing, as is the search for treatment modalities that will halt the degenerative processes of rheumatoid arthritis.

Orthopedic implants are now quite successful in the hip, sometimes successful in the knee, but otherwise not universally useful in elbows, fingers, toes, and other joints that can be destroyed by disease. This is an area that is being addressed.

Operating techniques and instrumentation improve constantly. Many procedures are now done with the aid of arthroscopic instruments. Rather than an extensive incision to reveal the joint and surrounding tissues, the surgeon works through a tiny hole, through which he or she can inspect the inflamed joint and even perform minor surgery.

Operations on prolapsed spinal disks once entailed long incisions and laborious, careful removal of disk tissue. Fusion of the involved vertebrae was often necessary, limiting spinal movement. Healing time could be extensive. Today, simpler, less painful procedures may be as successful and far less traumatic. In one procedure, an enzyme is injected into the prolapsed disk, causing it to shrink and reducing pressure on nearby nerves. In another procedure, disk material is removed with a needle inserted through the skin into the disk.

Overall, progress in the treatment of bone disorders has been significant: Many people who would have lived with deformities and disability are being helped with modern medical and surgical techniques, medications, and instrumentation. —*C. Richard Falcon*

See also Bone cancer; Dystrophy; Fracture and dislocation; Muscle sprains, spasms, and disorders; Muscular dystrophy; Osteoporosis; Paget's disease; Poliomyelitis; Scoliosis; Slipped disk; Spina bifida; Spinal disorders.

FOR FURTHER INFORMATION:

Cooper, Kenneth H. *Preventing Osteoporosis.* New York: Bantam Books, 1989. As the title suggests, Cooper's main interest is to advise women on how to avoid developing the brittle bones of osteoporosis. His text is clear, and the recommendations reflect contemporary practice.

Larson, David E., ed. *Mayo Clinic Family Health Book.* New York: William Morrow, 1990. Bones, muscles, and connective tissues are discussed, with disease conditions, symptoms, treatment, and outlook clearly explained. The text and illustrations are complete and easy to understand.

Schommer, Nancy. *Stopping Scoliosis.* Garden City, N.Y.: Avery Publishing Group, 1991. Schommer covers the condition of scoliosis with thoroughness and clarity.

Yates, George, and Michael B. Shermer. *Meeting the Challenge of Arthritis.* Los Angeles: Lowell House, 1990. A good treatment of the arthritic diseases, covering their causes and treatment. Concentrates on helping patients to help themselves.

BONE FRACTURES. *See* FRACTURE AND DISLOCATION.

BOTULISM

SYSTEMS AFFECTED: Gastrointestinal, muscular, nervous

SPECIALISTS: Emergency physicians, neurologists, public health specialists, toxicologists

DEFINITION: Botulism is food poisoning caused by eating incompletely cooked or contaminated canned foods; such foods may contain bacteria which produce a toxin that is absorbed by the digestive tract and spread to the central nervous system. Symptoms, which usually occur eighteen to thirty-six hours after eating the contaminated food, include blurred vision, drooping eyelids, dry mouth, slurred speech, vomiting, diarrhea, and weakness leading to paralysis; no fever or disturbance of mental ability occurs. In infants, symptoms may also include severe constipation, feeble cry, and an inability to suck. Botulism may require hospitalization and antitoxin injections; if left untreated, it can prove fatal.

See also Food poisoning.

BRAIN DISORDERS

SYSTEMS AFFECTED: Brain, psychic-emotional

SPECIALISTS: Embryologists, geriatric specialists, neurologists, neurosurgeons, psychiatrists

DEFINITION: Disorders of the brain can interfere with its role in the control of body functions, behavior, learning, and expression, while defects can also threaten life itself.

KEY TERMS:

anencephaly: a fatal congenital condition in which tissues that should have differentiated to form the brain failed to do so

coma: a condition of unconsciousness that may or may not be reversible; various degrees of coma are assessed by the presence or absence of reflex responses, such as pupil dilation when a light is shone into the eyes

dementia: a diseased state in which intellectual ability is ever decreasing; personality changes, decreased interest or ability to care for one's self, and long-term and short-term memory loss can indicate dementia

embolus: a clot or other piece of matter that may travel through the circulatory system to tiny blood vessels (as in the brain) and block the path that normally allows blood flow

hydrocephalus: a painful condition caused by excess cerebrospinal fluid within the spaces of the brain

ischemia: an inadequate blood flow to a region; may be caused by an incomplete blockage in or constriction of a blood vessel (as may occur with atherosclerosis or a blood clot)

seizure: a misfiring of cortical neurons that alters the patient's level of consciousness; the seizure may or may not involve muscular convulsions

stroke: a complete loss of blood flow to a region of the brain that is of sudden onset and causes abrupt muscular weakness, usually to one side of the body

thrombus: a blood clot that is attached to the interior wall of a blood vessel

CAUSES AND SYMPTOMS

The cerebral cortex acts as a processor for sensory information and as an integrator of memory, interpretation, creativity, intellect, and passion. Disorders of the brain or brain defects can disrupt these processing or integrating functions. Disorders of the brain include such commonly heard terms as stroke, ischemia, dementia, seizure, and coma. Brain disorders may also occur as a result of infection, various tumors, traumas leading to blot clots (hematomas) or lack of oxygen (hypoxia), and cancer. Brain defects include anencephaly, a congenital defect in which a newborn lacks a brain, and hydrocephaly, commonly called "water on the brain."

A stroke is any situation in which the blood supply to a region of the brain is lost. This can occur as a result of a cerebral hemorrhage, during which blood escapes from blood vessels to surround and compress brain tissue; cerebral thrombosis, whereby a clot attached to the wall of a blood vessel restricts the amount of blood flowing to a particular region; or an embolus, a foreign substance which may be a clot that migrates in the bloodstream, often to lodge in a smaller vessel in the brain. The embolus will block blood flow to some area. An embolus can originate from substances other than a blood clot, which is why health care staff often squirt fluid out of a needle before administering a shot or other therapy: to ensure that no air embolus, which could induce a stroke or prove fatal if it enters the brain, is injected.

Human Brain

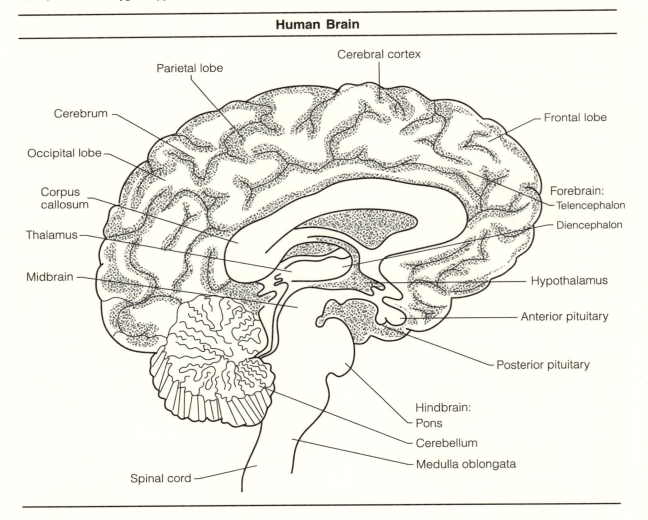

Transient ischemic attacks (TIAs) are often thought of as small strokes, but, technically, ischemia simply means that oxygen is not reaching the cells within a tissue. Basically, the mechanism is similar to a stroke, in that blood flow to a portion of the brain is compromised. Although blood actually reaches the brain tissue during ischemia, there is not a sufficient flow to ensure that all cells are receiving the oxygen necessary to continue cellular life. This condition is called hypoxia (low oxygen). If hypoxia is sustained over a sufficient period of time, cellular death occurs, causing irreversible brain damage.

The important differences between a stroke and a TIA are the onset and duration of symptoms, as well as the severity of the damage. Persons with atherosclerosis actually have fat deposits along the interior walls of their blood vessels. These people are vulnerable to experiencing multiple TIAs. Many TIAs are small enough to be dismissed and ignored; others are truly inapparent, causing no symptoms. This is unfortunate because TIAs often serve as a warning of an impending full-scale stroke. Action and treatments could be implemented, if medical advice is sought early, to decrease the likelihood of a stroke. Repeated TIAs also contribute to dementia.

Dementia is not the normal path for the elderly, nor is it a sign of aging. Dementia is a sign of neurological chaos and can be caused by diseases such as Alzheimer's disease or acquired immunodeficiency syndrome (AIDS). Although most elderly are not afflicted with dementia, nearly all have a slowing of reaction and response time. This slowing is believed to be associated with chemical changes within nerve cell membranes as aging occurs; slowing of reaction times is not necessarily indicative of the first steps on a path to dementia. In addition, forgetfulness may not be a sign of dementia, since it occurs at all ages. Forgetfulness is such a sign, however, if it is progressive and includes forgetting to dress or forgetting one's name or date of birth.

While it is incorrect to say that dementia is caused by aging, it is correct to say that dementia is age-related. It may first appear in a person any time between the late thirties and the mid-nineties, but it usually begins to appear in the late seventies. Patients with Alzheimer's disease are believed to account for about 20 percent of all cases of dementia. Other diseases cause dementia, including an autosomal-dominant genetic disease called Huntington's disease. Huntington's disease manifests itself with a distinct chorea, or dance, of the body that is neither solicited nor controlled. This genetic disease is particularly cruel in that its symptoms appear in midlife, often after the adult has had offspring and passed on the gene. The disease continues to alter the intellect and personality of the afflicted one and progresses to the point of complete debilitation of the body and mind.

A seizure occurs when a collection of neurons misfires, sending nerve impulses that are neither solicited nor con-

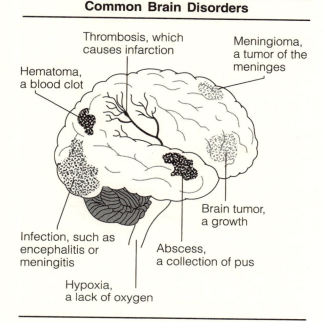

Common Brain Disorders

Thrombosis, which causes infarction

Meningioma, a tumor of the meninges

Hematoma, a blood clot

Brain tumor, a growth

Infection, such as encephalitis or meningitis

Abscess, a collection of pus

Hypoxia, a lack of oxygen

trollable. In the everyday use of the term, seizure describes a condition of epilepsy or convulsion. Medically speaking, a seizure is a sign of an underlying problem within the gray matter of the brain; it is the most common neurological disorder. Epilepsy is a term used to describe a condition of repeated seizures, while convulsion is a term generally applied to describe an isolated seizure. A seizure may occur as a consequence of extreme fever or a violent blow to the head. Seizures are also associated with metabolic disorders, such as hypoglycemia (low blood sugar); trauma causing a loss of blood or oxygen to a region, such as in a newborn after a traumatic birth; toxins, as seen in drug abuse or withdrawal; or bacterial or viral encephalitis or meningitis. In addition, about one-third of those persons who survive a gunshot wound to the head will experience seizures afterward. In closed head trauma, which can occur in a sporting or automobile accident, there is a 5 percent chance of post-trauma seizures.

Loss of consciousness can be caused by a violent impact to the head, a lack of oxygen or blood flow to the head, a metabolic imbalance, or the presence of a toxin such as alcohol. Usually, this is a transient event, but it may become a permanent condition. When this happens, a person is said to be in a coma. A comatose person exists in a nonresponsive state and may be assessed for brain death. Brain death is a legally defined term which means that no electrical activity in the brain is seen on an electroencephalogram (EEG). Thus some comatose patients may be determined to be brain-dead, particularly if the condition is deemed irreversible.

Brain defects are not common, but they do occur. One particularly tragic defect is the absence of a brain in a newborn, called anencephaly. Death usually occurs within a few hours of birth. Although anencephaly is rare and generally associated with a genetic factor, there have been cases in population clusters, such as one in the Rio Grande area of south Texas, suggesting that an environmental factor may contribute to these defects.

Another defect that may appear in newborns or in an infant's first months of life is hydrocephalus. Although the descriptive term "water on the brain" is often used, the condition does not involve a collection of water in the cranium; rather, it involves an accumulation of cerebrospinal fluid (CSF). CSF is the fluid that insulates the brain and allows it to "float" under the bony cranial encasement. As the ventricles, or spaces, in the brain fill with CSF, bulging occurs and pressure builds to the point of compressing the surrounding brain tissue. This can be very painful and is fatal if untreated. Hydrocephalus can be caused by an overproduction of CSF or a blockage of the CSF drainage from the ventricles of the brain. The symptoms often include a protrusion or abnormal shape of the cranium. In newborns, the skull bones have not yet sutured (fused) to one another, so the soft bones are pushed apart, causing unusual head shapes. This is a warning sign. Another sign is observed if a newborn's head has a circumference greater than 35.5 centimeters (14 inches); if that is the case, the newborn must be immediately checked for hydrocephalus. Adolescents and adults may also experience hydrocephalus. This can be a response to head trauma, infection, or the overproduction of CSF. The symptoms include lethargy, headache, dullness, blurred vision, nausea, and vomiting.

TREATMENT AND THERAPY

TIAs can progress to strokes. In fact, about 30 percent of those diagnosed with TIA will have a major stroke within the subsequent four years. One of the most prevalent causes of TIAs is hypertension. Hypertension is known as the "silent killer" because many persons with this problem ignore the subtle symptoms of fatigue, headache, and general malaise. Hypertension is also known as a good predictor of major strokes if left untreated. Thus, hypertensive persons need to be diagnosed as such in order to control their blood pressure. This allows them to avoid or delay either a major stroke or multiple TIAs. Management for the hypertensive's blood pressure may include taking diuretics and hypotensive drugs (to lower the blood pressure). If taken diligently, these drugs offer longevity and quality of life to the sufferer. Aside from hypertension, TIAs may be induced in some metabolic disorders, which should be corrected if possible, or by constricted blood vessels. Sometimes, surgery on such vessels can stop the ischemic attacks and prevent or delay the onset of a stroke.

Although TIAs lead to strokes, strokes are not necessarily preceded by a TIA. Nearly 90 percent of all major strokes occur without a TIA warning. Sadly, hypertension is the main contributor to this number. Measures can be taken to avoid strokes. This includes maintaining cardiovascular health by exercising, not smoking, and managing hypertension, diabetes mellitus, or other problems that may place stresses on the body's chemical balance.

Dementia is so poorly understood in terms of causes that a rational probe of drug therapy or a cure is nearly impossible. The drugs most often used in dementia treatment, the ergoloid mesylates, are used to manage the symptoms; namely, the confused mind. These drugs, however, do not stop or prevent the unexplained cellular degeneration associated with dementia. It is interesting to note that a tiny subgroup within those persons suffering from Alzheimer's disease have greatly improved in mental status with the drug tacrine. It is unfortunate that all patients are not responsive to this drug—a fact which suggests that Alzheimer's disease is a complex condition.

Seizures are treated pharmacologically according to type. Carbamazepine, phenobarbitol, phenytoin, and valproate are some of the drugs available to treat seizure disorders. Barbiturates may also be used in certain cases. Most of these drugs are highly effective when taken as prescribed, and patient noncompliance is the main cause of drug failure. Sometimes, two drugs are combined in therapy. It should be mentioned that pregnant women with epilepsy are urged to continue taking antiepilepsy drugs during pregnancy since a maternal seizure may be more damaging to the fetus than the drug itself.

Some forms of hydrocephalus can be corrected surgically by performing a CSF shunt from the cranium to the peritoneal (abdominal) region, where the fluid can be eliminated from the body as waste. This is not without risk, and the introduction of infection into the brain is a major concern.

PERSPECTIVE AND PROSPECTS

The therapies in use for brain diseases and disorders have been derived from the practical experience of physicians, the laboratory research of scientists, and the hopes of multitudes of doctors, patients, families, and friends. Medical science has done much to improve the lives of those who suffer with seizures, to reduce the risk of strokes to the hypertensive person and those with TIAs, and is making great progress in treating certain kinds of dementia. Yet much remains to be done.

While one can argue that much is known about the human brain, it would be erroneous to argue that the human brain is fully understood. Despite centuries of research, the brain, as it functions in health, remains largely a mystery. Since the healthy brain is yet to be understood, it is not surprising that the medical community struggles to determine what goes wrong in dementia, seizure, or mental illness or to discover drug therapies that can cross the blood-brain barrier. Thus, the human brain is the uncharted frontier in medicine. As technology improves to support researchers and medical practitioners in their pursuits of cures and treatments for brain diseases and disorders, one can only remain hopeful for the future ability to restore health to the damaged human brain. —*Mary C. Fields*

See also Alzheimer's disease; Amnesia and memory loss; Cerebral palsy; Cluster headaches; Concussion; Dementia; Encephalitis; Epilepsy; Guillain-Barré syndrome (GBS); Hallucinations; Headaches; Hemiplegia; Lead poisoning; Meningitis; Migraine headaches; Motor neuron diseases; Multiple sclerosis; Neuralgia, neuritis, and neuropathy; Numbness and tingling; Palsy; Paralysis; Paraplegia; Parkinsonism; Quadriplegia; Sciatica; Seizures; Tics; Unconsciousness.

FOR FURTHER INFORMATION:

Bannister, Roger. *Brain and Bannister's Clinical Neurology.* 7th ed. Oxford, England: Oxford University Press, 1992. Several chapters are dedicated to the topics of seizures, dementia, hydrocephalus, and loss of consciousness. Because the writing can be fairly technical, it is best used by someone with a background in human anatomy and physiology.

Kunz, Jeffrey R. M., and Asher J. Finkel, eds. *The American Medical Association Family Medical Guide.* Rev. ed. New York: Random House, 1987. An excellent reference for the beginner. The scientific accuracy of the text is not compromised by its accessibility.

Parsons, Malcolm. *Colour Atlas of Clinical Neurology.* 2d ed. St. Louis: Mosby Year Book, 1993. An excellent atlas that allows the pictures to tell the story. The color photographs and brief descriptions capture the essence of brain disorders and remind the reader that people are suffering from these maladies.

BREAST CANCER

SYSTEMS AFFECTED: Breasts, lymphatic, psychic-emotional

SPECIALISTS: Geneticists, gynecologists, oncologists, pathologists, plastic and reconstructive surgeons

DEFINITION: Malignancy occurring in breast tissue and possibly involving the associated lymph nodes.

KEY TERMS:

adjuvant therapy: therapy used in addition to surgery in order to control the growth of remaining cancer cells

benign: not cancerous

chemotherapy: adjuvant therapy which uses drugs to kill cancer cells

malignant: cancerous

metastasis: the spread of cancer cells from a tumor to other sites in the body

CAUSES AND SYMPTOMS

Genetic and familial risk factors. Some families have a clear history of breast cancer. It is estimated that nearly 10 percent of the 180,000 diagnosed cases of breast cancer in the United States have developed because of some heredi-

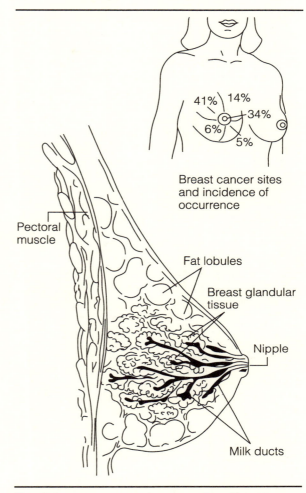

Female breast anatomy and common sites of breast cancer.

tary defect. Research efforts have intensified to isolate the breast cancer 1 (BRCA 1) gene. When this gene is isolated, clinicians will be able to use a simple blood test to screen women for the presence of the defective gene and therefore identify those with an increased risk of developing breast cancer. Any clustering of breast cancer within a family, especially among immediate family members, is probably indicative of hereditary or familial breast cancer. This is especially true when family members develop breast cancer at an early age, particularly at or before the mid-forties. Women with a family history of breast cancer should seek regular screening and counseling regarding the best-known methods of prevention and therapy. Current preventive methods include modification of diet and lifestyle, hormonal treatment with antiestrogens such as tamoxifen, and prophylactic (preventive) mastectomies.

Diet. Although the exact role that diet may play in the development of breast cancer is still unclear, there is evidence to indicate that factors such as dietary fat may increase the risk for the development of this disease. Comparison of the rates of breast cancer in different countries throughout the world show that certain populations, such as women in Japan and China, tend to have much lower rates of breast cancer than Caucasians in the United States. Not only is their total intake of fat much lower than that of American women (15 percent versus 40 percent of total calories), but as their intake of fat increases (as seen in Asian families that have moved to the United States and adopted Westernized diets) so have their rates of breast cancer. Since fat has also been linked to an increased risk for the development of colon cancer and heart disease, it has been recommended that the overall consumption of fat in the diet be limited to less than 30 percent of total calories. Vitamins and certain minerals may also be effective in helping to prevent breast cancer. Vitamins A, C, and E are antioxidants that have been shown to protect cells from cancer-causing chemicals. Some minerals such as selenium and zinc also appear to have a protective effect on cells. Adequate amounts of these nutrients should be included in the diet, either through consumption of vegetables, fruits, and grains, which supply these nutrients, or through supplements. Several studies have demonstrated a link between alcohol consumption and breast cancer. Alcohol consumption, even in moderate amounts, can increase a woman's risk for breast cancer, an effect which is even more evident in women who consumed alcohol at a young age. This causal relationship does not, however, appear to affect women who are close to the menopause. It seems that the main effect of alcohol, as with fat, may be during the period of a woman's reproductive lifetime, when breast cells are most vulnerable to genetic damage.

Reproductive and hormonal factors. Three major reproductive-related events influence a woman's risk for the development of breast cancer: the age when menstruation begins (menarche), the age at first full-term pregnancy, and the age when the menopause occurs. An increased risk of breast cancer has been found in women who have started menstruation before the age of twelve, who have had their first full-term pregnancy after the age of thirty, and/or who enter the menopause after the age of fifty-five. These findings indicate that reproductive hormones such as estrogen may play a role in the development of breast cancer. The apparent association between reproductive hormones and breast cancer raises concerns about potential risks associated with birth control pills (oral contraceptives) or postmenopausal estrogen replacement pills. Studies to date show some evidence that the use of oral contraceptives slightly increases the risk of developing breast cancer, but the risks depend upon many factors, including type of birth control pill used, age when use is started, and overall duration of use. The potential risk of using oral contraceptives must be weighed against other risks associated with alter-

native contraceptives, unwanted pregnancies, or abortion. Postmenopausal women have been treated with ovarian hormones (estrogen with or without progesterone) to alleviate the symptoms of the menopause and, more recently, to reduce the risks of osteoporosis and ischemic heart disease. There are few definitive data to establish a clear association between such hormone-replacement therapy and an increased risk for the development of breast cancer. Again, the potential risk associated with the use of these hormones, even by women who have had breast cancer or who are at high risk for the development of breast cancer, must be weighed against such factors as a potential high risk for osteoporosis or heart disease or against the severity of menopausal symptoms.

Psychosocial aspects. Findings from a number of studies have suggested an association between psychological factors and disease outcome in breast cancer patients. It has been shown that women who are described by their physicians as having a "fighting spirit" live significantly longer than more passive women. Recent studies have also demonstrated that participation of cancer patients in psychosocial support groups significantly increases survival time. These and other findings suggest that suppression of negative feelings, severe stress, and lack of social support predict a poorer outcome with cancer. Conversely, patient assertiveness and sense of control, especially when enhanced by social support, appear to improve the course of this disease. How these psychological factors influence the immune system is being investigated.

Mammography and breast self-examination. Two methods of screening for breast cancer are mammography (an X ray of the breast) and breast self-examination. Routine use of both of these screening methods can help to detect breast cancer at earlier stages, where surgery and chemotherapy have been shown to be highly effective. It is recommended that a breast self-examination be done once a month. If the woman is menstruating, the best time to perform the examination is two or three days after the end of the cycle, when the breasts are not swollen or tender. If a woman is not menstruating, she should pick one day per month, such as the first or last day of the month, to do a breast self-examination. Women learning how to examine their breasts may want to perform the examination once a week until they learn how their breast tissue changes over time. Once familiar with the changes in their breasts, they can check the tissue only once a month. In addition, doctors should examine the breasts during routine medical checkups. Although there is some controversy surrounding mammograms before the age of fifty, it is currently recommended that routine mammograms be scheduled between the ages of forty and fifty. After the age of fifty, women should have mammograms scheduled every year or every other year, coinciding with their routine physicals.

Following an unusual mammogram reading or the discovery of a suspicious lump, a biopsy is required to evaluate fully whether cancer is present. A biopsy may be done by one of the following techniques: a fine-needle aspirate (the collection of cells within a lump by a small needle, done on an outpatient basis); a needle biopsy (the removal of a core of tissue with a needle, done on an outpatient basis); an incisional biopsy (the removal of a wedge of tissue, done on an outpatient basis); or an excisional biopsy (the removal of the entire lump, which may require general anesthesia).

Most breast cancers (86 percent) begin within the ducts of the breast. A much smaller percentage (12 percent) develops within the lobules, with the remainder (2 percent) developing in surrounding tissue. A ductal or lobular cancer that has not grown outside the duct is called ductal or lobular carcinoma in situ, noninvasive carcinoma, or simply intraductal (intralobular) carcinoma. A ductal or lobular cancer that has grown outside the duct is called invasive or infiltrating carcinoma.

TREATMENT AND THERAPY

Treatment for breast cancer depends upon the age of the woman (pre- or postmenopausal), the extent of the local tumor invasion, the size of the tumor, the aggressiveness of the cancer cells, the number of regional lymph nodes involved, and whether cancer is detected in distant organs (metastasis). Standard treatment options include surgery, radiation therapy, and adjuvant therapy (chemotherapy and/or hormonal therapy).

Surgical options include lumpectomy (the removal of the tumor mass only), partial mastectomy (the removal of a wedge of breast tissue), quandrantectomy (the removal of at least 2 to 3 centimeters of normal tissue around the tumor and the excision of the overlying skin of that quadrant), mastectomy (the removal of all breast tissue, surrounding skin, and regional lymph nodes), and radical mastectomy (the removal of all breast tissue, skin, underlying pectoral muscle, and lymph nodes). New studies are indicating that the timing of surgery relative to the stage of the menstrual cycle in premenopausal women may affect long-term survival. It appears that having surgery during the luteal phase (the second half of the woman's menstrual cycle) favorably influences survival.

Radiation therapy is designed to treat a specific area (unlike chemotherapy, which travels through the bloodstream and affects the entire body). Radiation therapy is administered by a linear accelerator, which shoot radioactive particles directly at a clearly defined region of the body (the breast area and possibly the lymph nodes). Radiation therapy is usually administered one day a week for a given number of weeks. Breast conservation therapy, consisting of excision of the primary tumor and a limited amount of adjacent breast tissue followed by radiation therapy, has been proven to be as effective as mastectomy for early stage breast cancer.

Breast Self-Examination

Visual exam

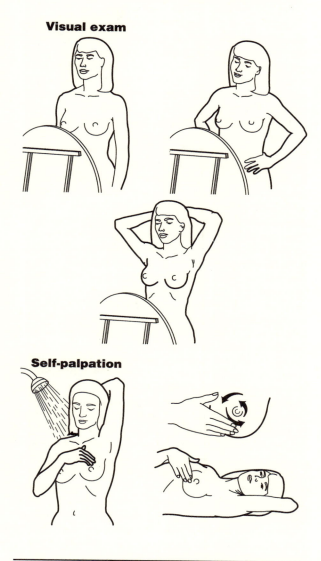

Self-palpation

Women should examine their breasts both visually, to detect any changes in appearance, such as size, asymmetries (one breast suddenly, as opposed to historically, larger than the other), "peau d'orange"—the appearance of dimpled skin resembling orange peel—and other unusual features. Women should also apply pressure to their breasts, working circularly from the nipple to the far periphery of the breast (including the underarms), to determine the presence of any lumps or other unusual nodules. Self-exam should be combined with routine visits to a physician and regular mammograms, which can detect cancer long before it develops into a palpable lump.

Adjuvant therapy, including chemotherapy and/or hormonal therapy, is indicated for all node-positive patients. Chemotherapy is the use of drugs designed to kill actively dividing cancer cells. More than one kind of drug is typically used because different drugs interfere with the process of cell division in different ways, making the overall treatment more effective. Since these toxic drugs act on dividing cells, they also kill actively dividing normal cells such as hair cells and bone marrow cells. It is important that the bone marrow, which gives rise to red blood cells and white blood cells (immune cells), be allowed to recover from the effects of chemotherapy. Giving chemotherapy in cycles rather than all at once not only helps the bone marrow to recover but also kills cancer cells that may be actively dividing at different times. Hormonal therapy is designed to alter the growth of hormone-sensitive cancer cells. Some cancer cells need estrogen to grow. It has been shown that either removing endogenous sources of estrogen (by removing the ovaries) or giving antiestrogens such as tamoxifen helps to control the growth of these cancer cells. Tamoxifen is frequently used in postmenopausal women, and the drug is being tested in a large clinical trial to help prevent breast cancer in healthy, but high-risk, women.

PERSPECTIVE AND PROSPECTS

Breast cancer is on the rise throughout the Western world. In the United States, it is the second leading cause of cancer deaths: In 1994, it was estimated that 180,000 women would be diagnosed with breast cancer and that nearly 50,000 would die from the disease that year. The overall lifetime risk of developing breast cancer in the United States is 11 percent, which means that one out of nine women will develop breast cancer by the age of eighty-five. Multiple environmental, lifestyle, and genetic factors are believed to be involved in the development of this disease, and the increase in risk has been associated with changing environmental and lifestyle patterns.

Clinicians and researchers are constantly evaluating new methods to control the growth of cancer cells. New treatments that are being tested in clinical trials throughout the United States include the use of monoclonal antibodies, the use of paclitaxel (Taxol), and the administration of cancer vaccines. Monoclonal antibodies are made in laboratories. These antibodies are similar to those that the body makes against foreign invaders (bacteria and viruses), except that monoclonal antibodies can be made to bind specifically to cancer cells. Monoclonal antibodies that have been tagged with chemicals detectable by a scanner can be used to find cancer cells in the body. Monoclonal antibodies can also be tagged with radioactive substances or poisons which directly kill cancer cells and spare normal cells. Taxol is a drug which has been isolated from the yew tree. This drug acts by preventing cancer cells from dividing and is being tested in patients with recurrent breast cancer. Several centers in the United States and Canada are testing vaccines designed to fight cancer cells. Specific molecules that are found on tumor cells and not on normal cells are being used as injectable vaccines to stimulate the production of antibodies against cancer cells. —*Sylvia Adams Oliver*

See also Breast disorders; Cancer.

FOR FURTHER INFORMATION:

Boston Women's Health Collective. *The New Our Bodies, Ourselves*. New York: Touchstone-Simon & Schuster, 1992.

Love, Susan, and Karen Lindsey. *Dr. Susan Love's Breast Book*. Reading, Mass.: Addison-Wesley, 1990.

BREAST DISORDERS

SYSTEMS AFFECTED: Breasts, lymphatic, psychic-emotional

SPECIALISTS: Geneticists, gynecologists, plastic and reconstructive surgeons

DEFINITION: A variety of breast conditions.

"Fibrocystic condition or disease" is an umbrella term which has been used to define these disorders, which include swelling and tenderness, cysts, mastalgia (breast pain), infections and inflammations (mastitis), nipple discharge, fibroadenomas, and epithelial proliferation of varying degrees. These conditions are known to occur in approximately 90 percent of women. Although a diagnosis of fibrocystic disease was previously thought to increase a woman's risk for the development of breast cancer, further studies and the reevaluation of older data have shown that only a small percentage of these women later develop carcinoma in either breast. The following are brief descriptions of commonly occurring, benign breast conditions.

Mastalgia. Also commonly termed mastodynia, mastalgia is defined as breast pain. Cyclic mastalgia has been associated with reproductive hormones such as estrogen and progesterone since breast tenderness and pain tend to occur just before menstruation with the symptoms becoming less intense once bleeding starts. The most promising therapies include hormonal treatment (birth control pills or progesterone ointments) and the modification of diet (avoiding fatty and fried foods, reducing the consumption of caffeine-containing beverages, and taking vitamin supplements, especially of vitamins E and B). Noncyclical pain occurs much less frequently than cyclical pain. The occurrence of this type of breast pain does not vary with the menstrual cycle and typically occurs in a single, localized spot. The cause of this pain is not fully understood.

Fibroadenomas. Lumps that typically develop during the teenage years through the twenties and that do not fluctuate during the menstrual cycle are called fibroadenomas. These benign lumps are smooth and round, and they move freely within the breast tissue. Although the lumps may last throughout a woman's lifetime once they appear, they can easily be removed surgically. The conditions that cause the growth of fibroadenomas are unknown.

Common Breast Disorders

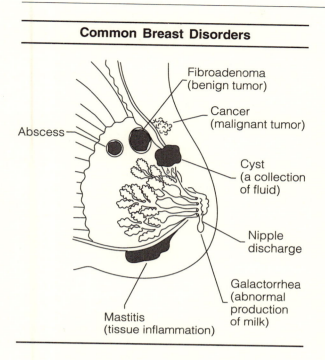

Abscess

Fibroadenoma
(benign tumor)

Cancer
(malignant tumor)

Cyst
(a collection
of fluid)

Nipple
discharge

Galactorrhea
(abnormal
production
of milk)

Mastitis
(tissue inflammation)

Cysts. Breast cysts are found in approximately 60 percent of premenopausal women. They occur most often in women who are approaching the menopause, but they also develop when a woman is in her thirties and forties. Cysts are fluid-filled sacs, much like blisters, that develop within the breast tissue. Cysts may feel pliable if they are near the surface of the breast or may feel hard, much like a lump, if they are located deep within the breast tissue. The fluid within the cyst can easily be removed by needle aspiration in a doctor's office. Cysts are almost never malignant and do not increase a woman's risk of developing breast cancer.

Infections and inflammations. The breast may become inflamed or infected because of lactational mastitis, non-lactational mastitis, or chronic subareolar abscesses. Lactational mastitis is the result of a localized bacterial infection which occurs most often within a blocked duct. Nonlactational mastitis typically occurs in a woman whose immune system is depressed; it is an infection which usually involves the skin of the breast and therefore covers a larger area of the breast than lactational mastitis. Both of these conditions can be treated with antibiotics. Chronic subareolar abscesses are infections of the small, dead-end glands that surround the nipple. These abscesses appear as localized hot areas on the border of the nipple, much like a boil. If caught early, they can be treated with antibiotics; if not, the abscess and gland must be surgically removed.

Nipple discharge. Discharge from the nipple is a common occurrence in women of all ages and reproductive histories. Although naturally occurring, nipple discharge should be checked if it is unilateral (occurring in one

breast), spontaneous, and persistent. These symptoms could be attributable to intraductal papilloma (wartlike growths), intraductal papillomatosis, intraductal carcinoma in situ, or invasive cancer. Only about 4 percent of spontaneous unilateral bloody discharges are the result of cancer. In galactorrhea, an increase in prolactin production causes the abnormal discharge of breast milk in a woman who is not lactating. Each of these conditions requires a different treatment, which can be discussed with a physician.

Epithelial dysplasia and hyperplasia. The abnormal, but benign, growth of the epithelial cells that form the ductal branching of the breast tissue is termed epithelial dysplasia, while epithelial hyperplasia refers to an abnormal increase in the number of nonmalignant cells in a normal tissue arrangement. The degree of abnormality of these cells can be determined through the histological (microscopic) examination of breast tissue obtained during a biopsy. Epithelial dysplasia can be divided into three main categories: non-proliferative (mild hyperplasia, cysts, epithelial-related calcifications, fibroadenomas), proliferative (mild-to-moderate hyperplasia, papillomas, sclerosing adenosis), and atypical hyperplasia. Biopsy-proven atypical hyperplasia of the breast tissue has been shown to increase a woman's risk of developing breast cancer significantly, especially if the woman has a family history of breast cancer.

—*Sylvia Adams Oliver*

See also Breast-feeding; Mastitis.

BREAST-FEEDING

SYSTEM AFFECTED: Breasts

SPECIALISTS: Gynecologists, obstetricians, perinatologists

DEFINITION: The preferred feeding method for infants, providing optimal nutrition for the infant (including immunologic protection), mother-infant bonding, and enhanced maternal health.

KEY TERMS:

alveoli: the milk-producing cells of the mammary gland

bifidus factors: factors in colostrum and breast milk that favor the growth of helpful bacteria in the infant's intestinal tract

bonding: a process in which a mother forms an affectionate attachment to her infant immediately after birth

colostrum: the secretion from the breast before the onset of milk

foremilk: the milk released early in a nursing session, which is low in fat and rich in nutrients

hindmilk: the milk released late in a nursing session, which is higher in fat content

lactoferrin: a breast milk factor that binds iron, preventing it from supporting the growth of harmful intestinal bacteria; it may also promote the ability to absorb dietary iron

let-down reflex: the reflex that forces milk to the front of the breast

oxytocin: the hormone secreted from the posterior pituitary gland that stimulates the mammary glands to eject milk; it also stimulates the uterus to contract after birth

prolactin: a hormone secreted from the anterior pituitary gland that signals the breast to start and sustain milk production

PROCESS AND EFFECTS

The terms "breast-feeding," "nursing," and "lactation" all refer to the best-known method of infant feeding. Although there are a few rare exceptions, almost every mother can breast-feed and thereby provide low-cost, nutritional support for her infant. Although it is often thought otherwise, the size of the mother's breast has no relationship to successful lactation. In fact, the physiology of successful lactation is determined by the maturation of breast tissue, the initiation and maintenance of milk secretion, and the ejection or delivery of milk to the nipple. This physiology is dependent on hormonal control, and all women have the required anatomy for successful lactation unless they have had surgical alteration of the breast.

Hormonal influence on breast development begins in adolescence. Increased estrogen causes the breast ducts to elongate and duct cells to grow. (The ducts are narrow tubular vessels that run from the segments of the breast into the tip of the nipple.) More fibrous and fatty tissue develops, and the nipple area matures. As adolescence progresses, regular menstrual cycle hormones cause further development of the alveoli, which are the milk-producing cells.

The elevated levels of estrogen present during pregnancy promote the growth and branching of milk ducts, while the increase in progesterone promotes the development of alveoli. Throughout pregnancy and especially during the first three months, many more milk ducts are formed. Clusters of milk-producing cells also begin to enlarge, while at the same time placental hormones promoted breast development.

Shortly before labor and delivery, the hormone prolactin is produced by the pituitary gland. Prolactin, which is necessary for starting lactation and sustaining milk production, reaches its peak at delivery. Another hormone, oxytocin, which is also produced by the pituitary, stimulates the breast to eject milk. This reaction is called the "let-down reflex," which causes the milk-producing alveoli to contract and force milk to the front of the breast. Oxytocin serves an important function after delivery by causing the uterus to contract. Initially, the let-down reflex occurs only when the infant suckles, but later on it may be initiated simply by the baby's cry. An efficient let-down reflex is critical to successful breast-feeding. Emotional upset, fatigue, pain, nervousness, or embarrassment about lactation can interrupt this reflex; these psychological factors, rather than breast size or physiology, are predictive of successful lactation.

Not only is breast-feeding a natural response to childbirth, but the nutrient content is tailor-made for the human infant as well. More than one hundred constituents of breast milk, both nutritive and nonnutritive, are known. Although the basic nutrient content is a solution of protein, sugar, and salts in which fat is suspended, those concentrations vary depending on the period of lactation and even within a given feeding.

Colostrum, often called "first milk," is produced in the first few days after birth. It is lower in fat and Calories (kilocalories) and higher in protein and certain minerals than is mature breast milk. Colostrum is opaque and yellow because it contains a high concentration of the vitamin A-like substances called carotenes. It also has a high concentration of antibodies and white blood cells, which pass on immunologic protection to the infant.

Within a few days after birth, the transition is made from colostrum to mature milk. There are two types of mature milk. Foremilk is released first as the infant begins to suckle. It has a watery, bluish appearance and is low in fat and rich in other nutrients. This milk accounts for about one-third of the baby's intake. As the nursing session progresses, the draught reflex helps move the hindmilk, with its higher fat content, to the front of the breast. It is important that the nutrient content of breast milk be determined from a sample of both types of milk in order to make an adequate assessment of all nutrients present.

Breast milk best meets the infant's needs and is the standard from which infant formulas are judged. Several nutrient characteristics make it the ideal infant food. Lactose, the carbohydrate content of breast milk, is the same simple sugar found in any milk, but the protein content of breast milk is uniquely tailored to meet infant needs. An infant's immature

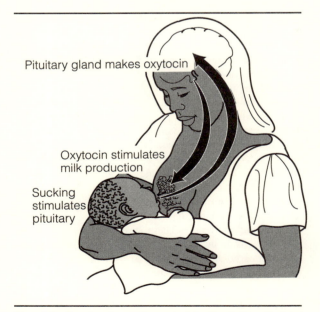

Pituitary gland makes oxytocin

Oxytocin stimulates milk production

Sucking stimulates pituitary

Breast-feeding involves a hormonal feedback loop that encourages milk production.

kidneys are better able to maintain water balance because breast milk is lower in protein than cow's milk. Most breast milk protein is alpha-lactalbumin, whereas cow's milk protein is casein. Alpha-lactalbumin is easier to digest and provides two sulphur-containing amino acids that are the building blocks of protein required for infant growth.

The fat (lipid) content of breast milk differs among women, and even from the same woman, from day to day. The types of fatty acids that make up most of the fat component of the milk may vary in response to maternal diet. Mothers fed a diet containing corn and cottonseed oil produce a milk with more polyunsaturated fatty acids, which are the predominant fatty acids in those oils. Breast milk is higher in the essential fatty acid called linoleic acid than is cow's milk, and it also contains omega-3 fatty acids. About 55 percent of human milk Calories come from fat, compared to about 49 percent of Calories found in infant formulas. In addition, enzymes in breast milk help digest fat in the infant's stomach. This digested fat is more efficiently absorbed than the products that result from digesting cow's milk.

Breast milk contains more cholesterol than cow's milk, which seems to stimulate development of the enzymes necessary for degrading cholesterol, perhaps offering protection against atherosclerosis in later life. Cholesterol is also needed for proper development of the central nervous system.

The vitamin and mineral content of breast milk from healthy mothers supplies all that is needed for growth and health except for vitamin D and fluoride, and these are easily supplemented. Breast milk and the infant's intestinal bacteria also supply all the necessary vitamin K, but since no bacteria are present at birth, an injection of vitamin K should be given to prevent deficiencies.

Breast milk mineral content is balanced to promote growth while protecting the infant's immature kidneys. Breast milk has a low sodium content, which helps the immature kidneys to maintain water balance. No type of milk is a good source of iron. Although breast milk contains relatively small amounts of iron, about 50 percent of this iron can be absorbed by the body, compared to only 4 percent from cow's milk. This phenomenon is called bioavailability. Because of the high bioavailability of breast milk iron, the introduction of solids, which are given to replace depleted iron stores, can be delayed until six months of age in most infants; this delay may help to reduce the incidence of allergies in susceptible infants. There is also evidence that zinc is better absorbed from breast milk.

The vitamin content of milk can vary and is influenced by maternal vitamin status. The water-soluble vitamin content of breast milk (the B vitamins and vitamin C) will change more because of maternal diet than the fat-soluble vitamin content (vitamins A, E, and K). If women have diets that are deficient in vitamins, their levels in breast milk will be lower. Yet even malnourished mothers can breast-feed, although the quantity of milk is decreased. As the maternal diet improves, the level of water-soluble vitamins in the milk increases. There is a level, however, above which additional diet supplements will not increase the vitamin content of breast milk.

There are many nonnutritive advantages to breast-feeding. A major advantage is the immunologic protection and resistance factors that it provides to the infant. Bifidus factors, found in both colostrum and mature milk, favor the growth of helpful bacteria in the infant's digestive tract. These bacteria in turn offer protection against harmful organisms. Lactoferrin, another resistance factor, binds iron so that harmful bacteria cannot use it. Lysozyme, lipases, and lactoperoxidases also offer protection against harmful bacteria.

Immunoglobulins are present in large amounts in colostrum and in significant amounts in breast milk. These protein compounds act as antibodies against foreign substances in the body called antigens. Generally, the resistance passed to the infant is from environmental antigens to which the mother had been exposed. The concentration of antibodies in colostrum is highest in the first hour after birth. Secretory IgA is the major immunoglobulin that provides protection against gastrointestinal organisms. Breast milk also contains interferon, an antiviral substance which is produced by special white blood cells in milk. Protection against allergy is another advantage of breast-feeding. It is not known, however, whether less exposure to the antigens found in formula or some substance in the breast milk itself provides this protection. Normally, a mucous barrier in the intestine prevents the absorption of whole proteins, the root of an allergic reaction. In the newborn, this barrier is not fully developed to allow whole immunologic proteins to be absorbed. The possibility that whole food proteins will be absorbed as well is greater if cow's milk or early solids are given, and this absorption increases the potential for allergic reactions.

Other possible benefits of breast-feeding are protection against the intestinal disorders Crohn's disease and celiac sprue and insulin-dependent diabetes. The reasons for this protection are not clear.

Breast-feeding encourages infant bonding, a process in which the mother forms an affectionate attachment to her baby. It is a matter of controversy whether breast-feeding mothers bond better than bottle-feeding mothers. If a mother has early and prolonged contact with her baby, however, the mother is more likely to breast-feed and to nurse her baby for more months.

Milk from mothers delivering preterm infants is higher in protein and nonprotein nitrogen, calcium, IgA, sodium, potassium, chloride, phosphorus, and magnesium. It also has a different fat composition and is lower in lactose than mature milk of mothers delivering after a normal term. These concentrations support more rapid growth of a preterm infant.

Breast-feeding is not only good for the baby but also good for the mother. There is an association between reduced breast cancer rates and breast-feeding, although the reason is not known. In addition, the hormonal influences caused by suckling the infant help to contract the uterus, returning it to pre-pregnancy size and controlling blood loss. Breast-feeding also helps to reduce the mother's weight. Calories required to make milk are drawn form the fat stores that were deposited during pregnancy. Nevertheless, breast-feeding should be viewed not as a quick weight loss program but as a healthful, natural weight loss process.

If a woman breast-feeds completely, which means that no supplements or solid foods are given until the baby is six months of age, often she will not menstruate. Many women find this lack of menstrual periods psychologically pleasant while not realizing the physiological benefit of restoring the iron stores that were depleted during pregnancy and delivery. An important advantage to breast-feeding in developing countries is that it can help to space pregnancies naturally. Most infant malnutrition occurs when the second child is born, because breast-feeding is stopped for the first child. The first child is weaned to foods that do not supply enough nutrients. By spacing pregnancies out, the first child has a chance to nurse longer.

Breast-feeding is very convenient and does not require time to mix and prepare formula or sterilize bottles. Breast milk is always sterile and at the proper temperature. The money needed for the extra food required to produce breast milk is much less than that required to purchase commercial formula. This can be a major benefit for women with low incomes and is critically important for the health of those babies born in developing countries.

COMPLICATIONS AND DISORDERS

Some special problems or circumstances can make breast-feeding difficult. The breasts may become engorged—so full of milk that they are hard and sore—making it difficult for the baby to latch onto the nipple. Gentle massaging of the breasts, especially with warm water or a heating pad, will allow release of the milk and reduce pain in the breast. This situation is common during the first few weeks of nursing but will occasionally recur if a feeding is missed or a schedule changes.

Sometimes a duct will become plugged and form a hard lump. Massaging the lump and continuing to nurse will remedy the situation. If influenza-like symptoms accompany a plugged duct, the cause is probably a breast infection. Since the infection is in the tissue around the milk-producing glands, the milk itself is safe. The mother must apply heat, get plenty of rest, and keep emptying the breast by frequent feedings. Stopping nursing would plug the duct further, making the infection worse.

Of concern to many mothers are reports of contaminants in breast milk. Drugs, environmental pollutants, viruses, caffeine, alcohol, and food allergens can be passed to the infant through breast milk. Drug transmission depends on the administration method, which influences the speed with which it reaches the blood supply to the breast. Whether that drug can remain functional after it is subjected to the acid in the baby's digestive tract varies. Large amounts of caffeine in breast milk can produce a wakeful, hyperactive infant, but this situation is corrected when the mother stops her caffeine consumption. Large amounts of alcohol produce an altered facial appearance which is reversible; however, some psychomotor delay in the infant may remain even after the mother's drinking has stopped. Nicotine also enters milk, but the impact of secondhand smoke may pose more of a health threat than the nicotine content of breast milk. Since the human immunodeficiency virus (HIV), the virus that causes acquired immunodeficiency syndrome (AIDS), can also pass through breast milk, HIV-positive mothers should not breast-feed their infants.

Of greater concern is the presence of contaminants that cannot be avoided, such as pesticide residues, industrial waste, or other environmental contaminants. Polychlorinated biphenyls (PCBs) and the pesticide DDT have received the most attention. Long-term exposure to contaminants promotes their accumulation in the mother's body fat, and the production of breast milk is one way to rid the body of these contaminants. Concentrations present in the breast milk vary. Ordinarily, these substances are in such small quantities that they pose no health risk. Women who have consumed large amounts of fish from PCB-contaminated waters or have had occupational exposure to this chemical, however, need to have their breast milk tested. It is also possible for these substances to enter the infant's food supply from other sources.

PERSPECTIVE AND PROSPECTS

Although breast-feeding is the best method of infant feeding, many women choose not to breast-feed. Before the 1700's, human milk was the only source for infant feeding. If a mother did not breast-feed, a woman called a wet nurse fed her baby. At the end of the nineteenth century, formula feeding became popular when bottles were developed and water sanitation improved. Breast-feeding declined to less than 20 percent by 1970 but dramatically increased to 60 percent in the early 1980's.

Breast-feeding used to be more prevalent among more-educated, higher-income mothers. Increased employment of women outside the home, however, has dramatically altered trends in breast-feeding. Although mothers may opt to breast-feed in the hospital, many quit because they are returning to work and believe that it would be too difficult to continue. A working mother needs four to six weeks at home to establish successful breast-feeding.

Formula use has increased in developing countries. Because formula is very expensive, it is often diluted with water and therefore does not provide enough nutritional support to the infant. The quality of water is often so poor in these countries that the infant is exposed to disease-causing organisms. In addition, formula-fed infants do not receive the immunologic protection of breast milk. The result is a higher infant mortality rate.

There are very few instance in which a woman should not breast-feed her infant. Babies with a rare genetic disorder called galactosemia cannot nurse since they lack the enzyme to metabolize milk sugar. Phenylketonuria (PKU), another genetic disorder, requires close monitoring of the infant's blood phenylalanine level, but the infant can be totally or at least partially breast-fed. Breast-feeding is contraindicated for women suffering from AIDS, alcoholism, drug addiction, malaria, active tuberculosis, or a chronic disease that results in maternal malnutrition. The presence of other conditions, from diabetes to the common cold, are not reasons to avoid breast-feeding.

Lactation, the secretion of milk, is a physiological process, but breast-feeding is a learned practice, a philosophy about nurturing an infant that goes beyond nutritional support. Society needs to foster this practice. Unfortunately, the etiquette of nursing in public areas is not clearly defined, often resulting in embarrassment that inhibits mothers from nursing their babies. The only remedy is for society to recognize that the normal function of breasts is to nurture infants. Breast-feeding represents a vital resource that improves the health and nutritional status of children, especially in underdeveloped countries.

—*Wendy L. Stuhldreher*

See also Breast disorders; Mastitis; Pregnancy and gestation.

FOR FURTHER INFORMATION:

Huggins, Kathleen. *The Nursing Mother's Companion*. Boston: Harvard Common Press, 1986. This personable book provides comprehensive information about breast-feeding. Topics include preparation, special situations, returning to work, and nursing the older infant.

Price, Anne, and Nancy Dana. *The Working Woman's Guide to Breastfeeding*. Deephaven, Minn.: Meadowbrook, 1987. This book provides information about pumping and storing milk and selecting a breast pump. Presents the nursing mother with several choices about the work situation and explains her legal rights.

Pryor, Karen. *Nursing Your Baby*. Rev. ed. New York: Harper & Row, 1973. This long-standing reference is considered to be a classic work on breast-feeding. Information about establishing successful nursing, the advantages of breast-feeding, and extensive chronicling of the breast-feeding experience throughout the infant's first year of life is laced with warmth and understanding toward women facing obstacles to nursing.

Raphael, Dana. *The Tender Gift: Breastfeeding*. New York: Schocken Books, 1976. Although this book provides basic information on breast-feeding, its unique feature is a survey of breast-feeding in many cultures. Emphasizes the need to give support to the mother who breast-feeds. Historical and cultural influences on infant feeding practices are documented.

Rolfes, Sharon Rady, and Linda Kelly DeBruyne. *Life Span Nutrition: Conception Through Life*. Edited by Eleanor Noss Whitney. St. Paul, Minn.: West, 1990. Chapter 5 of this textbook contains a comprehensive section on breast-feeding. Covers societal support, special medical conditions, physiology, the nutritional characteristics of breast milk, and the nutrient requirements for nursing mothers. An easy-to-read text with illustrations of the physiology of breast-feeding.

Stanway, Penny, and Andrew Stanway. *Breast Is Best*. London: Pan Books, 1980. Written by two doctors who are also parents, this book provides practical, yet medically sound information about many aspects of breast-feeding. Chapters on etiquette, working, special situations, and readers' questions and answers cover issues not discussed in other books.

The Womanly Art of Breastfeeding. 3d rev. ed. Franklin Park, Ill.: La Leche League International, 1981. This bible of breast-feeding covers preparation, the advantages of breast-feeding, and how to overcome problems. This illustrated manual provides the most up-to-date, comprehensive information, supported by an advisory board of medical experts. A must-read for all nursing mothers.

BREATHING DIFFICULTY. *See* HEART ATTACK; PULMONARY DISEASES.

BRONCHITIS

SYSTEM AFFECTED: Respiratory
SPECIALISTS: Family physicians, internists, pulmonologists
DEFINITION: An inflammation of the bronchial tree of the lungs.

CAUSES AND SYMPTOMS

The inflammation associated with bronchitis may be localized or diffuse, acute or chronic, and it is usually caused by infections or physical agents. In its infectious form, acute bronchitis is part of a general, acute upper-respiratory infection, sometimes brought on by the common cold. It can also develop from a virus infection of the nasopharynx, throat, or tracheobronchial tree. Acute bronchitis is most prevalent in winter. Factors contributing to the onset of the disease include exposure, chilling, malnutrition, fatigue, or rickets. The inflammation may be serious in debilitated patients and those with chronic pulmonary disease, and the real danger rests in the development of pneumonia. Certain physical and chemical irritants can bring on acute bronchitis. Such agents as mineral and vegetable dusts, strong acid fumes, volatile organic compounds, and tobacco smoke can trigger an attack.

The disease causes thickening of the bronchi and a loss of elasticity in the bronchial tree. Changes in the mucous

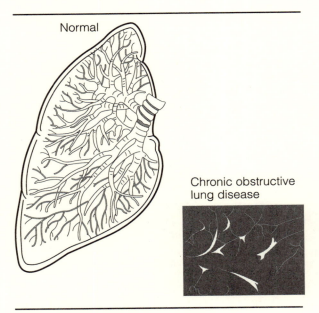

Normal

Chronic obstructive lung disease

Normal vs. obstructed bronchioles.

membranes occur, leukocytes infiltrate the submucosa, and a sticky, mucopurulent exudate is formed. The normally sterile bronchi are invaded by bacteria and cellular debris. A barking cough is often present, and this serves as an essential mechanism for eliminating bronchial secretions.

Chronic bronchitis is characterized by swollen mucous membranes, tenacious exudate, and spasms in the bronchiolar muscles. The result is dyspnea, the ventilatory insufficiency known as shortness of breath.

TREATMENT AND THERAPY

Acute bronchitis is treated with bed rest and medication to counteract the symptoms of inflammation. The room air should be kept warm and humid. Steam inhalation and cough syrup sometimes give relief from the severe, painful cough.

All surveys have demonstrated a high incidence of bronchitis in cigarette smokers when compared with nonsmokers, thus providing a good reason for the cessation of smoking. —*Jane A. Slezak*

See also Coughing; Pneumonia; Pulmonary diseases.

FOR FURTHER INFORMATION:

Beeson, Paul, Walsh McDermott, and James B. Wyngaarden, eds. *Textbook of Medicine*. 15th ed. Philadelphia: W. B. Saunders, 1979. A comprehensive textbook covering the diagnosis and treatment of diseases.

Berland, Theodore, and Gordon Snider. *Living with Your Bronchitis and Emphysema*. New York: St. Martin's Press, 1972. A reference for those with lung disease. Includes suggestions for clearing airways and helping oneself breathe.

Petty, Thomas, and Louise Nett. *For Those Who Live and Breathe with Emphysema and Chronic Bronchitis*.

Springfield, Ill.: Charles C Thomas, 1967. A book written for patients suffering from emphysema and bronchitis. The book covers medical facts, rehabilitation programs, and includes an extensive glossary.

Shayevitz, Myra, and Berton R. Shayevitz. *Living Well with Emphysema and Bronchitis*. Garden City, N.Y.: Doubleday, 1985. A book written to help those suffering from chronic lung disease. Provides an agenda for living with the disease.

BULIMIA

SYSTEMS AFFECTED: Gastrointestinal, psychic-emotional

SPECIALISTS: Gastroenterologists, psychiatrists, psychologists

DEFINITION: Bulimia is a compulsive eating disorder in which the patient (usually a young woman) goes on food binges and then intentionally purges herself, either through self-induced vomiting or by using laxatives. As with anorexia nervosa, the patient has a fear of gaining weight, but unlike anorectics, bulimics may or may not experience a significant weight loss. Nevertheless, there are medical dangers: Chronic laxative use can result in dehydration and other gastrointestinal disorders, and repeated vomiting may cause severe tooth decay from the gastric acids found in bile. Counseling is necessary to address the patient's underlying psychological illness.

See also Eating disorders; Malnutrition; Poisoning; Weight loss and gain.

BURNS AND SCALDS

SYSTEMS AFFECTED: Skin, most other tissues in severe cases

SPECIALISTS: Burn specialists, emergency physicians, general surgeons, physical therapists, plastic and reconstructive surgeons

DEFINITION: Injury to skin and other tissues caused by contact with dry heat (fire), moist heat (steam or hot liquid), chemicals, electricity, lightning, or radiation.

KEY TERMS:

burn: an injury to tissues caused by contact with dry heat (fire), moist heat (steam or a hot liquid), chemicals, electricity, lightning, or radiation

burn degrees: system of classification for burns based on the depth of damage to the skin

major (or severe) burn: a burn covering more than 20 percent of the body and any deep burn of the hands, face, feet, or perineum

minor burn: a superficial burn of less than 5 percent of the body that can be treated without hospitalization

moderate burn: a burn that requires hospitalization but not specialized care

rule of nines: a system used to designate areas of the body, represented by various body parts; used in determining the extent of a burn *skin graft:* a surgical graft of skin from one part of the body to another or from one individual to another

CAUSES AND SYMPTOMS

Burns are injuries to tissues caused by contact with dry heat (fire), moist heat (steam or a hot liquid, also called scalds), chemicals, electricity, lightning, or radiation. The word "burn" comes from the Middle English *brinnen* or *brennen* (to burn) and from the Old English *byrnan* (to be on fire) combined with *baernan* (to set afire). Each year in the United States, more than two million people are burned or scalded badly enough to need medical treatment, and about 70,000 require admission to a hospital. Burns are most common in children and older people, and many are caused by accidents in the home that are usually preventable.

The depth of the injury is proportional to the intensity of the heat of the causative agent and the duration of exposure. Burns can be classified according to the agent causing the damage. Some examples of burns according to this classification are brush burns, caused by friction of a rapidly moving object against the skin or ground into the skin; chemical burns, caused by exposure to a caustic chemical; flash burns, caused by very brief exposure to intense radiant heat (the typical burn of an atomic explosion); radiation burns, caused by exposure to radium, X rays, or atomic energy; and respiratory burns, caused by inhalation of steam or explosive gases.

Burns can also be classified as major or severe (involving more than 20 percent of the body and any deep burn of the hands, face, feet, or perineum), minor (a superficial burn involving less than 5 percent of the body that can be treated without hospitalization), and moderate (a burn that requires hospitalization but not specialized care, as with burns covering 5 to 20 percent of the body but without deep burns of hands, face, feet, or perineum).

While many domestic burns are minor and insignificant, more severe burns and scalds can prove to be dangerous. The main danger for a burn patient is the shock that arises as a result of loss of fluid from the circulating blood at the site of the burn. This loss of fluid leads to a fall in the volume of the circulating blood in the area. The maintenance of an adequate blood volume is essential to life, and the body attempts to compensate for this temporary loss by withdrawing fluid from the uninjured areas of the body into the circulation. In the first forty-eight hours after a severe burn is received, fluid from the blood vessels, salt, and protein pass into the burned area, causing swelling, blisters, low blood pressure, and very low urine output. The body loses fluids, proteins, and salt, and the potassium level is raised. Such low-fluid levels are followed by a shift of fluid in the opposite direction, resulting in excess urine, high blood volume, and low concentration of blood electrolytes. If carried too far, this condition begins to affect the viability of the body cells. As a result, essential body cells such as those of the liver and kidneys begin to suffer, eventually causing the liver and kidneys to cease proper function. Liver and renal failure are revealed by the development of jaundice and the appearance of albumin in the urine. In addition, the circulation begins to fail, with a resultant lack

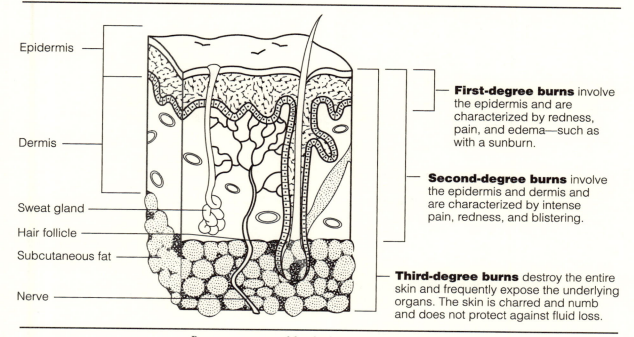

Epidermis

Dermis

Sweat gland

Hair follicle

Subcutaneous fat

Nerve

First-degree burns involve the epidermis and are characterized by redness, pain, and edema—such as with a sunburn.

Second-degree burns involve the epidermis and dermis and are characterized by intense pain, redness, and blistering.

Third-degree burns destroy the entire skin and frequently expose the underlying organs. The skin is charred and numb and does not protect against fluid loss.

Burns are measured by the layer(s) of skin affected.

Rule of Nines

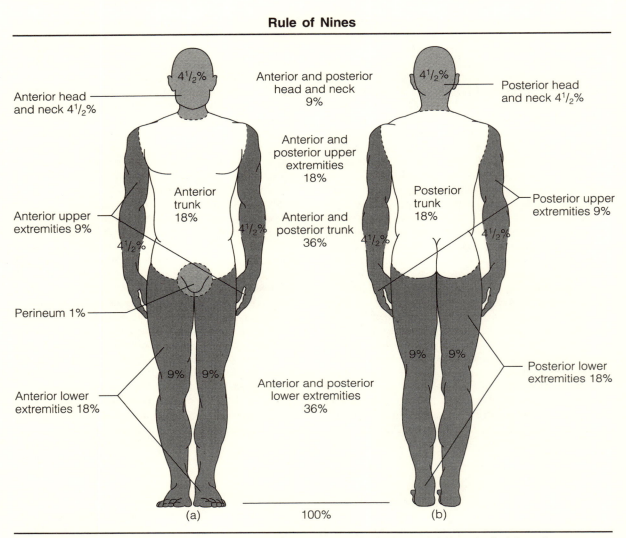

Anterior and posterior
head and neck
9%

Anterior head
and neck 4$^{1}/_{2}$%

Posterior head
and neck 4$^{1}/_{2}$%

4$^{1}/_{2}$%

4$^{1}/_{2}$%

Anterior and
posterior upper
extremities
18%

Anterior
trunk
18%

Posterior
trunk
18%

Posterior upper
extremities 9%

Anterior upper
extremities 9%

Anterior and
posterior trunk
36%

4$^{1}/_{2}$%

4$^{1}/_{2}$%

4$^{1}/_{2}$%

4$^{1}/_{2}$%

Perineum 1%

9%   9%

9%   9%

Posterior lower
extremities 18%

Anterior lower
extremities 18%

Anterior and posterior
lower extremities
36%

(a)   100%   (b)

The "rule of nines" specifies the extent and hence seriousness of a burn in relation to the body's surface area.

of oxygen in the tissues. The victim becomes cyanosed, restless, and collapsed, and in some cases death ensues. Other possible problems related to burns include collapse of the circulatory system; shutdown of the digestive and excretory systems, shock, pneumonia, and stress ulcers.

In addition, particularly with severe burns, there is a strong risk of infection. This type of burn can leave a large area of raw skin surface exposed and extremely vulnerable to any microorganisms. The infection of extensive burns may cause fatal complications if effective antibiotic treatment is not given. The combination of shock and infection can often be life-threatening unless expert treatment is immediately available.

The immediate outcome of a burn is more determined by its extent (amount of body area affected) than by its depth (layers of skin affected). The "rule of nines" is used to assess the extent of a burn in relation to the surface of a body. The head and each of the arms cover 9 percent of the body surface; the front of the body, the back, and each leg cover 18 percent; and the crotch accounts for the remaining 1 percent. The greater the extent of a burn, the more seriously ill the victim will become from loss of fluid. The depth of the burn (unless it is very great) is mainly of importance when the question arises as to how much surgical treatment, including skin grafting, will be required. An improvement over the rule of nines in the evaluation of the seriousness of burns is the Berkow formula, which takes into account the age of the patient.

A burn caused by chemicals differs from a burn caused by fire only in that the outcome of the chemical burn is usually more favorable, since the chemical destroys the bacteria on the affected part and reduces the chance of infection. Severe burns can also be caused by contact with electric wires. As current meets the resistance in the skin, high temperatures are developed and burning of the victim takes place. Exposure to 220 volts burns only the skin, but higher voltage can cause severe underlying damage to any tissue in its path. Electrical burns normally cause minimal external skin damage, but they can cause serious heart damage and require evaluation by a physician. Explosions and the action of acids and other chemicals also cause burns. Severe and extensive fire burns are most frequently produced by the clothes catching fire.

TREATMENT AND THERAPY

General treatment of a burn injury includes pain relief, the control of infection, the maintenance of the balance of fluids and electrolytes in the system, and a good diet. A high-protein diet with supplemental vitamins is prescribed to aid in the repair of damaged tissue. The specific treatment depends on the severity of the burn. Major burns should be treated in a specialized treatment facility, while minor burns can be treated without hospitalization. A moderate burn normally requires hospitalization but not specialized care.

In the case of minor burns or scalds, all that may be necessary is to hold the body part under cold running water until the pain is relieved, as cooling is one of the most effective ways of relieving the pain of a burn. If the burn involves the distal part of a limb—for example, the hand and forearm—one of the most effective ways of relieving the pain is to immerse the burned part in lukewarm water and add cold water until the pain disappears. If the pain does not return when the water warms up, the burn can be dressed in the usual way (a piece of sterile gauze covered by cotton with a bandage on top). The part should be kept at rest and the dressing dry until healing takes place. Blisters can be pierced with a sterile needle, but the skin should not be cut away. No ointment or oil should be applied, and an antiseptic is not always necessary. Even this type of burn can be serious if it covers as much as two-thirds of the body area. On a child, such burns are dangerous on an even smaller area of the skin, and special attention should be given to the patient.

In the case of moderate burns or scalds, it is advisable to use antiseptics (such as chlorhexidine, bacitracin, and neomycin), and the patient should be taken to a doctor. Treatment may consist of using a dressing impregnated with a suitable antibiotic or of applying a cream containing antiseptic and pain-relieving creams and covering the burn with a dressing sealed at the end. This dressing is left on for four to five days and removed if there is evidence of infection or if pain occurs.

For severe burns and scalds, the only sound rule is to go to the hospital. Unless there is a need for resuscitation,

or attention to other injuries, nothing should be done on the spot except to make sure that the patient is comfortable and warm and to cover the burn with a clean or sterile cloth. Clothing should be removed from the burned area only if this does not traumatize the skin further. Burned clothing should be sent to the burn center, as it may help determine the chemicals and other substances that either caused or entered the wound. Once the victim is in the hospital, the first thing to check is the extent of the burn and whether a transfusion is necessary. If the burn covers more than 9 percent of the body surface, a transfusion is required. It is essential to prevent infection or to bring it under control. A high-protein diet with ample fluids is needed to compensate for the protein that has been lost along with the fluid from the circulation. The process of healing is slow and tedious, including careful nursing, physiotherapy, and occupational therapy. The length of hospital stay can vary from a few days in some cases to many weeks in the case of severe and extensive burns.

In some cases depending on the extent of the burn, it will be necessary to consider skin grafting, in which a graft of skin from one part of the body (or from another individual) is implanted in another part. Skin grafting is done soon after the initial injury. The donor skin is best taken from the patient, but when this is not possible, the skin of a matched donor can be used. Prior to grafting, or in some cases as a substitute for it, the burn may be covered with either cadaver or pig skin to keep it moist and free from exogenous bacterial infection. Newly developed artificial skin holds great promise for treating severe burns.

In the case of chemical burns, treatment can be specific and depends on the chemical causing the burn. For example, phenol or lysol can be washed off promptly, while acid or alkali burns should be neutralized by washing with sodium bicarbonate or acetic acid, respectively, or with a buffer solution for either one. In many cases, flushing with water to remove the chemical is the first method of action.

Victims who have inhaled smoke may develop swelling and inflammation of the lungs, and they may need special care for burns of the eyes. People who have suffered an electrical burn may suffer from shock and may require artificial respiration; which should begin as soon as contact with the current has been broken.

PERSPECTIVE AND PROSPECTS

Burns have been traditionally classified according to degree. The French surgeon Guillaume Dupuytren divided burns into six degrees, according to their depth. A first-degree burn is one in which there is simply redness; it may be painful for a day or two. This level of burn is normally seen in cases of extended exposure to X rays or sunlight. A second-degree burn affects the first and second layers of skin. There is great redness, and the surface is raised up in blisters accompanied by much pain. Healing normally occurs without a scar. A third-degree burn affects all skin layers. The epidermis is entirely peeled off, and the true skin below is destroyed in part, so as to expose the endings of the sensory nerves. This is a very painful form of burn, and a scar follows on healing. With a fourth-degree burn, the entire skin of an area is destroyed with its nerves, so that there is less pain than with a third-degree burn. A scar forms and later contracts, and it may produce great deformity in the affected area. A fifth-degree burn will burn the muscles as well, and still greater deformity follows. In a sixth-degree burn, a whole limb is charred, and it separates as in gangrene.

In current practice, burns are referred to as superficial (or partial thickness), in which there is sufficient skin tissue left to ensure regrowth of skin over the burned site; and deep (or full thickness), in which the skin is totally destroyed and grafting will be necessary. It is difficult to determine the depth of a wound at first glance, but any burn involving more than 15 percent of the body surface is considered serious. As far as the ultimate outcome is concerned, the main factor is the extent of the burn—the greater the extent, the worse the outlook.

Unfortunately, burns are most common in children and older people, those for whom the outcome is usually the worst. Many of the burns are caused by accidents in the home, which are usually preventable. In fact, among the primary causes of deaths by burns, house fires account for 75 percent of the incidents. Safety measures in the home and on the job are extremely important in the prevention of burns. Severe and extensive burns most frequently occur when the clothes catch fire. This rule applies especially to cotton garments, which burn quickly. Particular care should always be exercised with electric fires and kettles or pots of boiling water in houses where small children or elderly people are present.

In the United States, most severely burned patients are given emergency care in a local hospital and are then transferred to a large burn center for intensive long-term care. The kind of environment provided in special burn units in large medical centers varies, but all have as their main objective avoiding contamination of the wound, as the major cause of death in burn victims is infection. Some special units use isolation techniques and elaborate laminar air flow systems to maintain an environment that is as free of microorganisms as possible.

The patient who has suffered some disfigurement from burns will have additional emotional problems in adjusting to a new body image. Burn therapy can be long and tedious for the patient and for family members. They will need emotional and psychological support as they work their way through the many problems created by the physical and emotional trauma of a major wound. —*Maria Pacheco*

See also Electrical shock; Heat exhaustion and heat stroke; Radiation sickness; Shock; Wounds.

FOR FURTHER INFORMATION:

Clayman, C. B., ed. *American Medical Association Encyclopedia of Medicine*. New York: Random House, 1989. A concise presentation of numerous medical terms and illnesses. A good general reference.

Glanze, Walter D., Kenneth N. Anderson, and Lois E. Anderson, eds. *The Mosby Medical Encyclopedia*. Rev. ed. New York: Plume, 1992. Excellent general reference for the layperson. Offers a concise but clear presentation of numerous medical topics.

Landau, Sidney, ed. *International Dictionary of Medicine and Biology*. New York: John Wiley & Sons, 1986. Contains a brief presentation of medical and biological terms. A good, easy-to-comprehend general reference.

Miller, Benjamin, and Claire B. Keane. *Encyclopedia and Dictionary of Medicine, Nursing, and Allied Health*. 5th ed. Philadelphia: W. B. Saunders, 1992. A good, concise presentation of the topic of burns.

Thomson, W. A., ed. *Black's Medical Dictionary*. 34th ed. Totowa, N.J.: Barnes & Noble Books, 1984. An excellent presentation of the topic can be found in this general medical reference work.

BURSITIS

SYSTEM AFFECTED: Joints
SPECIALISTS: Rheumatologists, internists
DEFINITION: An inflammation of a bursa, one of the membranes that surround joints.

CAUSES AND SYMPTOMS

Bursas are flattened, fibrous sacs that minimize friction on adjacent structures during activity involving a joint. The most well known bursas are around the knees, elbows, and shoulders. These protective joint sacs are lined with a fluid-producing membrane called the synovial membrane. Bursas are common in sites where ligaments, muscles, skin, or tendons overlie and may rub against bone. Most bursas are present at birth, but false bursas may develop at any site where there is excessive motion.

Bursitis is inflammation of a bursa, causing it to become warm, painful, and often swollen. Bursitis is usually caused by the inappropriate or excessive use of a joint. For example, pressure, friction, infections, or injury to a joint and surrounding tissues can cause membranes of the bursa to become inflamed.

Bursitis of the kneecap (prepatellar bursitis, or "housemaid's knee") is commonly caused by prolonged kneeling on a hard surface such as the floor. Similarly, olecranon bursitis ("student's elbow") is caused by pressure of the elbow against a table or desk. Perhaps the most common type of bursitis is of the shoulder joint, called subdeltoid bursitis.

TREATMENT AND THERAPY

The treatment for bursitis caused by overuse is usually rest and avoidance of the activity that resulted in the con-

dition. Several days of rest is typically all that is needed for the swelling to subside. Ice packs may help relieve some of the minor pain and inflammation. If the inflammation does not subside after a few days, a physician may prescribe anti-inflammatory drugs such as ibuprofen or naproxen to reduce the inflammation and pain. Occasionally, a doctor will inject the inflamed bursa with a corticosteroid such as triamcinolone. In rare cases, where the symptoms are recurrent, a physician may remove the bursa (bursectomy). If the bursitis is caused by an infection, the most appropriate treatment is antibiotic therapy. During and after medical or surgical treatment, physical therapy may be recommended to improve the strength and mobility of the joint.
—*Matthew Berria*

See also Arthritis; Gout; Osteoarthritis; Rheumatoid arthritis; Tendon disorders.

FOR FURTHER INFORMATION:

Clayman, Charles B., ed. *The American Medical Association Encyclopedia of Medicine.* New York: Random House, 1989.

Marieb, Elaine N. *Human Anatomy and Physiology.* 2d ed. Redwood City, Calif.: Benjamin/Cummings, 1992.

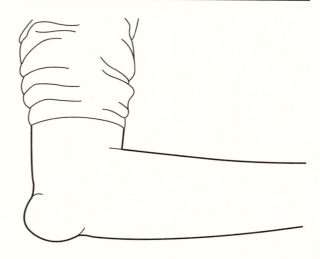

Bursitis produces a painful, fluid-filled swelling around a joint; bursitis may occur in the bursa at any joint, such as the elbow.

CALCULI. *See* STONES.

CANCER

SYSTEMS AFFECTED: All

SPECIALISTS: General surgeons, oncologists, orthopedic surgeons, radiation oncologists, radiologists

DEFINITION: Inappropriate and uncontrollable cell growth within one of the specialized tissues of the body, threatening normal cell and organ function and in serious cases traveling via the bloodstream to other areas of the body.

KEY TERMS:

carcinogen: a cancer-causing substance; usually a chemical that causes mutations

cell: the basic functional unit of the body, each of which contains a set of genes and all the other materials necessary for carrying out the processes of life

cell cycle: a stepwise process whereby one cell duplicates itself to form two cells; it is the way in which most growth occurs, and the cycle leads to cancer if it becomes defective

gene: a master molecule that encodes the information needed for the body to carry out one specific function; many thousands of genes working together are needed to sustain normal human life

initiation: the first abnormal change that starts a cell along the pathway to cancer

metastasis: the process whereby tumor cells spread from one part of the body to another

mutation: damage to a gene that changes how it works

oncogene: a gene that functions normally to allow cells to progress through the cell cycle; when mutated, such genes can cause cancer

promotion: the second step in tumor development, which causes initiated cells to begin growing into tumors

CAUSES AND SYMPTOMS

Cancer is a disease of abnormal growth. Growth is an important feature in the development of all living things, but it must be precisely controlled for life processes to occur properly. Much is known about how growth occurs and how it is regulated with such precision.

All growing cells pass through a strictly regulated series of events called the cell cycle. Most structures of the cell are duplicated during this sequence. At the end of the cycle, one cell is separated into two "daughter cells," each of which receives one copy of the duplicated cellular structures. The most important structures that must be exactly duplicated are the genes, the master blueprints that govern all cellular activities. Human life starts with a single microscopic cell—a fertilized egg. This cell divides again and again; the adult human body is composed of more than a trillion cells, each with a very specific job to perform.

After adulthood is reached, most cells of the body stop duplicating themselves. Some cell types, however, do need to continue dividing to replace worn-out cells; these include cells of the blood, skin, intestine, and some other tissues. Such growth is very accurately controlled so that excess cells are not produced. It is in these cell types, those that normally grow in the adult body, that cancer most often occurs. A small defect arises in one gene so that the cells are able to progress through the cell cycle even though more cells are not needed. This is the start of cancer. Such cancer cells do not need to grow faster than do their normal neighbors; their key feature is simply that they continue growing when no more cells should be produced. At first, these cells very closely resemble their neighbors. For example, newly altered blood cells still look very much like normal blood cells, and in most respects they are.

The first defect that gets cancer started is called initiation. It is typically the result of a mutation in one of the genes whose job it is to control some feature of the cell cycle. There are probably several hundred such genes, each of which regulates a different aspect of the cell cycle. These genes have perfectly normal jobs in the life of the cell until they become damaged. When there is a mutation in a controlling gene, the gene functions improperly: It does not govern the cell cycle quite right, and the cell cycle therefore proceeds when it should instead be halted. Such cancer-causing genes are called oncogenes.

After the initiation of cancer, additional mutations and other defects begin to pile up, and the defective cells become increasingly abnormal. Typically, a second change, called promotion, must take place before cancer cells begin really growing freely. The promotion step typically allows the initiated cell to escape some policing activity of the body. For example, various hormones provide cells with instructions about how to behave; a promotion-type change may allow a cell to ignore such instructions. Both initiation and promotion occur randomly. Many cells that are initiated, however, fail to grow into tumors. It is only those relatively few cells that happen to acquire both defects that become a problem.

At this point, the new cancer cell is dividing and collecting in large numbers. These excess cells make up a mass called a tumor (except in the blood and lymph cancers, in which the cancer cells circulate individually). Nevertheless, all these cells are fairly "normal." Indeed, at this early stage, cancer is relatively easy to control using methods such as surgery. The excess cells may not cause much harm—warts, for example, are excess numbers of growing cells. Such relatively harmless tumors are called benign. If the cancer is detected at this early stage, while it is still relatively harmless, effective treatment and even a cure are still quite possible, which is why early diagnosis is so important in cancer medicine.

Unfortunately, more and more defects accumulate in these cells as they grow, and some of these defects (again by chance) will be particularly harmful. The most harmful changes make the growing cells capable of causing damage to other parts of the body. For example, cancer cells may acquire the ability to digest their way through nearby tissues, a process called invasion. Eventually, the functions of organs containing such cells become impaired. Such an invasion of body parts can be extremely painful as well. Other cancer cells may come loose from the tumor and travel to other parts of the body in the circulatory or lymphatic system: This process is called metastasis. In advanced stages of cancer, a patient may actually have dozens or hundreds of tumors, all of which have developed from a single parent tumor. Cells that can invade or metastasize are called malignant. It becomes increasingly difficult to eradicate cancer cells as they become more malignant. Pathologists are highly skilled at distinguishing benign from malignant cancer cells based on their appearance in a microscope and can provide accurate diagnosis of how far a case of cancer has progressed. Such information is crucial for deciding how best to treat the cancer.

Most kinds of cancer typically occur during old age. Because each of the events that leads to tumor development is rather uncommon, it takes years for the several required mistakes to accumulate in a single cell, which then grows into a tumor. A few kinds of cancer occur most commonly in children. Such children usually have inherited one or more of the genetic defects that lead to cancer from their parents. It then takes less time before the additional required defects are likely to occur. Thus, a tendency toward certain kinds of cancer can be inherited in families, as with other genetic traits (such as hair and eye color, height, and nose shape).

Cancer occurs when anything causes oncogenes to function abnormally, allowing cells to continue growing when they should not. The delicate genes in an individual's cells can be modified chemically by a number of different highly active and dangerous chemicals known collectively as carcinogens. Several kinds of radiation also pose a threat to genes. The best-known example is ultraviolet radiation from the sun, which can damage genes of the skin and lead to skin cancer. Finally, certain kinds of viruses can cause oncogenes to function improperly.

TREATMENT AND THERAPY

Most people who live to an advanced age can expect to be faced with cancer. Because cancer is such a serious and widespread health problem, enormous efforts have gone into learning how the disease develops and then applying those discoveries to cure and prevent cancer.

The cancer treatments used most commonly are of three kinds: surgery, chemotherapy, and radiation therapy. First, and most straightforward, is the surgical removal of tumors. If done at an early stage, before cancer has spread, this method can be highly successful. Even so, surgery is much easier and less dangerous for some cancers (for example, skin cancer) than for others (such as brain tumors, which can be difficult to reach and remove safely). Naturally, sur-

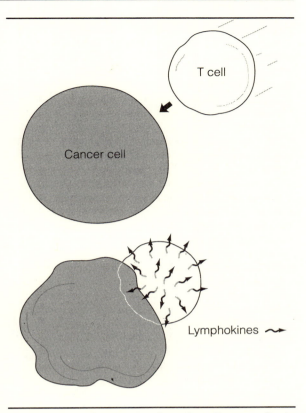

Cancer cells are fast-growing, irregular cells; normally, the body releases killer T cells that interact with antigens on the surface of the cancer cell, releasing lymphokines that are toxic to the cancer cell.

gery is much less successful with widely spread cancers such as leukemia (a cancer of blood cells) and in more advanced stages of cancer.

The second type of cancer treatment is chemotherapy. Patients are treated with chemicals that prevent cells from duplicating themselves, or at least limit or slow that process. Such drugs, which are usually injected, reach all parts of the body and so are much more effective than surgery when cancer has reached a later stage of spreading. Different kinds of chemicals work in very different ways to achieve this result. These chemicals can be roughly divided into four categories. First are chemicals that react directly with the substances required for cells to survive and function. Many such agents directly attack a cell's genes, preventing them from passing along information required for a cancer cell to stay alive. Second are antimetabolites, which prevent the chemical reactions that allow cells to produce energy (energy must also be available for cells to stay alive). The third category consists of steroid hormones. Cancer cells in some organs of the body respond to these hormones, which can therefore be used to regulate their growth. Thus estrogens, the female sex steroid hormones, are often used for treatment of breast cancer, whereas the male sex steroids, or androgens, may influence prostate cancer. Fourth are miscellaneous drugs, a few other chemicals that affect cancer cells in some different way. For example, drugs called vinca alkaloids stop the mechanical process of one cell dividing into two, in this way preventing growth. A derivative of the insecticide DDT (dichloro-diphenyl-trichloroethane) prevents unwanted steroid-hormone production and has been useful for treating tumors of the adrenal gland.

The most common and difficult problem with the chemotherapeutic approach to cancer management is that normal cells that happen to be growing are also affected by the same drugs that halt the growth of cancer cells. This reaction causes many difficulties for patients, some serious and some less so. Probably the most serious problems are in the immune system. The growth of blood cells that make antibodies, called lymphocytes, is necessary before antibodies can be produced in response to an infectious disease. Because these cells cannot grow, patients in chemotherapy are much more vulnerable to illnesses caused by bacteria and viruses. Other blood cells, including those that carry oxygen, are also affected, causing additional problems. Skin cells and cells lining the digestive tract stop dividing, causing additional difficulties for the patients. A less serious problem for such patients is hair loss, as hair cells also are prevented from growing.

Designing drug treatments that kill cancer cells while minimizing these problems is a demanding and precise task for oncologists (physicians who specialize in cancer research and treatment). Some drugs affect different cell types in somewhat different ways, allowing normal cells to continue their functions while killing tumor cells. Doses and timing of treatments can be adjusted to maximize the effect of the drugs. It is typical for several drugs that act in different ways to be given in the same treatment, to assure that all cancer cells are halted; this approach is called combination chemotherapy. It is of critical importance that all cancer cells be stopped because a single unaffected cancer cell at any place in the body can begin growing after chemotherapy and develop into a cancer, a process known as relapse.

Another useful approach for improving chemotherapy is drug targeting. The chemical structure of tumor cells is subtly different from that of normal cells, and it is sometimes possible to make use of this difference. For example, a drug can be attached to an antibody molecule that reacts with a tumor protein (antigen) that is not found on normal cells. In this way, most of the drug will be directed to the tumor cells, while normal cells will receive a much lower dose. Hormones and other molecules also attach to specific molecules on cells, and this fact can sometimes be exploited to target drugs if the tumor cells have a particularly high number of such molecules.

Another problem with drug delivery is that the most effective drugs are rapidly degraded by the body's defense systems and secreted from the body. The actual period of exposure to an active drug in the body can be quite brief (a few minutes) for this reason. Methods have been developed for hiding or disguising drugs so they are not removed so rapidly. For example, some drugs can be placed inside fat droplets, and in this way they can escape detection by the immune system and breakdown in the liver.

Because of the great importance of effective chemotherapy, thousands of new compounds are screened each year for their effectiveness against cancer. The first step in this process is the careful and extensive testing of such compounds on animals, usually mice and rats. Both the effectiveness of the drug against cancer and its effects on normal bodily functions are carefully measured. Drugs that pass the animal tests are then tried out in cautious human tests. Often, the first patients tested are those with advanced cancer conditions who volunteer for such treatment. Three further levels of human testing then follow before a new drug can be marketed. Only about one in five thousand drugs tested reaches clinical trials; one in fifty thousand becomes available for general use. The testing process is lengthy and expensive, but thousands of lives are saved each year because of the careful testing and development of new chemotherapies.

The third type of cancer treatment is radiation therapy. The radiation of choice is X rays, which can penetrate the body to reach a tumor and which can be produced at very high dosages using modern equipment. X rays can be focused on a specific small area or can be given over the whole body in the case of metastasized cancer. Therapeutic radiation damages genes to such an extent that they become physically fragmented and nonfunctional, ending the life of the target cell.

Radiation therapy has some of the same drawbacks as chemotherapy. Again, the most serious problem is that normal cells in the pathway of the radiation will also be killed. Bone marrow, the source of blood cells, is destroyed by whole-body cancer treatments. This problem can be overcome after radiation therapy by transplanting new bone marrow to the patient from close relatives, so that a treated patient can begin to remanufacture blood cells. Ironically, radiation designed to kill cancer cells can also turn normal cells into new cancer cells. Some normal cells can receive a reduced exposure of X rays. The dosage may be just sufficient to damage oncogenes of normal cells, causing them to become cancerous. Thus radiation therapy must be carried out with great care and precision.

PERSPECTIVE AND PROSPECTS

Cancer has plagued humankind for thousands of years. Fossils of humanoid ancestors show evidence of cancer, bone cancer is identifiable in Egyptian mummies, and the ancient Greek physician Hippocrates described many kinds of cancer that were common during his time. Animals and even plants develop abnormal growths comparable to cancer in people—the curse of cancer is inherent in the way that all organisms grow.

The first major insight into why cancer occurs was made by Percivall Pott, a British physician. In 1775, he reported his observations on scrotal cancer in young chimney sweeps. This cancer was unusually frequent in these boys. Pott suggested that repeated exposure to the irritating soot in chimneys was what started this cancer. He is credited with the first description of cancer initiation.

During the next 150 years, the major advances in fighting cancer were safer and more effective surgery procedures. These important improvements were made much easier by the development of effective anesthetics and antibiotics. Also, by the end of the nineteenth century, the principles of radiation therapy and chemotherapy were being established, based on fundamental research in physics and chemistry.

Progress in the battle against cancer was steady in the first half of the twentieth century. The principles of initiation and promotion became firmly established, and the features of most kinds of cancer were thoroughly described. It became clear that cancer is not a single disease, that each type has its own causes and potential cures. Cancer epidemics, for example among asbestos workers, drove home the lesson that substances in the environment can cause cancer and must be carefully monitored.

In the 1940's and 1950's, research on genes started a revolution in the understanding of biology and how the human body functions. These new advances were quickly related to cancer, and it was understood that defective genes could lead to abnormal growth. The exciting implication of this insight was that a solution to the cancer problem seemed within grasp: It was necessary either to prevent mutations in cancer-causing genes or to correct such errors after they happened.

In the 1970's and 1980's, the intense effort of scientists and physicians around the world resulted in the oncogene concept. Finally, cancer-cell growth was understood as resulting from defects in genes that have a perfectly normal function in the economy of the body. Meanwhile, new advances made it possible to analyze and manipulate genes in ways only dreamed of previously. Gene therapy became another weapon in the arsenal available to physicians.

Because of its nature and importance, the fight against cancer has involved an unusually broad spectrum of medical and scientific specialties. As a result, people are becoming increasingly protected from this disease. Cancer-causing agents are closely regulated, and new diagnostic procedures can detect abnormal cells at the earliest stages.

—*Howard L. Hosick*

See also Bone cancer; Breast cancer; Carcinoma; Cervical, ovarian, and uterine cancers; Colon cancer; Dental dis-

eases; Hodgkin's disease; Leukemia; Liver cancer; Lung cancer; Lymphadenopathy and lymphoma; Malignancy and metastasis; Prostate cancer; Sarcoma; Skin cancer; Stomach, intestinal, and pancreatic cancers; Tumors.

FOR FURTHER INFORMATION:

Cairns, John. *Cancer: Science and Society*. San Francisco: W. H. Freeman, 1978. Cairns is a prominent molecular biologist who has turned his attention to cancer. He writes eloquently but nontechnically about the biology and medical implications of cancer. Several chapters are designed specifically to introduce concepts to individuals with little background in science. An excellent and accessible overview of the basic features of this disease.

Levenson, Frederick B. *The Causes and Prevention of Cancer*. New York: Stein & Day, 1985. A very personal attempt to give an overview of cancer and how it fits into health maintenance in general. Presented as a storylike narrative with the emphasis ultimately on the author's unproved ideas about cancer prevention and its relationship to human life.

Levitt, Paul M., and Elissa S. Guralnick. *The Cancer Reference Book: Direct and Clear Answers to Everyone's Questions*. New York: Facts on File, 1983. A different format, structured as a series of specific questions and answers dealing mostly with practical, medically oriented questions about cancer. Contains a simple glossary, an honest discussion of treatments, and facts about many individual kinds of cancer.

Maugh, Thomas H., II, and Jane L. Marx. *Seeds of Destruction*. New York: Plenum Press, 1975. This book is by two science writers who are skilled at explaining complex facts and ideas. Although the book is not up to date on more recent findings, it is still an accurate and unusually clear summary of the basic biology of cancer.

Oppenheimer, Steven B. *Cancer: A Biological and Clinical Introduction*. Boston: Allyn & Bacon, 1982. A more rigorous treatment of the characteristics of cancer than are the other books listed. It is unusually well written, however, and those willing to expend the extra effort required will be rewarded with a deeper understanding of the characteristics of cancer.

Prescott, D. M., and Abraham S. Flexer. *Cancer: The Misguided Cell*. Sunderland, Mass.: Sinauer Associates, 1986. The authors focus primarily on how cells change during cancer. This book describes more basic biology than most of the other publications listed.

Siegel, Mary-Ellen. *The Cancer Patient's Handbook: Everything You Need to Know About Today's Care and Treatment*. New York: Walker, 1986. Siegel is a physician who explains concepts in simple terms. A very practical discussion of medical procedures related to cancer, including diagnosis and therapy. Provides descriptions of the various kinds of cancer and a useful glossary.

CANDIDIASIS

SYSTEMS AFFECTED: Blood, circulatory, gastrointestinal, immune, skin, urinary

SPECIALISTS: Family physicians, immunologists, infectious disease physicians, internists

DEFINITION: An acute or chronic fungal infection of humans and animals that can be superficial or deep-seated, caused by a species of the fungus *Candida*.

KEY TERMS:

acquired immunodeficiency syndrome (AIDS): a severe and usually fatal disease caused by infection with the human immunodeficiency virus (HIV); infection results in progressive impairment of the immune system

antifungal agents: drugs that can result in the inhibition of growth or killing of fungi; these drugs may be topical or systemic in application

cell-mediated immunity: protection mediated by thymus-derived lymphocytes; this type of immunity is particularly important for certain types of pathogenic organisms such as *Candida*

chlamydoconidia (chlamydospores): budding organisms that form directly from vegetative mycelia (molds); they differ from true spores, which are the result of sexual reproduction

culture: the propagation of organisms, such as fungi, on artificial media; *Candida* organisms grow in many kinds of media in both the yeast and mold forms

dimorphism: the ability of a fungus to exist in two forms, yeasts and molds; yeasts are unicellular round, oval, or cylindrical cells, and molds are branching tubular structures called hyphae

germ tube test: an initial laboratory test used to identify unknown yeasts and performed by microscopically examining a colony of yeast inoculated into rabbit or human plasma

histopathology: the study of the appearance and structure of abnormal or diseased tissue under the microscope

phagocytosis: the progress of ingestion and digestion by cells that are part of the immune system; this process is one of the ways that mammals use to defend themselves against infectious invaders, including *Candida* organisms

CAUSES AND SYMPTOMS

Candida is a genus of dimorphic fungi found widely in nature. This fungus may be found in soil, inanimate objects, plants, and most important, as a harmless parasite of humans and other mammals. It can exist in two forms: as a yeast and as a mold. In the yeast phase, this fungus exists as a normal inhabitant in and on human bodies. Nearly all infections are of such endogenous origin, but human-to-human transmission may occasionally occur from mother to newborn or between sexual partners. The yeasts reproduce asexually by budding, and a sexual stage has been recognized only in a few species. Pseudohyphae develop when yeasts and their progeny adhere to one another, forming chains. Hyphae, the branching tubular structures of molds, are formed in tissue invaded by the fungus.

Identification of *Candida* as the causative agent in clinical infections depends largely on the microscopic examination of infected tissue or secretions and on a culture of *Candida* prepared from infected material. Histopathological examination may reveal yeast forms and/or hyphal or pseudohyphal forms. The microscopic appearance of these organisms is similar to those of some other fungi, and a culture is necessary to confirm this fungus as the responsible pathogen. *Candida* will grow on many types of artificial microbiologic media and can usually be grown on the same media used to grow bacteria. With some types of infection, however, the use of special media or techniques may lead to a higher yield from cultures. After an unknown yeast is grown on artificial media, tests must be performed to determine its identity. Most laboratories initially use the germ tube test, in which yeast is introduced into rabbit or human plasma at 35 degrees Celsius for one to two hours. In this test, a structure called a germ tube is observed if the yeast is *Candida albicans, Candida stelloidea,* or rare strains of *Candida tropicalis.* If this test is positive (a germ tube is produced), then most laboratories assume that the microorganism is *C. albicans*—it is by far the most common species causing disease—and conduct no further, and usually more expensive, tests. Simple cultural tests may also be used to identify *C. albicans,* including the formation of spider-like colonies on eosin methylene blue agar or the production of chlamydoconidia on cornmeal agar. The identification of *Candida* antigens in the serum of patients with

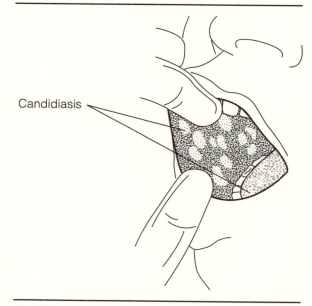

Candidiasis

Candidiasis of the mouth is a fungal infection characterized by white patches and commonly called "thrush mouth."

widespread or disseminated infection is sometimes used to assist in the diagnosis of candidiasis, but this test is neither sensitive nor specific.

The bodies of humans and other mammals possess multiple defense mechanisms against candidiasis. The skin and mucous membranes provide a protective wall, but breaks in the mucocutaneous barrier may occur in many ways, including trauma, surgery, and disease. A balanced microbial flora in the gastrointestinal tract prevents the overgrowth of *Candida* organisms, which can lead to penetration of this fungus into the lining of the gastrointestinal tract and its entrance into the bloodstream. When invasion occurs, phagocytic cells (including monocytes, neutrophils, and eosinophils) further protect the body by ingesting and killing *Candida* organisms. Phagocytosis is assisted by serum proteins called opsonins. Lymphocytes are also important defenders against this fungus and are part of the cell-mediated immune system. Candidiasis may result when cell-mediated immunity is defective, as is the case with the hereditary condition of chronic mucocutaneous candidiasis or with acquired immunodeficiency syndrome (AIDS). Approximately 80 percent of healthy people exhibit delayed hypersensitivity reactions to *Candida* antigens, indicating the presence of a previously induced cell-mediated immunity directed against such an infection.

Candidiasis may be divided into superficial mucocutaneous and deep-seated, tissue-invasive types. There are more than one hundred fifty species of this fungus, but only ten are recognized as human pathogens, and *C. albicans* is the most important. Oral candidiasis, or thrush, is a common infection characterized by white patches on the tongue and oral mucosal surfaces (oropharyngeal infection). Scrapings taken from these patches contain masses of yeasts, pseudohyphae, and hyphae. Culturing is not as useful as clinical appearance and microscopic examination, since *Candida* organisms can be grown from normal mouths. Thrush is particularly common when the immune system is impaired, as in patients with cancer or AIDS or in asthmatics treated with inhaled steroids. Infection of other parts of the gastrointestinal tract, especially the esophagus, may occur in patients with a variety of underlying conditions, including an impaired immune system, gastrointestinal surgery, and antibiotic treatment. Esophageal involvement often results in difficult or painful swallowing. Only about half of patients with esophageal candidiasis will also have the more easily diagnosed oropharyngeal infection. Some patients with gastrointestinal candidiasis will develop systemic or disseminated infection.

Vaginal candidiasis, the most common type of vaginitis, is a common form of the infection associated with an overgrowth of *Candida* organisms in the vagina followed by mucocutaneous invasion. The patient will have a thick, curdlike vaginal discharge and itching of the surrounding skin areas. Antibiotic therapy, pregnancy, birth control pills, diabetes, and AIDS all predispose women to this form of infection. Recurrent or chronic infection can occur and may be associated with tissue invasion or impaired response of lymphocytes to the infection in some patients.

Cutaneous infection is common with candidiasis. This fungus is often the cause of diaper rash in infants; the condition often results from infection of skin under wet diapers by *Candida* organisms from the gastrointestinal tract. Intertrigo is another skin condition produced by candidiasis in the warm, moist area of skin folds, and similar environments result in perianal or scrotal infections that cause intense itching (pruritus). A widespread eruption of infection involving the trunk, thorax, and extremities is occasionally seen in both children and adults. Disseminated candidiasis, usually in association with persistent candidemia (the presence of the fungus in the bloodstream), may be associated with widely distributed, nodular skin lesions. Candidiasis of the skin, mucous membranes, hair, and nails beginning early in life and associated with defective cell-mediated immunity has been called chronic mucocutaneous candidiasis. This disease is often associated with a variety of endocrine diseases, including diabetes mellitus and decreased function of the parathyroid, thyroid, and adrenal glands.

Deep-organ involvement with candidiasis is serious and often life-threatening. The placement in the body of foreign material used for medical therapy may provide the initial breeding ground for the infection. Examples of these devices are vascular catheters, artificial heart valves, artificial vascular grafts, and artificial joints and other orthopedic implants. The environment created by these foreign materials makes it impossible for the normal defense mechanisms of the body to function.

Urinary tract infection with *Candida* organisms is seen in association with urinary catheters, especially when usage is chronic. Colonization of the urine with *Candida* organisms may also occur following a course of antibiotics or in diabetic patients. Infection of the kidney can result if the candidiasis spreads upward from the bladder through the ureter or via the bloodstream. Renal involvement has been reported in up to 80 percent of patients with disseminated candidiasis. In disseminated disease, infection is spread to the kidney through the bloodstream, with the formation of renal abscesses. Primary renal infection occurs when the kidney is invaded directly without concomitant invasion through the blood. Such direct infection may occur in association with urinary catheters or following surgical procedures involving the genital and urinary tracts. A particularly severe form of ascending renal infection, more frequent in diabetic patients, causes necrosis of the renal papillae and renal failure.

Ocular candidiasis (endophthalmitis) may occur when the eye is infected with *Candida* organisms either by direct invasion or through the bloodstream. Virtually any portion or structure of the eye may be involved. Examination of the retina using an ophthalmoscope can reveal white spots, resembling cotton balls, indicating *Candida* organisms in the blood vessels of the eye. This finding may also be a clue to infection elsewhere in the body that has spread through the bloodstream to the eye.

Endocarditis (inflammation of the lining of the heart) occurs when a native or artificial heart valve becomes infected. Candidiasis is an increasingly frequent cause of endocarditis of the native valves of intravenous drug abusers and artificial valves of all varieties. Such endocarditis is presumptively diagnosed when the organism is grown from blood specimens in the presence of a heart murmur. Abnormal growth on the heart valves, called vegetation, can usually be demonstrated using echocardiography. Fragments of vegetation may break off and circulate in the bloodstream, leading to the obstruction of vessels in many organs of the body including the brain, eyes, lungs, spleen, and kidneys. Without treatment, this disease is uniformly fatal.

Disseminated candidiasis is seen in the most susceptible patients, including those with cancer, prolonged postoperative illness, and extensive burns. In these patients, further risk is associated with the use of central venous or arterial catheters, broad-spectrum antibiotic therapy, artificial feeding, or abdominal surgery. Dysfunction of neutrophils, or neutropenia, may increase the susceptibility of the patient to widespread infection with *Candida* organisms and can also be seen with AIDS. The kidney, brain, heart, and eye are the most common organs to be involved. Despite severe and extensive disease, specific diagnosis of disseminated candidiasis is difficult during life and is often only made at the time of postmortem examination.

TREATMENT AND THERAPY

Candidiasis may be prevented by avoiding or ameliorating the underlying predisposing factor or disease state and by decreasing or halting growth of the fungi. Dry or cracked skin can be treated with dermatologic lubricants. Invasive devices used for medical treatment should be placed in the body under the most sterile conditions and only employed when absolutely necessary. Care of these devices, including urinary catheters, intravascular lines, and peritoneal renal dialysis catheters must be performed by skilled personnel using the most sterile approach possible. If antibacterial therapy is used excessively, fungal overgrowth may occur; *Candida* organisms can grow with ease in the gastrointestinal tract and vagina when bacteria are inhibited or killed by antibiotics, and overgrowth can lead not only to local infection but also to bloodstream invasion and secondary infection elsewhere in the body. Moreover, the treatment of underlying disease states such as diabetes mellitus, neoplasia, and AIDS will lessen the detrimental effects of candidiasis on the immune system.

Growth of *Candida* organisms can be decreased by altering the local conditions that favor their proliferation. For example, changing a baby's diaper frequently and applying a drying powder can avoid the wet and warm conditions that can result in diaper rash. Obese patients can lose weight, which will minimize skin fold infections. Wearing non-occlusive clothing, especially cotton fabrics, is often helpful in discouraging candidiasis.

Antifungal agents are often used to prevent candidiasis. Hospitalized patients recovering from surgery who have received antibacterial agents are given nystatin, an oral, non-absorbed antifungal, to prevent the overgrowth of *Candida* organisms in the gastrointestinal tract. For cancer patients receiving chemotherapy, systemic antifungal drugs are often employed during the period when the cancer chemotherapy has had the most deleterious effects on the immune system.

Antifungals are employed by the topical, oral, parenteral (through a blood vessel or muscle), or irrigation routes for treatment of candidiasis. Among the many antifungal agents, nystatin, flucytosine, amphotericin B, and a variety of imidazole agents are the most commonly used. Antifungals utilize a number of different mechanisms that impede the metabolic activities of the organism or disrupt the integrity of the cell membrane on the outer surface of the fungus. Amphotericin B and fluconazole are useful in the treatment of systemic or deep-organ disease. Amphotericin B is produced by the fungus *Streptomyces nodosus* and is administered intravenously for systemic and deep-organ disease and by bladder irrigation for lower urinary tract infection (cystitis). When administered intravenously, amphotericin B has serious side effects, including fever, chills, kidney failure, liver abnormalities, and bone marrow suppression. Fluconazole has fewer adverse effects and can be administered by the oral or intravenous routes; for these reasons, it is now commonly used as the initial therapy for candidiasis. Amphotericin B remains the treatment of choice for serious or life-threatening infection or when a *Candida* species isolated from a patient has been demonstrated by laboratory testing to be resistant to other antifungal agents.

In addition to antifungals, removal of foreign material or infected tissue is often necessary to treat severe candidiasis. Catheters, vascular grafts, artificial heart valves, artificial joints, and other devices must be removed and then replaced, if necessary, while the patient is receiving antifungal therapy or after the infection is cured. In some cases, such as with endocarditis, the infected tissue must be surgically removed to ensure a cure.

As with prevention, treatment of the underlying disease state greatly assists other measures directed against candidiasis. Gaining control of hyperglycemia in diabetes mellitus patients, viral infection in AIDS patients, and bone marrow suppression in cancer patients will aid in the treatment of candidiasis when it is present.

PERSPECTIVE AND PROSPECTS

More than two thousand years ago, the Greek physicians Hippocrates and Galen described oral lesions that were probably thrush, but it was not until 1839 that fungi were found in such lesions. Deep-seated infection was first described in 1861, and endocarditis was identified in 1940. Candidiasis was recognized as an indicator disease in the 1987 surveillance definition for AIDS by the Centers for Disease Control in the United States. *Candida* ranks among the most common pathogens in hospital-acquired infections.

Candidiasis is on the increase largely because of increasingly sophisticated medical therapies and the worldwide epidemic of AIDS. Medical devices, immunosuppressive medical therapies, and organ transplantation are all becoming more common, and it is anticipated that candidiasis will increase in a corresponding manner. Likewise, as the number of patients infected with human immunodeficiency virus (HIV) progress to clinical illness, the cases of candidiasis are expected to rise dramatically.

More effective preventive and therapeutic measures will be necessary to combat such an increase in cases of candidiasis. New antifungal agents will need to be developed to treat resistant strains of *Candida*. Laboratory testing to determine whether various antifungal agents can kill or inhibit the growth of *Candida* species isolated from patients will need to be more widely available and more frequently performed if organisms resistant to antifungals are to be identified. Early identification of resistant organisms will benefit patients by providing more effective antifungal therapy early in the course of treatment. Testing procedures will need to employ better methodology that is standardized to enable laboratories in different locations to compare results and determine regional or national trends in antifungal resistance. —*H. Bradford Hawley*

See also Fungal infections.

FOR FURTHER INFORMATION:

De Vita, Vincent T., Jr., Samuel Hellman, and Steven A. Rosenberg. *AIDS: Etiology, Diagnosis, Treatment, and Prevention.* 3d ed. Philadelphia: J. B. Lippincott, 1992. The definitive reference text concerning acquired immunodeficiency syndrome. Contains excellent chapters describing the clinical types of candidiasis in these patients and their treatment.

Emmons, Chester W., Chapman H. Binford, John P. Utz, and K. J. Kwon-Chung. *Medical Mycology.* 3d ed. Philadelphia: Lea & Febiger, 1977. The finest text concerning fungal diseases. All aspects of these diseases, including their diagnosis and treatment, are covered. Excellent photographs of gross microscopic pathology and the appearance of the organisms are provided.

Holmberg, Kenneth, and Richard D. Meyer, eds. *Diagnosis and Therapy of Systemic Fungal Infections.* New York: Raven Press, 1989. This specialized text offers a thorough review of the various types of systemic fungal infections and appropriate preventive and therapeutic measures; the majority of this text concerns candidiasis.

Koneman, Elmer W., et al. *Color Atlas and Textbook of Diagnostic Microbiology.* 4th ed. Philadelphia: J. B. Lippincott, 1992. A practical text with excellent tables, charts, and photographs of microorganisms, including *Candida.* Also contains information on the collection of specimens from patients, the processing of cultures, and the interpretation of laboratory data.

Ledger, William J. *Infection in the Female.* 2d ed. Philadelphia: Lea & Febiger, 1986. An excellent treatise on gynecologic and obstetric infections. Offers information about the aspects of candidiasis in the female patient.

Mandell, Gerald L., R. Gordon Douglas, Jr., and John E. Bennett, eds. *Principles and Practice of Infectious Diseases.* 3d ed. New York: Churchill Livingstone, 1990. An outstanding textbook in infectious diseases, with chapters on the various diseases caused by Candida, illnesses and conditions associated with this fungus, and antifungal agents.

Reese, Richard E., and Robert F. Betts, eds. *A Practical Approach to Infectious Diseases.* 3d ed. Boston: Little, Brown, 1991. A well-written and very popular text. This clinically oriented, multiauthor book on infectious diseases, including candidiasis, contains carefully chosen, annotated references at the end of each of the twenty-eight chapters. Offers a very good section on antifungal chemotherapy.

CARCINOMA

SYSTEMS AFFECTED: All

SPECIALISTS: Dermatologists, internists, oncologists, plastic and reconstructive surgeons

DEFINITION: A carcinoma is a malignant neoplasm, or cancer, arising from the epithelial cells that make up the surface layers of skin or other membranes; by contrast, sarcomas are malignant neoplasms that arise from the mesodermal cells of connective tissue, bone, and muscle. Carcinomas commonly occur in the skin, the large intestine, the lungs, the breasts and cervix in women, and the prostate gland in men. The term "carcinoma" is often used as a synonym for "cancer."

See also Breast cancer; Cancer; Liver cancer; Lung cancer; Lymphadenopathy and lymphoma; Malignancy and metastasis; Skin cancer; Stomach, intestinal, and pancreatic cancers; Tumors.

CARIES, DENTAL

SYSTEM AFFECTED: Teeth

SPECIALISTS: Dentists

DEFINITION: Commonly known as tooth decay or cavities, dental caries are disintegrations of tooth enamel, allowing injury to the dentin below the enamel and eventually allowing injury to the pulp, which contains nerves and blood vessels. Dental caries are caused by bacteria in the mouth that produce acid. Food debris and sugars provide the fuel for bacteria development. Risk of dental caries

Development of Dental Caries

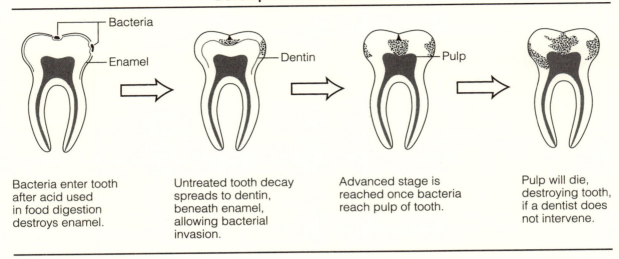

Bacteria enter tooth after acid used in food digestion destroys enamel.

Untreated tooth decay spreads to dentin, beneath enamel, allowing bacterial invasion.

Advanced stage is reached once bacteria reach pulp of tooth.

Pulp will die, destroying tooth, if a dentist does not intervene.

increases with poor nutrition and improper diet, as well as with poor dental hygiene. Existing caries can be stopped by a dentist by removing all decay and filling the space left with a metal or ceramic substance.

See also Dental diseases; Endodontic disease; Gingivitis; Periodontitis; Toothache.

CATARACTS

SYSTEM AFFECTED: Visual
SPECIALISTS: Ophthalmologists
DEFINITION: Dark regions in the lens of the eye that cause gradual loss of vision.
KEY TERMS:

artificial lens implant: a plastic lens inserted permanently into the eye to replace a defective natural lens that has been removed

cornea: the transparent front surface of the eye; its curvature produces about 60 percent of the focusing power needed to produce an image on the retina

extracapsular cataract extraction: a procedure in which the lens is emulsified (broken up) with an ultrasonic probe and the pieces are suctioned out

intracapsular cataract extraction: a procedure in which the faulty lens is removed in one piece while still inside its capsule

iris: the colored portion of the eye that regulates the amount of light entering the pupil at its center

laser: an intense light beam, used in eye surgery to reattach a detached retina or to open a secondary cataract

microsurgery: surgery performed with the aid of a microscope

retina: the dark membrane on the inside rear surface of the eye, where light is converted into nerve signals sent to the brain

CAUSES AND SYMPTOMS

Cataracts are imperfections in the clarity of the eye lens that reduce its ability to transmit light. They are a very common medical problem. In the United States, cataract removal is the most frequently performed surgery and the largest line-item cost in the Medicare budget. There are many misconceptions about cataracts. Cataracts are not an infection, a growth, a disease, or a film on the surface of the lens. They do not cause pain, redness, teardrops, or other discomforts of the eye. The initial symptom is a gradual deterioration of vision, usually in one eye at a time. There is no known treatment other than to remove the lens surgically. After surgery, neither the lens nor the cataracts can grow back. The formation of cataracts is a normal part of aging, like gray hair or hardening of the arteries. All people would develop cataracts eventually if they lived long enough.

In a discussion of cataracts, it is helpful to review the structure of the human eye. The eye is often compared to a camera, with its lens and film. The camera lens, however, can be moved back and forth slightly to focus on objects at different distances, whereas the eye lens is squeezed into a thicker shape by muscular action to change its focus. Both camera and eye have a variable-size diaphragm to regulate the amount of light that is admitted.

When light enters the eye, it first encounters a transparent, tough outer skin called the cornea. There are no blood vessels in the cornea, but many nerve cells make it sensitive to touch or other irritation. Immediately behind the cornea is the clear aqueous fluid that carries oxygen and nutrients for cell metabolism. Next comes the colored portion, the iris of the eye, with a variable-size opening at its center called the pupil. The pupil has no color, but looks black, like the opening of a cave. A person looking at his or her own eye in a mirror and then shining a flashlight on it can see the black pupil quickly shrink in size.

Next comes the lens of the eye, surrounded by an elastic membrane called the capsule. The lens is suspended by short strands, or ligaments, which are attached to a sphincter muscle. When the muscle contracts, the lens becomes thicker in the middle, thus increasing its focusing strength. The transparent lens has no blood vessels, so its metabolism is provided by the aqueous fluid. Behind the lens is the vitreous fluid, which fills about two-thirds of the eyeball and maintains its oval shape. At the back of the eye is the retina, where special visual cells convert light into electrical signals that travel to the brain via nerve fibers.

The lens of the eye is not simply a homogeneous fluid, but has a unique, internal structure and growth pattern. It continues to grow larger throughout the life of the individual. New cells originate at the front surface of the lens, just inside the capsule enclosure. These cells divide and grow into fibers that migrate toward the middle, or nucleus, of the lens. The whole structure has been compared to the layers of an onion, with the oldest cells at the center. The protein molecules in the nucleus are less soluble and more rigid than those in the outer part of the lens. By the age

of forty, in most people the firm nucleus has enlarged until the lens has lost much of its elasticity. Even with considerable muscular strain, the curvature of the lens surface will no longer bulge enough to focus on nearby objects. The eye loses its power of accommodation, and reading glasses will be needed.

The mechanism by which cataracts form in the lens is not yet clearly understood. Like the loss of accommodation, however, it is a normal part of the aging process. One proposed biochemical explanation is the Maillard reaction, in which glucose and protein molecules combine when heated to form a brown product. The Maillard reaction is responsible for the browning of bread or cookies during baking. The same process is thought to occur even at body temperature, but very slowly over a period of years. Some scientists have theorized that wrinkled skin, hardening of the arteries, and other normal features of aging may be caused by this reaction. The biochemistry of aging is an active area of research, in which the deterioration of the eye lens is only one example.

The most common symptom of cataracts is a loss of clear vision that cannot be corrected with eyeglasses. Brighter lighting can partially help to overcome the blockage of light

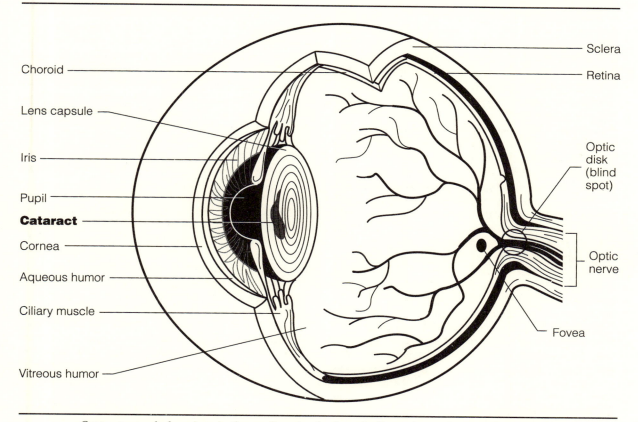

Cataracts are dark regions in the eye lens that lead gradually to obscured vision and blindness.

transmission. There is one paradoxical situation reported by some patients, however, whose vision becomes worse in bright light. The explanation for this problem is that brightness causes the pupil to become smaller. If the cataract is centered right in the middle of the lens, it will block a larger fraction of the incoming light. In dimmer light, the pupil opening is larger, so light can pass through the clear periphery of the lens.

By far the most common cataracts are those attributable to normal aging, called senile cataracts. (This has nothing to do with the common use of the term "senility" to describe declining mental ability.) So-called secondary cataracts can also develop in special circumstances. For example, exposure to X rays or nuclear radiation will increase the probability of cataracts, and the eye lens seems to be particularly sensitive to the effects of ionizing radiation. Certain medications such as cortisone, which is used in arthritis treatment, increase the risk of cataracts. A diet deficient in protein, especially in developing countries, has been associated with cataract formation. A blow to the eye from a sports injury or an accident can lead to a cataract. Diabetics are more likely to develop cataracts than the general public. Some studies have suggested that electric shock, ultraviolet rays, or certain environmental pollutants may be other causes.

Some babies are born with cataracts. These are called congenital and are frequently associated with the mother having had German measles (rubella) during the first three months of pregnancy. Surgery on the infant's eye must be done with little delay. Otherwise, the nerve connections between eye and brain will not develop, and permanent blindness can result.

Cataracts are much more prevalent in Israel and India than in Western Europe. It is not clear yet whether race or different diets and life habits are the determining factors. Some ophthalmologists believe that cataracts run in families, suggesting a genetic influence. The evidence is not conclusive, and further studies are needed. What causes cataracts is much less understood than how to treat them surgically.

TREATMENT AND THERAPY

When cataracts begin to form in the eye lens, no medication can remove them and they will not get better on their own. The patient's vision will continue to deteriorate as the cataracts mature, although the process may be quite slow. Fortunately, modern techniques of surgery for cataract removal have a success rate of better than 95 percent.

Consider a typical middle-aged man who believes that his vision is getting worse. When he goes to an optometrist, he is informed that his eye examination has revealed the onset of senile cataracts (as a result of aging). He is referred to an ophthalmologist, who finds no need for surgery at this time, but recommends more frequent, semiannual checkups. The patient is told that reading or other eye-straining activities will not accelerate cataract growth, but that brighter lighting will help him to see more clearly. During the next several years, the cataracts slowly darken and increase in size. Eventually, distant vision in one eye (even with glasses) may deteriorate to 20/160, which means that what he is able to see at 20 feet can be seen by a normal person at 160 feet. The ability of the patient to drive a car is seriously impaired, and surgery is indicated. It is not a medical emergency, but operating on one eye while the other one is still fairly clear is recommended.

Once the decision has been made to go ahead with surgery, it is necessary for the patient to have a thorough physical examination. The doctor checks for possible health problems that could complicate cataract surgery. Among these are diabetes, high blood pressure, kidney disease, anemia, and glaucoma (excess pressure in the eye). Normally, extracting the cataractous lens and implanting an artificial, plastic one are done at the same time. Before proceeding with surgery, the ophthalmologist must determine what the proper strength of the implant lens should be, so that light will focus properly on the retina. An accurate measurement is made by reflecting a beam of high-frequency sound waves (ultrasound) from the back of the eye. Measuring the time for an echo to return gives the needed data for calculating the strength of the implant lens.

On the day of the surgery, the patient is given an injection to make him drowsy and eyedrops to dilate the pupil. Gradually, more eyedrops are administered to produce a large dilation, so that access to the lens is easier. In the operating room, local anesthetic is injected to keep the eyelids from closing and to deaden the normally very sensitive surface of the cornea. To prepare for surgery, a microscope is moved into place above the eye. Making an incision in the cornea, removing the defective lens, inserting and fastening the artificial lens, and finally closing the incision with a very fine needle and thread are all performed by the surgeon while looking through the microscope. Its magnification and focus controls are operated using foot pedals, so that both of the surgeon's hands are free.

There are three basic types of cataract extraction. Each method has its advantages and disadvantages. The first method is called intracapsular extraction. The capsule is the membrane that surrounds the lens. Intracapsular means that the lens and capsule are removed together, that is, with the lens still inside its capsule. The advantage of this method is that no part of the lens is left behind to cause possible problems with infection or swelling later. The disadvantage is that the incision at the edge of the cornea must be fairly large to allow the lens and capsule to be pulled out together. Five to ten stitches are needed to close the incision. The patient must avoid strenuous activity for about a month to permit thorough healing. Before 1962, forceps were used to bring the lens and capsule out of the eye. Then Charles D. Kelman introduced the cryoprobe, which uses a freezing process. When the rather slippery lens is touched by the cold probe, it freezes to the probe and can be pulled out in one piece. Most eye surgeons have adopted the cryo-probe for intracapsular extraction.

A second method of cataract surgery is called extracapsular extraction, in which the lens is removed, while the capsule is left in the eye. The advantage is that the unbroken back surface of the capsule can prevent leakage of fluid from the rear of the eye and therefore can decrease the chances for damage to the retina. A disadvantage is that small fragments of the lens may remain behind, causing infection or irritation. The size of the incision and the recuperation period are about the same as for the intracapsular method.

The third method of cataract surgery is an improvement of extracapsular extraction, first developed by Kelman in 1967. An ultrasonic probe is used to emulsify, or break up, the lens. The small pieces are then suctioned out of the capsule while fluid is washed into the opening. The main advantage of emulsification is that the incision can be very small, because the lens is brought out in fragments, not as a whole. The incision may be only 3 millimeters long, and a single suture to close it would heal rapidly. This method requires very specialized training, however, because surgeons must learn to operate the microscope, the ultrasonic generator, and the suction apparatus with their feet while manipulating the probe with their hands.

After the eye lens has been extracted, an artificial lens is inserted in its place. The implant is made of clear plastic, about the size of an aspirin tablet. Two spring loops embedded in the plastic are used to center the implant and to keep it there permanently. A variety of different spring loop attachments has been designed by ophthalmologists. In the United States, if a particular design is prone to failure, the Food and Drug Administration (FDA) has the authority to ban its use.

To complete the surgery, the incision in the cornea is closed. During the recuperation period, the patient is instructed to avoid strenuous exercise and to protect the eye from any hard contact. Normally there is little pain, although some eye irritation should be expected during the healing process. A plastic implant lens has a fixed focal length, with no power of accommodation for different distances. It is like a box camera that gives a good picture at a set distance, while near and far objects are somewhat blurry. After the eye has healed thoroughly, the patient is fitted with prescription glasses for reading and for distant vision, respectively.

A number of minor complications can develop after cataract surgery. About one-third of the patients develop a so-called secondary cataract, which is a clouding of the capsule membrane just behind the implant. This condition is easily corrected with a laser beam to open the membrane, requiring no surgery. Another potential complication is astigmatism. The eye is squeezed and flattened slightly, and the curvature of the surface will differ between the flattened and the more rounded regions. During surgery, the symmetry of the corneal surface can be distorted if some sutures are tighter than others. Astigmatism is relatively easy to correct with prescription glasses.

All operations have some risks, and a small percentage of cataract surgeries can lead to serious complications. Among these are a detached retina, glaucoma caused by scar tissue, and hemorrhage into the vitreous fluid in front of the retina. Fortunately, such problems are rare, and the percentage of successful eye surgeries continues to improve.

PERSPECTIVE AND PROSPECTS

In the history of medicine, surgery for cataracts has been traced back to Roman times. The method was called "couching." The physician would insert a needle through the white of the eye into the lens and he would try to push the lens down out of the line of vision, leaving it in the eyeball. The procedure must have been painful, with a high chance for infection. The complete extraction of a lens from the eye was done for the first time in 1745. A French ophthalmologist named Jacques Daviel was performing a couching operation, but was unable to push the lens out of the line of sight. On the spur of the moment, he decided to make a small cut in the cornea, through which he was able to extract the lens. The operation was successful. During the following ten years, he repeated his procedure more than four hundred times with only fifty failures, a much better result than with couching.

A major advance in eye surgery was the discovery of local anesthesia by Carl Koller in 1884. Together with the famous psychiatrist Sigmund Freud, Koller had been investigating the psychological effects of cocaine. He noticed that his tongue became numb from the drug and wondered if a drop of cocaine solution locally applied to the eyes might work as an anesthetic. He tried it first on a frog's eye and then on himself, and the cocaine made his eye numb. He published a short article, and the news spread to other physicians. Synthetic substitutes such as novocaine were developed and came into common use, thereafter making eye surgery virtually painless.

When the lens of the eye is surgically removed, it becomes impossible to focus light on the retina. A strong replacement lens is needed. For example, the French painter Claude Monet had cataract surgery in the 1920's, and photographs show him with the typical thick cataract glasses of that time. Today, contact lenses or artificial lens implants are much better alternatives to restore good vision.

The recovery period after cataract surgery used to be several weeks of bed rest, with the head kept absolutely still, because the cut in the cornea had to heal itself without any stitches. The development of microsurgery made it possible for the surgeon to see the extremely fine thread and needle that can be used for closing the cut. With stitches in place, the patient can usually carry on normal activities within a day after surgery.

In the 1960's, the cryoprobe and the ultrasound probe were developed to replace forceps for removing an eye lens. The size of the required incision was smaller and the healing time correspondingly shorter. In the 1980's, reliable lens implants became available, making near-normal vision possible again. In the future, perhaps drugs can be found that will prevent or delay the onset of cataracts, so that surgery will not be necessary. Further research is needed to obtain a better understanding of biochemical changes in the eye lens that occur with aging.

—*Hans G. Graetzer*

See also Aging; Blindness; Visual disorders.

FOR FURTHER INFORMATION:

Eden, John. *The Physician's Guide to Cataracts, Glaucoma, and Other Eye Problems*. Yonkers, N.Y.: Consumers Reports Books, 1992. The author, an ophthalmologist, describes the medical history of a typical cataract patient in her sixties: the original diagnosis, gradually deteriorating vision, surgery with the insertion of an artificial lens implant, postoperative care, and the fitting of prescription glasses. Informative and reassuring.

Houseman, William. "The Day the Light Returned." *New Choices for Retirement Living* 32 (April, 1992): 54-58. A personal account of a patient who had successful cataract surgery. Under local anesthetic, his faulty eye lens was removed and a plastic lens was inserted. The whole procedure took only half a day. The initial eye examination and follow-up care after surgery are described.

Kelman, Charles D. *Cataracts: What You Must Know About Them*. New York: Crown, 1982. The author is one of the world's leading cataract surgeons. In the 1960's, he invented the cryogenic probe and later the ultrasonic procedure for removing a faulty lens. This book describes cataract formation, eye surgery, lens implantation (with enlarged photographs), and possible medical complications. Highly recommended.

Lerman, Sidney. "Cataracts." *Scientific American* 206 (March, 1962): 106-114. An informative, basic article on the structure of the normal eye and the formation of cataracts as a result of aging, radiation exposure, or other factors. Excellent illustrations and accompanying explanations.

Ravin, James G. "Monet's Cataracts." *Journal of the American Medical Association* 254 (July, 1985): 394-399. Monet was a famous French painter who had cataract surgery in 1922. The article gives interesting details about the operation, his recovery (lying immobilized with sandbags for ten days), and his difficulty with the thick eyeglasses of that era. A fascinating story.

Shulman, Julius. *Cataracts: The Complete Guide—from Diagnosis to Recovery—for Patients and Families*. New York: Simon & Schuster, 1984. A concise, well-written book by an ophthalmologist to educate patients who may need cataract surgery. Using nontechnical language and helpful diagrams, Shulman explains several methods for extracting the eye lens. Authoritative and highly recommended. Printed in large type for easier reading.

Van Heyningen, Ruth. "What Happens to the Human Lens in Cataract." *Scientific American* 233 (December, 1975): 70. The structure of the human eye is described, with a labeled cutaway drawing. Mechanical stress, a high blood sugar level, and other factors are identified as potential causes for the deteriorating transparency within the lens. Offers good explanations.

CEREBRAL PALSY

SYSTEMS AFFECTED: Muscular, skeletal, nervous

SPECIALISTS: Embryologists, neurologists, orthopedic surgeons, physical therapists, speech pathologists

DEFINITION: Cerebral palsy is a term applied to a variety of nonprogressive muscular and nervous system disorders caused by brain damage occurring to a child during pregnancy or birth. Risks to the newborn increase with prematurity and the mother's alcohol consumption during pregnancy. The symptoms of cerebral palsy include lack of muscle tone, slow development, unusual body posture, stiffness, and muscle spasms. More severe cases include widespread loss of muscular control, seizures, and mental retardation, as well as deficiencies in speech, vision, and hearing. Treatment may include orthopedic braces, surgical correction of some deformities, physical and speech therapy, and medication to control seizures and relieve spasms.

See also Hemiplegia; Palsy; Paraplegia; Quadriplegia.

Spastic Cerebral Palsy

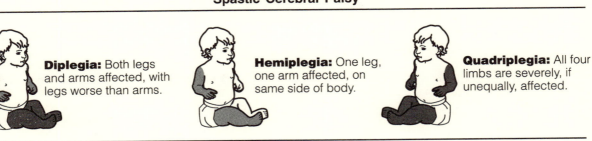

Diplegia: Both legs and arms affected, with legs worse than arms.

Hemiplegia: One leg, one arm affected, on same side of body.

Quadriplegia: All four limbs are severely, if unequally, affected.

CERVICAL, OVARIAN, AND UTERINE CANCERS

SYSTEM AFFECTED: Reproductive (female)

SPECIALISTS: Gynecologists, obstetricians, oncologists

DEFINITION: The primary cancers of the female reproductive system.

KEY TERMS:

benign: referring to a tumor made of a mass of cells which do not leave the site where they develop

cancer: one of a group of diseases in which cells divide uncontrollably; cancerous tissues do not contribute to the function of the body

cervix: the narrowest part of the uterus, which opens into the vagina

endometrium: the inner lining of the uterus, which normally thickens and then is sloughed off during each menstrual cycle; estrogens cause its growth and development, and progesterone prepares it for possible pregnancy

malignant: referring to a tumor which is capable of losing cells, which can travel via blood or lymph fluid to other sites

metastasis: the process by which malignant tumors invade other tissues either locally or distally

neoplasm: the new and abnormal formation of a tumor

ovary: the female gonad located in the pelvic cavity, where egg production occurs; the principal organ that produces the hormones estrogen and progesterone

tumor: a mass of cells characterized by uncontrolled growth; it can be either benign or malignant

uterus: the female organ in which the embryo develops; it is located in the pelvic cavity and is connected to the ovaries by the uterine tubes

CAUSES AND SYMPTOMS

Although people commonly talk about cancer as a single disease, it actually includes more than one hundred different diseases. These diseases do appear to have a common element to them. All cancer cells divide without obeying the normal control mechanisms. These abnormal cells have altered deoxyribonucleic acid (DNA) that causes them to divide and form other abnormal cells, which again divide and eventually form a neoplasm, or tumor.

If the neoplasm has the potential to leave its original site and invade other tissues, it is called malignant. If the tumor stays in one place, it is benign. One major difference between these tumors is that malignant cells seem to have lost the cellular glue that holds them to one another. Therefore, they can metastasize, leaving the tumor and infiltrating nearby tissues. Metastatic cells can also travel to distant sites via the blood or lymph systems.

Medical scientists do not know exactly what causes a cell to become cancerous. In fact, it is likely that several different factors in some combination cause cancer. Genetic, viral, hormonal, immunological, toxic, and physical factors may all play a role. Whatever the cause, cancer is

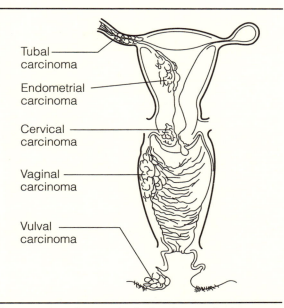

Common sites of cancer in the female reproductive system.

a common disease, resulting in one out of five deaths in the United States. Tumors of the reproductive tract occur in relatively high rates in women. Cervical cancer accounts for 6 percent, ovarian cancer 5 percent, and cancer of the lining of the uterus (endometrial cancer) 7 percent of all cancers in women.

Cervical cancer is most frequently found in women who are between forty and forty-nine years of age, but the incidence has been steadily increasing in younger women. Several factors appear to be involved in initiating this cancer: young age at first intercourse, number of sexual partners (as well as the number of the partner's partners), infection with sexually transmitted diseases such as herpes simplex type 2 and human papilloma virus, and cigarette smoking. Since most patients do not experience symptoms, regular checkups are necessary. The Pap (Papanicolaou) smear performed in a physician's office will detect the presence of cervical cancer. In this procedure, the physician obtains a sample of the cervix by swabbing the area and placing the cells on a microscope slide for examination.

Ovarian cancer accounts for more deaths than any other cancer of the female reproductive system. While the cause of ovarian cancer is unknown, the risk is greatest for women who have not had children. Ovarian cancer does not appear to run in families, and its incidence is slightly decreased in women who use oral contraceptives for many years. Ovarian tumors generally affect women over fifty years of age.

There are two major types of ovarian cancer: epithelial and germ cell neoplasms. About 90 percent of ovarian cancers are epithelial and develop on the surface of the ovary.

These tumors often are bulky and involve both ovaries. Germ cell tumors are derived from the eggs within the ovary and, if malignant, tend to be highly aggressive. Malignant germ cell neoplasms tend to occur in women under the age of thirty.

Ovarian cancer is generally considered a silent disease, as the signs and symptoms are vague and often ignored. Abdominal pain is the most obvious symptom, followed by abdominal swelling. Some patients also report gastrointestinal disorders such as changes in bowel habits. Abnormal vaginal bleeding may occur but like the other symptoms is not specific for the disease. Diagnosis is made using imaging techniques such as ultrasound, computed tomography (CT) scanning, and magnetic resonance imaging (MRI).

Uterine cancer, also known as endometrial cancer, most frequently affects women between the ages of fifty and sixty-five. Like most cancers, the cause of endometrial cancer is not clear. Nevertheless, relatively high levels of estrogens have been identified as a risk factor. For example, obese women, women who have an early onset of their first period (menarche), and women who never became pregnant tend to have high estrogen levels for longer durations than those without these conditions. Medical scientists believe not only that it is estrogens that are important but also that the other ovarian hormone, progesterone, must be lower than normal for the cancer to develop. Therefore, progesterone appears to have a protective effect in endometrial cancer. Detection of endometrial cancer is accomplished by having a physician take a small tissue sample (biopsy) from the lining of the uterus. The sample can be examined under the microscope to determine if the cells are cancerous.

TREATMENT AND THERAPY

A variety of treatments are available for patients with cancers of the reproductive tract: surgical removal of the organ, hormonal therapy, chemotherapy, or radiation therapy.

The treatment of cervical cancer depends on the size and location of the tumor and whether the cells are benign or malignant. If the patient is no longer capable of or interested in childbearing, then she may choose to have her uterus, including the cervix, removed in the procedure known as hysterectomy. The physician may also use a laser, cryotherapy (use of a cold instrument), or electrocautery (use of a hot instrument) to destroy the tumor without removing the uterus. Malignant tumors may require a total hysterectomy and removal of associated lymph nodes, which can trap metastatic cells. This surgery may be followed by radiation or chemotherapy if there is a possibility that all cancer cells have not been removed.

Cervical cancer diagnosed in a pregnant patient can complicate the treatment. Fortunately, only about 1 percent of cervical cancers are found in pregnant women. If the cancer is restricted to the cervix (that is, it has not metastasized), treatment is usually delayed until after childbirth. It is in-teresting to note that a normal vaginal delivery may occur without harming the mother or the infant. Malignant cervical cancer must be treated in a similar way as in non-pregnant women. If the cancer is found in the first trimester, a hysterectomy or radiation therapy or both is used to help eradicate the malignancy. Obviously, these approaches terminate the pregnancy. During the second trimester, the uterus must be emptied of the fetus and placenta, followed by radiation therapy or removal of the affected reproductive organs. In the third trimester, the physician will typically try to delay treatment until he or she believes that the fetus has developed sufficiently to stay alive when delivered by cesarean section. A vaginal delivery is not recommended, as it has been shown to lower the cure rate of malignant cervical cancer. Treatment after delivery consists of surgery, radiation therapy, and chemotherapy.

The prognosis in patients who have elected surgical removal of the tumor is a five-year survival rate of up to 90 percent. Cure rates for patients undergoing radiation therapy are between 75 and 90 percent. Chemotherapeutic agents have not had as much effect, as they significantly reduce only 25 percent of tumors. It is important to note that the best outcomes are achieved with early diagnosis.

Ovarian cancers are treated with a similar approach. Surgery may involve the removal of the ovaries, uterine tubes, and uterus, as well as associated lymph nodes depending upon the extent of malignancy. Radiation and chemotherapy are usually employed but oftentimes are not effective. The drug taxol is a relatively new agent which shows some promise in treating ovarian cancers. This drug was isolated from the bark of the yew tree and shows some specificity for ovarian tumors. Taxol prevents cell division in ovarian tumors, slowing the progression of the disease.

The outcome for ovarian cancer is usually not as good as for cervical and endometrial cancers, since the disease is usually in an advanced stage by the time that it is diagnosed. The overall survival rate without evidence of recurrence in patients with epithelial ovarian cancers is between 15 and 45 percent. The more uncommon germ cell ovarian cancers have a much more variable prognosis. With early diagnosis, aggressive surgery, and the use of newer chemotherapeutic agents, the long-term survival rate for all ovarian cancer patients approaches 70 percent.

Surgery is often the treatment of choice for endometrial cancer. As with cervical cancer, however, treatment depends upon the extent of the disease and the patient's wishes relative to reproductive capabilities and family planning. A hysterectomy—removal of the uterine tubes, ovaries, and surrounding lymph nodes—is usually indicated. Chemotherapy and radiation therapy are occasionally utilized as adjunctive therapy, as is progesterone. Progesterone (medroxyprogesterone or hydroxyprogesterone) may benefit patients with advanced disease, as it seems to cause a decrease in tumor size and regression of metastases. In fact, progesterone therapy in patients with advanced or recurrent endometrial cancer leads to regression in about 40 percent of cases. Progesterone therapy also has produced regression in tumors that have metastasized to the lungs, vagina, and chest cavity.

The outcome of endometrial cancer is influenced by the aggressiveness of the tumor, the age of the woman (older women tend to have a poorer prognosis), and the stage at which the cancer was detected. Almost two-thirds of all patients live without evidence of disease for five or more years after treatment. Unfortunately, 28 percent die within five years. For cancer identified and treated early, almost 90 percent of patients are alive five years after treatment.

PERSPECTIVE AND PROSPECTS

Even though medical science has advanced the ability to detect and treat cancers much earlier, many lives are still lost to cancer each year. Therefore, as with most diseases, prevention may be a significant way to reduce one's chances of getting cancer, as well as of reducing the effects of cancer itself.

The National Institutes of Health and the American Cancer Society have made several suggestions which can be followed to reduce the risk of cancer. The dietary guidelines include reducing fat intake to less than 30 percent of total calories, eating more high-fiber foods such as whole-grain breads and cereals, and eating more fruits and vegetables in general and in particular those high in vitamins A, C, and E.

Scheduling regular checkups with a health care provider may increase the likelihood of detecting cervical, ovarian, and uterine cancers early, even if no symptoms are present. Pelvic examinations should be performed every three years for women under the age of forty and yearly thereafter. Pap smear tests for cervical cancer should be undertaken yearly from the time that a woman becomes sexually active. Some physicians will take an endometrial tissue biopsy from women at high risk and at the time of the menopause.

Some data suggest that modifying lifestyle may help reduce the incidence of cervical cancer. The cervix is exposed to a variety of factors during intercourse, including infections and physical trauma. Multiple sexual partners increases the risk of sexually transmitted diseases which may predispose the cervix to cancer. This factor is compounded by the fact that infectious agents and other carcinogens can be transmitted from one individual to another. Therefore, theoretically the cervix can be exposed to carcinogens from a partner's sexual partners. Regular intercourse begun in the early teens also predisposes one to cervical cancer, as the tissue of the cervix may be more vulnerable at puberty. Barrier methods of contraception, mainly the condom, reduce the risk of developing cervical cancer by reducing the exposure of the cervix to potential carcinogens. Smoking also increases the risk of cervical cancer, perhaps because carcinogens in tobacco enter the blood which in turn has access to the cervix. Thus, such lifestyle changes as safer sexual practices, quitting smoking, and dietary changes would be beneficial to someone wanting to reduce the chance of having cervical cancer.

Women who are twenty or more pounds over ideal body weight are twice as likely to develop endometrial cancer, and the risk increases with increased body fat. Some estrogens are produced in fat tissue, and this additional estrogen may play a role in the development of endometrial cancer. Therefore, reduction of excess body fat through diet and exercise would be important for a woman who wished to reduce her chances of developing uterine cancer.

—*Matthew Berria*

See also Cancer; Female genital disorders; Malignancy and metastasis.

FOR FURTHER INFORMATION:

Clayman, Charles B., ed. *The American Medical Association Encyclopedia of Medicine*. New York: Random House, 1989. This encyclopedia lists in alphabetical order medical terms, diseases, and medical procedures. It does an excellent job of explaining the different types of cancer and their treatments.

Fox, Stuart I. *Perspectives on Human Biology*. Dubuque, Iowa: Wm. C. Brown, 1991. Chapter 14 provides the nonscientist with a basic understanding of cancer biology. Fox explains how oncogenes are thought to act in the formation of neoplasms and how antioxidant vitamins may protect against certain forms of cancer.

Hales, Dianne. *An Invitation to Health*. 4th ed. Redwood City, Calif.: Benjamin/Cummings, 1989. This text should be read by anyone who wishes an overview of health topics. Particularly important reading for those interested in the prevention of cancer.

Mader, Sylvia S. *Human Biology*. 3d ed. Dubuque, Iowa: Wm. C. Brown, 1992. Chapter 20 is devoted to a discussion of cancer and provides an excellent overview of cancer biology. This text was written for the nonscientist yet details contemporary theories on cancer formation and treatment.

Rosenfeld, Isadore. *Modern Prevention: The New Medicine*. New York: Linden Press/Simon & Schuster, 1986. An easy-to-read book. The author is a practicing physician with the ability to communicate to patients in a down-to-earth style. Rosenfeld addresses the causes and prevention of cancer in chapter 23.

CHEST PAIN. *See* HEART ATTACK; PAIN, TYPES OF.

CHICKENPOX

SYSTEMS AFFECTED: Skin, respiratory, mucous membranes

SPECIALISTS: Dermatologists, family physicians, infectious disease physicians, internists

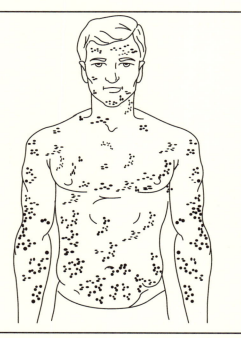

Chickenpox causes skin eruptions that form blisters and itch; although children are the most common victims of the disease, adults may also catch it (often if they did not have it as children), and the results can be more serious, including longer recovery periods and greater risk of complications, such as male sterility.

DEFINITION: Chickenpox is a very contagious though mild disease caused by the herpes zoster virus. Affecting all ages, but mostly children between the ages of five and ten, chickenpox causes fever, abdominal pain, and skin eruptions almost anywhere on the body, including the scalp, mouth, nose, throat, penis, or vagina. Blisters erupt every three to four days and collapse within twenty-four hours, forming scabs. Recovery for children usually occurs in seven to ten days. Adults take longer to recover, have more severe symptoms, and are more likely to develop complications, such as sterility in men and pneumonia. Symptoms may be treated with wet compresses and a cool environment to reduce itching; bed rest, fluids, and medication may be used to reduce fever.

See also Childhood infectious diseases; Herpes; Shingles.

CHILD ABUSE. *See* DOMESTIC VIOLENCE.

CHILDBIRTH

SYSTEMS AFFECTED: Reproductive (female), psychic-emotional

SPECIALISTS: Gynecologists, neonatologists, obstetricians, perinatologists

DEFINITION: The process whereby a fetus moves from the uterus to the outside of the mother's body—a natural event that normally requires no, or minimal, medical intervention.

KEY TERMS:

birth canal: the passageway from the uterus to the outside of the mother's body formed by the fully opened cervix in continuity with the vagina

cervix: a ring of tissue at the lowest and narrowest part of the uterus forming a canal that opens into the vagina

contraction: a squeezing action of the uterus that results in birth

dilation: the opening of the cervix to allow passage of the fetus through the birth canal

hormone: a chemical carried in the blood that acts as a messenger between two or more body parts

labor: the period in the birth process in which forceful and rhythmic uterine contractions are present

parturition: the process or action of giving birth

placenta: a structure located inside the uterus during pregnancy that provides oxygen to the fetus, removes fetal wastes, and produces hormones; also known as the afterbirth

prostaglandins: chemical messengers that are not carried in the blood and that function only locally

uterus: the organ in the female pelvis that supports the fetus during pregnancy and expels it during birth; also known as the womb

vagina: the stretchy tubular structure that leads from the uterus to the outside of the mother's body; part of the birth canal

PROCESS AND EFFECTS

In humans, pregnancy lasts an average of forty weeks, counting from the first day of the woman's last menstrual cycle. Actually, ovulation, and therefore conception and the start of pregnancy, does not normally occur until about two weeks after the beginning of the last menstrual period, but because there is no good external indicator of the time of ovulation, obstetricians typically count the weeks of pregnancy using the easily observed last period of menstrual bleeding as a reference point. Because of the uncertainty about the actual time of ovulation and conception, the calculated due date for an infant's birth may be inaccurate by as much as two weeks in either direction.

There is incomplete understanding of the processes that determine the timing and initiation of childbirth. Near the end of pregnancy, the uterus undergoes changes that prepare it for the birth process: The cervix softens and becomes stretchy, the cells in the uterus acquire characteristics that enable them to contract in a coordinated fashion, and the uterus becomes more responsive to hormones that cause contractions.

A number of substances are involved in the preparation of the uterus for birth, including the hormones estrogen and progesterone (produced within the placenta), the hormone relaxin (from the maternal ovary and/or uterus), and prostaglandins (produced within the uterus). The fetus participates in this preparation, since it provides precursors necessary for the uterine synthesis of estrogens. In addition, the amnion and chorion, two membranes surrounding the fetus, are capable of producing prostaglandins that assist in the preparation of the uterus.

Once labor begins, the hormone oxytocin (from the maternal pituitary gland) and uterine prostaglandins cause uterine contractions. It is not known what triggers the onset of labor or how the preparatory hormones and prostaglandins work together.

In humans, the onset of labor is indicated by one or more of three signs: the beginning of regular, rhythmic uterine contractions; the rupture of the amniotic membrane, a painless event that is usually accompanied by the leakage of clear fluid from the vagina; and the expulsion of a slightly bloody mucus plug from the cervix, which is an indication that the cervix is beginning to dilate. These signs may appear in any order, or occasionally one sign may be absent or unnoticed. For example, the amniotic membrane may fail to rupture spontaneously; in this case, the attendant will usually pierce the membrane in order to facilitate the birth.

Uterine contractions are the most prominent indication of labor, which is divided into three stages. In the first stage of labor, the contractions have the effect of dilating the cervix from its initial size of only a few millimeters to full dilation of 10 centimeters, large enough to permit the passage of the fetus. When the first stage of labor starts, the contractions may be up to twenty minutes apart, with each contraction of relatively short duration. As the first stage progresses, the contractions become longer and closer together, so that by the end of the first stage there may be

Stages of Childbirth

Stage one

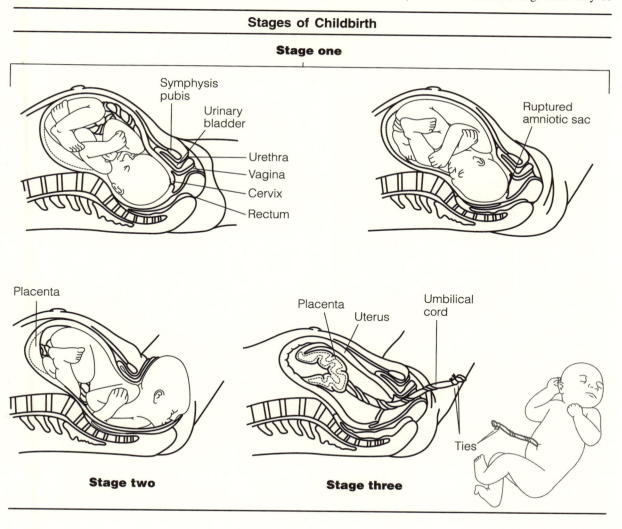

Symphysis pubis
Urinary bladder
Urethra
Vagina
Cervix
Rectum

Ruptured amniotic sac

Placenta

Stage two

Placenta
Uterus
Umbilical cord
Ties

Stage three

only a minute between contractions. There is no downward movement of the fetus during the first stage of labor, but the contractions do force the fetus against the cervix, and this force is important in causing cervical dilation. This first stage lasts for an average of eleven hours in women giving birth for the first time, but up to twenty hours is considered normal. The average length of the first stage of labor in women who have previously delivered is reduced to seven hours, with a norm of up to fourteen hours.

In the second stage of labor, the fetus moves downward through the fully dilated cervix and then into the vagina as a result of the force exerted by the continuing uterine contractions. Voluntary contractions of the abdominal muscles by the mother can help shorten this stage of labor by applying additional force, but in the absence of voluntary contractions (as with an anesthetized mother), the uterine contractions are usually sufficient to cause delivery. In 96 percent of human births, the fetus is situated so that the head is downward and thus is first to pass through the birth canal. Because the vagina does not lie in the same line as the cervix and uterus, the head of the fetus must flex and rotate as the fetus progresses downward past the mother's pelvic bones. The final barrier to the birth of the fetus is the soft tissue surrounding the vaginal opening; once the head of the fetus passes through and stretches this opening, the rest of the body usually slips out readily. The average duration of this second stage of labor in women delivering for the first time is slightly more than one hour; the average duration is shortened to twenty-four minutes in women who have previously delivered. Most women agree that the actual birth of the child during the second stage is less uncomfortable than the strong uterine contractions that occur at the very end of the first stage of labor, when the cervix is dilating the last centimeter or so.

Most infants begin to take regular, deep breaths immediately upon delivery. These breaths serve to inflate the lungs with air for the first time. The infant now becomes dependent on breathing to supply oxygen to the blood, whereas oxygen had been supplied to the fetal blood by circulation through the placenta.

Following delivery of the infant, the mother enters the third stage of labor, during which continued uterine contractions serve to reduce the size of the uterus and expel the placenta. The placenta usually separates from the uterus and is expelled five to fifteen minutes after the birth of the infant.

Uterine contractions do not end with the delivery of the placenta; they continue, with decreasing frequency and intensity, for as long as six weeks following childbirth. These later contractions, known as afterpains, serve to reduce bleeding from the site of placental attachment and to return the uterus and cervix to their pre-pregnancy condition.

Another significant process that occurs in the mother's body following delivery is the onset of milk production.

During pregnancy, the breasts are prepared for later milk production by a number of hormones, but actual milk production does not begin until about the second day after delivery. It appears that the decrease in progesterone levels caused by the removal of the placenta at birth allows milk production to commence.

Most obstetrical attendants agree that the ideal childbirth situation is a labor and delivery with a minimum of medical intervention. If all goes well, the role of the attendant will be primarily that of a support person. Most women are admitted to a hospital or birthing center during the first stage of labor. The mother's blood pressure and temperature will be frequently checked. In addition, the strength and timing of contractions will be assessed either by a hand placed lightly on the abdomen or by an electronic monitor that detects uterine activity through a sensor belt placed around the abdomen. The fetal heart rate will be measured with a stethoscope or by an electrical lead placed on the fetus' scalp through the cervix. Cervical dilation can be assessed by a vaginal examination: The attendant will insert one or more fingers into the cervix to determine its state of dilation. It is also important that the attendant provide emotional support and reassurance to the mother throughout the delivery.

During the second stage of labor, the attendant will monitor the progress of the fetus through the birth canal. By inserting a hand into the vagina and feeling for the fetal skull bones, the attendant can determine the exact placement of the fetus within the birth canal. As the infant's head appears at the vaginal opening, an incision called an episiotomy is usually performed to prevent accidental tearing of these tissues. Many physicians believe that episiotomy should be done to prevent possible vaginal tearing, since a planned incision is easier to repair than an accidental tear. Another advantage of episiotomy is that it tends to speed the expulsion of the infant, which may be an advantage to both the mother and the child at this stage. The episiotomy incision is made after the injection of a local anesthetic to numb the area, and the incision is stitched closed following the delivery of the placenta.

Once the infant's head has emerged from the vagina, the attendant uses a suction device to clear the infant's nose and mouth of fluid. As the rest of the infant emerges, the attendant supports the body; a quick examination is conducted at this time to determine whether the infant has any major health problems. The umbilical cord that joins the infant to the placenta is usually cut within a few minutes after birth. When the placenta is delivered, the attendant will examine it for completeness and then will perform a thorough examination of the mother and child to ensure that all is well.

COMPLICATIONS AND DISORDERS

If the labor and delivery do not progress normally, the attendant has available a number of medical interventions that will promote the safety of both the mother and the baby. For example, labor may be induced by administration of oxytocin through an intravenous catheter. Such induction is performed if the amniotic membrane ruptures without the spontaneous onset of uterine contractions or if the pregnancy progresses well beyond the due date. The induction of labor has been found to be safe, but careful monitoring of the progress of labor is required.

Another fairly common procedure is the use of forceps to assist delivery. These tonglike instruments have two large loops that are placed on the sides of the fetal head when the head is in the birth canal. Forceps are not used to pull the fetus from the birth canal; instead, they are used to guide the fetus through the birth canal and to assist in the downward movement of the fetus during contractions. The use of forceps can help to speed the second stage of labor, and injury to the fetus or the mother is minimal when the forceps are not applied until the fetal head is well within the birth canal, as is the convention. Some type of anesthesia is always used with a forceps delivery. In some areas, vacuum extraction of the fetus is preferred. As the name implies, vacuum extraction makes use of a suction cup on the end of a vacuum hose; the suction cup is affixed to the fetal scalp.

Many women require some type of pain relief during labor, although this need can be reduced by thorough education and preparedness during the pregnancy. A wide range of pain-reducing drugs (analgesics), sedatives, and tranquilizers is available for use during the first stage of labor. These are typically administered by injection; they work at the level of the brain to alter the perception of pain and to promote relaxation. The goal is to use the minimum drug dose that allows the woman to be comfortable. The main danger is that these drugs reach the fetus through the placental circulation; side effects in the infant, which can persist for many hours after delivery, may include depressed respiration, irregular heart rhythm or rate, and sleepiness accompanied by poor suckling response.

Anesthetics that numb pain-carrying nerves in the mother may also be used during the first and second stages of labor. Two routes of delivery are in common use: epidural and spinal, both of which involve the injection of anesthetic drugs into or near the membranes around the mother's spinal cord. The epidural route of injection places the anesthetic in a space that lies outside the spinal cord membranes; with spinal anesthesia, the injection is made slightly deeper into the membranous layers. An advantage of both methods is that the mother remains awake during the delivery and can assist by pushing during the second stage. There are no direct effects of the anesthetics on the infant, since the drugs are not carried in the blood. Nevertheless, the use of such anesthesia is associated with a prolongation of the second stage of labor and with increased need for forceps to assist delivery. Headaches and other side effects

may also result in the mother following the use of spinal anesthesia.

General anesthesia refers to the use of drugs that induce sleep; they may be administered by inhalation or by injection. Because of profound side effects in both the mother and child, most physicians use general anesthesia only in an emergency situation requiring an immediate cesarean section.

Cesarean section refers to the delivery of the fetus through an incision made in the mother's abdominal and uterine walls. (The name derives from an unsubstantiated legend that Julius Caesar was delivered in this way.) Cesarean deliveries may be planned in advance, as when a physician notes that the fetus is in a difficult-to-deliver position, such as breech (buttocks downward) or transverse (sideways). Multiple fetuses may also be delivered by cesarean section in order to spare the mother and her infants excessive stress. Alternatively, cesarean delivery may be performed as an emergency measure, perhaps after labor has started. One indication of the need for emergency cesarean delivery is fetal distress, a condition characterized by an abnormal fetal heart rate and rhythm. Fetal distress is thought to be an indication of reduced blood flow to the placenta, which may be life-threatening to the fetus. Cesarean section may be performed using spinal or epidural anesthesia, as well as general anesthesia. A woman who delivers one child by cesarean section does not necessarily require a cesarean for later deliveries; each pregnancy is evaluated separately.

PERSPECTIVE AND PROSPECTS

Prior to 1800 in the United States, most women were attended during childbirth by female midwives. In some areas, a midwife was provided a salary by the town or region; her contract might stipulate that she provide services to all women regardless of financial or social status. In other areas, midwives worked for fees paid by the clients. Midwives of this time had little, if any, formal training and learned about birth practices from other women. Because birth was considered a natural event requiring little intervention on the part of the attendant, the midwife's medical role was limited and the few doctors available were consulted only in difficult cases. Although birth statistics were not kept at the time, anecdotal accounts from the diaries of midwives and doctors suggest that the births were most often successful, with rare cases of maternal or infant deaths.

The nineteenth century saw a gradual shift away from the use of midwives to a preference for formally trained male doctors. This shift was made possible by the establishment of medical schools that provided scientific training in obstetrics. Because these schools were generally closed to women, only men received this training and had access to the instruments and anesthesia that were coming into use.

Maternity hospitals came into being during the 1800's but were at first used primarily by poor or unmarried women. Women of higher social status still preferred to deliver their children in the privacy of their homes. Indeed, home birth was safer than hospital birth, since the building of hospitals had outpaced the knowledge of how to sanitize them. Rates of infection and maternal and infant death were higher in hospitals than in homes.

By the 1930's, the situation had reversed: Hospital births had become safer than home births, because sanitation and surgical procedures had improved. There followed an increasing trend for women to enter hospitals for delivery, so that the percentage of women giving birth in hospitals increased from about 25 percent in 1930 to almost 100 percent by 1960. In the same period, maternal and infant mortality showed a dramatic reduction. The shift to hospital birth had coincided with an interventionist philosophy: Most women were anesthetized during delivery, and forceps deliveries and episiotomy became more common.

By the 1960's, the older idea of "natural" childbirth—that is, a birth with as little medical intervention as possible—had regained popularity. This change in attitude was brought about in part by recognition that analgesic and anesthetic drugs often had profound effects on the infant. Psychologists also pointed out the need for maternal-infant bonding in the immediate hours after delivery. By the latter part of the twentieth century, a compromise between the more radical approaches of the past seemed to have been reached, with common practice in obstetrics being to allow the birth to proceed naturally when possible, but with the advantage of having refined drugs, diagnostics, and surgical techniques available if needed. The midwife had been reinstated as a specially trained nurse who could supervise normal births and provide educated assistance at difficult ones. —*Marcia Watson-Whitmyre*

See also Birth defects; Breast-feeding; Childbirth, complications of; Conception; Miscarriage; Postpartum depression; Pregnancy and gestation; Premature birth; Stillbirth.

FOR FURTHER INFORMATION:

Chestnut, David H., ed. *Obstetric Analgesia and Anesthesia*. Philadelphia: Harper & Row, 1987. Noteworthy for its completeness, this volume contains individual chapters covering specialized aspects of obstetric anesthesia. One chapter covers prepared childbirth as a technique for pain management.

Creasy, Robert K., and Robert Resnik, eds. *Maternal-Fetal Medicine: Principles and Practice*. 2d ed. Philadelphia: W. B. Saunders, 1989. This complete text covers all aspects of pregnancy and delivery, from conception to medical care of the newborn. Chapters cover normal physiology as well as problems and their treatment.

Cunningham, F. Gary, Paul C. MacDonald, and Norman F. Gant. *Williams Obstetrics*. 18th ed. Norwalk, Conn.: Appleton and Lange, 1989. This standard medical school text is still named in honor of its first author, J. Whitridge Williams, who was a professor of obstetrics at The Johns Hopkins Medical School at the beginning of the twenti-

eth century. Although written for the medical specialist, this work is fairly easy to read.

Lieberman, Adrienne B. *Giving Birth*. New York: St. Martin's Press, 1987. Written by a natural-childbirth instructor, this guide for expectant parents contains twelve first-hand accounts of birth experiences. Medical issues are well explained. Contains a chapter on home birth.

Quilligan, Edward J., and Frederick P. Zuspan, eds. *Current Therapy in Obstetrics and Gynecology*. Philadelphia: W. B. Saunders, 1990. Short sections cover the treatment of most reproductive and infant health problems. This compact book contains a wealth of information, such as charts showing fetal weight at different points in pregnancy, the responsibilities of various members of the obstetrical team, and the criteria used in determining specific treatments.

Simkin, Penny, Janet Whalley, and Ann Keppler. *Pregnancy, Childbirth, and the Newborn: A Complete Guide for Expectant Parents*. Deephaven, Minn.: Meadowbrook Books, 1984. This comprehensive guide is written in easy-to-understand language and is medically accurate and up to date. Contains many excellent illustrations and charts. The authors are associated with the Childbirth Education Association of Seattle.

Wertz, Richard W., and Dorothy C. Wertz. *Lying-in: A History of Childbirth in America*. Expanded ed. New Haven, Conn.: Yale University Press, 1989. Written in a style accessible to the general reader, this book charts the social history of childbirth practices in the United States. The authors suggest reasons for all the major changes that have occurred in obstetrical practice. Well illustrated with pictures showing instruments and procedures of bygone times.

CHILDBIRTH, COMPLICATIONS OF

SYSTEMS AFFECTED: Reproductive (female), circulatory
SPECIALISTS: Neonatologists, obstetricians
DEFINITION: The difficulties that can occur during childbirth, either for the mother or for the baby.

With medical monitoring and diagnostic tests, about 5 to 10 percent of pregnant women can be diagnosed as high-risk pregnancies, and appropriate precautions and preparations for possible complications can be made prior to labor. Yet up to 60 percent of complications of labor, childbirth, and the postpartum period (immediately after birth) occur in women with no prior indications of possible complications. Difficulties in childbirth can be placed into two general categories—problems with labor and problems with the child—and encompass a wide range of causes and possible treatments.

Complications of labor. Cesarean birth (also called cesarean section, C-section, or a section) is the surgical removal of the baby from the mother. About one in ten infants is delivered by cesarean birth. In this procedure, one incision is made through the mother's abdomen and a second through her uterus. The baby is physically removed from the mother's uterus, and the incisions are closed. This type of surgery is very safe but carries with it the general risks of any major surgery and requires approximately five days of hospitalization. In some cases, diagnosed preexisting conditions suggest that a cesarean birth is necessary and can be planned; in the majority of cases, unexpected difficulties during labor dictate that an emergency cesarean section be performed.

Some conditions leave no question about the necessity of a cesarean section. These absolute indications include a variety of physical abnormalities. Placenta previa is a condition in which the placenta has implanted in the lower part of the uterus instead of the normal upper portion, thereby totally or partially blocking the cervix. The baby could not pass down the birth canal without dislodging or tearing the placenta, thereby interrupting its blood and oxygen supply. Placenta previa is frequently the cause of bleeding after the twentieth week of pregnancy, and it can be definitively diagnosed by ultrasound. For women with this condition, bed rest is prescribed, and the baby will be delivered by cesarean birth at the thirty-seventh week of pregnancy.

Placental separation, also known as placenta abruptio, is the result of the placenta partially or completely separating from the uterus prior to the normal separation time after birth. This condition results in bleeding, with either mild or extreme blood loss depending on the severity of the separation. If severe, up to four pints of blood may be lost, and the mother is given a blood transfusion. If the pregnancy is near term, an emergency cesarean section will deliver the child.

Occasionally, as the baby begins traveling down the birth canal, the umbilical cord slips and lies ahead of the baby. This condition, called prolapsed cord, is very serious because the pressure of the baby against the cord during a vaginal delivery would compress the cord to the extent that the baby's blood and oxygen supply would be cut off. This condition necessitates an emergency cesarean section.

Some conditions that occur during labor are judged for their potential for causing harm to either the mother or the baby. The physician's decision to proceed with vaginal delivery will be based on the severity of the complication and consideration of the best option for the mother and baby. A few of the more common indicators for possible cesarean section which occur during labor include a fetal head size that is too large for the mother's birth canal; fetal distress, evidenced by insufficient oxygen supply reaching the baby; rupturing of the membranes without labor commencing or prolonged labor after membranes burst (usually twenty-four hours); and inelasticity of the pelvis in first-time mothers over forty years of age.

Other maternal conditions are diagnosed prior to the onset of labor, and the physician may or may not recommend a cesarean birth based on the severity of the complication. These include postmaturity, in which the onset of labor is at least two weeks overdue and degeneration of the placenta may compromise the health of the baby; maternal diseases, such as diabetes mellitus and toxemia, in which the stress of labor would be highly risky to the mother; and previous cesarean section.

Complications with the baby. Premature labor can occur between twenty and thirty-six weeks gestation, and a premature infant is considered to be any infant whose birth weight is less than 5.5 pounds. Certain maternal illnesses or abnormalities of the placenta can lead to premature birth, but in 60 percent of the cases there is no identifiable cause. If labor begins six weeks or more prior to the due date, the best chance of infant survival is to be delivered and cared for at a hospital with a perinatal center and specialized intensive care for premature infants. Prior to twenty-four weeks development, a premature infant will not survive as a result of inadequate lung development. The survival rate of premature infants increases with age, weight, and body system maturity.

In about 4 percent of births, the baby is in the breech position—buttocks first or other body part preceding the head—rather than in the normal head-down position. Delivery in this position is complicated because the cervix will not dilate properly and the head may not be able to pass through the cervix. Other complications of breech position are prolapse or compression of the umbilical cord and trauma to the baby if delivered vaginally. Manual tech-

Breech Birth

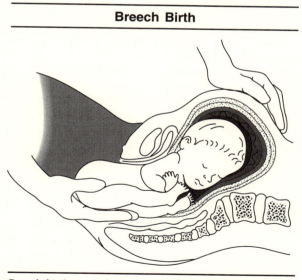

Breech birth, one of several complications that may occur during childbirth, is the emergence of the infant buttocks-first rather than head-first; such a birth is risky for the child, and often birth is accomplished by cesarean section, a surgical procedure to eliminate that risk.

niques may be used to rotate the baby into the correct position. Vaginal delivery may be attempted, frequently aided by gentle forceps removal of the baby. Breech babies are frequently born by cesarean section.

Cephalopelvic disproportion is a condition in which the baby's head is larger than the pelvic opening of the mother. This can only be determined after labor has begun, because the mother's muscles and joints expand to accommodate the baby's head. If at some point during labor the doctor determines that the baby will not fit through the mother's pelvic opening, a cesarean section will be performed.

—*Karen E. Kalumuck*

See also Birth defects; Breast-feeding; Childbirth; Conception; Eclampsia; Ectopic pregnancy; Miscarriage; Postpartum depression; Pregnancy and gestation; Premature birth; Stillbirth.

FOR FURTHER INFORMATION:

Hotchner, Tracy. *Pregnancy and Childbirth*. 2d ed. New York: Avon Books, 1990.

Sears, William, and Martha Sears. *The Birth Book*. Boston: Little, Brown, 1994.

Stoppard, Miriam. *Conception, Pregnancy, and Birth*. London: Dorling Kindersley, 1993.

CHILDHOOD INFECTIOUS DISEASES

SYSTEMS AFFECTED: Gastrointestinal, respiratory, muscular

SPECIALISTS: Epidemiologists, family physicians, immunologists, infectious disease physicians, internists, pediatricians, public health specialists

DEFINITION: A group of diseases including diphtheria, tetanus, measles, polio, rubella (German measles), mumps, and pertussis (whooping cough).

KEY TERMS:

anorexia: diminished appetite or aversion to food

conjunctivitis: inflammation of the conjunctiva, which lines the back of the eyelid, extends into the space between the lid and the globe of the eye, and goes over the globe to the transparent tissue covering the pupil

erythematous: related to or marked by reddening

malaise: a general feeling of discomfort, of being "out of sorts"

nuchal rigidity: stiffening of the back of the neck

oophoritis: inflammation of the ovary

orchitis: inflammation of the testis

photophobia: dread or avoidance of light

prodrome: a forewarning symptom of a disease

rhinitis: inflammation of the nasal mucous membrane

salivary glands: the glands that produce saliva

CAUSES AND SYMPTOMS

Acute communicable diseases occur primarily in childhood because most adults have become immune to such diseases, either by having acquired them as children or by having been inoculated against them. For example, prior to the use of vaccine for measles—a highly contagious disease found in most of the world—the peak incidence of the disease was in five- to ten-year-olds. Most adults were immune. Before a vaccine was developed and used against measles, epidemics occurred at two- to four-year intervals in large cities. Today, most cases are found in nonimmunized preschool children or in teenagers or young adults who have received only one dose of the vaccine.

A person infected with red measles (also known as rubeola) becomes contagious about ten days after exposure to the disease virus, at which time the prodromal stage begins. Typically, the infected person experiences three days of slight to moderate fever, a runny nose, increasing cough, and conjunctivitis. During the prodromal stage, Koplik's spots appear inside the cheeks opposite the lower molars. These lesions—grayish white dots about the size of sand particles with a slightly reddish halo surrounding them that are occasionally hemorrhagic—are important in the diagnosis of measles.

After the prodrome, a rash appears, usually accompanied by an abrupt increase in temperature (sometimes as high as 104 or 105 degrees Fahrenheit). It begins in the form of small, faintly red spots and progresses to large, dusky-red confluent areas, often slightly hemorrhagic. The rash frequently begins behind the ears but spreads rapidly over the entire face, neck, upper arms, and upper part of the chest within the first twenty-four hours. During the next twenty-four hours, it spreads over the back, abdomen, entire arms, and thighs. When it finally reaches the feet after the second or third day of the rash, it is already fading from the face. At this point, the fever is usually disappearing as well.

The chief complications of measles are middle-ear infections, pneumonia, and encephalitis (a severe infection of the brain). There is no correlation between the severity of the case of measles and the development of encephalitis, but the incidence of the infection of the brain runs to only one or two per every thousand cases. Measles can also exacerbate tuberculosis.

The incubation period for rubella (German measles) lasts between fourteen and twenty-one days, and the disease occurs primarily in children between the ages of two and ten. Like the initial rash of measles, the initial rash of rubella usually starts behind the ears, but children with rubella normally have no symptoms save for the rash and a low-grade fever for one day. Adolescents may have a three-day prodromal period of malaise, runny nose, and mild conjunctivitis; adolescent girls may have arthritis in several joints that lasts for weeks. The red spots begin behind the ears and then spread to the face, neck, trunk, and extremities. This rash may coalesce and last up to five days. Temperature may be normal or slightly elevated. Complications from rubella are relatively uncommon, but if pregnant women are not immune to the disease and are exposed to the rubella virus during early pregnancy, severe congenital anomalies may result. Because similar symptoms and rashes develop in many viral diseases, rubella is difficult to diagnose clinically. Except in known epidemics, laboratory confirmation is often necessary.

The patient with mumps is likely to have fever, malaise, headache, and anorexia—all usually mild—but "neck swelling," a painful enlargement of the parotid gland near the ear, is the sign that often brings the child to a doctor. Maximum swelling peaks after one to three days and begins in one or both parotid glands, but it may involve other salivary glands. The swelling pushes the earlobe upward and outward and obscures the angle of the mandible. Drinking sour liquids such as lemon juice may increase the pain. The opening of the duct inside the cheek from the affected parotid gland may appear red and swollen.

The painful swelling usually dissipates by seven days. Abdominal pain may be caused by pancreatitis, a common complication but one that is usually mild. The most feared complication, sterility, is not as common as most believe. Orchitis rarely occurs in prepubertal boys and occurs in only 14 to 35 percent of older males. In 30 percent of patients with orchitis, both testes are involved, and a similar percentage of affected testes will atrophy. Surprisingly, impairment of fertility in males is only about 13 percent; absolute infertility is rare. Ovary involvement in women, with pelvic pain and tenderness, occurs in only about 7 percent of postpubertal women and with no evidence of impaired fertility.

Measles, rubella, and mumps are all viral illnesses, but *Hemophilus influenzae* type B is the most common cause of serious bacterial infection in the young child. It is the leading cause of bacterial meningitis in children between the ages of one month and four years, and it is the cause of many other serious, life-threatening bacterial infections in the young child. Bacterial meningitis, especially from *Hemophilus influenzae* and pneumococcus, is the major cause of acquired hearing impairment in childhood.

Poliomyelitis (polio), an acute viral infection, has a wide range of manifestations. The minor illness pattern accounts for 80 to 90 percent of clinical infections in children. Symptoms, usually mild in this form, include slight fever, malaise, headache, sore throat, and vomiting but do not involve the central nervous system. Major illness occurs primarily in older children and adults. It may begin with fever, severe headache, stiff neck and back, deep muscle pain, and abnormal sensations, such as of burning, pricking, tickling, or tingling. These symptoms of aseptic meningitis may go no further or may progress to the loss of tendon reflexes and asymmetric weakness or paralysis of muscle groups. Fewer than 25 percent of paralytic polio patients suffer permanent disability. Most return in muscle function occurs within six months, but improvement may continue for two years. Twenty-five percent of paralytic patients have mild residual symptoms, and 50 percent recover completely. A long-term study of adults who suffered the disease has documented

slowly progressive muscle weakness, especially in patients who experienced severe disabilities initially.

Tetanus is a bacterial disease which, once established in a wound of a patient without significant immunity, will build a substance that acts at the neuromuscular junction, the spinal cord, and the brain. Clinically, the patient experiences "lockjaw," a tetanic spasm causing the spine and extremities to bend with convexity forward; spasms of the facial muscles cause the famous "sardonic smile." Minimal stimulation of any muscle group may cause painful spasms.

Diphtheria is another bacterial disease that produces a virulent substance, but this one attacks heart muscle and nervous tissue. There is a severe mucopurulent discharge from the nose and an exudative pharyngitis (a sore throat accompanied by phlegm) with the formation of a pseudomembrane. Swelling just below the back of the throat may lead to stridor (noisy, high-pitched breathing) and to the dark bluish or purplish coloration of the skin and mucous membranes because of decreased oxygenation of the blood. The result may be heart failure and damaged nerves; respiratory insufficiency may be caused by diaphragmatic paralysis.

Clinically, pertussis (whooping cough) can be divided into three stages, each lasting about two weeks. Initial symptoms resembling the common cold are followed by the characteristic paroxysmal cough and then convalescence. In the middle stage, multiple, rapid coughs, which may last more than a minute, will be followed by a sudden inspiration of air and a characteristic "whoop." In the final stage, vomiting commonly follows coughing attacks. Almost any stimulus precipitates an attack. Seizures may occur as a result of hypoxia (inadequate oxygen supply) or brain damage. Pneumonia can develop, and even death may occur when the illness is severe.

Varicella (chickenpox) produces a generalized itchy, blisterlike rash with low-grade fever and few other symptoms. Minor complications, such as ear infections, occasionally occur, as does pneumonia, but serious complications such as infection in the brain are thankfully rare. It is a very inconvenient disease, however, requiring the infected person to be quarantined for about nine days or until the skin lesions have dried up completely. Varicella, a herpes family virus, may lie dormant in nerve linings for years and suddenly emerge in the linear-grouped skin lesions identified as herpes zoster. These painful skin lesions follow the distribution of the affected nerve. Herpes zoster is popularly known as "shingles."

Hepatitis type B is much more common in adults than in children, except in certain immigrant populations in which hepatitis B viral infections are endemic. High carrier rates appear in certain Asian and Pacific Islander groups and among some Inuits in Alaska, in whom perinatal transmission is the most common means of perpetuating the disease. Having this disease in childhood can cause problems later in life. An estimated five thousand deaths in the United

States per year from cirrhosis or liver cancer occur as a result of hepatitis B. Carrier rates of between 5 and 10 percent result from disease acquired after the age of five, but between 80 and 90 percent will be carriers if they are infected at birth. The serious problems of hepatitis B occur most often in chronic carriers. For example, 50 percent of carriers will ultimately develop liver cancer. The virus is fifty to one hundred times more infectious than human immunodeficiency virus (HIV), the virus that causes acquired immunodeficiency syndrome (AIDS). Health care workers are at high risk of contracting hepatitis B, but virtually everyone is at risk for contracting this disease because it is so contagious.

TREATMENT AND THERAPY

The Immunization Practices Advisory Committee of the U.S. Public Health Service recommends immunizing all infants and some adolescents against hepatitis B, but the Committee on Infectious Diseases of the American Academy of Pediatrics recommends extending hepatitis B immunization to all adolescents, if possible. Based on field trials, the hepatitis B vaccine appears to be between 80 and 90 percent effective. The plasma-derived vaccine is protective against chronic hepatitis B infection for at least nine years. Newer, yeast-derived vaccines appear to be safe for administration to all, including pregnant women and infants: Both the vaccine and a placebo evoke the same incidence of reactions. These yeast-derived vaccines will be monitored to see if a booster dose is needed.

The incidence of infection with hepatitis B increases rapidly in adolescence, but teenagers are less likely to comply with immunization than are infants. Asking adolescents to participate in a three-dose immunization program over a six-month period is likely to result in high dropout rates. Therefore, the American Academy of Pediatrics' committee has recommended combining vaccination at birth with vaccination of teenagers. Two states, Alaska and Hawaii, have implemented universal immunization of infants with hepatitis B vaccine, and so have twenty nations.

Primary vaccination with DPT (diphtheria, pertussis, and tetanus) vaccine is recommended at two months, four months, and six months of age, followed by boosters with a new vaccine, DTaP, at fifteen months and upon entry into school (at four to six years of age). The last two vaccinations once used the DPT vaccine. The newer DTaP vaccine includes an acellular pertussis component manufactured in Japan, as well as the traditional diphtheria and tetanus toxoids. This Japanese acellular pertussis component contains various pertussis antigens but much less of the pertussis toxic products than the older, whole-cell vaccine. The substitution of the DTaP for the older DPT vaccine decreases the incidence of local and febrile reactions, but its effectiveness for the primary vaccinations has yet to be established.

Once a child reaches fifteen months of age, only one dose of the *Hemophilus influenzae* type B vaccine is nec-

essary, but vaccination should begin at two months of age. Two vaccines are licensed for use in infants, HbOC and PRP-OMP. HbOC is given on a four-dose schedule at two, four, six, and fifteen months of age, whereas PRP-OMP is given on a three-dose schedule at two, four, and twelve months of age. These vaccines are safe and at least 90 percent effective in preventing serious illness, such as sepsis and meningitis, from influenza B.

At two and four months of age, infants should receive an oral polio vaccination, with boosters at fifteen months and upon entry into school (four to six years of age). TOPV, the polio vaccine, contains a live virus that is excreted and may infect close contacts. Therefore, children who have close contact with someone who is immunocompromised (or who are themselves immunocompromised) should receive EIPV, an enhanced, inactivated polio virus vaccine.

MMR (measles, mumps, rubella) vaccination should take place at fifteen months and at four to six years of age. If the infant lives in a high-risk area, the first dose should occur at twelve months of age. While women who are pregnant or plan to become pregnant in the next three months should not receive MMR vaccination, children may receive the vaccine even if the mother is pregnant, since the viruses are not shed by immunized individuals.

In the 1990's, researchers announced that they had developed a vaccine to prevent chickenpox. Preliminary trials show the vaccine to be safe and effective even in immunocompromised patients.

Other available vaccines to prevent serious infections in children are recommended only in special circumstances. These include vaccines to prevent classic viral flu and pneumococcal disease. (The viral flu is to be distinguished from the bacterial vaccine to prevent influenza B.) Vaccination with the viral influenza vaccine is recommended especially for elderly and high-risk persons, their household contacts, and health care personnel who may come in contact with such patients. Any child who has a heart disease, lung disease, diabetes, or other serious chronic disease should receive the vaccine. This includes the child who is immunocompromised, even if he or she is HIV-positive.

Pneumococcal vaccine is not routinely given to children and is not recommended for use in children under two years of age, but it is given to children who are at risk of overwhelming pneumococcal infections. For example, children without spleens and children with sickle-cell anemia should be considered for vaccination against pneumococcal disease.

Some parents refuse to have their children vaccinated against pertussis because of concerns about the vaccine's safety. Media focus on the safety of pertussis vaccines, as well as legal suits, has frightened many physicians as well, the result being that they may be overly cautious in interpreting vaccine contraindications. Yet primary care physicians have also been sued for failing to give timely immunizations, which may result in complications from preventable disease. The Tennessee Medicaid Pertussis Vaccine Data should reassure them of the vaccine's safety. Other pertussis vaccine safety information is also available, including reports from the American Academy of Pediatrics' Task Force on Pertussis and Pertussis Immunization.

The means exist to prevent many serious illnesses from infectious diseases in childhood, but both parents and health care professionals must make the effort to vaccinate all children at the appropriate times in their lives.

PERSPECTIVE AND PROSPECTS

Some vaccines are more protective than others; effectiveness may hinge on a number of factors. In 1989, for example, 40 percent of people who developed measles had been vaccinated correctly under the old guidelines of one dose. Recommendations were therefore revised to include a booster dose. In the case of the hepatitis B vaccine, initial recommendations for administration of the vaccine established no injection site (only intramuscular), but studies revealed that there were fewer vaccine failures in recipients who were vaccinated in the deltoid region of the arm as opposed to the buttocks. The recommendation for injection site was therefore revised.

In the United States, vaccine coverage become woefully inadequate during the 1980's: One state's department of health, in a 1987 study, discovered that only 64 percent of children who were two years old were adequately vaccinated with DPT, oral polio, and MMR vaccines. Undoubtedly, multiple and interacting factors have inhibited adequate vaccine coverage, including physicians' attitudes and practice behaviors. For parents, the cost of vaccination, lack of health insurance, and other barriers to health care frustrate their efforts to get their children immunized. Some parents, for ideological or other reasons, may even be disinterested in or opposed to vaccination. In today's highly mobile society, however, all persons should keep a standard personal immunization record to facilitate immunization coverage. —*Wayne R. McKinny*

See also Bacterial infections; Chickenpox; Common cold; Hepatitis; Herpes; Influenza; Measles, red; Mononucleosis; Mumps; Pertussis; Poliomyelitis; Rabies; Rheumatic fever; Rhinitis; Roseola; Roundworm; Rubella; Rubeola; Scarlet fever; Smallpox; Strep throat; Tapeworm; Tetanus; Tonsillitis; Tuberculosis; Typhoid fever and typhus; Viral infections; Worms.

FOR FURTHER INFORMATION:

Behrman, Richard E., ed. *Nelson Textbook of Pediatrics.* 14th ed. Philadelphia: W. B. Saunders, 1992. This standard pediatrics textbook contains complete discussions of all common (and uncommon) causes of infectious disease in children. Many chapters are well written and easily understood by the nonspecialist.
Berkow, Robert, ed. *The Merck Manual.* 15th ed. Rahway, N.J.: Merck, 1987. Published since 1899, this classic work is well indexed and easy to use. Discussions of the various infectious diseases of childhood are usually brief but thorough.
Burg, Fredric D., ed. *Treatment of Infants, Children, and Adolescents.* Philadelphia: W. B. Saunders, 1990. One can quickly find specific information about vaccine dosages and other valuable information in this text.
Cotran, Ramzi S., ed. *Robbins Pathologic Basis of Disease.* 4th ed. Philadelphia: W. B. Saunders, 1989. An excellent textbook that combines the clinical and the pathological beautifully.
Korting, G. W. *Diseases of the Skin in Children and Adolescents.* Philadelphia: W. B. Saunders, 1970. An older textbook that contains color photographs of skin lesions in many childhood infectious diseases, matched by brilliant discussions of clinical patterns and signs.

CHLAMYDIA

SYSTEMS AFFECTED: Eyes, reproductive, joints, mucous membranes
SPECIALISTS: Family physicians, gynecologists, infectious disease physicians, neonatologists
DEFINITION: Chlamydia is a common sexually transmitted disease caused by the transfer of viruslike intracellular parasites during vaginal, rectal, or oral sexual intercourse, or by vaginal infection during the delivery of a newborn, which may infect the baby's eyes. Following infection through sexual contact, there is an incubation period of five to twenty-eight days. Vaginal and urethral discharges as well as anal swelling, pain, and reddening of the vagina or tip of the penis may occur. Elsewhere in the body, the infection leads to fever, joint pain, blisters, and conjunctivitis in infants. Early treatment with medication cures the infection and prevents further complications.
See also Conjunctivitis; Female genital disorders; Gonorrhea; Sexually transmitted diseases; Syphilis; Warts.

CHOKING

SYSTEM AFFECTED: Respiratory
SPECIALISTS: Emergency physicians
DEFINITION: A condition in which the breathing passage (windpipe) is obstructed.

CAUSES AND SYMPTOMS

A person who is choking may cough, turn red in the face, clutch his or her throat, or any combination of the above. If the choking person is coughing, it is probably best to do nothing; the coughing should naturally clear the airway. The true choking emergency occurs when a bit of food or other foreign object completely obstructs the breathing passage. In this case, there is little or no coughing—the person cannot make much sound. This silent choking calls for immediate action.

TREATMENT AND THERAPY

An individual witnessing a choking emergency should first call for emergency help and then perform the Heimlich

Heimlich Maneuver

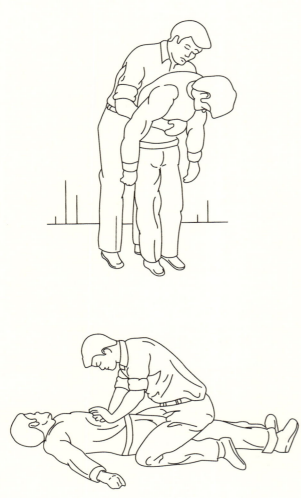

The Heimlich maneuver is ideally performed on a standing or seated victim who has indicated consent that this maneuver be performed by nodding or another gesture of affirmation; if unconscious, the victim may be lying on his or her back, and abdominal thrusts are administered using the heel of the hand. NOTE: *The illustration depicts only part of the procedure, which is not fully detailed above; for full information on the protocols for first aid for persons with obstructed airways, such as CPR, refer to the American Heart Association's* Heartsaver Manual, *which is periodically updated.*

maneuver. The choking person should never be slapped on the back. The Heimlich maneuver is best performed while the choking victim is standing or seated. If possible, the person performing the Heimlich maneuver should ask the victim to nod if he or she wishes the Heimlich maneuver to be performed. If the airway is totally blocked, the victim will not be able to speak and may even be unconscious.

The individual performing the Heimlich maneuver positions himself or herself behind the choking victim and places his or her arms around the victim's waist. Making a fist with one hand and grasping that fist with the other hand, the rescuer positions the thumb side of the fist toward the stomach of the victim—just above the navel and below the ribs. The person performing the maneuver pulls his or her fist upward into the abdomen of the victim with several quick thrusts. This action should expel the foreign object from the victim's throat, and he or she should begin coughing or return to normal breathing.

The Heimlich maneuver is not effective in dislodging fish bones and certain other obstructions. If the airway is still blocked after several Heimlich thrusts, a finger sweep should be tried to remove the obstruction. First the mouth of the victim must be opened: The chin is grasped, and the mouth is pulled open with one hand. With the index finger of the other hand, the rescuer sweeps through the victim's throat, pulling out any foreign material. One sweep should be made from left to right, and a second sweep from right to left. The Heimlich maneuver may then be repeated if necessary. —*Steven A. Schonefeld*

See also Coughing; Unconsciousness.

FOR FURTHER INFORMATION:

Castleman, Michael. "Emergency! Fifty-four Ways to Save Your Life." *Family Circle* 107, no. 4 (March 15, 1994): 37.

Glanze, Walter D., et al., eds. *Mosby's Medical and Nursing Dictionary.* 2d ed. St. Louis: Mosby Year Book, 1986.

Heimlich, H. J., and E. A. Patrick. "The Heimlich Maneuver: The Best Technique for Saving Any Choking Victim's Life." *Postgraduate Medicine* 87, no. 6 (May 1, 1990): 38-48, 53.

Stern, Loraine. "Your Child's Health: Mom, I Can't Breathe!" *Woman's Day* 57, no. 6 (March 15, 1994): 18.

CHOLECYSTITIS

SYSTEM AFFECTED: Gallbladder

SPECIALISTS: Family physicians, gastroenterologists, general surgeons, internists

DEFINITION: Cholecystitis is the inflammation or bacterial infection of the gallbladder, which is usually caused by gallstones or blockage of the bile ducts. Signs may include an indigestion-like cramping pain in the upper-right abdomen, symptoms in the chest resembling a heart attack, or pain in the upper-right back and shoulder following fatty meals. More severe cases include abdominal

Cholecystitis

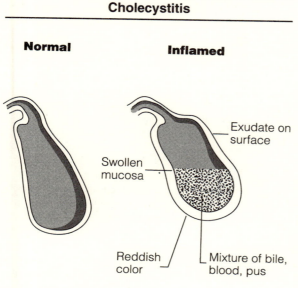

Normal

Inflamed

Exudate on surface

Swollen mucosa

Reddish color

Mixture of bile, blood, pus

A normal gallbladder and one inflamed by cholecystitis.

spasms and tenderness, nausea and vomiting, fever, and sometimes jaundice, pale stools, and skin irritation. Cholecystitis can be prevented by avoiding foods that trigger indigestion or by having gallstones surgically removed. Surgery to remove an infected gallbladder may be necessary in chronic cases.

See also Gallbladder diseases.

CHOLERA

SYSTEM AFFECTED: Gastrointestinal

SPECIALISTS: Epidemiologists, gastroenterologists, infectious disease physicians, pediatricians, public health specialists, tropical medicine physicians

DEFINITION: An infection of the small intestine caused by *Vibrio cholerae*, a comma-shaped bacterium.

CAUSES AND SYMPTOMS

The symptoms of cholera begin one to three days after the patient has ingested contaminated food or water. In mild cases, the patient experiences a brief episode of diarrhea. In severe cases, the symptoms progress quickly to include vomiting and a profuse watery diarrhea. The effects of *Vibrio cholerae* are caused by the production of a toxin that attacks the cells of the small intestine. Up to one liter of water and essential electrolytes such as sodium, potassium, and bicarbonate can be lost each hour.

TREATMENT AND THERAPY

The patient with cholera must be treated quickly with fluid and electrolyte replacement. A solution of salts, bicarbonate, and sugar in water can be given orally or intravenously. Antibiotic treatment shortens the duration of the dis-

ease. Without treatment, death can occur within twenty-four hours, and the death rate has exceeded 60 percent in some epidemics. With treatment, however, the death rate is less than 1 percent. A patient who recovers from cholera has some immunity in subsequent epidemics.

PERSPECTIVE AND PROSPECTS

The disease is often called Asiatic cholera because it was first reported in India. As travel increased, cholera spread to other areas of the world. During one epidemic in 1854, British physician John Snow systematically mapped the cases of cholera in London and determined that a single water pump was the source of the epidemic. Robert Koch discovered *Vibrio cholerae* as the cause of the disease in 1884. It was also determined that drinking water contaminated by human waste was the most common source of the disease. Modern sewer and water purification systems have virtually eliminated cholera in developed areas of the world.

Epidemics are still possible, especially when sanitary systems break down. In the early 1990's, an epidemic occurred in seven South American countries, resulting in more than 342,000 cases and 3,600 deaths. *Vibrio cholerae* occurs naturally in the Gulf of Mexico, and each year several cases in the United States result from eating shellfish taken from those waters. To avoid becoming ill, travelers to areas where cholera occurs are warned to eat only cooked food and drink only sterilized beverages. —*Edith K. Wallace*

See also Bacterial infections.

FOR FURTHER INFORMATION:

Berkow, Robert, ed. "Cholera." In *The Merck Manual of Diagnosis and Therapy.* 16th ed. Rahway, N.J.: Merck Sharp & Dohme Research Laboratories, 1992.

Jensen, Marcus M., and Donald N. Wright. *Introduction to Microbiology for the Health Sciences.* 3d ed. Englewood Cliffs, N.J.: Prentice Hall, 1993.

McNeill, William H. *Plagues and Peoples.* Garden City, N.Y.: Anchor Press, 1976.

CHOLESTEROL

SYSTEM AFFECTED: Circulatory

SPECIALISTS: Cardiologists, family physicians, internists, registered dietitians, vascular surgeons

DEFINITION: Found in animal oils and fats, tissues, bile, blood, and egg yolk, cholesterol is used by the body in the production of steroids, including sex hormones and hormones of the adrenal glands. Excessive amounts of cholesterol in the blood have been shown to increase the risk of atherosclerosis, which is the deposit of fatty plaques on the inside of blood vessels that can lead to heart disease. The replacement of animal fat in the diet with vegetable oil containing polyunsaturated fats will cause blood cholesterol levels to fall. Cholesterol is also responsible for the development of gallstones in the majority of such cases.

See also Hyperlipidemia.

CHROMOSOMAL ABNORMALITIES. *See* BIRTH DEFECTS; GENETIC DISEASES.

CHRONIC FATIGUE SYNDROME

SYSTEMS AFFECTED: Immune, muscular, psychic-emotional

SPECIALISTS: Family physicians, hematologists, immunologists, internists, psychiatrists

DEFINITION: Chronic fatigue syndrome is a multifaceted disease state characterized by debilitating fatigue.

KEY TERMS:

adenopathy: the enlargement of any gland (often the lymph gland)

Burkitt's lymphoma: a tumor in the lower jaw of children that is believed to be caused by the Epstein-Barr virus, usually occurring in Africa

cell-mediated immune response: an immune response that involves cells rather than antibodies, particularly T lymphocytes rather than B lymphocytes

delayed hypersensitivity: an abnormal cell-mediated immune reaction caused by an exogenous agent and resulting in tissue destruction

infectious mononucleosis: acute self-limiting infection of lymphocytes by the Epstein-Barr virus

interleuken II: a protein messenger that regulates T cell activity and differentiation during the immune response

lymphocytes: agranular leukocytes that differentiate into B lymphocytes and T lymphocytes and play a fundamental role in the immune response

polymerase chain reaction: a laboratory method used to increase the amount of DNA found in small quantities

Spumavirus: a virus found in humans, primates, and cats that gives a foamy appearance to the lymphocyte tissue culture

suppressor T cell: a type of T lymphocyte that is believed to modulate the immune response

CAUSES AND SYMPTOMS

Chronic fatigue syndrome is a heterogenous disease state that has been difficult to define, diagnose, and treat because of poorly understood cause-and-effect relationships. The disease can be best described in terms of long-lasting and debilitating fatigue, the etiology of which has been linked to such external factors as microbial agents, stress, and lifestyle as well as such internal factors as genetic makeup and the body's immune response. The fact that it is a physical disease with psychological components has also caused confusion in the medical community.

Among the many names that have been used for the disease, the three that demonstrate the many factors that contribute to chronic fatigue syndrome are chronic Epstein-Barr virus syndrome, chronic fatigue immune dysfunction syndrome, and "Yuppie flu." Because of the marked immunological aspects of the disease and the fact that different viruses have been found in patients with chronic fatigue,

the disease is referred to as chronic fatigue immune dysfunction syndrome by many involved in the study. The Centers for Disease Control (CDC) continues to refer to it as chronic fatigue syndrome (CFS).

Although the disease is not specific by race, sex, or age group, there is demographic evidence that young white females make up two-thirds of the known cases. It is estimated by the CDC that between 1 and 10 of every 10,000 people in the United States have CFS. The disease has also been identified as a problem in Europe and Australia.

CFS can manifest itself in acute and chronic phases, although some patients do not remember an acute phase presentation. Acute phase symptoms are general and flulike, with a low-grade fever, sore throat, headache, muscle pain, painful lymph nodes, and overall fatigue. Unlike with a bout of influenza, the symptoms do not subside with time, instead intensifying into a chronic phase. The fatigue can become disabling, with severe muscle and joint pain, swollen and painful lymph nodes, and the inability to develop proper sleep patterns. Some researchers blame psychological and emotional stress, with a viral infection having triggered the initial acute phase. Although the psychological description does not fit all cases, problems of concentration, attention, and depression have been implicated to the point that researchers recognize both psychological and physical components. The working definition from both a research and a clinical perspective requires that the fatigue cause at least 50 percent incapacitation and last at least six months. The ineffectiveness of treatment, compounded by the inability to provide a concrete diagnosis, further complicates the psychological aspects of the disease for the patient.

Although the environment provides an array of agents that could trigger the physical condition of CFS, the hypothesis for a viral cause is supported by the flulike symptoms, occasional clustering of cases, and the presence of antiviral antibodies in the patient's serum. The involvement of the Epstein-Barr virus in CFS seems likely because of its role as the etiological agent of mononucleosis and Burkitt's lymphoma, which are similar diseases. In both of these diseases, the Epstein-Barr virus has a unique and harmful effect on the immune system because it directly invades B lymphocytes, the antibody-producing cells of the body, using them to grow new virus particles while disrupting the proper functioning of the immune system. Like CFS, mononucleosis is characterized by flulike symptoms and fatigue, but the disease is self-limiting and the patient eventually recovers.

Despite this seeming difference in outcome, the Epstein-Barr virus can cause a chronic condition. The viruses that infect humans can become dormant within the cells that they infect. The nucleic acid of a virus can become incorporated into the DNA of its host cell, and the body no longer shows physical signs of their presence. A virus can become active at times of physical or emotional stress and can once again trigger the physical symptoms of disease. For example, herpes simplex virus 1 remains dormant in its host cell but periodically, in response to environmental factors, causes a cold sore lesion.

Some patients with CFS have also been infected with two retroviruses, human T-cell lymphotropic virus type II (HTLV-II) and a Spumavirus. Both are related to the human immunodeficiency virus (HIV), the causative agent of acquired immunodeficiency syndrome (AIDS). Retrovirus genes are made of ribonucleic acid (RNA) rather than deoxyribonucleic acid (DNA), as are the genes of herpes-type viruses such as Epstein-Barr and herpes simplex virus 1. Retroviruses must convert their RNA into complementary DNA (cDNA) when they infect a host cell in order to incorporate their genes into the host cell genes. Although the two viruses are associated with some CFS patients, diagnostic tests developed to detect their presence have not confirmed that the CFS condition depends on their presence. This same finding is true of herpesvirus 6 and other viruses. Although viruses may play a role in CFS, they are not the only factors involved and are not substantive evidence to define a clinical or research case.

Immunological dysfunction has been observed in CFS patients because they demonstrate increased allergic sensitivity to skin tests when compared to normal individuals. Cells and cellular chemicals directly involved with protective immunity and the regulation of the immune response have been found in these patients in abnormal concentrations. For example, they have abnormal numbers of the natural killer cells and suppressor T cells that are essential to cell-mediated immunity. Cellular chemicals such as gamma interferon and interleuken II that regulate the activities of the cells in the cell-mediated and humeral immune responses are seen in abnormal concentrations in some CFS patients. Infectious agents, bacteria, viruses, yeasts, parasites, and even cancer cells are eliminated from the body when humeral and cell-mediated immune systems are operating properly. When the immune system is not working properly, however, not only is the body more susceptible to a variety of infectious agents but the immune system can actually begin to destroy normal body tissues, such as the thyroid gland and other vital organs, as well. Such disease states are referred to as autoimmune diseases. Allergic reactions are also examples of uncontrolled immune responses. The component immune dysfunction of CFS is thought to be significant enough for some researchers to recommend that new and worsening allergies be added as minor criteria to the case definition for the disease.

The psychological and emotional aspects of CFS are also in question. Some studies indicate that the brain is physically affected by inflammation and hormonal changes. Other studies demonstrate that some of the known viral infective agents can have neurological effects. Psychiatric studies give ample evidence that depression, memory loss, and concentration are significant problems for some CFS patients. The extent to which stress is a factor in the disease is unknown.

TREATMENT AND THERAPY

Defining and treating chronic fatigue syndrome has been difficult because it manifests itself as a systemic disease with confusing cause-and-effect relationships involving external factors such as infectious viruses, internal factors such as the immune response, and a psychological component that is difficult to assess in the light of the biological changes occurring in the body. The symptoms, provided by patient histories, physical examinations, and laboratory findings, involve neuromuscular, psychoneurological, and immunological changes that vary between patients. The variety of factors to consider has caused difficulty in establishing diagnostic criteria for primary care in a clinical setting or further definition of the disease and treatments in a research setting.

In 1988, the CDC established diagnostic criteria that are divided into two major criteria, eleven minor symptom criteria, and three minor physical criteria. The first major criterion defines chronic fatigue as lasting at least six months and causing debilitation to 50 percent of the patient's normal activity. The second major criterion requires that all other disease conditions that could fit the patient history, physical examination, and appropriate laboratory tests be ruled out. The categories of disease that might be similar to CFS are cancers, chronic degenerative disease, autoimmune disorders, microbial and parasitic disease, and chronic psychiatric disease. Combinations of some minor criteria that would fit a general flulike condition must be demonstrated.

In 1993, a meeting at the CDC attempted to evaluate what had been learned over the previous five-year period and to make recommendations regarding a case definition. It was suggested that the case definition format involve inclusion and exclusion criteria that would increase the number and range of cases being studied because of the heterogenous nature of the disease. The cases should also be subcategorized to provide a homogeneity that would allow for subgroup identification and comparison. The inclusion evidence should be simple, with a descriptive interpretation of the fatigue being essential and having objective criteria to define a 50 percent reduction of physical activity. Symptoms that are specific to unexplained fatigue should be used, while the physical exam information should not be included. It was also suggested that exclusion of any cases should involve an in-depth history (both medical and psychiatric), a physical examination, and standardized testing that would involve medical, laboratory, and psychiatric information.

Because it appears that CFS overlaps with many other medical and psychiatric conditions that can be identified and treated, there is debate as to how to interpret CFS as it relates to patient care and research. Some believe that an in-depth history is fundamental to the understanding of CFS and that CFS could be the final pathway that occurs from a variety of biological and psychosocial insults to the body.

The minor criteria used to define CFS involve both symptom and physical criteria that have not been proved adequate to validate or define the condition. In fact, the conflicting data have only served to emphasize further the clinical heterogeneity of the disease and suggest a heterogeneity of cause. Suggestions have been made to drop the concept of minor criteria, use symptoms that are specific for the unexplained fatigue, and drop all physical examination criteria. The argument for eliminating physical criteria is that more specific criteria exist for a case definition. Because physical symptoms are inconsistent or periodic, it is believed that a documented patient history would provide more case-specific information.

Although symptom criteria have widespread support in the case definition of CFS, symptoms with the greatest sensitivity and specificity are also being debated. Night sweats, cough, gastrointestinal problems, and new and worsening allergies are not presently considered and are believed by some to be more specific than fever or chills and sore throat. Others have proposed that symptoms should be reduced to chills and fever, sore throat, neck or axilla adenopathy, and sudden onset of a main symptom complex. The most prevalent symptoms are believed to be muscle weakness and pain, problems in concentration, and sleep disturbance.

The importance of the psychiatric component in CFS continues to be a problem in case definition. Some believe that the neurological component is a major criterion in case definition and that behavior symptoms, including stress and psychiatric illness, must be emphasized in clinical diagnosis as well as in therapy. It has been recommended that objective neuropsychological testing be used to determine cognitive dysfunction and depression. There is agreement that CFS patients have impaired concentration and attention, but forgetfulness and memory problems are questioned. There is also evidence that the duration and severity of myalgia are closely associated with psychological distress and that psychotherapy improves physical symptoms. Finally, it has been argued that the psychiatric component of the case definition is essential because there is evidence that the disease directly affects the brain and that CFS can cause both isolation and limitation of the patient's normal lifestyle.

Whatever the case definition, the second major criterion will be expressed in some form. Proper patient care necessitates extensive evaluation in order to identify the biological or psychological reasons for the problem. Proper CFS patient care demands the elimination of other serious disease possibilities that may appear superficially similar. Primary care physicians may find it difficult to make a diagnosis without a team of specialists in the areas of hematology,

immunology, and psychiatry. Numerous laboratory tests must be made available. Although there are no specific recommended tests, those that must be performed should be tailored to specific patients and used by the team of specialists for their care.

The possibility of infectious disease, either as part of CFS (as in the case of certain viral agents) or as an autonomous infection having no relation to CFS, requires a variety of antibody tests to detect such viruses as Epstein-Barr or HIV. Skin tests such as the purified protein derivative (PPD) test for tuberculosis are used. Polymerase chain reaction and tissue culture for cytopathic effects have been developed to detect certain retroviruses for ultimate use in diagnosis at the clinical level.

The immune system is so intimately interactive with the entire body that most disease conditions are affected by or affect its function. The measure of its components provides a clue to the identity of the disease that is operating because they indicate whether normal protection activity or immune dysfunction (or a combination) is occurring in the patient.

The components of the immune system can be measured in numerous ways, from methodologies used in standard clinical laboratory procedures to research protocols used to study immune function and disease treatment. Tests are available that can measure total antibody concentration and the various subgroups IgG, IgM, IgA, IgE, IgD; cytokines such as interleuken II and gamma interferon; cellular components such as T cells and their subtypes (such as suppressor T cells and natural killer cells), and B cells.

Autoimmune diseases and allergies are immune dysfunction diseases in their own right. Because there is an immune dysfunction component to CFS, tests for these conditions are important considerations. An antinuclear antibody (ANA) test determines the presence of antibodies that attack the tissues of the patient, as in systemic lupus erythematosus. The type and extent of allergic reactions can be measured using the radioimmunosorbent (RIST) tests for total IgE concentration and radioallergosorbent (RAST) tests for IgE concentration for particular antigens.

Systemic disease states, including CFS, often involve generalized inflammation that is considered part of the body's protective response. While inflammation is important to the elimination of various infective agents, it is also involved in neurological and muscle tissue damage. C-reactive protein (CRP) and the erythrocyte sedimentation rate (ESR) tests measure the intensity of the inflammatory response. A variety of other tests provide information that indicates the extent of muscle, liver, thyroid, and other vital organ damage.

Although a diagnosis can be made for CFS, there is no standard treatment. Clinical treatment essentially takes the form of alleviating the symptoms. Antidepressants such as doxepin (Sinequan) are useful in the treatment of depression and are also used to control muscle pain, lethargy, and sleeping problems. Nonsteroidal anti-inflammatory drugs (NSAIDs) provide relief for headache and muscle pain. Two drugs that have demonstrated antiviral activities are acyclovir and ampligen; ampligen can also modulate the immune response.

An example of research to develop therapies that might alleviate other symptoms of CFS involves the treatment of a number of patients with dialyzable leukocyte extract and psychologic treatment in the form of cognitive-behavioral therapy. The patients' cell-mediated immune response after therapy was evaluated by peripheral blood T cell subset analysis and delayed hypersensitivity skin testing. Psychologic analysis was performed using numerous cognitive tests. Both therapies proved to be inconclusive.

Because of the systemic nature of the disease, including its psychoneurological component, consideration must be given to holistic medical treatment. Any treatment protocol must be able to address the interactive factors of CFS that are still being defined in terms of cause and effect. Some researchers believe that therapeutic treatment should comprise diet, exercise, vitamins, and homeopathic medicine. They further believe that psychoemotional treatment should allow patients to be responsible for their own recovery and help them to develop a personal lifestyle that provides general good health.

PERSPECTIVE AND PROSPECTS

It is believed that chronic fatigue syndrome is not a new phenomenon but a disease condition that is in the process of being defined. For several centuries, the medical community has described a disease condition involving fatigue, with fever, neuromuscular, and brain involvement. The condition was called little fever, vapors, neurasthenia or nervous exhaustion, and benign myalgic encephalomyelitis. The infectious nature of the condition resulted in names such as chronic brucellosis, chronic Epstein-Barr virus infection, chronic candidiasis, and postviral fatigue syndrome.

Since being linked with the Epstein-Barr virus, CFS has been the subject of many studies that support its definition as a heterogenous illness. The case definition provided by the CDC in 1988 has allowed the disease to be diagnosed and treated at the clinical level and to be identified and compared at the research level. The disease state has proven to be elusive, however, and the case definition too complex and open to interpretation. It is believed that the refinement of the case definition proposed by the CDC in 1993 will promote greater understanding of the problem at both clinical and research levels, particularly because more objective criteria to validate and define CFS have not emerged.

As indicated by its very definition, CFS has presented the health care system with a challenge whereby the primary care physician receives information provided by a team of specialists. Continued technological advances and research into both the immune system and the nature of viral infection will provide new insights into more tradi-

tional treatment protocols. Nevertheless, the multicausal nature of CFS may require holistic medical treatment that can only be provided by personalized patient care. The neuro-psychological components of the disease, as well as evidence demonstrating intimate ties between these components and the immune system, require a personal, active approach by the patient to achieving a healthy state. CFS provides a challenge to the patient to adapt to a personal lifestyle that will create a healthy mind and body.

CFS must also be considered in terms of the society in which it is manifest as a serious and genuine illness. Medical treatment and diagnostic testing can be costly as well as useless, particularly as the health care community continues to refine its understanding of the condition. Patients must remain vigilant regarding phony or trendy treatments that have no correlation to acceptable research findings; such treatments not only can be expensive but also could lead to deteriorating health. Furthermore, the definition and diagnosis of CFS have legal ramifications that have an impact on insurance and other forms of medical care compensation. —*Patrick J. DeLuca*

See also Fatigue; Mononucleosis.

FOR FURTHER INFORMATION:

Collinge, William. *Recovering from Chronic Fatigue Syndrome: A Guide to Self-Empowerment.* New York: Body Press/Perigee, 1993. An excellent book written for the general public that speculates on the multifaceted nature of the disease. Offers information for those who have CFS, such as suggested diets and treatments. Also provides addresses for support groups.

Holmes, Gary P., et al. "Chronic Fatigue Syndrome: A Working Case Definition." *Annals of Internal Medicine* 108, no. 3 (March, 1988): 387-389. An article of historical significance that gave credibility to the disease. Served as a starting point for organized data collecting about CFS in both research and clinical settings.

National Institutes of Health. *Chronic Fatigue Syndrome: A Pamphlet for Physicians.* Bethesda, Md.: Author, 1990. NIH Publication 90-484. A brief, concise description of what is known about CFS. Although printed for physicians, this pamphlet can be read and understood by an educated reader.

Stoff, Jesse A., and Charles Pellegrino. *Chronic Fatigue Syndrome.* Rev. ed. New York: HarperPerennial, 1992. An excellent book describing the biological aspects of the disease in layperson's terms. Essential reading for anyone suffering from the disease because of its diary-like accounts, anecdotal data, emphasis on holistic treatment, and inspirational tone.

CIRRHOSIS

SYSTEM AFFECTED: Liver

SPECIALISTS: Family physicians, general surgeons, internists, psychologists

Cirrhosis

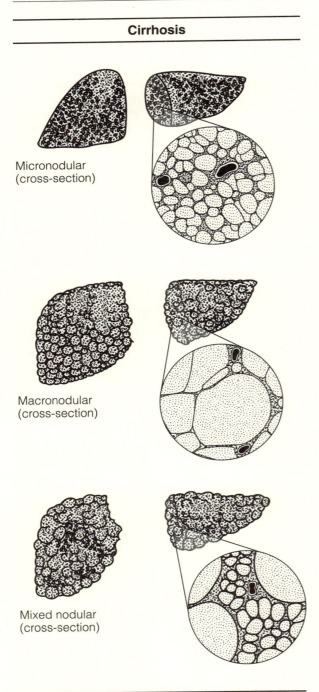

Micronodular
(cross-section)

Macronodular
(cross-section)

Mixed nodular
(cross-section)

Cirrhosis appears in three forms, detectable under the microscope, each depending primarily on the cause of the liver damage. All, however, are characterized by the replacement of normally soft, spongy tissue with hard, fibrous scarring. Alcohol-related cirrhosis usually produces the micronodular form.

DEFINITION: The formation of scar tissue in the liver, which interferes with its normal function.

CAUSES AND SYMPTOMS

The liver is a large, spongy organ that lies in the upper-right abdomen. Regarded as primarily part of the digestive system because it manufactures bile, the liver has many other functions, including the synthesis of blood-clotting factors and the detoxification of such harmful substances as alcohol.

Cirrhosis describes the fibrous scar tissue (or nodules) that replaces the normally soft liver after repeated long-term injury by toxins such as alcohol or viruses. The liver may form small nodules (micronodular cirrhosis), large nodules (macronodular cirrhosis), or a combination of the two types (mixed nodular cirrhosis). Cirrhosis is a frequent cause of death among middle-aged men, and increasingly among women. While alcoholism is the most common cause, chronic hepatitis and other rarer diseases can also produce the irreversible liver damage that characterizes cirrhosis. The resulting organ is shrunken and hard, unable to perform its varied duties. Because of its altered structure, the cirrhotic liver causes serious problems for surrounding organs, as blood flow becomes difficult. The barrier to normal circulation leads to two serious complications: portal hypertension (the buildup of pressure in the internal veins) and ascites (fluid leakage from blood vessels into the abdominal cavity).

TREATMENT AND THERAPY

Diagnosis is usually made from a history of alcoholism; a physical examination revealing a small, firm liver; a fluid-filled abdomen (ascites); and laboratory studies that show low concentrations of the blood products that the liver manufactures. A definitive diagnosis can only be made by biopsy, although radiographic methods such as computed tomography (CT) scanning and magnetic resonance imaging (MRI) can be quite conclusive.

The mortality rate is very high, as the damage is irreversible. Deaths from internal vein rupture and hemorrhage (the results of portal hypertension) and from kidney failure are most common. Repeated hospitalizations attempt to control the variety of complications that arise with agents that stop bleeding, bypass tubes that relieve pressure, the removal of the ascitic fluid, and nutritional support for malnutrition. Eventually, kidney failure ensues or one of these control measures fails, and death rapidly follows. Cases of mild cirrhosis, where sufficient normal tissue remains, have a clearly better course. *—Connie Rizzo*

See also Alcoholism; Jaundice; Liver cancer; Liver disorders.

FOR FURTHER INFORMATION:

Fishman, Mark, et al. *Medicine.* 3d ed. Philadelphia: J. B. Lippincott, 1991.

Mulvihill, Mary. *Human Diseases: A Systemic Approach.* 3d ed. Norwalk, Conn.: Appleton and Lange, 1991.

Wyngaarden, James B., et al., eds. *Cecil Textbook of Medicine*. 19th ed. Philadelphia: W. B. Saunders, 1992.

CLAUDICATION

SYSTEMS AFFECTED: Circulatory, muscular, nervous
SPECIALISTS: Internists, neurologists, vascular surgeons
DEFINITION: Claudication describes a cramplike pain in one or both legs while walking, which eventually may develop into a limp. It is caused by atherosclerosis in the legs, in which the arteries become blocked or narrowed, restricting blood flow. Another, more rare form of claudication involves spinal stenosis, in which the spinal cord is constricted, putting pressure on the nerve roots going toward the legs. People suffering intermediate claudication are able to walk short distances, with rests in between to alleviate the pain.

See also Atherosclerotic disease; Thrombosis and thrombus.

CLEFT PALATE

SYSTEM AFFECTED: Skeletal
SPECIALISTS: Pediatricians, plastic and reconstructive surgeons, speech therapists
DEFINITION: A fissure in the midline of the palate so that the two sides fail to fuse during embryonic development; in some cases, the fissure may extend through both hard and soft palates into the nasal cavities.
KEY TERMS:
alveolus: the bony ridge where teeth grow
ectrodactyly: a congenital anomaly characterized by the absence of part or all of one or more of the fingers or toes
hard palate: the bony portion of the roof of the mouth, contiguous with the soft palate
Logan's bow: a metal bar placed, for protection and tension removal, on the early postoperative cleft lip
obturator: a sheet of plastic shaped like a flattened dome which fits into the cleft and closes it well enough to permit nursing
soft palate: a structure of mucous membrane, muscle fibers, and mucous glands suspended from the posterior border of the hard palate
syndactyly: a congenital anomaly characterized by the fusion of the fingers or toes
uvula: the small, cone-shaped process suspended in the mouth from the posterior of the soft palate

CAUSES AND SYMPTOMS

Cleft palate is a congenital defect characterized by a fissure along the midline of the palate. It occurs when the two sides fail to fuse during embryonic development. The gap may be complete, extending through the hard and soft palates into the nasal cavities, or may be partial or incomplete. It is often associated with cleft lip or "hare lip." About one child in eight hundred live births is affected with some degree of clefting, and clefting is the most common of the craniofacial abnormalities.

Cleft palate is not generally a genetic disorder; rather, it is a result of defective cell migration. Embryonically, in the first month, the mouth and nose form one cavity destined to be separated by the hard and soft palates. In addition, there is no upper lip. Most of the upper jaw is lacking; only the part near the ears is present. In the next weeks, the upper lip and jaw are formed from structures growing in from the sides, fusing at the midline with a third portion growing downward from the nasal region. The palates develop in much the same way. The fusion of all these structures begins with the lip and moves posteriorly toward, then includes, the soft palate. The two cavities are separated by the palates by the end of the third month of gestation.

If, as embryonic development occurs, the cells that should grow together to form the lips and palate fail to move in the correct direction, the job is left unfinished. Clefting of the palate generally occurs between the thirty-fifth and thirty-seventh days of gestation. Fortunately, it is an isolated defect not usually associated with other disabilities or with mental retardation.

If the interference in normal growth and fusion begins early and lasts throughout the fusion period, the cleft that results will affect one or both sides of the top lip and may continue back through the upper jaw, the upper gum ridge, and both palates. If the disturbance lasts only part of the time that development is occurring, only the lip may be cleft, and the palate may be unaffected. If the problem begins a little into the fusion process, the lip is normally formed, but the palate is cleft. The cleft may divide only the soft palate or both the soft and the hard palate. Even the uvula may be affected; it can be split, unusually short, or even absent.

About 80 percent of cases of cleft lip are unilateral; of these, 70 percent occur on the left side. Of cleft palate cases, 25 percent are bilateral. The mildest manifestations of congenital cleft are mild scarring and/or notching of the upper lip. Beyond this, clefting is described by degrees. The first degree is incomplete, which is a small cleft in the uvula. The second degree is also incomplete, through the soft palate and into the hard palate. Another type of "second-degree incomplete" is a horseshoe type, in which there is a bilateral cleft proceeding almost to the front. Third-degree bilateral is a cleft through both palates but bilaterally through the gums; it results in a separate area of the alveolus where the teeth will erupt, and the teeth will show up in a very small segment. When the teeth appear, they may not be normally aligned. In addition to the lip, gum, and palate deviations, abnormalities of the nose may also occur.

Cleft palate may be inherited, probably as a result of the interaction of several genes. In addition, the effect of some environmental factors that affect embryonic development

Forms of Cleft Palate

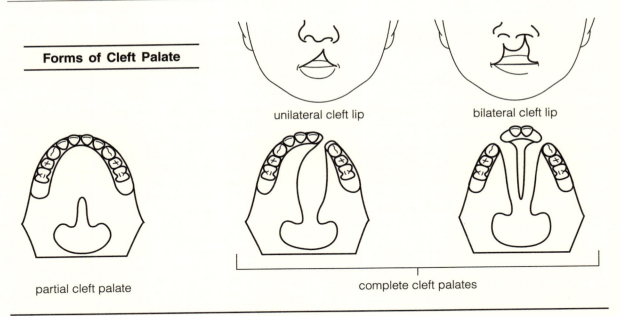

unilateral cleft lip

bilateral cleft lip

partial cleft palate

complete cleft palates

may be linked to this condition. They might include mechanical disturbances such as an enlarged tongue, which prevents the fusion of the palate and lip. Other disturbances may be caused by toxins introduced by the mother (drugs such as cortisone or alcohol) and defective blood. Other associated factors include deficiencies of vitamins or minerals in the mother's diet, radiation from X rays, and infectious diseases such as German measles. No definite cause has been identified, nor does it appear that one cause alone can be implicated. It is likely that there is an interplay between mutant genes, chromosomal abnormalities, and environmental factors.

There are at least 150 syndromes involving oral and facial clefts. Four examples of cleft syndromes that illustrate these syndromes are EEC (ectrodactyly, ectodermal dysplasia, cleft lip/palate), popliteal pterygium syndrome, van der Woude's syndrome, and trisomy 13 syndrome. EEC and trisomy 13 both result in mental retardation as well as oral clefts, plus numerous other disabilities more serious than clefting. Popliteal pterygium has as its most common feature skin webbing (pterygium), along with clefts and skeletal abnormalities. Van der Woude's syndrome usually shows syndactyly as well as clefting and lower-lip pitting.

Problems begin at birth for the infant born with a cleft palate. The most immediate problem is feeding the baby. If the cleft is small and the lip unaffected, nursing may proceed fairly easily. If the cleft is too large, however, the baby cannot build up enough suction to nurse efficiently. To remedy this, the hole in the nipple of the bottle can be enlarged, or a plastic obturator can be fitted to the bottle.

Babies with cleft palate apparently are more susceptible to colds than other children. Since there is an open con-

nection between the nose and mouth, an infection that starts in either location will easily and quickly spread to the other. Frequently, the infection will spread to the middle ear via the Eustachian tube. One end of a muscle is affixed to the Eustachian tube opening and the other end is attached to the middle of the roof of the mouth (palate). Normal contraction opens the tube so that air can travel through the tube and equalize air pressure on both sides of the eardrum. As long as the eardrum has flexibility of movement, the basics for good hearing are in place. Children with cleft palates, however, do not have good muscle reactions; therefore, air cannot travel through the tube. If the tube remains closed after swallowing, the air that is trapped is absorbed into the middle-ear tissue, resulting in a vacuum. This pulls the eardrum inward and decreases its flexibility, and hearing loss ensues. The cavity of the middle ear then fills with fluid, which often breeds bacteria, causing infection. The infection may or may not be painful; if there is no pain, the infection may go unnoticed and untreated. The accumulated fluid can cause erosion of the tiny bones, which would decrease sound transmission to the auditory nerve. This conductive hearing loss is permanent. Persistent and prolonged fluid buildup can also cause accumulation of dead matter, forming a tumorlike growth called a cholesteotoma.

Other problems associated with cleft palate are those related to dentition. In some children there may be extra teeth, while in others the cleft may prevent the formation of tooth buds so that teeth are missing. Teeth that are present may be malformed; those malformations include injury during development, fusion of teeth to form one large tooth, teeth lacking enamel, and teeth that have too little calcium in the enamel. If later in development and growth the teeth are misaligned, orthodontia may be undertaken. Another possible problem met by patients with a cleft palate is maxillary (upper-jaw) arch collapse; this condition is also remedied with orthodontic treatment.

TREATMENT AND THERAPY

One of the first questions a parent of a child with a cleft palate will pose regards surgical repair. The purpose of surgically closing the cleft is not simply to close the hole—although that goal is important. The major purpose is to achieve a functional palate. Whether this can be accomplished depends on the size and shape of the cleft, the thickness of the available tissue, and other factors. When the child is scheduled for surgery, it is a tangible sign that the condition is correctable. When the lip is successfully closed, it is positive affirmation that a professional team can help the family. The goals of both the team and the family are extremely similar: Both want the patient to look as normal as possible and to have a functional palate.

Cleft lip surgery is performed when the healthy baby weighs at least seven pounds; it is done under a general anesthetic. If the cleft is unilateral, one operation can accomplish the closure, but a bilateral cleft lip is often repaired in two steps at least a month apart. When the lip is repaired, normal lip pressure is restored, which may help in closing the cleft in the gum ridge. It may also reduce the gap in the hard palate, if one is present. Successive operations may be suggested when, even years after surgery, scars develop on the lip.

Surgery to close clefts of the hard and soft palate is typically done when the baby is at least nine months of age, unless there is a medical reason not to do so. Different surgeons prefer different times for this surgery. The surgeon attempts to accomplish three goals in the repair procedure. The surgeon will first try to ensure that the palate is long enough so that function and movement will result (this is essential for proper speech patterns). Second, the musculature around the Eustachian tube should work properly in order to cut down the incidence of ear infections. Finally, the surgery should promote the development of the facial bones and, as much as possible, normal teeth. This goal aids in eating and appearance. All this may be accomplished in one operation, if the cleft is not too severe. For a cleft that requires more procedures, the surgeries are usually spaced at least six months apart so that complete healing can occur. This schedule decreases the potential for severe scarring.

At one time, it was thought that if surgery were performed before the child began talking, speech problems would be avoided. In reality, not only did the surgery not remedy that problem but the early closure often resulted in a narrowing of the upper jaw and interference with facial growth as well. Thus the trend to put off the surgery until the child was four or five years of age developed; by this age, more than 80 percent of the lateral growth of the upper

jaw has occurred. Most surgeons can perform the corrective surgery when the child is between one and two years of age without affecting facial growth.

Successful repair greatly improves speech and appearance, and the physiology of the oral and nasal cavities is also improved. Additional surgery may be necessary to improve appearance, breathing, and the function of the palate. Sometimes the palate may partially reopen, and surgery is needed to reclose it.

When the baby leaves the operating room, there are stitches in the repaired area. Sometimes a special device called a Logan's bow is taped to the baby's cheeks; this device not only protects the stitches but also relieves some of the tension on them. In addition, the baby's arms may be restrained in order to keep the baby's hands away from the affected area. (The child has been fitted for elbow restraints before surgery; the elbows are encased in tubes which prevent them from bending.) A parent of a child that has just undergone cleft palate repair should not panic at the sight of bleeding from the mouth. To curb it, gauze may be packed into the repaired area and remain about five days after surgery. As mucous and other body fluids accumulate in the area, they may be suctioned out.

During the initial recovery, the child is kept in a moist, oxygen-rich environment (an oxygen tent) until respiration is normal. The patient will be observed for signs of airway obstruction or excessive bleeding. Feeding is done by syringe, eyedropper, or special nipples. Clear liquids and juices only are allowed. The child sits in a high chair to drink, when possible. After feeding, the mouth should be rinsed well with water to help keep the stitches clean and uncrusted. Peroxide mixed with the water may help, as well as ointment. Intake and output of fluids are measured. Hospitalization may last for about a week, or however long is dictated by speed of healing. At the end of this week, stitches are removed and the suture line covered and protected by a strip of paper tape.

An alternative to surgery is the use of an artificial palate known as an obturator. It is specially constructed by a dentist to fit into the child's mouth. The appliance, or prosthesis, is carefully constructed to fit precisely and snugly, but it must be easily removable. There must be enough space at the back so the child can breathe through the nose. While speaking, the muscles move back over this opening so that speech is relatively unaffected.

Speech problems are likely the most residual of the problems in the cleft palate patient. The speech of the untreated, and sometimes the treated, cleft palate patient is very nasal. If the soft palate is too short, the closure of the palate may leave a space between the nose and the throat, allowing air to escape through the nose. There is little penetrating quality to the patient's voice, and it does not carry well. Some cleft palate speakers are difficult to understand because there are several faults in articulation. Certainly not all cleft lip or palate patients, however, will develop communication problems; modern surgical procedures help ensure that most children will develop acceptable speech and language without necessitating the help of a speech therapist.

Genetic counseling may help answer some of the family's questions about why the cleft palate occurred, whether it will happen with future children, and whether there is any way to prevent it. There are no universal answers to these questions. The answers are dependent on the degree and type of cleft, the sex of the child, the presence of other problems, the family history, and the history of the pregnancy. Genetic counseling obtained at a hospital or medical clinic can determine whether the condition was heritable or a chance error and can establish the risk level for future pregnancies.

PERSPECTIVE AND PROSPECTS

Oral clefts, as well as other facial clefts, have been a part of historical record for thousands of years. Perhaps the earliest recorded incidence is a Neolithic shrine with a two-headed figurine dated about 6500 B.C. The origination and causative agent of such clefts remain mysterious today.

Expectant parents are rarely alerted prior to birth that their child will be born with a cleft, so it is usually in the hospital, just after birth, that parents first learn of the birth defect. Even if it is suspected that a woman is at risk for producing a child with a cleft palate, there is no way to determine if the defect is indeed present, as neither amniocentesis nor chromosomal analysis reveals the condition. When the baby is delivered, the presence of the cleft can evoke a feeling of crisis in the delivery room. Shocklike reactions may be caused by the unexpectedness of the event or can occur because the doctors and medical personnel in the room have had little exposure to the defect. The parents may feel personal failure.

The problems accompanying clefting may alter family morale and climate, increasing the complexity of the problem. A team of specialists usually work together to help the patient and the family cope with these problems. This team may include a pediatrician, a speech pathologist, a plastic surgeon, an orthodontist, a psychiatrist, a social worker, an otologist, an audiologist, and perhaps others. The formation and cooperation of a team of professionals and the emotional support that they provide for an affected family hopefully will enable that family to perceive the baby more positively, to focus on the child's potential rather than on the disability.

The cooperating team should monitor these situations: feeding problems, family and friend reactions to the baby's appearance, how parents encourage the child to talk or how they respond to poor speech, and whether the parents are realistic about the long-term outcome for their child. The grief, guilt, and shock that the parents often feel can be positively altered by how the professional team tackles the problem and by communication with the parents. Usually the team does not begin functioning in the baby's life until he or she is about a month old. Some parents have confronted their feelings, while others are still struggling with the negative feeling that the birth brought to bear. Therefore, the first visit that the parents have with the team is important, because it establishes the foundation of a support system which should last for years.

If the cleft was only a structural defect, the solution would simply be to close the hole. Yet, since there are problems concerning feeding and health, facial appearance, communication, speech, dental functioning, and hearing loss, as well as the potential for psychosocial difficulties, additional surgical, orthodontic, speech, and otolaryngological interventions may be necessary. In other words, after the closure has been made, attention is focused on aesthetic, functional, and other structural deficits.

—Iona C. Baldridge

See also Birth defects; Genetic diseases.

FOR FURTHER INFORMATION:

Batshaw, Mark L., and Yvonne M. Perret. *Children with Handicaps*. Baltimore: Paul H. Brookes, 1981. This book first takes the reader through the basics of genetics. Based on this information, diagnoses and descriptions of birth defects are made relative to the various organ systems. Concludes by examining the emotional aspects of living with a handicapped child.

Clifford, Edward. *The Cleft Palate Experience*. Springfield, Ill.: Charles C Thomas, 1987. This author writes from the perspective of a cleft-palate team participant and incorporates the value of the team in his chapters. Much space is given to the child's development of a positive self-image and the parents' role, from birth, in forming this image.

Dronamraju, Krishna R. *Cleft Lip and Palate*. Springfield, Ill.: Charles C Thomas, 1986. A compilation of research emphasizing population genetics, dental genetics, evolution, teratology, reproductive biology, and epidemiology. The purpose is to provide a basis for genetic counseling. An extensive bibliography is included.

Johnson, Wendell, and Dorothy Moeller, eds. *Speech Handicapped School Children*. 3d ed. New York: Harper & Row, 1967. Although this is a text for courses in speech pathology, the development and treatment of cleft palate are addressed. Psychological factors are considered, along with physical factors and associated problems with several speech handicaps.

Stengelhofen, Jackie, ed. *Cleft Palate*. Edinburgh: Churchill Livingstone, 1989. Explores the various communication problems met by those with a cleft palate. An appeal to the entire team of professionals treating the patient and their partnership with parents. Case histories are discussed.

Wynn, Sidney K., and Alfred L. Miller. *A Practical Guide to Cleft Lip and Palate Birth Defects*. Springfield, Ill.:

Charles C Thomas, 1984. A very readable book that is actually a series of dialogues between the parents and doctors of affected children. The tone is a reassuring one, and most physical and psychological aspects are addressed forthrightly.

CLUSTER HEADACHES
SYSTEM AFFECTED: Brain
SPECIALISTS: Family physicians, internists, neurologists
DEFINITION: Cluster headaches are characterized by intense pain behind one eye. They are generally recurrent in nature and are of such severity that they may wake the sufferer nightly for periods of weeks or months. Some researchers have suggested that cluster headaches are one category of migraine headache. Cluster headaches may be precipitated by the injection of histamine, a vasodilator that causes a fall in blood pressure; they are sometimes termed histaminic headaches or cephalalgia.

See also Brain disorders; Head and neck disorders; Headaches; Migraine headaches.

COLITIS
SYSTEM AFFECTED: Gastrointestinal
SPECIALISTS: Gastroenterologists, internists
DEFINITION: A potentially fatal but manageable disease of the colon which inflames and ulcerates the bowel lining, occurring in both acute and chronic forms.
KEY TERMS:
diarrhea: persistent liquid or mushy, shapeless stool
dysentery: bloody diarrhea caused by infectious agents affecting the colon
ileum: the last section of the small bowel, which passes food wastes to the colon through the ileocecal valve
inflammation: swelling caused by the accumulation of fluids and chemical agents
mucosa: the membrane of cells that lines the bowel; admits fluids and nutrients but also serves as the first-line protection against infectious agents and other materials foreign to the body
procedure: any medical treatment that entails physical manipulation or invasion of the body
stoma: an opening, formed by surgery, from the bowel to the exterior surface of the body
stool: the food wastes mixed with fluid, bacteria, mucus, and dead cells that exit the body upon defecation
ulcer: an area of the mucosa that has been abraded or dissolved by infection or chemicals, creating an open sore

CAUSES AND SYMPTOMS
The colon is the section of the lower bowel, or intestines, extending from the ileocecal valve to the rectum. It is wider in diameter than the small bowel, although shorter in length at about one meter. From behind the pelvis, the colon rises along the right side of the body (ascending colon), turns left to cross the upper abdominal cavity (transverse colon),

and then turns down along the left side of the body (descending colon) until it joins the sigmoid (S-shaped) colon. The sigmoid colon empties into the rectum, a pouch that stores the waste products of digestion that are excreted through the anus. The colon absorbs most of the fluid passed to it from the small bowel, so that wastes solidify; meanwhile, bacteria in the colon break down undigested proteins and carbohydrates, creating hydrogen, carbon dioxide, and methane gases in the process.

A key structure in colonic activity is its mucosa. This thin sheet of cells lining the bowel wall permits passage of fluids and certain nutrients into the bloodstream but resists bacteria and toxins (poisonous chemical compounds). When the mucosa is torn or worn away, bacteria and toxins enter, infecting the bowel wall. The body responds to infection by rushing fluids and powerful chemicals to the endangered area to confine and kill the infecting agents. In the process, the tissues of the bowel wall swell with the fluids; this is known as inflammation. The medical suffix denoting this response is *-itis;* when it occurs in the colon, physicians call it colitis.

A variety of agents can cause colitis, which is divided into two major types depending on the duration of the disease: acute colitis and chronic ulcerative colitis. Acute colitis is a relatively brief, single episode of inflammation. It is often caused by bacteria or parasites. For example, *Giardia lamblia,* a bacterium in many American streams, is a common infectious agent in colitis, and the amoebas in polluted water supplies are responsible for the type of colitis known as amebic dysentery. Some medicines, however, especially antibiotics, can also induce colitis. Acute colitis either disappears on its own or can be cured with drugs. Untreated, however, it may be fatal.

Chronic ulcerative colitis and Crohn's disease constitute a category of serious afflictions called inflammatory bowel disease (IBD) whose primary physical effects include swelling of the bowel lining, ulcers, and bloody diarrhea. Although some medical researchers think that these afflictions may be two aspects of the same disease, ulcerative colitis affects only the colon, whereas Crohn's disease can involve the small bowel as well as the colon. Moreover, colitis chiefly involves the colonic mucosa, but Crohn's disease delves into the full thickness of the bowel wall.

Chronic ulcerative colitis is a permanent disease that manifests itself either in recurring bouts of inflammation or in continuous inflammation that cannot be cleared up with drugs. It is commonly called ulcerative colitis because ulcers, open sores in the mucosa, spread throughout the colon and rectum, where the disease usually starts. Researchers have not yet discovered the causes of chronic ulcerative colitis, although there are many theories, of which three are prominent. The first is bacterial or viral infection, and many agents have been proposed as the culprit. Because such a multitude of organisms commonly reside in or pass through the colon, researchers have enormous difficulty separating out a specific kind in order to show that it is always present during colitis attacks. Second is autoimmune reaction. Research in other diseases has shown that sometimes the body's police system, enforced by white blood cells, mistakes native, healthy tissue for a foreign agent and attacks that tissue in an attempt to destroy it. Yet no testing in chronic ulcerative colitis has yet proven the theory. Third is a combination of foreign infection and autoimmune response; it is as if the immune system overreacts to an infectious agent and continues its attack even after the agent has been neutralized. Many researchers have suspected that the disease is inherited, because certain families have higher rates of the disease than others. This genetic theory is not universally accepted, however, because it is just as likely that family members share infection rather than having passed on a genetic predisposition for the disease. Other theories propose food allergies as the cause; even toothpaste has been considered.

Regardless of the cause, there is no doubt that colitis is a painful, disabling, bewildering disease. When the bowel inflames, the tissues heat up and fever results. Cramps are common, and sufferers feel an urgent, frequently uncontrollable urge to defecate. When they reach the toilet (if they do so in time), they have soft, loose stool or diarrhea, which can seem to explode from the anus. They may have as many as ten to twenty bowel movements a day. Because ulcers often erode blood vessels, blood can appear in the stool, as well as mucus and pus from the bowel wall. Severe weight loss, anemia, lack of energy, dehydration, and anorexia often develop as the colitis persists. The symptoms may clear up on their own only to recur months or years later; attacks may come with increasing frequency thereafter. The first attack, if it worsens rapidly, is fatal in about 5 to 10 percent of patients, although the death rate can rise to 25 percent among first-time sufferers who are more than sixty years old.

Complications from colitis can be life-threatening. These include perforation of the bowel wall, strictures, hemorrhaging, and toxic megacolon (hyperinflation of the colon, an emergency medical condition). Furthermore, studies show that patients who have had ulcerative colitis for more than ten years have about a 20 percent chance of developing cancer in the colon or rectum.

Because colitis is a relapsing, embarrassing disease, patients often suffer psychological turmoil. In *Colitis* (1992), Michael P. Kelly reports the results of his study of forty-five British colitis patients. According to Kelly, they typically denied that early symptoms were the signs of serious illness, passing them off as the result of overeating or influenza. The denial continued until the continual, desperate urge to defecate made them despair of controlling their bowels without help. Often, they suffered embarrassment because they had to flee family gatherings or work in order

to find a toilet or because they passed stool inadvertently in public. Many feared being beyond easy access to a toilet, shunned public places, and felt humiliated. Only then did some visit a physician, and even after chronic ulcerative colitis was diagnosed, a portion hoped they could still cope on their own. When they could not, they grew depressed, insomniac, angry at their fate, or antisocial. Even with treatment, the strain of enduring the disease can be debilitating.

TREATMENT AND THERAPY

Fortunately, medical science has several well-tested methods of controlling or curing colitis. In the case of acute colitis, patients usually resume normal bowel functions on their own and emerge as healthy as they were before the onset of symptoms. For chronic ulcerative colitis patients, however, the body is rarely the same again, and they must adjust to the effects of medication, surgery, or both—an adjustment that some authors claim is essentially a redefinition of the self.

After interviewing a patient and assessing the reported symptoms, the physician suspecting colitis orders a stool sample to check for blood, bacteria, parasites, and pus. If any of these are present, the physician directly examines the rectum and colon by inserting a fiberoptic endoscope into the rectum and up the colon. Early in the disease, the mucosa looks granular with scattered hemorrhages and tiny bleeding points. As the disease progresses, the mucosa turns spongy and has many ulcers that ooze blood and pus. An X ray often helps determine the extent of inflammation, and tissue samples taken by endoscopic biopsy can establish if it is ulcerative colitis or infection, and not Crohn's disease, that is present.

There is no easy treatment for chronic ulcerative colitis. Dietary restrictions—especially the elimination of fibrous foods such as raw fruits and vegetables or of milk products—may reduce the irritation to the inflamed colon, and symptoms then may improve if the disease is mild. Antidiarrheal drugs can firm the stool and reduce the patient's urgency to defecate, although such drugs must be used very cautiously to avoid dangerous dilation of the bowels.

Such nonspecific measures are seldom more than delaying tactics, and drugs are needed to counteract the colon's inflammation. Two types are most common. The first, sulfasalazine, is a sulfa drug developed in the 1940's. It is an anti-inflammatory agent that is most effective in mild to moderate ulcerative colitis and helps prevent recurrence of inflammation. Corticosteroids, the second type, behave like the hormones produced by the adrenal gland that suppress inflammation. The drug works well in relieving the symptoms of moderate to moderately severe attacks. Both types of drugs have serious side effects, so physicians must carefully tailor dosages for each patient and check repeatedly for reactions. In some patients, sulfasalazine induces nausea, vomiting, joint pain, headaches, rashes, dizziness, and hepatitis (liver inflammation). The effects of corticosteroids include sleeplessness, mood swings, acne, high blood pressure, diabetes, cataracts, thinning of the bones (especially the spine), and fluid retention and swelling of the face, hands, abdomen, and ankles. Women may grow facial hair; adolescents may have delayed sexual maturation. In most cases, the side effects clear up when patients stop taking the drugs.

With medication, people who suffer mild or moderate chronic ulcerative colitis can control it for years, often for the rest of their lives. Severe colitis requires surgery, and sometimes patients with milder forms choose to have surgery rather than live with the disease's unpredictable recurrence or the ever-present side effects of drugs. In any case, surgery is the one known cure for chronic ulcerative colitis, although fewer than one-third of patients undergo surgical procedures. Several types of these surgeries have high success rates.

Because ulcerative colitis eventually spreads throughout the colon, complete removal of the large bowel and rectum is the surest way to eliminate the disease. This "total proctocolectomy" takes place in three steps. The surgeon first cuts through the wall of the abdomen, the incision extending from the mid-transverse colon to the rectum, and removes the colon. Next, the end of the ileum is pulled through a hole in the abdomen to form a stoma (a procedure called an ileostomy). Finally, the rectum is removed and the anus sutured shut. Thereafter the patient defecates through the stoma. Either of two arrangements prevents stool from simply spilling out unchecked. Most patients affix plastic bags around their stomas into which stool flows without their control; when full, the bag is either emptied and reattached or thrown away and replaced. To avoid external bags, some patients prefer a "continent ileostomy," so called because it allows them to control defecation. The surgeon constructs a pouch out of a portion of the ileum and attaches it right behind the stoma, a procedure called a Kock pouch after its inventor, Nils Kock of Sweden. When this pouch is full, the patient empties it with a catheter inserted through the stoma. Some patients can choose to have an ileoanal anastomosis. In this procedure, the surgeon forms the end of the ileum into a pouch, which is attached to the anus and collects wastes in place of the rectum. The patient continues to defecate through the anus rather than through a stoma.

None of these surgical procedures is free of problems, and all require extensive recovery in the hospital and rehabilitation. Moreover, both infections and mechanical failures can occur. If healthy portions of the colon are left intact, they often flare with colitis later, and more operations become necessary. Patients with stomas are vulnerable to bacterial inflammation of the small intestine, resulting in diarrhea, vomiting, and dehydration. Stomas and pouches sometimes leak or close up, and even after successful operations patients lose some capacity to absorb zinc, bile salts, and vitamin B_{12}, although food supplements can make up for these deficiencies.

Any major surgery is an emotional trial. One that leaves a basic function of the body permanently altered, as with proctocolectomy or ileostomy, is difficult to accept afterward, even when the surgery was an emergency to save the patient's life. Patients must live with a bag of stool on their abdomen or a pouch that they must empty with a plastic straw—bags and pouches that sometimes leak stool or gas and that, even when functioning smoothly, are not pleasant to handle. They must pay close attention to body functions that they rarely had to think about before the ulcerative colitis began. The changes can severely depress patients, who then may need psychiatric help and antidepressant drugs to recover their spirits. Patients with anastomoses, who continue to defecate through their anus, also find their bowel functions changed, although not so severely. For example, it takes many months before normal stool forms, and diarrhea plagues these patients.

After their operations, patients have access to considerable help in addition to physicians and surgeons. Special nurses train patients to care for their stomas, check regularly for infection or malfunction, and generally ease them into their new lives. Formal support groups and informal networks are common, through which the afflicted can get information and reassurance. In the United States, the National Foundation for Ileitis and Colitis arranges many support groups, as well as sponsoring medical research and education programs.

PERSPECTIVE AND PROSPECTS

Acute forms of colitis, especially amebic dysentery, have long been recognized as among the endemic diseases of polluted water, and until the development of antibiotics, they regularly killed significant portions of local populations, especially the young and elderly. Chronic ulcerative colitis was first described in 1859, but no effective treatment for it existed until the 1940's. At that time, Nana Svartz of Sweden noticed that when rheumatoid arthritis patients were given sulfasalazine, the bowel condition of those who had colitis improved as well. J. Arnold Bargen, an American physician, confirmed Svartz's observation in a formal clinical trial, and sulfasalazine soon was mass-produced for distribution in the United States and later throughout the world. Since the 1940's, medications and surgical techniques for ulcerative colitis have proliferated, although none restores a patient's original state of health.

Because the agents causing ulcerative colitis are unknown, the historical and geographical origin of the disease likewise cannot be determined. Nevertheless, three somewhat odd social facets of the disease are recognized.

Evidence suggests that ulcerative colitis is a disease of urban industrial society. Along with Crohn's disease, colitis appears to be entrenched in Scandinavia, the United States, Western Europe, Israel, and England. It rarely occurs in rural Africa, Asia, or South America, despite the poor nutrition and sanitation in some of these areas. Yet the disease does not appear to vary solely by racial type or nationality, although Jewish people tend to fall ill with it more often than any other group. For example, African Americans, whether from families long-established in the United States or recently immigrated, show an incidence of colitis as high as residents of European descent.

Furthermore, ulcerative colitis strikes the young. It most often begins between the ages of fifteen and thirty; men and women are equally likely to come down with it. This fact, taken with the high rate of inflammatory bowel disease (IBD) sufferers who have family members also with the disease (20 to 25 percent), has led some researchers to believe that a genetic factor creates a susceptibility for IBD.

Finally, IBD patients bear some social stigma, or at least believe they do. Ulcerative colitis involves bowel incontinence and often ends with surgical replacement of the anus with a stoma; in such cases, bowel movements can dominate a patient's life and become obvious to family members, coworkers, and even strangers. Because the subject of stool is taboo to many and the odor offends most people, patients can feel severe embarrassment and come to see themselves as pariahs. Even though the causes of ulcerative colitis remain obscure and the treatment is often distressing, modern medicine saves people who otherwise would die.

—Roger Smith

See also Colon cancer; Crohn's disease; Diarrhea and dysentery; Diverticulosis and diverticulitis; Gastrointestinal disorders; Intestinal disorders.

For Further Information:

Berkow, Robert, and Andrew J. Fletcher. *The Merck Manual of Diagnosis and Therapy*. 15th ed. Rahway, N.J.: Merck, 1987. This is a reference work for physicians, and the nomenclature can be daunting. It is best consulted after more general introductory reading. The sections on colitis describe the physical symptoms, tests, and treatments systematically and thoroughly.

Brandt, Lawrence J., and Penny Steiner-Grossman, eds. *Treating IBD: A Patient's Guide to the Medical and Surgical Management of Inflammatory Bowel Disease*. New York: Raven, 1989. The most thorough introduction to ulcerative colitis and Crohn's disease. Writing for patients, the authors, who are all medical experts, present technical information and guidelines on symptoms, drugs, surgical procedures, nutritional management, psychotherapy, and counseling. Illustrations, tables, and very helpful glossaries accompany the text.

Kelly, Michael P. *Colitis*. New York: Routledge, 1992. Kelly begins his book with a description of symptoms and treatments, but his is primarily a sociological study. Based on interviews with forty-five patients, the work discusses typical effects that the disease had on their lives and how they coped with the treatments, especially sur-

gical procedures. Essential reading for anyone diagnosed as having chronic ulcerative colitis.

Oppenheim, Michael. *The Complete Book of Better Digestion: A Gut-Level Guide to Gastric Relief*. Emmaus, Pa.: Rodale Press, 1990. Oppenheim's discussion of colitis is brief, but it provides a good generalized guide to symptoms and treatment. The book is most valuable as an introduction to the entire digestive tract's functions and maladies.

Plaut, Martin E. *The Doctor's Guide to You and Your Colon*. New York: Harper & Row, 1982. Although somewhat out of date, this guide is a simple and often-humorous survey of the colon and its diseases, including ulcerative colitis. Adorned with illustrations and cartoons and supplemented with recipes, it is useful as background for more specific literature about colitis.

Steiner-Grossman, Penny, Peter A. Banks, and Daniel H. Present, eds. *People . . . Not Patients: A Source Book for Living with Inflammatory Bowel Disease*. New York: National Foundation for Ileitis and Colitis, 1985. Written to help IBD patients live with their diseases, this book combines very practical information—about support groups and patients' rights, for example—with overviews of symptoms and treatments. Its main strength, however, lies in case histories of patients from different walks of life.

Colon cancer

System affected: Gastrointestinal

Specialists: Colorectal surgeons, gastroenterologists, general surgeons, internists, oncologists

Definition: Cancer occurring in the large intestine, which is the second deadliest type of this disease.

Causes and Symptoms

With an estimated 60,000 deaths per year in the United States, cancer of the colon and rectum (also called large bowel or colorectal cancer) is the second most deadly cancer, ranking only behind lung cancer. About 90 percent of colorectal cancers arise from the glandular epithelium lining the inner surface of the large bowel and are termed adenocarcinomas. The cells of this layer are constantly being replaced by new cells. This fairly rapid cell division, along with the relatively hostile environment within the bowel, promotes internal cellular errors that lead to the formation of aberrant cells. These cells can become disordered and produce abnormal growths or tumors. Often, colorectal tumors protrude into the lumen (the spaces within the bowel), forming growths called polyps. Some polyps are benign and do not spread to other parts of the body, but they may still disturb normal bowel functions. Other polyps become malignant by forming more aggressive cell types, which allows them to grow larger and spread to other organs. The cancer can grow through the layers of the colon wall and extend into the body cavity and nearby organs such as the urinary bladder. Cancer cells can also break away from the main tumor and spread (metastasize) through the blood or lymphatic vessels to other organs, such as the lungs or liver. If not controlled, the spreading cancer eventually causes death by impairment of organ and system functions.

The risk of colorectal cancer is increased by certain hereditary and environmental factors. The dietary intake of fat and fiber also influences colorectal cancer risk. Researchers believe that fiber reduces the exposure of colon cells to cancer-causing chemicals (carcinogens) by diluting them and causing them to move more rapidly through the colon. Fats may promote colorectal cancer by triggering the excess secretion of bile, which is known to be carcinogenic in animals. In addition, fat may be converted to carcinogens by bacteria that live in the colon. Diets high in protein or low in fruit and vegetables may also elevate the risk. The tendency to develop colorectal polyps and cancer can be inherited; this genetic predisposition may be responsible for about 5 to 7 percent of all colorectal cancers. One example is an inherited disorder called familial adenomatous polyposis (FAP), in which multiple polyps develop in the colon; it often leads to colorectal cancer. Some of the defective genes that cause this and other types of colorectal cancers have been identified and are being studied to determine their role. Irritable bowel syndrome (IBS) and exposure to certain occupational carcinogens are also known to increase the risk.

TREATMENT AND THERAPY

The chances for survival are greatly increased when colorectal cancer is detected and treated at an early stage. Early detection in the general population is possible with the use of three common medical tests: digital rectal examination, in which the physician checks the inner surface of the rectal wall with gloved finger for abnormal growths; fecal occult blood test, in which a stool sample is tested for hidden blood that may have emanated from a cancerous growth; and sigmoidoscopy, in which the physician examines the rectal and lower colon inner lining with a narrow tubular optical instrument inserted through the anus. If cancer is suspected, further tests will be done to arrive at a diagnosis. This may include a computed tomography (CT) scan, double-contrast barium enema X-ray series, and colonoscopy. The CT scan and contrast X rays reveal abnormal growths, and colonoscopy is similar to sigmoidoscopy but uses a longer, flexible tube in order to inspect the entire colon. During sigmoidoscopy and colonoscopy, the physician can remove polyps and obtain tissue samples for biopsy. Microscopic examination of the tissue samples by a pathologist can determine the stage or extent of growth of the cancer. This is important because it helps determine the type of treatment. In one type of staging, the following criteria are used: stage 0 (cancer confined to epithelium lining of the bowel), stage 1 (cancer confined to the bowel wall), stage 2 (cancer penetrating through all layers of the bowel wall and possibly invading adjacent tissues), stage 3 (cancer invading

lymph nodes and/or adjacent tissues), and stage 4 (cancer spreading to distant sites, forming metastases).

Surgery is the primary treatment for colorectal cancer. Very small tumors in stage 0 can be removed surgically with the colonoscope. Tumors in more advanced stages require abdominal surgery in which the tumor is removed along with a portion of the bowel and possibly some lymph nodes. For cases in which the bowel cannot be reconnected, an opening is created through the abdominal wall (colostomy). This is usually a temporary procedure, and the hole will be closed when the bowel can be rejoined. Some advanced cancers cannot be cured by surgery alone. Adjuvant therapies—chemotherapy, radiation therapy, and biological therapy—may be used in combination with surgery. Chemotherapy drugs kill spreading cancer cells. The most common is 5-fluorouracil (5-FU), a chemical that interferes with the production of deoxyribonucleic acid (DNA) in dividing cells. 5-FU is more effective when given together with leucovorin (a compound similar to folic acid) and levamisole (an immune system stimulant). Levamisole and other treatments that reinforce the immune system are forms of biological therapy. Radiation therapy, given either before or after surgery, is helpful in killing undetected cancer cells near the site of the tumor.

PERSPECTIVE AND PROSPECTS

More than 150,000 new cases of colorectal cancer are diagnosed in the United States each year, or roughly 15 percent of all cancers. The incidence of colorectal cancer is lower among females than males and rises dramatically after the age of fifty. Colorectal cancer is more common in developed countries such as the United States and in densely populated, industrialized regions. American mortality rates from colorectal cancer are higher in the Northeast and north-central regions of the country than in the South and Southwest. Populations moving from low-risk parts of the world, such as Asia or Africa, to high-risk areas, such as the United States or Europe, take on the higher risk within a generation or two, and vice versa.

—*Rodney C. Mowbray*

See also Cancer; Intestinal disorders; Stomach, intestinal, and pancreatic cancers.

FOR FURTHER INFORMATION:

Cooper, Geoffrey M. *Elements of Human Cancer.* Boston: Jones and Bartlett, 1992.

DeVita, Vincent T., Jr., Samuel Hellman, and Steven A. Rosenberg, eds. *Cancer: Principles and Practice of Oncology.* 4th ed. Philadelphia: J. B. Lippincott, 1993.

Holleb, Arthur I., ed. *The American Cancer Society Cancer Book.* Garden City, N.Y.: Doubleday, 1986.

U.S. Department of Health and Human Services. Public Health Service. National Institutes of Health. *Cancer of the Colon and Rectum.* Bethesda, Md.: Author, 1991.

_____. *What You Need to Know About Cancer of the Colon and Rectum.* Bethesda, Md.: Author, 1987.

COLOR BLINDNESS

SYSTEM AFFECTED: Visual
SPECIALISTS: Geneticists, ophthalmologists
DEFINITION: Color blindness is a genetic condition of the eye in which the patient is unable to distinguish between some colors. Common forms involve an inability to distinguish between red and green; red and green color blindness affects about 10 percent of men and is very rare in women. Total color blindness is the inability to perceive any color at all and is extremely rare. Both conditions are sex-linked disorders inherited from the mother, who carries a defective gene on one of her X chromosomes but is not affected herself.

See also Genetic diseases; Visual disorders.

COMA

SYSTEM AFFECTED: Brain
SPECIALISTS: Emergency physicians
DEFINITION: A loss of consciousness from which a person cannot be aroused; a symptom signifying a variety of causes.

KEY TERMS:

alcoholic coma: coma accompanying severe alcohol intoxication

apoplectic coma: coma induced by cerebrum, cerebellar, or brain-stem hemorrhage, as well as by embolism or cerebral thrombosis

brain death: irreversible brain damage so extensive that the organ enjoys no potential for recovery and can no longer maintain the body's internal functions

coma: a loss of consciousness from which the patient cannot be aroused

conscious: having an awareness of one's existence

hepatic coma: coma accompanying cerebral damage caused by the degeneration of liver cells (especially that associated with cirrhosis of the liver)

traumatic coma: coma following a head injury

CAUSES AND SYMPTOMS

Consciousness is defined by the normal wakeful state, with its self-aware cognition of past events and future anticipation. Disease or dysfunction that impairs this state usually causes readily identifiable conditions such as coma. The self-aware. cognitive aspects of consciousness depend largely on the interconnected neural networks of the cerebral hemispheres. Normal conscious behavior depends on the continuous, effective interaction of these systems. Loss of consciousness from medical causes can be brief (a matter of minutes to an hour or so) or it can be sustained for many hours, days, or sometimes even weeks. The longer the duration of the comatose state, the more likely it is to reflect structural damage to the brain rather than a transient alteration in its function.

The word "coma" comes from the Greek *koma*, meaning to put to sleep or to fall asleep. This state of unarousable

unresponsiveness results from disturbance or damage to areas of the brain involved in conscious activity or the maintenance of consciousness—particularly parts of the cerebrum (the main mass of the brain), upper parts of the brain stem, and central regions of the brain, especially the limbic system. A wide spectrum of specific conditions can injure the brain and cause coma. The damage to the brain may be the result of a head injury or of an abnormality such as a brain tumor, brain abscess, or intracerebral hemorrhage. Often there has been a buildup of poisonous substances that intoxicates brain tissues. This buildup can occur because of a drug overdose, advanced kidney or liver disease, or acute alcoholic intoxication. Encephalitis (inflammation of the brain) and meningitis (inflammation of the brain coverings) can also cause coma, as can cerebral hypoxia (lack of oxygen in the brain, possibly attributable to the impairment of the blood flow to some areas). Whatever the underlying mechanism, coma indicates brain failure, and the high degree or organization of cerebral biochemical systems has been disrupted. Coma is easily distinguishable from sleep in that the person does not respond to external stimulation (such as shouting or pinching) or to the needs of his or her body (such as a full bladder).

Comas are classified according to the event or condition that caused the comatose state. Some of the most frequently encountered types of comas are traumatic coma, alcoholic coma, apoplectic coma, deanimate coma, diabetic coma, hepatic coma, metabolic coma, vigil coma, pseudo coma, and irreversible coma. Traumatic coma follows a head injury. It enjoys a somewhat more favorable outcome than that of comas associated with medical illness. About 50 percent of patients in a coma from head injuries survive, and the recovery is closely linked to age: The younger the patient, the greater the chance for recovery. Alcoholic coma refers to the coma accompanying severe alcohol intoxication, usually more than 400 milligrams alcohol per 100 milliliters of blood. This coma is marked by rapid, light respiration, usually with tachycardia and hypotension. Apoplectic coma is induced by cerebrum, cerebellar, or brain-stem hemorrhage, as well as by embolism or cerebral thrombosis. The term "deanimate coma" refers to a deep coma with loss of all somatic and autonomic reflex activity. The maintenance of life depends wholly upon such supportive measures as assisted respiration, and cardiac arrest will quickly follow if the respirator is stopped; this may be a transient or irreversible state. Diabetic coma is the coma of severe diabetic acidosis. Hepatic coma is the coma accompanying cerebral damage resulting from degeneration of liver cells, especially that associated with cirrhosis of the liver. "Metabolic coma" is the term applied to the coma occurring in any metabolic disorder in the absence of a demonstrable macroscopic physical abnormality of the brain. Vigil coma is defined as a state of stupor in which the patient is mute and shows no verbal or motor responses to stimuli although the eyes are open and give a false impression of alertness. Pseudo coma refers to states resembling acute unconsciousness but with self-awareness preserved. Irreversible coma, or brain death, occurs when irreversible brain damage is so extensive that the organ enjoys no potential for recovery and can no longer maintain the body's internal functions.

TREATMENT AND THERAPY

Of the acute problems in clinical medicine, none is more difficult than the prompt diagnosis and effective management of the comatose patient. The difficulty exists partly because the causes of coma are so many and partly because the physician possesses only a limited time in which to make the appropriate diagnostic and therapeutic judgment.

Measurements of variations in the depth of coma are important in its assessment and treatment. Varying depths of coma are recognized. In less severe forms, the person may respond to stimulation by, for example, moving an arm. In severe cases, the person fails to respond to repeated vigorous stimuli. Yet even deeply comatose patients may show some automatic responses, as they may continue to breathe unaided, may cough, yawn, blink, and show roving eye movement. These actions indicate that the lower brain stem, which controls these responses, is still functioning.

Assessment of the patient in coma includes an evaluation of all vital signs, the level of consciousness, neuromuscular responses, and reaction of the pupils to light. In most hospitals, a printed form for neurologic assessment is used to measure and record the patient's responses to stimuli in objective terms. The Glasgow coma scale also provides a standardized tool that aids in assessing a comatose patient and eliminates the use of ambiguous and easily misinterpreted terms such as "unconscious" and "semicomatose." Additional assessment data should include evaluation of the gag and corneal reflexes. Abnormal rigidity and posturing in response to noxious stimuli indicate deep coma.

The definitive treatment of altered states of consciousness requires removing, correcting, or halting the specific process responsible for the state to whatever degree possible. Often, accurate diagnosis and specific therapy require time, and the first priority is to protect the brain from permanent damage.

General treatment measures that apply to all patients include the following: ensurance of an adequate airway passage and oxygenation; maintenance of proper circulation; intravenous administration of glucose or thiamine if the patient is undernourished; any measures necessary to stop generalized seizures; the restoration of the blood acid-base and osmolar balance; the treatment of any detected infection; the treatment and control of extreme body temperatures; the administration of specific antidotes for situations such as drug overdoses; control of agitation; and the protection of the corneas.

In the absence of the gag reflex, regurgitation and aspiration are potential problems. Tube feeding, if necessary, must be done slowly and with the head of the bed raised during the feeding and for about half an hour later. Absence of the corneal reflex can inhibit blinking and natural moistening of the eye. The cornea cannot be allowed to dry, since blindness can result; therefore, artificial tears are instilled in the eyes to keep them moist.

Once the cause leading to the comatose state has been determined, the appropriate steps should be taken to minimize or eliminate it whenever possible. For many causes of coma, rapid intervention and treatment can mean recuperation for the patient, such as in the cases of diabetes, removable hematomas, and drug overdose.

Comatose patients are predisposed to all the hazards of immobility, including impairment of skin integrity and the development of ulcers, contractures and joint disabilities, problems related to respiratory and circulatory status, and alterations in fluid and electrolyte balance. All these factors must be taken into consideration when dealing with the comatose patient.

The outcome from severe medical coma depends on its cause and, with the exception of depressant drug poisoning, on the initial severity and extent of neurologic damage. Depressant drug poisoning reflects a state of general anesthesia, and, barring severe complications, almost all patients who survive drug intoxication can recover physically unscathed.

The clinical tests most valuable for estimating the capacity for recovery after medical coma are identical to those used in making the initial diagnosis. Within a few hours or days after the onset of coma, many patients show neurologic signs that can differentiate, with a high probability, the future extremes of either no improvement or the capacity for good recovery. After a period of about six hours (except for patients on drugs), certain neurological findings begin to correlate with the potential for neurologic recovery and can predict the outcome of about one-third of patients who will do badly. By the end of the first day, tests can predict the two-thirds of the patients who will do well. With each successive day, the signs develop greater predictive power. Persistence of coma in an adult for more than four weeks is almost never associated with later complete recovery.

PERSPECTIVE AND PROSPECTS

Attempts to define coma must give at least brief consideration to the concepts of consciousness. Consciousness involves not only the reception of stimuli but also the emotional implications of such stimuli, as well as the construction of intricate mental images.

Since the days of the ancient Greeks, people have known that normal conscious behavior depends on intact brain function and that disorders of consciousness are a sign of cerebral insufficiency. The range of awake and intelligent behavior is so rich and variable, however, that clinical abnormalities are difficult to recognize unless there are substantial deviations from the norm. Impaired, reduced, or absent conscious behavior implies the presence of severe brain dysfunction and demands urgent attention if recovery is to be expected. The brain can tolerate only a limited amount of physical or metabolic injury without suffering irreparable harm, and the longer the failure lasts, the narrower the margin between recovery and the development of permanent neurologic invalidism.

Since such researchers as Pierre Mollaret and Maurice Goulon first examined the question in 1959, many others have tried to establish criteria that would accurately and unequivocally determine that the brain is dead, or about to die no matter what therapeutic measures one undertakes. In 1968, the Harvard Medical School Ad Hoc Committee to Examine the Definition of Brain Death established criteria for determining irreversible coma, or brain death. These criteria are often used to complement the traditional criteria for determining death. All other existing guidelines, such as the Swedish, British, and United States Collaborative Study Criteria, include nearly identical clinical points but contain some differences as to the duration of observation necessary to establish the diagnosis as well as the emphasis to be placed on laboratory procedures in diagnosis.

Techniques such as computed tomography (CT) scanning and electroencephalography (EEG) have transformed the process of diagnosis in clinical neurology, with technology sometimes replacing clinical deduction. The art of diagnosis, however, is to comprehend the whole picture—where the lesion is, what it comprises, and above all, what it is doing to the patient.

Advances in resuscitative medicine have made obsolete the traditional clinical definition of death, that is, the cessation of heartbeat. Cardiac resuscitation can salvage patients after periods of asystole lasting up to several minutes. Cardiopulmonary bypass machines permit the patient's heartbeat to cease for several hours with full clinical recovery after resuscitation. While respiratory depression formerly meant death within minutes, modern mechanical ventilators can maintain pulmonary oxygen exchange indefinitely. Such advances have permitted many patients with formerly lethal cardiac, pulmonary, and neuromuscular disease to return to relatively full and useful lives. Abundant clinical evidence, however, demonstrates that severe damage to the brain can completely destroy the organ's vital functions and capacity to recover, even when the other parts of the body still live. The result has been to switch the emphasis in defining death to a cessation of brain function. Brain death occurs when brain damage is so extensive that the organ has no potential for recovery and cannot maintain the body's internal functions. Countries worldwide have adopted the principle that death occurs when either the brain or the heart irreversibly fails in its functions. In the United States, the time of brain death has been accepted as the time of the person's death in legal terms.

The determination of whether a comatose patient is brain-dead or can possibly recuperate is extremely important. Issues such as organ transplant programs that require donation of healthy organs and the economic and emotional expense involved in the treatment and care of a comatose patient make it critical to know when to fight for life and when to diagnose death.

In carrying out the many details of the physical care and assessment of the comatose patient, health care personnel must not lose sight of the fact that the patient is a fellow human being and a member of a family. One cannot always be sure exactly how much the patients are aware of what is being said or done as care is given. Whatever the level of awareness and response, comatose patients are told what will be done to and for them, as they deserve the same respect afforded alert and aware patients.

—*Maria Pacheco*

See also Concussion; Unconsciousness.

FOR FURTHER INFORMATION:

Clayman, C. B., ed. *The American Medical Association Encyclopedia of Medicine.* New York: Random House, 1989. A concise presentation of numerous medical terms and illnesses. A very good general reference.

Fazekas, J. F., and Ralph W. Alman. *Coma: Biochemistry, Physiology, and Therapeutic Principles.* Springfield, Ill.: Charles C Thomas, 1962. A good basic reference work that presents eight different types of comas, their causes and treatment, as well as a general introduction to the subject.

Landau, Sidney I., et al., eds. *International Dictionary of Medicine and Biology.* 3 vols. Vol. 1. New York: John Wiley & Sons, 1986. Offers a brief presentation of medical and biological terms. A useful general reference work.

Miller, Benjamin Frank. *Encyclopedia and Dictionary of Medicine, Nursing, and Allied Health.* 5th ed. Philadelphia: W. B. Saunders, 1992. Contains a concise presentation of the topic of coma.

Plum, Fred, and J. B. Posner. *The Diagnosis of Stupor and Coma.* 3d ed. Philadelphia: F. A. Davis, 1980. An excellent book dealing in detail with the diagnosis, treatment, and management of the comatose patient. Well organized and easy to read, it also includes an excellent bibliography for individuals who are interested in more specific presentations of the topic.

Wyngaarden, J. B., Lloyd H. Smith, Jr., and J. Claude Bennett, eds. *Cecil Textbook of Medicine.* 19th ed. 2 vols. Philadelphia: W. B. Saunders, 1992. Offers in-depth coverage of numerous medical conditions and a comprehensive presentation of the comatose state. The discussion is very technical, however, and requires a good science background.

COMMON COLD

SYSTEM AFFECTED: Respiratory

SPECIALISTS: Family physicians, infectious disease physicians, internists, otolaryngologists

DEFINITION: A class of viral respiratory infections that form the world's most prevalent illnesses.

KEY TERMS:

acute: referring to a disease process of sudden onset and short duration

chronic: referring to a disease process of long duration and frequent recurrence

coronavirus: a microorganism causing respiratory illness; one of the most prevalent causes of the common cold

pathogen: any disease-causing microorganism

rhinovirus: a microorganism causing respiratory illness; one of the most prevalent causes of the common cold

virus: an extremely small pathogen that can replicate only within a living cell

CAUSES AND SYMPTOMS

One of the reasons that no cure has ever been found for the common cold is that it is caused by literally hundreds of different viruses. More than two hundred distinct strains from eight genera have been identified, and no doubt more will be discovered. Infection by one of these viruses may confer immunity to it, but there will still be scores of others to which that individual is not immune. The common cold is usually restricted to the nose and surrounding areas—hence its medical name, rhinitis (*rhin-* meaning "nose" and *-itis* meaning "inflammation").

Children get the most colds, averaging six to eight per year until they are six years old. From that age, the number diminishes until, for adults, the rate is three to five colds per year. Colds and related respiratory diseases are the largest single cause of lost workdays and school days. Colds and related respiratory diseases are probably the world's most expensive illnesses. In the United States, about a million and a half person-years are lost from work each year; this figure accounts for one-half of all absences. Worldwide, the costs of lost workdays, medications, physician's visits, and the complications that may require extensive medical care are incalculable.

Among the virus types that cause the common cold are rhinovirus, coronavirus, influenza virus, parainfluenza virus, enterovirus, adenovirus, respiratory syncytial virus, and coxsackie virus. They are not all equally responsible for cold infections. Rhinoviruses and coronaviruses between them are thought to cause 25 to 60 percent of all colds. Rhinoviruses appear to be responsible for colds that occur in the peak cold seasons of late spring and early fall. Coronaviruses appear to be responsible for colds that occur when rhinovirus is less active, such as in the late fall, winter, and early spring.

A respiratory syncitial virus can cause the common cold in adults; in children it causes much more severe diseases, including pneumonia and bronchiolitis (inflammation of the bronchioles, small air passages in the lungs). Similarly, influenza and parainfluenza viruses, adenoviruses, and enteroviruses can be responsible for rhinitis and sore throat, but they are also capable of more serious illnesses such as pneumonia and influenza.

Viruses are the smallest of the invading microorganisms that cause disease, so small that they are not visible using ordinary microscopes. They can be seen, however, with an electron microscope, and their presence in the body can be detected through various laboratory tests.

Viruses vary enormously in their size and structure. Some consist of three or four proteins with a core of either deoxyribonucleic acid (DNA) or ribonucleic acid (RNA); some have more than fifty proteins and other substances. Viruses can only replicate within living cells. They invade the body and produce disease conditions in different ways. Some travel through the body to find their target host cells. A good example is the measles virus, which enters through the mucous membranes of the nose, throat, and mouth and then finds its way to target tissues throughout the body. Some, such as the viruses that cause the common cold, enter the body through the nasal passages and settle directly into nearby cells.

Rhinoviruses are members of the Picornaviridae family (*pico-* from "piccolo," meaning "very small"; *rna* from RNA, the genetic material that it contains; and *viridae* denoting a virus family). Coronaviruses are members of the Coronaviridae family, and they also contain RNA. Most viruses that are pathogenic to humans can thrive only at the temperature inside the human body, 37 degrees Celsius (98.6 degrees Fahrenheit). Rhinoviruses prefer the cooler temperatures found in the nasal passages, 33 to 34 degrees Celsius (91.4 to 93.2 degrees Fahrenheit). More than one hundred different rhinovirus types have been identified.

Exactly how a patient contracts a cold is better understood than it once was. Exposure to a cold environment—for example, getting a chill in winter weather—does not cause a cold unless the individual is exposed to the infecting virus at the same time. Fatigue or lack of sleep does not increase susceptibility to the cold virus, and even the direct exposure of nasal tissue to cold viruses does not guarantee infection.

A group in England, the Medical Research Council's Common Cold Unit, studied the disease from 1945 to 1990 and made many fundamental discoveries—even though the researchers never found a cure, or for that matter, any effective methods to prevent the spread of the disease. As part of their research, they put drops containing cold virus into the noses of volunteers. Only about one-third of the subjects thus inoculated developed cold symptoms, showing that direct exposure to the infecting agent does not necessarily bring on a cold.

What appears to be essential in the spread of the disease is bodily contact, particularly handshaking or touching. The infected individual wipes his or her nose or coughs into his or her hand, getting nasal secretions on the fingers. These infected secretions are then transferred to the hand of another person who, if susceptible, can become infected by bringing the hand up to the mouth or nose. Sneezing and coughing also spread the disease. Many viral and bacterial diseases are transmissible through nasopharyngeal (nose and throat) secretions; these include measles, mumps, rubella, pneumonia, influenza, and any number of other infections.

One or more individuals in a group become infected and bring the disease to a central place, such as a classroom, office, military base, or day-care center. In the case of the common cold, transferring infected particles by touch exposes another person to the infection. In other respiratory diseases, breathing, sneezing, or coughing virus-laden particles into the air will spread the disease. The infected individual then becomes the means by which the disease is brought into the home. By far, the largest number of colds are brought into the family by children who have contracted the infection in classrooms or day-care centers.

The pathogenesis of the common cold—that is, what happens when an individual is exposed to the cold virus—is not fully understood. It is believed that the virus enters the nasal passages and attaches itself to receptors on a cell of the nasal mucous membrane and then invades the cell. Viruses traveling freely in the blood or lymphatic system are subject to attack by white blood cells called phagocytes in what is part of the body's nonspecific defense system against invading pathogens.

Once inside the host cell, the virus replicates itself by stealing elements of the protoplasm of the cell and using them to build new viruses under the direction of the RNA component. These new viruses are released by the host cell to infect other cells. This process can injure or kill the host cell, activating the body's specific immune response system and starting the chain of events that will destroy the invading virus and create immunity to further infection from it.

In response to cell death or injury, certain chemicals are released that induce inflammation in the nasal passages. Blood vessels in the nasal area enlarge, increasing blood flow to the tissues and causing swelling. The openings in capillary walls enlarge and deliver lymphocytes, white blood cells that produce antibodies to fight the virus, as well as other specialized white blood cells.

Nasal mucosa swell and secretions increase, a condition medically known as rhinorrhea (-*rrhea* meaning "flowing," denoting the runny nose of the common cold). During the first few days of infection, these secretions are thin and watery. As the disease progresses and white blood cells are drawn to the area, the secretions become thicker and more purulent, that is, filled with pus. A sore throat is common, as is laryngitis, or inflammation of the larynx or voice box. Fever is not a usual symptom of the common cold, but a cough will often develop as excess mucus or phlegm builds up in the lungs and windpipe.

As mucus accumulates and clogs nasal passages, the body attempts to expel it by sneezing. In this process, im-

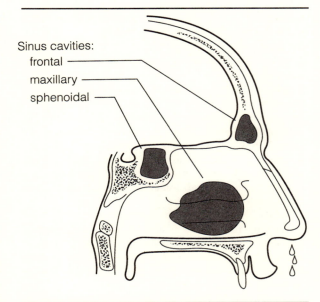

Sinus cavities:
frontal
maxillary
sphenoidal

The sinus cavities typically become congested with mucus as the body fights the virus that has caused the cold.

pulses from the nose travel to the brain's "sneeze reflex center," where sneezing is triggered to help clear nasal passages. Similarly, as phlegm accumulates in the windpipe and bronchial tree of the lungs, a message is sent to the "cough reflex center" of the brain, where coughing is initiated to expel the phlegm.

The common cold is self-limiting and usually resolves within five to ten days, but there can be complications in some cases. Patients who have asthma or chronic bronchitis frequently develop bronchoconstriction (narrowing of the air passages in the lungs) as a result of a common cold. If severe, purulent tracheitis and bronchitis develop, there may be a concomitant bacterial infection. In some patients, the infection may spread to other organs, such as the ears, where an infection called otitis media can develop. Sinusitis, infection of the cavities in the bone of the skull surrounding the nose, is common. If the invading organism spreads to the lungs, bronchitis or pneumonia may develop.

Other possible complications of the common cold depend on the individual virus. Rhinoviruses, usually limited to colds, may infrequently cause pneumonia in children. Coronaviruses, also usually limited to colds, infrequently cause pneumonia and bronchiolitis. A respiratory syncitial virus causes pneumonia and bronchiolitis in children, the common cold in adults, and pneumonia in the elderly. Parainfluenza virus, which causes croup and other respiratory diseases in children, can cause sore throat and the common cold in adults and, rarely, may cause tracheobronchitis in these patients. Influenza B virus, an occasional cause of the common cold, also causes influenza and, infrequently, pneumonia.

Another condition that can closely resemble the common cold, but which is not caused by a virus, is allergic rhinitis. The major form of allergic rhinitis is hay fever. It has many of the same symptoms as the common cold: sneezing, runny nose, nasal congestion, and sometimes, sore throat. In addition, the hay fever victim may suffer from itching in the eyes, nose, mouth, and throat. Hay fever is an allergic reaction to certain pollens. Because the pollens that cause hay fever are abundant at certain times of the year, it may be prevalent at the same times as some colds. Spring is a peak season for the common cold and also for hay fever, because of the many tree pollens that are carried in the air. In the fall, weed pollens, such as ragweed, affect hay fever sufferers during another peak period for colds. Colds occur less frequently in summer, but summer is another peak season for hay fever.

TREATMENT AND THERAPY

The nose is the first barrier of defense against the bacteria and viruses that cause upper respiratory infections. The nasal cavity is lined with a thin coating of mucus, a thick liquid that is constantly replenished by the mucous glands. Inner nasal surfaces are filled with tiny hairs, or cilia. Dust, bacteria, and other foreign matter are trapped by the mucus and moved by the cilia toward the nasopharynx to be expectorated or swallowed.

The blood vessels in the nasopharyngeal bed respond automatically to stimulation from the brain. Certain stimuli cause the vessels to constrict, widening air passages and at the same time reducing the flow of mucus. Other stimuli, such as those that are sent in response to a viral infection, allergen, or other irritant, cause blood vessels to dilate and increase the flow of mucus. Nasal passages become swollen, and airways are blocked.

The mucus-covered lining of the nasal passages contains various substances that help ward off infection and irritation by allergens. Lysozyme (lyso- meaning "dissolution" and -zyme from "enzyme," a catalyst that promotes an activity) attacks the cell walls of certain bacteria, killing them. It also attacks pollen granules. Mucus also contains glycoproteins that temporarily inhibit the activity of viruses. Mucus has small amounts of the antibodies immunoglobulin IgA and IgC that also may inhibit the activity of invading viruses.

Bed rest is usually the first element of treatment. Limiting physical stress may help keep the cold from worsening and may avoid secondary infections. The medications used to treat the common cold are directed at relieving individual symptoms: There is nothing available that will kill the viruses that cause it. Most cases of the common cold are treated at home with over-the-counter cold preparations. Children's colds and the complications that may arise from colds, such as bacterial and viral superinfection, may require the services of a physician.

Many medications for the common cold contain antihistamines. Histamine is a naturally occurring chemical in the body that is released in response to an allergen or an infection. It is a significant cause of the inflammation, swelling, and runny nose of hay fever. When these symptoms are seen with the common cold, however, they are probably caused by the body's inflammatory defense system rather than by histamine.

When antihistamines were first discovered, it was thought that they could inhibit the inflammatory defense against a cold. Patients were advised to take antihistamines at the first sign of a cold, in the hope of avoiding a full infection. Current thinking is that antihistamines have little value in the treatment of the common cold. They may have a minor effect on a runny nose, but there are better agents for this purpose. Antihistamines are usually highly sedative—most over-the-counter sleeping pills are antihistamines—so they may cause drowsiness. Patients taking many antihistamines are cautioned to avoid driving or operating machinery that could be dangerous.

The mainstays of therapy for the common cold are the decongestants that are applied topically (that is, directly to the mucous membranes in the nose) or taken orally. They are also called sympathomimetic agents because they mimic the effects of certain natural body chemicals that regulate many body processes. A group of these, called adrenergic stimulants, regulate vasoconstriction and vasodilation—in other words, they can narrow or widen blood vessels, respectively. Their vasoconstrictive capability is useful in managing the common cold, because it reduces the size of the blood vessels in the nose, reduces swelling and congestion, and inhibits excess secretion.

Topical decongestants are available as nasal sprays or drops. The sprays are squirted up into each nostril. The patient is usually advised to wait three to five minutes and then blow his or her nose to remove the mucus. If there is still congestion, the patient is advised to take another dose, allowing the medication to reach further into the nasal cavity. Nose drops are taken by tilting the head back and squeezing the medication into the nostrils through the nose-dropper supplied with the medication. Clearance of nasal congestion is prompt, and the patient can breathe more easily. Nasal irritation is reduced, so there is less sneezing. Some nasal sprays and drops last longer than others, but none works around-the-clock, so applications must be repeated throughout the day.

Patients who use nasal sprays and drops are advised to follow the manufacturer's directions exactly. Applied too often or in too great a quantity, these preparations can cause unwanted problems, such as rhinitis medicamentosa, or nasal inflammation caused by a medication (also called rebound congestion). As the vasoconstrictive effect of the drugs wears down, the blood vessels dilate, the area becomes swollen, and secretions increase. This reaction may be attributable to the fact that the drug's vasoconstrictive effect has deprived the area of blood, and thus excited an increased inflammatory state, or it may simply be attributable to irritation by the drug. Use of sprays or drops should be limited to three or four days.

Oral decongestants are also effective in reducing swelling and relieving a runny nose, although they do not have as great a vasoconstrictive effect concentrated in the nasal area as sprays or drops. Because they circulate throughout the body, their vasoconstrictive effects may be seen in other vascular beds. There are many patients who are warned not to use oral decongestants unless they are under the care of a physician. These people include patients with high blood pressure, diabetics, heart patients, and patients taking certain drugs such as monoamine oxidase (MAO) inhibitors, guanethidine, bethanidine, or debrisoquin sulfate.

Three kinds of coughs may accompany colds: coughs that produce phlegm or mucus; hyperactive nagging coughs, which result from overstimulation of the cough reflex; and dry, unproductive coughs. If the phlegm or mucus collecting in the lungs is easily removed by occasional coughing, a soothing syrup, cough drop, or lozenge may be all that the patient requires. If the cough reflex center of the brain is overstimulated, there may be hyperactive or uncontrollable coughing and a cough suppressant, such as dextromethorphan, may be needed. Dextromethorphan works in the brain to raise the level of stimulus that is required to trigger the cough reflex. Some antihistamines, such as diphenhydramine hydrochloride, are effective cough suppressants. If coughing is unproductive—that is, if the mucus has thickened and dried and is not easily removed—an expectorant should be taken. Currently, the only expectorant used in over-the-counter drugs is guaifenesin. It helps soften and liquefy mucus deposits, so that coughs become productive. When a cough of a cold is serious enough for a physician to be consulted, prescription drugs may have to be used, such as codeine to stop hyperactive coughing and potassium iodide for unproductive coughs.

For allergic rhinitis or hay fever, avoidance of allergens is recommended but is not always possible. For hay fever outbreaks, antihistamines are the mainstays of therapy, with other agents added to relieve specific symptoms. For example, topical and oral decongestants may be required to relieve a runny nose.

PERSPECTIVE AND PROSPECTS

Viruses are among the most intriguing and baffling challenges to medical science. Great progress has been made in preventing some virus diseases, such as by immunization against smallpox and hepatitis B. There has been only limited success, however, in finding agents to cure virus diseases, and so far nothing has been found to prevent or cure the common cold. Vaccines have been developed against certain rhinoviruses, and no doubt many more could be developed. Yet because the common cold is caused by so many different types of virus—more than two hundred—and vaccines against one virus are not necessarily effective

against others, it is questionable whether such vaccines would ever be useful. A helpful vaccine would be one that could immunize against an entire family of viruses such as rhinoviruses or coronaviruses, the two leading causes of the common cold.

The search goes on for agents to cure the common cold. Substances, such as interferons, have been found that are effective against a wide range of viruses. One of the interferons was used by the British Medical Research Council's Common Cold Unit. They reported that interferon applied as an intranasal spray was highly effective in protecting subjects from cold infection. After some years, however, experimentation with interferon in the common cold was abandoned because the agent had significant side effects, nasal congestion among them.

The science of virology only began in the 1930's, so it is not surprising that viruses continue to hide their mysteries. Nevertheless, many fundamental discoveries have been made and one can predict increasing success. As scientists unravel the intricacies of viral infections, they find clues that help them devise ways of interfering with virus life processes. In some cases, effective drugs have been developed, such as the interferons, acyclovir for herpes simplex, and amantadine for the influenza virus. It is likely that the cure for the common cold will continue to be elusive, unless a broad-spectrum antiviral agent could be developed that works against multiple viral infections in the way that broad-spectrum antibiotics work against multiple bacterial infections. —*C. Richard Falcon*

See also Allergies; Bacterial infections; Bronchitis; Coughing; Fever; Influenza; Nasopharyngeal disorders; Nausea and vomiting; Pneumonia; Rhinitis; Sinusitis; Sore throat; Staphylococcal infections; Streptococcal infections; Viral infections.

FOR FURTHER INFORMATION:

American Pharmaceutical Association. *Handbook of Nonprescription Drugs*. 9th ed. Washington, D.C.: Author, 1990. The section on drugs for colds, coughs, and allergies contains a thorough background discussion of these conditions. All major over-the-counter medications are listed.

Gallo, Robert. *Virus Hunting*. New York: Basic Books, 1991. Gallo gives a good general account of viruses—how they live and how modern medical science is trying to combat them.

Larson, David E., ed. *Mayo Clinic Family Health Book*. New York: William Morrow, 1990. One of the most thorough and accessible medical texts for the lay reader.

Scott, Andrew. *Pirates of the Cell*. Oxford, England: Basil Blackwell, 1985. A superior text on viruses for the lay reader, this book is particularly successful in clarifying the enormous range of pathogenic viruses, describing the infective process, and outlining the state of antiviral vaccines, medications, and procedures.

Young, Stuart H., Bruce S. Dobozin, and Margaret Miner. *Allergies*. Yonkers, N.Y.: Consumer Reports Books, 1992. A useful book that covers the treatment of allergic coldlike conditions, such as hay fever, and gives advice on how to manage them.

CONCEPTION

SYSTEM AFFECTED: Reproductive

SPECIALISTS: Gynecologists, obstetricians

DEFINITION: The process of creating new life, encompassing all the events from deposition of sperm into the female to the first cell divisions of the fertilized ovum.

KEY TERMS:

cervix: the lowest part of the uterus in contact with the vagina; contains an opening filled with mucus through which sperm can pass

ejaculation: the reflex activated by sexual stimulation that results in sperm mixed with fluid being expelled from the male's body

fertilization: the union of the sperm and the ovum, which usually occurs in the female's oviduct

menstruation: the process of shedding the lining of the uterus that occurs about once a month

oviduct: the thin tube that leads from near the ovary to the upper part of the uterus; also called the Fallopian tube

ovulation: the process by which the mature ovum is expelled from the ovary

ovum: the round cell produced by the female that carries her genetic material; also called the egg

sperm: the motile cells produced within the male that carry his genetic material

uterus: the organ above the vagina through which the sperm must pass on their way to the ovum; also called the womb

vagina: the stretchy, tube-shaped structure into which the male's penis is inserted during intercourse; the site of sperm deposition

PROCESS AND EFFECTS

The process of conception begins with the act of intercourse. When the male's penis is inserted into the female's vagina, the stimulation of the penis by movement within the vagina triggers a reflex resulting in the ejaculation of sperm. During ejaculation, involuntary muscles in many of the male reproductive organs contract, causing semen, a mixture of sperm and fluid, to move from its sites of storage out through the urethra within the penis.

The average volume of semen in a typical human ejaculation is only 3.5 milliliters, but this small volume normally contains 200 million to 400 million sperm. Other constituents of semen include prostaglandins, which cause contractions of involuntary muscles in both the male and the female; the sugar fructose, which provides energy to the sperm; chemicals that adjust the activity of the semen; and a number of enzymes and other chemicals.

In a typical act of intercourse, the semen is deposited high up in the woman's vagina. Within a minute after ejaculation, the semen begins to coagulate, or form a clot, because of the activation of chemicals within the semen. Sperm are not able to leave the vagina until the semen becomes liquid again, which occurs spontaneously fifteen to twenty minutes after ejaculation.

Once the semen liquefies, sperm begin moving through the female system. The path to the ovum (if one is present) lies through the cervix, then through the hollow cavity of the uterus, and up through the oviduct, where fertilization normally occurs. The sperm are propelled through the fluid within these organs by the swimming movements of their tails, as well as by female organ contractions that are stimulated by the act of intercourse and by prostaglandins contained in the semen. It is not necessary for the woman to experience orgasm, a pleasurable climax, in order for these contractions to occur. The contractions allow sperm to reach the oviduct within five minutes after leaving the vagina, a rate of movement that far exceeds their own swimming abilities.

Although some sperm can reach the oviduct quite rapidly, others never enter the oviduct at all. Of the two hundred million to four hundred million sperm deposited in the vagina, it is estimated that only one hundred to one thousand enter the oviducts. Some of the other millions of sperm may be defective, lacking the proper swimming ability. Other apparently normal sperm may become lost within the female's organs, possibly trapped in clefts between cells in the organ linings. The damaged and lost sperm will even-

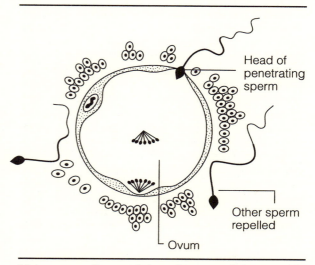

Male sperm cells propel themselves toward the ovum (female egg) by the swimming movements of their tails; fertilization occurs when a sperm cell penetrates the layers surrounding the ovum and fuses its membrane with the membrane of the ovum.

tually be destroyed by white blood cells produced by the female.

Sperm movement through the female system is enhanced around the time of ovulation. For example, at the time of ovulation, the hormones associated with ovulation cause changes in the cervical mucus that aid sperm transport. The mucus at that time is extremely liquid and contains fibers that align themselves into channels, which are thought to be used by the sperm to ease their passage through the cervix. The hormones present at the time of ovulation also increase the contractions produced by the uterus and oviduct, and thus sperm transport through the structures is enhanced as well.

During transport through the female, sperm undergo a number of important chemical changes, collectively called capacitation, that enable them to fertilize the ovum successfully. Freshly ejaculated sperm are not capable of penetrating the layers surrounding the ovum, a fact that was uncovered when scientists first began to experiment with in vitro fertilization (the joining of sperm and ovum outside the body). Capacitation apparently occurs during transport of the sperm through the uterus and possibly the oviduct, and it is presumably triggered by some secretion of the female. With in vitro fertilization, capacitation is achieved by adding female blood serum to the dish that contains the sperm and ovum. Capacitation is not instantaneous; it has been estimated that this process requires an hour or more in humans. Thus, even though the first sperm may arrive in the vicinity of the ovum within twenty minutes after ejaculation, fertilization cannot take place until capacitation is completed.

The site where ovum and sperm typically come together is within the oviduct. At the time of ovulation, an ovum is released from the surface of the ovary and drawn into the upper end of the oviduct. Once within the oviduct, the ovum is propelled by contractions of the oviduct and possibly by wavelike motions of cilia, hairlike projections that line the inner surface of the oviduct. It takes about three days for the ovum to travel the entire length of the oviduct to the uterus, and since the ovum only remains fertilizable for twelve to twenty-four hours, successful fertilization must occur in the oviduct.

Upon reaching the ovum, the sperm must first penetrate two layers surrounding it. The outermost layer, called the corona radiata, consists of cells that break away from the ovary with the ovum during ovulation; the innermost layer, the zona pellucida, is a clear, jellylike substance that lies just outside the ovum cell membrane. Penetration of these two layers is accomplished by the release of enzymes carried by the sperm. Once through the zona pellucida, the sperm are ready to fertilize the ovum.

Fertilization occurs when a sperm fuses its membrane with the membrane of the ovum. This act triggers a protective change in the zona pellucida that prevents any additional sperm from reaching the ovum and providing it with extra chromosomes. Following fusion of the fertilizing sperm and ovum, the chromosomes of each become mingled; the resulting one-celled zygote contains a complete set of chromosomes, half contributed by the mother and half by the father.

It is at the moment of fertilization that the sex of the new child is decided. Genetic sex is determined by a pair of chromosomes denoted X and Y. Female body cells contain two X's, and each ovum produced contains only one X. Male body cells contain an X and a Y chromosome, but each sperm contains either an X or a Y chromosome. Men usually produce equal numbers of X- and Y-type sperm. The sex of the new individual is determined by which type of sperm fertilizes the ovum: If it is a Y-bearing sperm, the new individual will be male, and if it is an X-bearing sperm, the new individual will be female. Since entry of more than one sperm is prohibited, the first sperm to reach the ovum is the one that will fertilize it.

Following fertilization, the zygote or early embryo begins a series of cell divisions while it travels down the oviduct. When it arrives at the uterus about three days after ovulation, the zygote will be in the form of a hollow ball of cells. Initially, this ball of cells floats in the fluid-filled cavity of the uterus, but two or three days after its arrival in the uterus (five to six days after ovulation), it will attach to the uterine lining. Over the next nine months, the body of the embryo will take on a human form and develop the ability to live independently outside the uterus.

COMPLICATIONS AND DISORDERS

Three factors limit the time frame in which conception is possible: the fertilizable lifetime of the ovulated ovum, estimated to be between twelve and twenty-four hours; the fertilizable lifetime of ejaculated sperm in the female tract, usually assumed to be about forty-eight hours; and the time required for sperm capacitation, which is one hour or more. The combination of these factors determines the length of the fertile period, the time during which intercourse must occur if conception is to be achieved. Taking the three factors into account, the fertile period is said to extend from forty-eight hours prior to ovulation until perhaps twenty-four hours after ovulation. For example, if intercourse occurs forty-eight hours before ovulation, the sperm will be capacitated in the first few hours and will still be within their fertilizable lifetime when ovulation occurs. On the other hand, if intercourse occurs twenty-four hours after ovulation, the sperm will still require time for capacitation, but the ovum will be near the end of its viable period. Thus the later limit of the fertile period is equal to the fertilizable lifetime of the ovum, minus the time required for capacitation.

Obviously, a critical factor in conception is the timing of ovulation. In a typical twenty-eight-day menstrual cycle, ovulation occurs about halfway through the cycle, or fourteen days after the first day of menstrual bleeding. In actuality, cycle length varies widely, both among individual women and in a single woman from month to month. It appears that generally the first half of the cycle is more variable in length, with the second half more stable. Thus, no matter how long the entire menstrual cycle is, ovulation usually occurs fourteen days prior to the first day of the next episode of menstrual bleeding. Therefore, it is relatively easy to determine when ovulation occurred by counting backward, but difficult to predict the time of ovulation in advance.

Assessment of ovulation time in women is notoriously difficult. There is no easily observable outward sign of ovulation. Some women do detect slight abdominal pain about the time of ovulation; this is referred to as *Mittelschmerz*, which means, literally, pain in the middle of the cycle. This slight pain may be localized on either side of the abdomen and is thought to be caused by irritation of the abdominal organs by fluid released from the ovary during ovulation. Other signs of ovulation are an increased volume and stretchiness of the cervical mucus and a characteristic fernlike pattern of the mucus when it is dried on a glass slide. There is also a slight rise in body temperature after ovulation, which again makes it easier to determine the time of ovulation after the fact rather than in advance. It is also possible to measure the amount of luteinizing hormone (LH) in urine or blood; this hormone shows a marked increase about sixteen hours prior to ovulation. Home test kits to detect LH levels are available for urine samples. There are additional signs of the time of ovulation, such as a slight opening of the cervix and a change in the cells lining the vagina, that can be used by physicians to determine the timing and occurrence of ovulation.

Since ovulation time is so difficult to detect in most women on an ongoing basis, most physicians would counsel that, to achieve a pregnancy, couples should plan on having intercourse every two days. This frequency will ensure that sperm capable of fertilization are always present, so that the exact time of ovulation becomes unimportant. A greater frequency of intercourse is not advised, since sperm numbers may be reduced when ejaculation occurs often. Approximately 85 to 90 percent of couples will achieve pregnancy within a year when intercourse occurs about three times a week.

Couples often wonder if it is possible to predetermine the sex of their child by some action taken in conjunction with intercourse. Scientists have found no consistent effect of parental diet, position assumed during intercourse, timing of intercourse within the menstrual cycle, or liquids that are introduced into the vagina to kill one type of sperm selectively. In the laboratory, it is possible to achieve partial separation of sperm in a semen sample by subjecting the semen to an electric current or other procedure. The separated sperm can then be used for artificial insemination (the introduction of semen through a tube into the uterus). This method is not 100 percent successful in producing offspring of the desired sex and so is available only on an experimental basis.

Some couples have difficulty in conceiving a child, in a few cases as a result of some problem associated with intercourse. For example, the male may have difficulty in achieving erection or ejaculation. The vast majority of these cases are caused by psychological factors such as stress and tension rather than any biological problem. Fortunately, therapists can teach couples how to overcome these psychological problems.

About 15 percent of couples in the United States suffer from some type of biological infertility—that is, infertility that persists when intercourse occurs successfully. In 10 percent of the cases of infertility, doctors are unable to establish a cause. In another 20 percent of couples, both partners are infertile. In the remaining 70 percent of cases, about half the problems are in the male and half in the female.

In men, the most commonly diagnosed cause of infertility is low sperm count. Sometimes low sperm count is caused by a treatable imbalance of hormones. If not treatable, this problem can sometimes be circumvented by the use of pooled semen samples in artificial insemination or through in vitro fertilization. In vitro fertilization may also be a solution for men who produce normal numbers of sperm but whose sperm lack swimming ability. Another cause of male infertility is blockage of the tubes that carry the semen from the body, which may be caused by a previous infection. Surgery is sometimes successful in removing such a blockage.

In women, a common cause of infertility is a hormonal problem that interferes with ovulation. Treatment with one of a number of so-called fertility drugs may be successful in promoting ovulation. Fertility drugs, however, have some disadvantages: They have a tendency to cause ovulation of more than one ovum, thus raising the possibility of multiple pregnancy, which is considered risky; and they may alter the environment of the uterus, making implantation of a resulting embryo less likely.

Another common cause of female infertility is blockage of the oviducts resulting from scar tissue formation in the aftermath of some type of infection. Because surgery is not always successful in opening the oviducts, this condition may require the use of in vitro fertilization or the new technique of surgically introducing ova and sperm directly into the oviduct at a point below the blockage.

Finally, some cases of infertility result from biological incompatibility between the man and the woman. It may be that the sperm are unable to penetrate the cervical mucus, or perhaps that the woman's body treats the sperm cells as invaders, destroying them before they can reach the ovum. Techniques such as artificial insemination and in vitro fertilization offer hope for couples experiencing these problems.

PERSPECTIVE AND PROSPECTS

For most of history, the events surrounding conception were poorly understood. For example, microscopic identification of sperm did not occur until 1677, and the ovum was not identified until 1827 (although the follicle in which the ovum develops was recognized in the 1600's). Prior to these discoveries, people held the belief espoused by early writers such as Aristotle and Galen that conception resulted from the mixing of male and female fluids during intercourse.

There was also confusion about the timing of the fertile period. Some early doctors thought that menstrual blood was involved in conception and therefore believed that the fertile period coincided with menstruation. Others recognized that menstrual bleeding was a sign that pregnancy had not occurred; they assumed that the most likely time for conception to result was immediately after the menstrual flow ceased. It was not until the 1930's that the first scientific studies on the timing of ovulation were completed.

Since there was little scientific understanding of the processes involved in conception, medical practice for most of human history was little different from magic, revolving around the use of rituals and herbal treatments to aid or prevent conception. Gradually, people rejected these practices, often because of religious teachings. By the 1900's, conception had been established as an area of intense privacy, thought by physicians and the general public to be unsuitable for medical intervention.

In the early part of the twentieth century, the role of physicians in aiding conception was mostly limited to educating and advising couples finding difficulty in conceiving. There were few techniques, other than artificial insemination and fertility drug treatment, available to assist in conception at that time.

The situation changed with the first successful in vitro fertilization in 1978. This event ushered in an era of intense medical and public interest in assisting conception. Other methods to aid conception were soon introduced, including embryo transfer, frozen storage of embryos, and surgical placement of ova and sperm directly into the oviduct.

Paralleling the development of these techniques has been demand on the part of society for medicine to apply them. Infertility rates in the United States have been gradually increasing. One reason for increased infertility has been the increasing age at which couples decide to start a family, since the fertility of women appears to undergo a decline past the age of thirty. Another factor affecting fertility rates of both men and women has been an increased incidence of various sexually transmitted diseases, which can result in chronic inflammation of the reproductive organs and infertility caused by scar tissue formation.

People's attitudes toward medical intervention in conception have also changed. The earlier religious taboos against interference in conception have been somewhat relaxed, although some churches still do not approve of certain methods of fertility management. Although there remain ethical issues to be resolved, the general public seems to have accepted the idea that medicine should provide assistance to those who wish to, but cannot, conceive children.

—*Marcia Watson-Whitmyre*

See also Childbirth; Infertility in females; Infertility in males; Pregnancy and gestation.

FOR FURTHER INFORMATION:

Birke, Lynda, Susan Himmelweit, and Gail Vines. *Tomorrow's Child: Reproductive Technologies in the Nineties*. London: Virago Press, 1990. Written for the general reader, this book is unique in its multifaceted coverage of medically assisted conception. Provides accurate information on the procedures involved and also covers ethical issues.

Hafez, E. S. E., ed. *Human Reproduction: Conception and Contraception*. Hagerstown, Md.: Harper & Row, 1980. Written by expert scientists, this text provides complete coverage of human conception. The first two sections cover male and female anatomy and physiology.

Harkness, Carol. *The Infertility Book*. San Francisco: Volcano Press, 1987. Presents a comprehensive guide to problems of infertility and combines both a medical and an emotional perspective. Contains anecdotal accounts in the patients' own words.

Jones, Richard E. *Human Reproductive Biology*. San Diego: Academic Press, 1991. This college-level textbook provides comprehensive coverage of all biological aspects of human reproduction. There is a separate chapter on fertilization, and information on the timing of ovulation, contraception, and infertility treatment is also presented.

Liebman-Smith, Joan. *In Pursuit of Pregnancy*. New York: Newmarket Press, 1987. This well-written book presents the stories of three couples as they discover and cope with their infertility. Contains good descriptions of diagnostic and treatment procedures.

McLaren, Angus. *Reproductive Rituals: The Perception of Fertility in England from the Sixteenth Century to the Nineteenth Century*. London: Methuen, 1984. Provides an account of practices surrounding fertility management using a combination of historical and cultural anthropological analyses. The author rejects the contention of many historians that couples in this period did little to control births.

Silber, Sherman J. *How to Get Pregnant*. New York: Charles Scribner's Sons, 1980. Written by a physician, this text is as straightforward as its title implies. Accurate, comprehensive, and easy to read.

CONCUSSION

SYSTEM AFFECTED: Brain

SPECIALISTS: Emergency physicians, neurologists

DEFINITION: The most common injury to the head is the concussion. When the head is struck by a hard blow or shaken violently, the brain is jostled, striking the inside of the skull. The result is temporary neural dysfunction, which may cause confusion, dizziness, nausea, headache, lethargy, changes in character, and amnesia for the time just before or after the injury. These symptoms are normal for a concussion and are not usually serious; some may last for weeks. Any worsening of these symptoms following the injury, however, may require further medical care and could indicate more severe damage to the brain, such as a cerebral contusion.

See also Brain disorders; Coma; Head and neck disorders; Unconsciousness.

CONGENITAL HEART DISEASE

SYSTEM AFFECTED: Heart

SPECIALISTS: Cardiologists, neonatologists, vascular surgeons

DEFINITION: Conditions resulting from malformations of the heart that occur during embryonic and fetal development, accounting for about 25 percent of all congenital defects.

KEY TERMS:

atrium: one of two heart chambers that receive blood, the left from the lungs and the right from the body

great arteries and veins: large vessels channeling blood into and out of the heart, including the aorta (to the body), the pulmonary artery (to the lungs), the vena cava (from the body), and the pulmonary veins (from the lungs)

heart failure: the inability of the heart to pump adequate amounts of blood to maintain the organs and tissues of the body; often results in tissue fluid retention and congestion

murmur: a sound made by the heart other than the normal two-step beat; murmurs are caused by the turbulent movement of blood and may indicate a heart defect

septum: a membrane which serves as a wall of separation; in the heart, the interatrial septum divides the two atria and the interventricular septum divides the two ventricles

ventricles: heart chambers that pump blood, the left to the body and the right to the lungs

CAUSES AND SYMPTOMS

Congenital heart disease collectively includes various structural and functional defects of the heart and blood vessels resulting from errors that occur during embryonic development. The defects may cause heart murmurs, high or low blood pressure, congestive heart failure, cyanosis (blue skin), abnormal heart rhythms and rates, and incidences of low oxygen (hypoxia). Congenital heart disease is detected in about 0.7 percent of live births and 2.7 percent of still births. Babies born with congenital heart disease have the most difficulty during the first few weeks of life. Some problems, however, are not easily detected at the time of birth and are discovered at various stages of life. Heart defects may be inherited from parents, induced by environmental agents such as drugs, or caused by an interaction

of genetic and environmental factors. Defects are more common in children with genetic disorders such as Down syndrome. With intensive treatment, including surgery, many forms of congenital heart disease can be corrected, allowing those affected to lead normal lives.

Knowledge of normal heart development will help in understanding how congenital heart disease occurs and will provide a means for categorizing these defects. Near the end of the third week of embryonic development, the heart begins to form from two cords of tissue that hollow out and fuse to form a primitive heart tube. This tube undergoes some constrictions and dilations to form the early divisions of the heart, including a receiving chamber, the atrium, and a pumping chamber, the ventricle, which exits into a muscular tube called the truncus arteriosus. At about twenty-two days, the heart begins to contract and pump blood. A day later, it bends or loops upon itself to form an S shape, with the atrium on one side, the truncus arteriosus on the other side, and the ventricle in the middle. If it bends to the left instead of to the right, a rare heart defect called dextrocardia results. The heart will be displaced to the right side of the body and may have some accompanying abnormalities.

During the fourth and fifth week of development, the heart begins to divide into four chambers by first forming a septum (dividing membrane) in the canal between the atrium and the ventricle. This septum is formed by heart tissue called the endocardial cushions. Failure of this septum to form properly causes atrioventricular canal defects. These are often associated with Down syndrome. During the fifth week of development, a spiral septum forms in the truncus arteriosus which divides it into two vessels: the pulmonary artery, which connects to the right ventricle, and the aorta, which connects to the left ventricle. The formation of this septum and the ventricular connections are subject to error and may result in a group of anomalies called conotruncal defects.

As these large arteries are forming, a shunt (bypass) develops between them called the ductus arteriosus. This short vessel allows the blood to be diverted away from the nonfunctional fetal lungs into the aorta and on to the placenta, where it will receive oxygen and nutrients. Persistence of this shunt after birth is responsible for a defect called patent ductus. A septum dividing the atrium into right and left halves also forms during the fourth and fifth weeks of development; however, blood is allowed to pass from the right atrium to the left atrium through a small hole in this septum called the foramen ovale. This hole normally closes after birth but is necessary during fetal life to shunt blood away from the fetal lungs and toward the placenta in a manner similar to that of the ductus arteriosus. At about the same time, a septum forms from the floor of the ventricle and divides it into right and left halves. Failure of the atrial and ventricular septa to form properly and to close at the time of birth results in septal defects.

After the appearance of the four chambers, two pairs of valves form in the heart to prevent the back flow of blood and to ensure greater efficiency in pumping. The semilunar valves (also called the pulmonary and aortic valves) form between the ventricles and their respective outlet arteries (pulmonary artery and aorta), and the atrioventricular valves (bicuspid or mitral on the left and tricuspid on the right) form between the atria and the ventricles. Improperly formed valves can lead to flow defects. During development, the heart also makes connections with veins returning from the general circulation and the lungs. Errors in these connections and other structural errors cause several other less common congenital heart defects.

The most common congenital heart defects are the septal defects and patent ductus, which together account for about 37 percent of all heart defects. After birth, because the pressure becomes higher in the left side of the heart, blood moves from left to right through the openings in the heart that come with such defects, causing too much to flow to the lungs and a mixing of systemic and pulmonary blood. The child's lungs will be congested, causing difficulty in breathing and eventually heart failure.

About 29 percent of congenital heart defects are categorized as right-heart and left-heart flow defects. These defects impede the flow of blood from either the right or the left side of the heart to its normal destination. Right-heart flow defects include bicuspid pulmonary valve (a valve with two cusps instead of three), pulmonary valve stenosis (a narrowing of the valve), dysplastic pulmonary valve (a malformed valve), peripheral pulmonary stenosis (a narrowing of the walls of the pulmonary artery), infundibular pulmonary stenosis (a narrowing below the valve), and hypoplastic right ventricle (incomplete formation of the valve). These defects impede blood flow to the lungs, which results in poor oxygenation of the blood (cyanosis). Left-heart flow defects include bicuspid aortic valve, aortic valve stenosis, coarctation of the aorta (narrowing), aortic atresia (a blocked aorta), and hypoplastic left ventricle. These defects impede blood flow to the body and often result in altered blood pressure, hypoxia of body tissues, and congestive heart failure.

The principal conotruncal defects, which account for about 17 percent of heart defects, are tetralogy of Fallot and transposition of the great arteries. Tetralogy of Fallot includes a group of four defects which results in cyanosis; they are pulmonary stenosis, a ventricular septal defect, an overriding or displaced aorta, and hypertrophy or enlargement of the right ventricle. With transposition of the great arteries, the aorta connects to the right ventricle and the pulmonary artery to the left ventricle, the opposite of the normal formation. The blood is not properly oxygenated, and survival is not possible without medical intervention or a natural shunt such as patent ductus. Other rare conotruncal defects include double outlet right ventricle

Tetralogy of Fallot

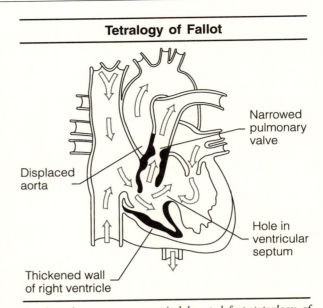

A relatively common congenital heart defect, tetralogy of Fallot comprises four defects: an overriding or displaced aorta, pulmonary stenosis (a narrowed pulmonary valve), a ventricular septal defect (a hole in the ventricular septum), and a thickened, or enlarged, right ventricle. These together result in cyanosis: poor blood oxygenation.

(the aorta and the pulmonary artery attached to right ventricle), truncus arteriosus (failure of the truncus to separate into the aorta and the pulmonary artery), and aortopulmonary window (an opening between the aorta and the pulmonary artery).

Defects resulting from improper fusion of the endocardial cushions and surrounding tissues cause atrioventricular defects, which affect about 9 percent of patients with congenital heart disease. Complete atrioventricular canal defect occurs in about 20 percent of Down syndrome cases, but it is rare outside this group. The defect produces a large open space in the center of the heart, allowing blood to intermix freely between the right and left sides of the heart. The defect is sometimes accompanied by hypoplastic ventricle. If the condition is not treated, the heart will fail. Patent foramen primum or ostium primum is a milder form of atrioventricular canal defect in which the atrial septum fails to fuse with the endocardial cushions, resulting in a problem similar to atria septal defect. In addition, the mitral valve is usually deformed.

Other less common defects include looping defects such as dextrocardia, in which the apex of the heart points to the right instead of to the left. This change in symmetry normally does not affect heart function, but some looping defects are associated with other problems such as transposition of the great arteries. Another less common defect is anomalous venous return, in which the veins returning blood to the heart from the lungs attach to the left atrium or return to the left atrium by attaching to other large veins rather than to the right atrium. Errors in the coronary artery connections may also occur, causing poor circulation of blood to the heart muscles. Very rarely, the heart may protrude through the chest wall at birth, causing a difficult-to-treat problem called ectopia cordis.

TREATMENT AND THERAPY

Congenital heart disease can often be diagnosed shortly after birth, especially if the baby experiences certain symptoms such as cyanosis, shortness of breath, fatigue and sweating while eating, and inability to gain weight. A physical examination by a physician will include checking the heart and breathing rates for abnormalities and listening to the heart for possible murmurs. Heart murmurs are whooshing sounds caused by turbulent movement of blood that may indicate faulty valves, patent ductus, and other heart defects. A cardiologist will make the definitive diagnosis by administering such tests as the electrocardiogram, Doppler-echocardiogram, and cardiac catheterization. The electrocardiogram measures the rhythmic electrical signal that passes through the heart with each beat. An abnormal signal will often indicate problems with a particular region of the heart and is especially useful in identifying rhythm disorders. The echocardiogram produces visual images of the heart by sending out ultrasound waves that bounce off and return to a receiving device. Most structural heart defects can be detected with this technique, and many are discovered prenatally with routine fetal ultrasound monitoring. At the same time, a second receiving device (the Doppler) analyzes ultrasound signals from blood moving through the heart and is able to provide information about the speed and direction of blood flow within the heart. This helps detect abnormal functions such as reverse blood flow. The Doppler-echocardiogram has revolutionized congenital heart disease diagnosis and in most cases provides enough information to define the patient's problem accurately.

If the cardiologist believes that it is necessary, further tests can be done. A chest X ray may be taken to determine if there is any lung involvement in the disorder. Cardiac catheterization can add information about the internal heart blood pressures and blood oxygen levels and can help visualize some defects better with the administration of contrast dyes in combination with X-ray analysis. Special monitors can be used to record the electrocardiogram for one or two days to check for intermittent rhythm irregularities, and older children can be monitored while exercising to see how the heart performs under stress. These and other tests allow physicians to assess the seriousness of the problem and to recommend timely and appropriate treatment.

Serious heart malformations need to be treated immediately upon diagnosis. Often these include defects that cause cyanosis, including transposition of the great arteries, left-heart flow defects such as coarctation of the aorta, and defects that cause heart failure such as truncus arteriosus. Immediate emergency surgery may be needed to save the life of the newborn infant. Additional follow-up surgeries may also be required to correct the defect completely. For example, one way of correcting transposition of the great arteries is by performing an atrial switch operation in which systemic blood returning from the body is diverted to the left side of the heart (so it can be pumped to the lungs) and pulmonary blood from the lungs is diverted to the right side of the heart (so it can be pumped to the body). This is accomplished by first enlarging the foramen ovale with a balloon catheter, a procedure called Rashkind balloon atrial septostomy, followed by a second operation several months later to enlarge the opening between the two atria further and to install a flap to enhance the cross flow of blood, which is known as a Mustard or Senning atrial switch operation. A more recently developed procedure for correcting this defect requires only one operation. The misplaced aorta and pulmonary artery are both cut and then reattached to the correct heart chamber; this is called a Jatene arterial switch operation. At the same time, the coronary arteries are moved to the new aorta.

Some defects require no surgery but can be treated with drugs and other less traumatic procedures, such as the balloon catheter. Drugs are also used to help improve heart performance before and after surgery. When fluid accumulates in the lungs or other body tissues, the heart has problems pumping all the blood that returns to it because of the congestion. The overworked heart suffers under this stress, and thus the condition is called congestive heart failure. Diuretics such as Lasix (furosemide) improve the kidneys' ability to remove the excess fluid and relieve the congestion. Another drug, digitalis, can be helpful in treating congestive heart failure by slowing the heart rate and causing it to beat more forcefully. An open ductus is beneficial to children born with cyanotic heart defects because it allows a more even distribution of oxygenated blood. Treatment with prostaglandin E1 helps keep the ductus open until corrective surgery can be performed. Indomethacin has the opposite effect and is often used to promote closing of a patent ductus in premature babies. As in adults, drugs such as digitalis, beta-blockers, and calcium channel blockers can be used to treat abnormal heart rhythms (arrhythmia) in children with congenital heart disease. The balloon catheter is a nonsurgical technique that is used to enlarge narrow vessels and passages and has been used successfully to treat pulmonary and aortic valve stenosis in a technique called balloon valvuloplasty.

Types of surgery done later in infancy or childhood include closed heart operations such as repair of a patent ductus and partial treatment of some types of cyanosis with a Blalock-Taussig shunt (connecting the subclavian artery to the pulmonary artery to bring more blood to the lungs). Open heart surgery is used to repair defects inside the heart such as septal defects. A heart-lung machine is used to by-pass the heart and lungs while the operation is underway, and the body is cooled so that the brain and other tissues require less oxygen. Children with very serious heart defects such as hypoplastic right or left ventricles may require a series of corrective surgical operations, and for some the only hope is a heart transplant. For example, children with hypoplastic right ventricle are given a Blalock-Taussig shunt shortly after birth to improve blood flow to their lungs and then are later given the Fontan operation, which involves closing off the Blalock-Taussig shunt and connecting the pulmonary artery to the right atrium so that blood returning from the body will flow directly to the lungs, completely bypassing the defective right ventricle.

Some heart defects require no treatment. For example, most small septal defects close on their own during the first one or two years of life. Also, mild disorders such as benign valve defects usually require no treatment, and many children with heart murmurs have no detectable problems.

PERSPECTIVE AND PROSPECTS

In the late nineteenth and early twentieth centuries, physicians were beginning to understand that certain congenital heart defects such as patent ductus could be diagnosed by listening to the heart. Treatment, however, was not possible at that time. The *Atlas of Congenital Cardiac Disease* was published in 1936 by Maude Abbot of McGill University. This work greatly assisted other physicians in recognizing and diagnosing congenital heart disease. In 1939, Robert Gross of Boston repaired a patent ductus, and in 1944, Alfred Blalock and Helen Taussig developed and performed their famous shunt operation in order to treat children with tetralogy of Fallot. Open heart surgery had to wait until the mid-1950's, when the heart-lung machine was perfected. Even then, open heart surgery could only be performed on older children. These operations were pioneered by Walton Lillehei of the University of Minnesota and John Kirlin of the Mayo Clinic. Open heart surgery on newborn infants was developed in the 1970's by Brian Barratt-Boyes of New Zealand.

During the period while heart surgery was being developed, cardiac catheterization was also advancing. It was used primarily for diagnosis, but in 1966, William Rashkind of Philadelphia began to use the balloon catheter to enlarge openings in the atrial septum in order to treat transposition of the great arteries. Microsurgical catheters are currently being developed to repair patent ductus and other heart defects without the need for major surgery. The echocardiogram was pioneered by Inge Edler in the 1950's, and the Doppler-echocardiogram came into widespread use as a diagnostic tool in the 1980's. This instrument has greatly reduced the need for other diagnostic tests that were used in the past.

The modern strategy for treatment of congenital heart defects is to perform the corrective surgery as early in in-fancy as possible. This eliminates the need for numerous hospitalizations and diagnostic tests and reduces the need for extensive drug treatment. Children with multiple defects will still need more than one surgery. Modern treatment also emphasizes the roles of the child, the family, and health care personnel in fostering an understanding of the condition, treatment, and outcome. Even children who have been successfully treated will sometimes have physical limitations. These children need to be encouraged and supported by their families and allowed to pursue their goals to the fullest extent possible. Overcoming congenital heart disease is now possible for the vast majority of those who are afflicted. *—Rodney C. Mowbray*

See also Arrhythmias; Genetic diseases; Heart disease; Heart failure; Hemophilia; Mitral insufficiency.

FOR FURTHER INFORMATION:

Berkow, Robert, ed. *The Merck Manual of Diagnosis and Therapy*. 16th ed. Rahway, N.J.: Merck Sharp & Dohme Research Laboratories, 1992. Chapter 25, "Disease of the Heart and Pericardium: Congenital Heart Disease," contains complete medical descriptions of the common congenital heart defects and appropriate methods of diagnosis and treatment. This reference work is found in most libraries.

Johnson, Robert Arnold, Edgar Haber, and W. Gerald Austen, eds. *The Practice of Cardiology*. Boston: Little, Brown, 1980. A thorough discussion of congenital heart disease is provided in two chapters: chapter 29, "Heart Disease in the Infant and Young Child," and chapter 30, "Congenital Heart Disease in the Child, Adolescent, and Adult Patient." Written for physicians, but much information can be gleaned by the layperson.

Mackintosh, Alan. *The Heart Disease Reference Book*. London: Harper & Row, 1984. A comprehensive reference book of heart problems, including congenital heart disease, written for the nonphysician seeking more in-depth information than provided by books written for the general public. Contains excellent line diagrams and descriptions of congenital heart defects.

Moore, Keith L. *The Developing Human*. 4th ed. Philadelphia: W. B. Saunders, 1988. An outstanding textbook on human embryonic development. Chapter 14 deals with the development of the circulatory system. The diagrams and descriptions allow the reader to compare normal and abnormal development and to see exactly how errors in development result in congenital heart defects.

Neill, Catherine A., Edward B. Clark, and Carleen Clark. *The Heart of a Child*. Baltimore: The Johns Hopkins University Press, 1992. A comprehensive, up-to-date work on heart disease affecting children written for the layperson by medical professionals. The authors give a thorough description of all congenital heart defects and explain their developmental basis. In addition to diagnosis, treatment, and rehabilitation, the book deals with the special problems of children with heart disease. The best reference for the general reader.

Roberts, William C., ed. *Adult Congenital Heart Disease.* Philadelphia: F. A. Davis, 1987. A medical text that focuses on adults with congenital heart defects. This book will be of interest to those that have survived congenital heart disease and now need follow-up medical care as adults.

CONGESTIVE HEART FAILURE. *See* HEART FAILURE.

CONJUNCTIVITIS

SYSTEM AFFECTED: Visual

SPECIALISTS: Infectious disease physicians, ophthalmologists

DEFINITION: One of the most common eye disorders, conjunctivitis is an inflammation of the white part of the eye, the conjunctiva. In addition to the redness caused by the presence of excess blood, symptoms often include pain and discharge; the patient's vision remains unaffected. Conjunctivitis is highly contagious and is usually spread from one eye to the other by the patient. The condition has many possible causes, ranging from bacterial infections to viral infections, from allergies to the sexually transmitted disease chlamydia. Acute bacterial conjunctivitis, commonly known as pinkeye, generally lasts two weeks and is characterized by itching and burning as well.

See also Chlamydia.

CONSTIPATION

SYSTEM AFFECTED: Gastrointestinal

SPECIALISTS: Family physicians, gastroenterologists, internists

DEFINITION: The slow passage of feces through the bowels or the presence of hard feces.

CAUSES AND SYMPTOMS

People of every age group, from infants to the elderly, can experience the unpleasant symptoms of constipation, which is characterized primarily by discomfort. Certain disease states such as diabetes mellitus, paralysis of the legs, colon cancer, and hypothyroidism predispose a person to constipation. Possible causes of constipation are medications, iron supplements, toilet training procedures, pregnancy, lack of adequate fluids, a low-fiber diet, and lack of physical activity.

TREATMENT AND THERAPY

Most cases of constipation can be treated by the patient at home. Drinking adequate fluids makes it easier for fecal material to pass through the large intestine. Without adequate hydration, a person may experience small, pellet-like stools. Eight to ten glasses of liquids per day are recommended, including water, milk, cocoa, fruit juice, herbal

tea, and soup. Once adequate hydration is achieved, a high-fiber diet can gradually be started. Without enough fluids, a high-fiber diet can worsen the problems of constipation. A high-fiber diet adds bulk to the bowel movement (increasing stool volume, decreasing pressure within the colon, and decreasing the intestinal transit time of foods) and thus can lead to more regular bowel habits and partial relief of the symptoms. One can increase fiber in the diet by eating prunes, high-fiber breakfast cereals, beans or legumes, raw fruits and vegetables, and whole-grain breads. In order to minimize gastrointestinal discomforts such as increased flatulence (gas), it is recommended to increase one's fiber consumption gradually.

In addition to adequate liquids and a high-fiber diet, exercise is important in treating constipation. Any sort of physical activity, such as walking, running, tennis, or swimming, can help to stimulate the activity of the large intestine.

Laxatives and enemas should not be used until after a discussion with a physician. Mineral oil should also not be used because many essential fat-soluble vitamins (such as vitamins A, D, E, and K) may be excreted as well. Persistent constipation should be evaluated by a physician.
—*Martha M. Henze*

See also Diarrhea and dysentery; Gastrointestinal disorders; Indigestion; Intestinal disorders; Renal failure.

COUGHING

SYSTEM AFFECTED: Respiratory

SPECIALISTS: Family physicians, internists, pulmonologists

DEFINITION: A cough is produced when air is suddenly forced through the glottis, the vocal apparatus of the larynx; this response is triggered by irritation of the trachea or the bronchi in the lungs. Such irritation can be caused by environmental factors, such as smoke or dust, or by infections or disease of the throat or the lungs themselves. Coughing is commonly seen with the common cold, bronchitis, pneumonia, croup, influenza, lung cancer, and tuberculosis. The nature of a cough may provide information for diagnosing a condition, such as the barking cough of croup, and coughing is often beneficial in removing secretions from the lungs, as with cystic fibrosis.

See also Bronchitis; Choking; Common cold; Diphtheria; Pertussis; Pneumonia; Pulmonary diseases; Tuberculosis.

CROHN'S DISEASE

SYSTEM AFFECTED: Gastrointestinal

SPECIALISTS: Gastroenterologists, general surgeons, internists

DEFINITION: A serious, chronic inflammatory disease of the gastrointestinal tract.

CAUSES AND SYMPTOMS

Crohn's disease, one of the two inflammatory bowel diseases (IBDs), can cause inflammation and ulceration within any region of the digestive tract. Though a break in the mucous membrane of the digestive tract can occur anywhere from the mouth to the anus, in this disease the inflammation occurs primarily in the ileum, the section of the small intestine that meets the large intestine. (Ulcerative colitis, the other IBD, occurs only in the colon or rectum.) Because of the patchy, nonuniform distribution of the inflamed areas in the small intestine, Crohn's disease is also known as regional enteritis.

Crohn's Disease

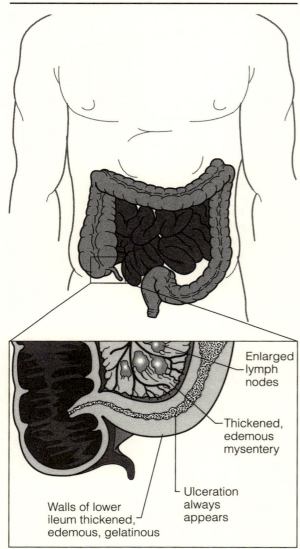

Enlarged lymph nodes

Thickened, edemous mysentery

Ulceration always appears

Walls of lower ileum thickened, edemous, gelatinous

Crohn's disease can cause inflammation and ulceration within any region of the digestive tract, but most often in the ileum.

Crohn's disease affects not only the mucosa or surface layer of the digestive tract but also often progresses so that all three layers of the intestinal wall become inflamed. Frequently, fistulas (connections) between the digestive tract and other body structures develop, causing further physical complications. Mechanical obstructions and stricture formation, in which the bowel abnormally narrows, can also occur.

The common symptoms of Crohn's disease are diarrhea, abdominal pain, nausea, and vomiting. These symptoms can lead to systemic complications of weight loss, dehydration, anemia, and fever. Malnutrition often also occurs because of the inability of the small intestine to absorb nutrients properly.

TREATMENT AND THERAPY

Since no medical cure exists for Crohn's disease, the goal of treatment is to decrease the inflammation of the diseased intestinal segment. This can be done by rest, nutritional therapy, and medication. In severe cases, surgical resection may be done; however, this procedure is not recommended because of the high rate of recurrence of Crohn's disease. The disease is characterized by periods of exacerbations and remissions. For acute flare-ups, bed rest is recommended and oral feeding may be stopped. Though nutritional management of Crohn's disease needs to be individualized, often a low-fiber, low-fat, high-protein, and high-carbohydrate diet is tolerated best. Immunosuppressive and anti-inflammatory medications are the most commonly prescribed drugs for treatment. —*Martha M. Henze*

See also Colitis; Colon cancer; Diarrhea and dysentery; Diverticulosis and diverticulitis; Gastrointestinal disorders; Intestinal disorders.

FOR FURTHER INFORMATION:

Steiner-Grossman, Penny, Peter A. Banks, and Daniel H. Present, eds. *People . . . Not Patients: A Source Book for Living with Inflammatory Bowel Disease*. New York: National Foundation for Ileitis and Colitis, 1985.

CUSHING'S SYNDROME

SYSTEMS AFFECTED: All

SPECIALISTS: Endocrinologists, internists

DEFINITION: Cushing's syndrome is an endocrine disorder that consists of a group of abnormalities; it usually strikes women. The result of excessive levels of adrenocortical hormones in the body, the syndrome causes characteristic fatty deposits in the face, neck, and trunk. Various other disorders may result, including diabetes mellitus, muscle wasting, bone fractures, peptic ulcers, insomnia, hypertension, a compromised immune system, and amenorrhea (cessation of menstruation), acne, and hirsutism (excessive hairiness) in women. Treatment of the syndrome may include radiation, drug therapy, or surgery, depending on the source of the hormone secretions, such as a tumor.

See also Addison's disease; Endocrine disorders.

Cushing's Syndrome

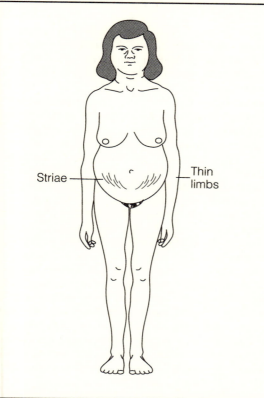

Striae — Thin limbs

An adrenal disorder, Cushing's syndrome causes symptomatic fatty deposits, striae, and thin limbs and may be associated with a variety of mild to serious conditions.

CYSTIC FIBROSIS

SYSTEMS AFFECTED: Respiratory, most bodily systems
SPECIALISTS: Pediatricians, pulmonologists
DEFINITION: A disease that affects the exocrine glands and, secondarily, most physical systems, resulting in death usually between the ages of sixteen and thirty.
KEY TERMS:

chloride transport: the movement of one of the ions found in ordinary salt across a membrane from the inside of a cell to the outside; this transport is common in human cells and is critical for many important metabolic functions

cystic fibrosis transmembrane-conductance regulator (CFTR): the protein product of the cystic fibrosis gene and a chloride transport channel

meconium ileus: the puttylike plug found in the intestines of some cystic fibrosis babies when they are born

mutation: an alteration in the deoxyribonucleic acid (DNA) sequence of a gene, which usually leads to the production of a nonfunctional enzyme or protein and thus a lack of a normal metabolic function

recessive genetic disease: a disease caused by mutated genes that must be inherited from both parents in order for that individual to show its symptoms

secretory epithelium: tissues or groups of cells that have the ability to move substances, such as chloride ions, from the inside of cells to a duct or tube

CAUSES AND SYMPTOMS

Genetic diseases are inherited, rather than caused by any specific injury or infectious agent. Thus, unlike many other types of diseases, genetic diseases rage throughout a person's entire lifetime and often begin to exert their debilitating effects prior to birth. Since in many cases the primary defect or underlying cause of the disease is unknown, treatment is difficult or impossible and is usually restricted to treating the symptoms of the disease. Genetic diseases include sickle-cell anemia; thalassemia; Tay-Sachs disease; some forms of muscular dystrophy, diabetes, and hemophilia; and cystic fibrosis.

In each disease, a specific normal function is missing because of a defect in the individual's genes. Genes are sequences of deoxyribonucleic acid (DNA) contained on the chromosomes of an individual that are passed to the next generation via ova and sperm. Usually, the primary defect in a genetic disease is the inability to produce a normal enzyme, the class of proteins used to speed up, or catalyze, the chemical reactions that are necessary for cells to function. A defective gene, also called a mutation, may not allow the production of a necessary enzyme; therefore, some element of metabolism is missing from an individual with such a mutation. This lack of function leads to the symptoms associated with a genetic disease, such as the lack of insulin production in juvenile diabetes or the inability of the blood to clot in hemophilia. In the 1940's and 1950's, when the understanding of basic cellular metabolism made clear the relationship between genes, enzymes, mutant genes, and lack of enzyme function, the modern definition of genetic disease came into routine medical use.

Cystic fibrosis, one such genetic disease, has several major effects on an individual. These effects begin before birth, extend into early childhood, and become progressively more serious as the affected individual grows. The primary diagnosis for the disease is a very simple test which looks for excessive saltiness in perspiration. Although the higher-than-normal level of salt in the perspiration is, of itself, not life-threatening, the associated symptoms are. Because these other symptoms may vary from one individual to the next, the perspiration test is a very useful early diagnostic tool.

Major symptoms of cystic fibrosis include the blockage of several important internal ducts. This blockage occurs because the cystic fibrosis mutation has a critical effect on the ability of certain internal tissues called secretory epithelia to transport normal amounts of salt and water across their surfaces. These epithelia are often found in the ducts that contribute to the digestive and reproductive systems.

The blockage of ducts resulting from the production and export of overly viscous secretions reduces the delivery of digestive enzymes from the pancreas to the intestine; thus proteins in the intestine are only partly digested. Fat-emulsifying compounds, called bile salts, are often blocked as well on their route from the pancreas to the intestine, so the digestion of fats is often incomplete. These two conditions often occur prior to birth. Approximately 10 percent of newborns with cystic fibrosis have a puttylike plug of undigested material in their intestines called the meconium ileus. This plug prevents the normal movement of foods through the digestive system and can be very serious.

Because of their overall inefficiency of digestion, young children with cystic fibrosis can seem to be eating quite normally yet remain severely undernourished. They often produce bulky, foul-smelling stools as a result of the high proportion of undigested material. This symptom serves as an indicator of the progress of the disease, as such digestive problems often increase as the affected child ages.

As individuals with cystic fibrosis grow older, their respiratory problems increase because of the secretion of a thick mucus on the inner lining of the lungs. This viscous material traps white blood cells that release their contents when they rupture, which makes the mucus all the more thick and viscous. The affected individuals constantly cough in an attempt to remove this material. Of greater importance is that the mucus forms an ideal breeding ground for many types of pathogenic bacteria, and the affected individual suffers from continual respiratory infections. Male patients are almost always infertile as a result of the blockage of the ducts of the reproductive system, while female fertility is sometimes reduced as well.

Traditional treatments for cystic fibrosis have improved an individual's chance of survival and have dramatically affected the quality of life. In the 1950's, a child afflicted with cystic fibrosis usually lived only a year or two. Thus, cystic fibrosis was originally described as a children's disease and was intensively studied only by pediatricians. Today, aggressive medical intervention has changed survival rates dramatically. Affected individuals are treated by a package of therapies designed to alleviate the most severe symptoms of the disease, and taken together, they had extended the median age of survival of cystic fibrosis patients to twenty-nine years by the early 1990's. In fact, since this figure contains many individuals who were born before many of the effective treatments were developed and so did not benefit from them throughout their entire lifetimes, the true average life expectancy may be as high as forty years.

The available treatments, however, do not constitute a cure for the disease. The major roadblock to developing a cure was that the primary genetic defect remained unknown. All that was clear until the mid-1980's was that many of the secretory epithelia had a salt and water transport problem. By the late 1980's, the defect was further restricted to a problem in the transport of chloride ions, one of the two constituents of ordinary salt and a critical chemical in many important cellular processes. Because individuals who had severe forms of cystic fibrosis could still live, however, this function was deemed important but not absolutely essential for survival. Furthermore, only certain

Cystic Fibrosis

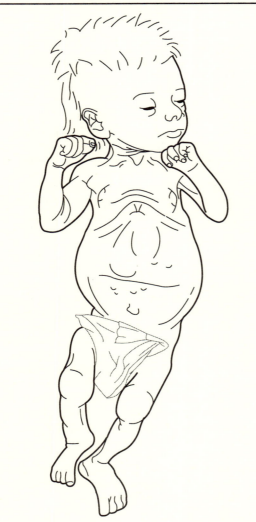

Approximately 10% of newborns with cystic fibrosis have a puttylike plug of undigested material in their intestines called the meconium ileus, which results in emaciation with a distended abdomen.

tissues and organs in the body seemed to show abnormal functions in a cystic fibrosis patient, while other organs—the heart, brain, and nerves—seemed to function normally. Thus, the defect was not uniform.

The pattern of inheritance of cystic fibrosis was relatively easy to determine. The disease acts as a recessive trait. Humans, like most animals, have two copies of each gene: one that is inherited on a chromosome from the egg, and the other on a similar chromosome from the sperm. There is a gene in all humans that controls some normal cellular function related to the transport of chloride from the inside of a cell to the outside. If this function is missing or impaired, the individual shows the symptoms of cystic fibrosis.

A recessive trait is one that must be inherited from both the mother and the father in order to take effect. Inheriting only a single copy of the mutation from one parent does not have a deleterious effect on an individual, who would not demonstrate any of the disease symptoms. Such a person, however, is a carrier of the disease and can still pass that mutation on to his or her own children. Thus genetic diseases caused by recessive mutations, such as cystic fibrosis, can remain hidden in a family for many generations. Only when two carriers of the disease marry are some of their children at risk. The rules of genetics, as first described by Gregor Mendel in the nineteenth century, predict that in such a marriage, approximately one in four children will have cystic fibrosis. Another one-fourth will be normal, and the remaining half will be carriers of the disease like their parents. Because the production of eggs and sperm involves a random shuffling of genes and chromosomes, however, the occurrence of normal individuals, carriers, and affected individuals cannot be predicted; only average probabilities can be discussed.

TREATMENT AND THERAPY

The traditional treatments for cystic fibrosis usually include dietary supplements which contain the digestive enzymes and bile salts that cannot pass through the blocked ducts; this is a daily requirement. Individuals with cystic fibrosis are also placed on special balanced diets to ensure proper nutrition despite their difficulties in digesting fats and proteins. One characteristic of cystic fibrosis treatment is the long daily ritual of backslapping, which is designed to help break up the thick mucus in the lungs. Aggressive antibiotic therapy can keep infections of the lungs from forming or spreading. In the 1990's, an additional therapy was begun using a special enzyme which when inhaled can break down DNA in the lung mucus. Many white blood cells rupture while trapped in the thick mucus lining of the lungs, and the release of their DNA adds to the high viscosity of the mucus. Genetically engineered deoxyribonuclease (DNse), an enzyme produced from bacteria, has been found to be helpful in degrading this extra DNA, thus making it easier to break up and cough out the mucus found in the lungs of affected patients.

Another treatment approach for cystic fibrosis focused on determining the nature of the primary genetic defect. The ultimate goal was to determine which of the thousands of human genes was the one that, when defective, led to cystic fibrosis. Once accomplished, the next step would be to determine the normal function of this gene so that therapies designed to replace this function could be developed.

The classic approach to studying any genetic phenomenon involves mapping the gene. First, it must be determined which of a human's twenty-three chromosomes contains the DNA that makes up the gene. By studying the inheritance of the disease, along with other human traits, the gene was located on chromosome number 7. To localize the gene more precisely, however, modern molecular techniques had to be applied. Success came when two independent groups announced that they had identified the location of the gene in 1989. The groups were led by Lap-Chee Tsui of the Hospital for Sick Children in Toronto, Canada, and Francis Collins of the University of Michigan in Ann Arbor. The groups not only located the exact chromosomal location of the gene but also purified the gene from the vast amount of DNA in a human cell so that it could be studied in isolation. Then the structure of the normal form of the gene was compared to the DNA structure found in individuals with the disease.

DNA from more than thirty thousand individuals with cystic fibrosis was analyzed, and to the surprise of most, more than 230 differences between these defective cystic fibrosis genes and normal genes were found. Although about 70 percent of the affected individuals did have a single type of DNA difference or mutation, the other 30 percent had a tremendous variety of differences. Thus unlike sickle-cell anemia, which seems to be attributable to the same defect in every affected individual, cystic fibrosis is a widely varying group of differences, which accounts for the range in severity of its symptoms. More important, this enormous diversity of defects makes developing a single, simple DNA-based screening procedure difficult. The only thing that all these individuals had in common was that, in each case, the same gene and gene product were affected.

Tsui's and Collins' groups, as well as several others, tried to determine the normal function of the protein that was coded by the cystic fibrosis gene. This protein was called cystic fibrosis transmembrane-conductance regulator (CFTR) because it was soon shown to create a channel or passage by which cells move chloride ions across their membranes. In an individual afflicted with cystic fibrosis, this channel does not work properly; both the salt and the water balance of the affected cell, and ultimately of the whole tissue, is disturbed. The thick mucus buildup in the lungs is a direct consequence of this disturbance, as is the higher-than-normal salt concentration in the patient's perspiration.

Remarkably, CFTR is an enormous protein that is embedded in the membrane of cells found in the lungs, pancreas, and the reproductive tracts. CFTR contains 1,480 amino acids linked end to end. The CFTR found in 70 percent of individuals with cystic fibrosis contains the same amino acids as normal genes, with one exception: The 508th amino acid found in a normal individual is missing. Thus, the extensive debilitating symptoms of this disease result from the mere omission of one amino acid from a long chain containing 1,479 identical ones. The other mutations affect different parts of this protein and, in all cases, reduce the ability of the CFTR protein to carry out its normal function.

In the cases of several other genetic diseases, screening programs have been developed to help patients make informed choices about having children. For Tay-Sachs disease, a fatal neurological disease found in 1 in 3,600 Ashkenazi Jews, a screening program coupled with a strong educational program has combined to reduce the incidence of the disease from approximately 100 births a year in the 1970's to an average of 13 by the early 1980's. Similar screening programs have been developed for a rare genetic disease called phenylketonuria (PKU). A screening program for cystic fibrosis, however, would be much more difficult for several reasons.

First, the population at risk for cystic fibrosis is much larger; hence the costs and scope of the program would be enormous. Second, since there are many different mutations that can affect the gene responsible for causing cystic fibrosis, it may not be easy to develop a simple test which could detect this enormous variation accurately without missing affected individuals or falsely concluding that some normal individuals are affected. Finally, the symptoms shown by individuals affected with cystic fibrosis range from quite severe to nearly normal, thus making it even more difficult to provide definitive genetic counseling. For such counseling to be truly effective, large numbers of individuals from groups known to be at risk for the disease would have to undergo screening and counseling. Furthermore, a prenatal diagnostic test would need to be available to allow couples at risk to ascertain with some degree of certainty whether any particular child is going to be born with the disease. Developing these tests and coupling them with widely available, low-cost counseling remain major challenges to the medical community.

Therapies for cystic fibrosis, like those of any genetic disease, once consisted solely of ways to treat the symptoms. Since every cell in the affected individual lacked a particular metabolic function as a result of the disease, there was no easy way to replace these functions. For cystic fibrosis, this problem was exacerbated by the lack of understanding of the primary defect. The work of Tsui's and Collins' teams allowed a more direct assault on the actual defect. Gene therapy involves either replacing a defective gene with a normal one in affected cells, or adding an additional copy or copies of the normal gene to affected cells,

in an attempt to restore the same functional enzymes and thus reestablish a normal metabolic process. In the case of cystic fibrosis, animal studies have shown that it is possible to produce normal lung function when either genes or genetically engineered viruses containing normal genes are sprayed into the lungs of affected animals. Yet since there is no similar direct route for getting engineered viruses or purified genes to the pancreas or reproductive system, because of their location deep within the body, other procedures will need to be developed. In the case of the lung cells, only those cells that actually receive the purified gene change, becoming normal. Since the cells lining the lung are continuously being replenished, lung gene therapy would need to be an ongoing process.

PERSPECTIVE AND PROSPECTS

Patients with the symptoms of cystic fibrosis were first described in medical records dating back to the eighteenth century. The disease was initially called mucoviscidosis and later cystic fibrosis of the pancreas. It was not clear that these symptoms were related to a single specific disease, however, until the work of Dorothy Anderson of Columbia University in the late 1930's. Anderson studied a large number of cases of persons who died with similar lung and pancreas problems. She noticed that siblings were sometimes affected and thus suspected that the disease had a genetic cause. Anderson was responsible for naming the disease on the basis of the fibrous cysts on the pancreas that she often saw in autopsies performed on affected individuals.

In the United States, cystic fibrosis is the most prevalent lethal genetic disease among Caucasians. Estimates vary, but most are in the range of 1 affected child in every 2,000 births. In the early 1990's, there were approximately 25,000 affected Americans and more than 50,000 affected people worldwide. The incidence of cystic fibrosis among Asian American or African American populations is considerably lower, ranging from 1 in 17,000 births for African Americans and less than 1 in 80,000 births for certain Asian American groups. What is particularly striking about this disease is that approximately 1 in 25 Caucasians is a carrier. Such individuals do not show disease symptoms but can have affected children if they marry another carrier.

Since this rate is so high, a premium has been placed on the development of inexpensive and accurate diagnostic procedures, which along with good genetic counseling, could greatly reduce the incidence of cystic fibrosis in the population. Yet, since carriers are perfectly normal and often do not realize that they are indeed carrying the gene, conventional genetic counseling cannot easily reduce the incidence of the mutation in human populations at risk. Only the widespread use of a DNA-based diagnostic procedure could serve to identify the large population of carriers, but even then, since three-fourths of the children of a marriage between two carriers would be normal, counseling would be fraught with severe ethical problems. Why such a deleterious gene remains in such high frequencies in the population remains a mystery.

—*Joseph G. Pelliccia*

See also Genetic diseases.

FOR FURTHER INFORMATION:

Boat, T. F., M. J. Welsh, and A. L. Beaudet. "Cystic Fibrosis." In *The Metabolic Basis of Inherited Disease*. 6th ed. New York: McGraw-Hill, 1989. Offers a full description of how the primary defect in chloride-ion transport leads to the various symptoms associated with cystic fibrosis.

Garber, Edward B., ed. *Genetic Perspectives in Biology and Medicine*. Chicago: University of Chicago Press, 1985. Clearly written essays that cover some of the basic issues of human genetics, genetic disease, birth defects, and the molecular diagnosis of genetic disease.

Harris, Ann, and Maurice Super. *Cystic Fibrosis: The Facts*. Oxford, England: Oxford University Press, 1987. An excellent overview of the disease, its symptoms, and its treatment in a readable text.

Pierce, Benjamin A. *The Family Genetic Sourcebook*. New York: John Wiley & Sons, 1990. Contains good background reading on genetics and genetic diseases. Cystic fibrosis is not the main focus of the text, but it is discussed.

Tsui, Lap-Chee. "Cystic Fibrosis, Molecular Genetics." In *The Encyclopedia of Human Biology*, edited by Renato Dulbecco. Vol. 2. New York: Academic Press, 1991. The pursuit of the cystic fibrosis gene is documented, along with some discussion of the function of the CFTR. Readable by someone with a strong high school science background.

U.S. Congress. Office of Technology Assessment. *Cystic Fibrosis and DNA Tests: Implications of Carrier Screening*. OTA-BA-532. Washington, D.C.: Government Printing Office, 1992. An excellent overview of the scientific, ethical, social, economic, and political issues involved with screening for cystic fibrosis or for any genetic disease.

U.S. Congress. Office of Technology Assessment. *Genetic Counseling and Cystic Fibrosis Carrier Screening: Results of a Survey-Background Paper*. OTA-BP-BA-97. Washington, D.C.: Government Printing Office, 1992. A survey that looks at issues related to genetic screening for cystic fibrosis.

CYSTITIS

SYSTEM AFFECTED: Urinary

SPECIALISTS: Gynecologists, infectious disease physicians, urologists

DEFINITION: An inflammation of the bladder, primarily caused by bacteria and resulting in pain, a sense of urgency to urinate, and sometimes hematuria (blood in the urine).

KEY TERMS:

cytoscopy: a minor operation performed so that the urologist can examine the bladder

dysuria: painful urination, usually as a result of infection or an obstruction; the patient complains of a burning sensation when voiding

Escherichia coli: bacteria found in the intestines that may cause disease elsewhere

hematuria: the abnormal presence of blood in the urine

perineum: the short bridge of flesh between the anus and vagina in women and the anus and base of the penis in men

ureters: the two tubes that carry urine from the kidneys to the bladder

urethra: the tube carrying urine from the bladder to outside the body

CAUSES AND SYMPTOMS

The term "cystitis" is a combination of two Greek words: *kistis*, meaning hollow pouch, sac, or bladder, and *itis* meaning inflammation. Cystitis is often used generically to refer to any nonspecific inflammation of the lower urinary tract. Specifically, however, it should be used to refer to inflammation and infection of the bladder. Three true symptoms denote cystitis: dysuria, frequent urination, and hematuria. In a given year, about two million people are afflicted with cystitis; most of them are women. Fifteen percent of those affected will be struck again.

The symptoms of cystitis may appear abruptly and, often, painfully. One of the trademark symptoms signaling an onset is dysuria (burning or stinging during urination). It may precede or coincide with an overwhelming urge to urinate, and very frequently, although the amount passed may be extremely small. In addition some sufferers may experience nocturia (sleep disturbance because of a need to urinate). In many cases there may be pus in the urine. Origination of hematuria (blood in the urine), which often occurs with cystitis, may be within the bladder wall, in the urethra, or even in the upper urinary tract. These painful symptoms should be enough to spur one to seek medical attention; if left untreated, the bacteria may progress up the ureters to the kidneys, where a much more serious infection may develop. Pyelonephritis can cause scarring of the kidney tissue and even life-threatening kidney failure. Usually kidney infections are accompanied by chills, high fever, nausea and/or vomiting, and back pain that may radiate downward.

Acute cystitis can be divided into two groups. One is when infection occurs with irregularity and with no recent history of antibiotic treatments. This type is commonly caused by the bacteria *Escherichia coli*. Types of bacteria other than *E. coli* that can cause cystitis are *Proteus*, *Klebsiella*, *Pseudomonas*, *Streptococcus*, *Enterobacter*, and, rarely, *Staphylococcus*. The second group of sufferers have undergone antibiotic treatment; those bacteria not affected by the antibiotics can cause infection. Most urinary tract

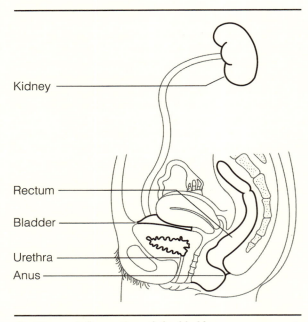

Kidney

Rectum

Bladder

Urethra

Anus

Cystitis, an inflammation of the bladder, may progress to the kidneys if left untreated.

infections are precipitated by the patient's own rectal flora. Once bacteria enter the bladder, whether they will cause infection depends on how many bacteria invade the bladder, how well the bacteria can adhere to the bladder wall, and how strongly the bladder can defend itself. The bladder's inherent defense system is the most important of the factors.

One of the natural defense mechanisms employed by the bladder is the flushing provided by regular urination at frequent intervals. If fluid intake is sufficient—most urologists consider this amount to be eight 8-ounce glasses daily—there will be regular and efficient emptying of the bladder, which can wash away the bacteria that have entered. This large volume of fluid also helps dilute the urine, thereby decreasing bacterial concentration. Another defense mechanism is the low pH of the bladder, which also helps control bacterial multiplication. It may be, too, that the bladder lining employs some means to repel bacteria and to inhibit their adherence to the wall. Others theorize that genetic, hormonal, and immune factors may help determine the defensive capability of the bladder.

Many women experience their first episode of cystitis as they become sexually active. So-called honeymoon cystitis, that related to sexual activity, comes about because intercourse may massage bacteria into the bladder, as can repeated thrusts of the penis, penetration of the vagina by fingers or other objects, or manual stimulation of the clitoris. Bacteria are boosted into and forced upward through the urethra. Also, a change in position—from back to front but not from front to back—may precede an attack of cys-

titis. When intercourse from the rear occurs, the penis may be contaminated with bacteria from the anal region, which then are transferred to the urethra. From the urethra, it is a short trip to the bladder for the bacteria. Unless they are voided upon conclusion of intercourse, they may multiply, causing inflammation and infection. Sex late in the day may be particularly hazardous if the perineal area has not been thoroughly cleansed after a bowel movement. Bathing after intercourse is too late to prevent the *E. coli* from being pushed into the urethral opening. Some instances of cystitis may be reduced if there is adequate vaginal lubrication prior to intercourse and avoidance of vaginal sprays and douches.

Women who use a diaphragm as birth control are more than twice as likely to develop urinary tract infections than other sexually active women. The reason for this increased likelihood may be linked to the more alkaline vaginal environment in diaphragm users, or perhaps to the spring in the rim of the diaphragm that exerts pressure on the tissue around the urethra. Urine flow may be restricted, and the stagnant urine is a good harbor for bacterial growth.

When urine remains in the bladder for an extended period of time, its stagnation may allow for the rapid growth of bacteria, thereby leading to cystitis. Besides the use of a diaphragm, urine flow may be restricted by an enlarged prostate or pregnancy. Diabetes mellitus may also lead to cystitis, as the body's resistance to infection is lowered. Infrequent voiding for whatever reason is associated with a greater likelihood of cystitis.

Less frequently, cases have been linked to vaginitis as a result of *Monilia* or *Trichomonas*. Yeasts such as these change the pH of the vaginal fluid, which will allow and even encourage bacterial growth in the perineal region. Sometimes, it is an endless cycle: A patient takes antibiotics for cystitis, which kills her protective bacteria and allows the overgrowth of yeasts. The yeasts cause vaginitis, which may promote another case of cystitis, and the cycle continues. In fact, recurrent cystitis may be a result of an inappropriate course of antibiotic treatment; the antibiotic is not specific to the bacteria. More rarely, recurrent cases may be a result of constant seeding by the kidneys or a bowel fistula. The most common cause of recurrent cystitis, however, is new organisms from the rectal area that invade the perineal area. This new pool may be inadvertently changed by antibiotic treatment.

A less common but often more severe kind of cystitis is interstitial cystitis, an inflammation of the bladder caused by nonbacterial causes, such as an autoimmune or allergic response. With this type of cystitis, there may be inflammation and/or ulceration of the bladder, which may result in scarring. These problems usually cause frequent and painful urination and possible hematuria. What separates interstitial cystitis from acute cystitis is that it primarily strikes women in their early to mid-forties and that, while urine output is normal, soon after urination, the urge to void again is overwhelming. Delaying urination may cause a pink tinge to appear in the urine. This minimal bleeding is most often a result of an overly small bladder being stretched so that minute tears in the bladder wall bleed into the urine. This form is often hard to diagnose, as the symptoms may be mild or severe and may appear and disappear or be constant.

TREATMENT AND THERAPY

Medical students are typically underprepared to deal with the numerous cases of cystitis. The student is told to test urine for the presence of bacteria, prescribe a ten-day course of antibiotics, sometimes take a kidney X ray and/or perform a cytoscopy, and then perhaps prescribe more antibiotics. If the patient continues to complain, perhaps a painful dilation of the urethra or cauterizing (burning away) of the inflamed skin is performed. None of these procedures guarantees a cure.

Diagnosis of cystitis should be relatively easy; however, in a number of cases it is misdiagnosed because the doctor has failed to identify the type of bacteria, the patient's history of past cases, and possible links between cystitis and life factors (sexual activity, contraceptive method, and diet, for example). A more appropriate antibiotic given at this point might lower the risks of frequent recurrences. Diagnosis of urinary tract infection takes into account the medical history, a physical examination of the patient, and performance of special tests. The history begins with the immediate complaints of the patient and is completed with a look back at the same type of infections that the patient has had from childhood to the present. The physician should conduct urinalysis but be cognizant that, if the urine is not examined at the right time, the bacteria may not have survived and thus a false-negative reading may occur.

One special test, a cytoscopy, is used to diagnose some of the special characteristics of cystitis. These include redness of the bladder cells, enlarged capillaries with numerous small hemorrhages, and in cases of severe cystitis, swelling of bladder tissues. Swelling may be so pronounced that it partially blocks the urethral opening, making incomplete emptying of the bladder likely to occur. Pus pockets may be visible.

In a woman who first experiences cystitis when she becomes sexually active, the doctor usually instructs the patient to be alert to several details. She should wash or shower before intercourse and be warned that contraceptive method and position during intercourse may increase her chances of becoming infected. To decrease the chance of introducing the contamination of bowel flora to the urethra, wiping after urination and defecation from front to back is advised.

Children are not immune to attacks of cystitis; in fact, education at an early age may aid children in lowering their chances of developing cystitis. Some of the following may be culprits in causing cystitis and maintaining a hospitable environment for bacteria to grow: soap or detergent that is too strong, too much fruit juice, overuse of creams and ointments, any noncotton underwear, shampoo in the bath water, bubble bath, chlorine from swimming pools, and too little fluid intake. Once children reach the teenage years, many of the above remain causes. Added to them are failure to change underwear daily, irregular periods, use of tampons, and the use of toiletries and deodorants. Careful monitoring of these conditions can greatly reduce the risk of recurrent infections.

The symptoms of cystitis are often urgent and painful enough to alert a sufferer to visit a physician as quickly as possible. Such a visit not only makes the patient feel better but also decreases the chances that the bacteria will travel toward and even into the kidney, causing pyelonephritis. Antibiotic therapy is the typical mode of treating acute or bacterial cystitis. The antibiotics chosen should reach a high concentration in the urine, should not cause the proliferation of drug-resistant bacteria, and should not kill helpful bacteria. Some antibiotics used to treat first-time sufferers of cystitis with a high success rate (80 to 100 percent) are TMP-SMX, sulfisoxazole, amoxycillin, and ampicillin. Typically, a three-day course of therapy not only will see the patient through the few days of symptoms but, also will not change bowel flora significantly. When *E. coli* cause acute cystitis, there is a greater than 80 percent chance that one dose of an antibiotic such as penicillin will effectively end the bout, and again, the bowel flora will not be upset. Such antibiotics, when chosen carefully by the physician to match the bacteria, are useful in treating cystitis because they act very quickly to kill the bacteria. Sometimes, enough bacteria can be killed in one hour that the symptoms begin to abate immediately.

Yet antibiotics are not without their drawbacks: They may cause nausea, loss of appetite, dizziness, diarrhea, and fatigue and may increase the likelihood of yeast infections. The most common problem is the one posed by antibiotics that destroy all bacteria of the body. When the body's normal bacteria are gone, yeasts may proliferate in the body's warm, moist places. In one of the areas, the vagina, vaginitis causes a discharge which can seep into the urethra. The symptoms of cystitis may begin all over again.

For those suffering from recurrent cystitis, the treatment usually is a seven-to-ten-day course of antibiotic treatment that will clear the urine of pus, indicating that the condition should be cured. If another bout recurs fairly soon, it is probably an indication that treatment was ended too quickly, as the infective bacteria were still present. To ensure that treatment has been effective, the urine must be checked and declared sterile.

Because cystitis is so common, and because many are frustrated by the inadequacies of treatment, self-treatment has become very popular. Self-treatment does not cure the infection but certainly makes the patient more comfortable while the doctor cultures a urine specimen, determines the type of bacteria causing the infection, and prescribes the appropriate antibiotic. Monitoring the first signs that a cystitis attack is imminent can save a victim from days of intense pain.

Those advocating home treatment do not all agree, however, on the means and methods that reduce suffering. All agree that once those first sensations are felt, the sufferer should start to drink water or water-based liquids; there is some disagreement on whether this intake should include fruit juice, especially cranberry juice. Some believe that the high acidic content of the juice may act to kill some of the bacteria, while others believe that the acid will only decrease the pH of the urine, causing more intense burnings as the acidic urine passes through the inflamed urethra. Through an increased fluid intake, more copious amounts of urine are produced. The excess urine acts to leach the bacteria from the bladder and, by diluting the urine, decreases its normal acidity. More dilute urine will relieve much of the burning discomfort during voiding. If a small amount of sodium bicarbonate is added to the water, it will aid in alkalinizing the urine. The best self-treatment is to drink one cup of water every twenty minutes for three hours; after this period, the amount can be decreased. A teaspoonful of bicarbonate every hour for three or four hours is safe (unless the person suffers from blood pressure problems or a heart condition). Additionally, the patient may wish to take a painkiller, such as acetaminophen. If lifestyle permits, resting will enhance the cure, especially if a heating pad is used to soothe the back or stomach. After the frequent visits to the toilet, cleaning the perineal area carefully can reduce continued contamination.

Diagnosis of interstitial cystitis can only be made using a cytoscope. Since the cause is not bacterial, antibiotics are not effective in treating this type of cystitis. To enhance the healing process of an inflamed or ulcerated bladder as a result of interstitial cystitis, the bladder may be distended and the ulcers cauterized; both procedures are done under anesthesia. Corticosteroids may be prescribed to help control the inflammation.

PERSPECTIVE AND PROSPECTS

Writings throughout history indicate that people have always suffered from bladder problems, including cystitis, although the prevalence probably was not as high. The first urologists likely were the Hindus of the Vedic era, about 1500 B.C. They were considered experts in removing bladder stones and relieving obstructions of the urinary tract.

The recorded incidence of cystitis was possibly lower because the topic would have been taboo; women in particular would not have mentioned the problem. Couples of generations past would not have participated in intercourse as frequently; both sexes wore so many clothes and had so many children underfoot or servants around that daytime sexual activity would have been rare. Without contracep-

tion, intercourse was often for procreation; once there were several children, the couple might choose to inhabit separate bedrooms. Life spans were clearly shorter; women frequently died in childbirth. Thus, the primary causes of cystitis were not common until the twentieth century.

Those forebears did not have antibiotics, but apparently those who suffered from cystitis recovered. The treatment they did use, though, has some merit. They drank copious amounts of herb teas—chamomile, mint, and parsley. They probably added some belladonna for pain relief. All this fluid would have served to help quench the "fire." It would also have had the benefit of helping flush the bacteria from the bladder.

Infection in males is far less frequent than in females; in fact, cystitis occurs ten times more often in females than in males, and it affects about 30 percent of women at some time in their lives. Unfortunately, most urologists are versed in male problems. Female specialists, gynecologists, treat the reproductive system but may not have studied female urinary dysfunction. If a male suffers from urinary dysfunction, he should seek the services of a urologist. A woman who has interstitial cystitis should also see a urologist, specifically one who knows about this form of cystitis. If a female is experiencing recurrent cystitis, she is probably already seeing a gynecologist or an internist; however, if she is not getting relief, she should avail herself of a urologist, especially one specializing in female urology, if possible.

A strong social stigma is associated with bladder dysfunction, which may create an obstacle when treatment is necessary. From the time of infancy, some children are taught that anything to do with bladder or bowel function is shameful or dirty. Therefore, when dysfunction occurs, self-esteem may be decreased. As a result, the sufferer may fail to ask for help. Such a reaction must be overcome if there is to be significant progress in treating and conquering cystitis. —*Iona C. Baldridge*

See also Urethritis; Urinary disorders.

FOR FURTHER INFORMATION:

Chalker, Rebecca, and Kristene E. Whitmore. *Overcoming Bladder Disorders*. New York: HarperCollins, 1990. This book was written to inform the general public about bladder disorders. It is meant to aid in diagnosis and in the selection of the right physician. Diagrams and a glossary help make this work easy to read.

Dalton, John R., and Erick J. Bergquist. *Urinary Tract Infections*. London: Croom Helm, 1987. One of a series written to update clinicians' and epidemiologists' knowledge of urinary infections. Included are clinical, epidemiological, and bacteriological aspects of infection that can be used for diagnosis and treatment. To understand this text, some knowledge of the subject is helpful.

Kilmartin, Angela. *Cystitis*. New York: Warner Books, 1980. A layperson's view of coping with cystitis. This easy-to-read book takes the reader through the steps that can help assuage and control recurring attacks of cystitis. Many case histories are quoted, and the seeking of knowledgeable medical help is strongly advised.

Memmler, Ruth Lundeen, Barbara J. Cohen, and Dena L. Wood. *The Human Body in Health and Disease*. 7th ed. Philadelphia: J. B. Lippincott, 1992. This textbook offers a clear presentation of how human systems maintain homeostasis through their interactions. Integral to the discussion of each system is a detailed list of the conditions that produce disease.

Yalla, Subbarao V., Edward J. McGuire, Ahmed Elbadawi, and Jerry G. Blaivas, eds. *Neurourology and Urodynamics*. New York: Macmillan, 1988. A complicated volume compiled to answer specific questions regarding urodynamics. The sections are designed to lead one from physiology through diagnostic tools and treatment. Not for the general reader.

CYSTS AND GANGLIONS

SYSTEMS AFFECTED: Skin, nervous, reproductive (female), muscular

SPECIALISTS: Colorectal surgeons, dermatologists, gastroenterologists, gynecologists, nephrologists, neurosurgeons

DEFINITION: A cyst is a swelling or nodule containing fluid or soft material that results from a blocked duct from a gland or abnormal growth in tissue that produces fluid. Cysts can occur in any tissue of the body. When surrounding a tendon, usually in the wrists, fingers, or feet, they are called ganglions. Cysts in the skin form when sebaceous glands become blocked. Ganglions and sebaceous cysts are benign but may be removed surgically if

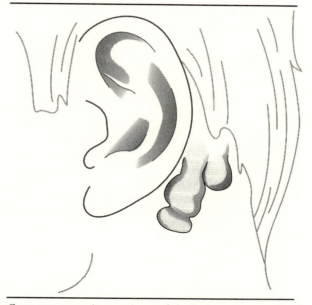

Cysts can occur in any tissue of the body; common sebaceous cysts may appear, among other places, behind the ears and at the base of the neck.

they become painful or unsightly. Such swellings occurring in body organs, where fluid cannot escape, may be more serious. For example, polycystic ovaries are enlarged from the presence of hundreds of tiny cysts, which can rupture and cause considerable pain.

See also Abscesses; Acne; Ovarian cysts; Pimples; Skin disorders.

DEATH AND DYING

SYSTEMS AFFECTED: Psychic-emotional, all bodily systems

SPECIALISTS: Family physicians, geriatric specialists, internists, neurologists, psychologists

KEY TERMS:

anticipatory depression: a depressive reaction to the awaited death of either oneself or a significant other; also called anticipatory grieving, preparatory grieving, or preparatory depression

bereavement: the general, overall process of mourning and grieving; considered to have progressive stages which include anticipation, grieving, mourning, postmourning, depression, loneliness, and reentry into society

depression: a general term covering mild states (sadness, inhibition, unhappiness, discouragement) to severe states (hopelessness, despair); typically part of normal, healthy grieving; considered the fourth stage of death and dying, between bargaining and acceptance

grief: the emotional and psychological response to loss; always painful, grieving is a type of psychological work and requires some significant duration of time

mourning: the acute phase of grief; characterized by distress, hopelessness, fear, acute loss, crying, insomnia, loss of appetite, anxiety, guilt, and restlessness

reactive depression: depression occurring as a result of overt events that have already taken place; it universally occurs in the bereaved

uncomplicated bereavement: a technical psychiatric label describing normal, average, and expectant grieving; despite an experience of great psychological pain, it is considered normal and healthy unless it continues much beyond one year

thanatology: the study and investigation of life-threatening actions, terminal illness, suicide, homicide, death, dying, grief, and bereavement

CAUSES AND SYMPTOMS

Medicine determines that death has occurred by assessing bodily functions in either of two areas. Persons with irreversible cessation of respiration and circulation are dead; persons with irreversible cessation of ascertainable brain functions are also dead. There are standard procedures used to diagnose death, including simple observation, brain-stem reflex studies, and the use of confirmatory testing such as electrocardiography (ECG or EKG), electroencephalography (EEG), and arterial blood gas analysis (ABG). The particular circumstances—anticipated or unanticipated, observed or unobserved, the patient's age, drug or metabolic intoxication, or suspicion of hypothermia—will favor some procedures over others, but in all cases both cessation of functions and their irreversibility are required before death can be declared.

Between 60 and 75 percent of all people die from chronic terminal conditions. Therefore, except in sudden death (as in a fatal accident) or when there is no evidence of consciousness (as in a head injury which destroys cerebral, thinking functions while leaving brain-stem, reflexive functions intact), dying is both a physical and a psychological process. In most cases, dying takes time, and the time allows patients to react to the reality of their own passing. Often, they react by becoming vigilant about bodily symptoms and any changes in them. They also anticipate changes that have yet to occur. For example, long before the terminal stages of illness become manifest, dying patients commonly fear physical pain, shortness of breath, invasive procedures, loneliness, becoming a burden to loved ones, losing decision-making authority, and facing the unknown of death itself.

As physical deterioration proceeds, all people cope by resorting to what has worked for them before: the unique means and mechanisms which have helped maintain a sense of self and personal stability. People seem to go through the process of dying much as they have gone through the process of living—with the more salient features of their personalities, whether good or bad, becoming sharper and more prominent. People seem to face death much as they have faced life.

Medicine has come to acknowledge that physicians should understand what it means to die. Indeed, while all persons should understand what their own deaths will mean; physicians must additionally understand how their dying patients find this meaning. Physicians who see death as the final calamity coming at the end of life, and thus primarily as something that only geriatric medicine has to face, are mistaken. Independent of beliefs about "life after life," the life process on this planet inexorably comes to an end for everyone, whether as a result of accident, injury, or progressive deterioration.

In 1969, psychiatrist Elisabeth Kübler-Ross published the landmark *On Death and Dying*, based on her work with two hundred terminally ill patients. Technologically-driven, Western medicine had come to define its role as primarily dealing with extending life and thwarting death by defeating specific diseases. Too few physicians saw a role for themselves once the prognosis turned grave. In the decades that followed *On Death and Dying*, the profession has reaccepted that death and dying are part of life and that, while treating the dying may not mean extending the length of life, it can and should mean extending its quality.

Kübler-Ross provided a framework which explained how people cope with and adapt to the profound and terrible news that their illness is going to kill them. Although other physicians, psychologists, and thanatologists have shortened, expanded, and adapted her five stages of the dying process, neither the actual number of stages nor what they are specifically called is as important as the information and insight that any stage theory of dying yields. As with any human process, dying is complex, multifaceted, multidimensional, and polymorphic.

Well-intentioned, but misguided, professionals and family members may try to help move dying patients through each of the stages only to encounter active resentment or passive withdrawal. Patients, even dying patients, cannot be psychologically moved to where they are not ready to be. Rather than making the terminally ill die the "right" way, it is more respectful and helpful to understand any stage as a description of normal reactions to serious loss, and that these reactions normally vary among different individuals and also within the same individual over time. The reactions appear, disappear, and reappear in any order and in any combination. What the living must do is respect the unfolding of an adaptational schema which is the dying person's own. No one should presume to know how someone else should die.

COMPLICATIONS AND DISORDERS

Denial is Kübler-Ross' first stage, but it is also linked to shock and isolation. Whether the news is told outright or gradual self-realization occurs, most people react to the knowledge of their impending death with existential shock: Their whole selves recoil at the idea, and they say, in some fashion, "This cannot be happening to me. I must be dreaming." Broadly considered, denial is a complex cognitive-emotional capacity which enables temporary postponement of active, acute, but in some way detrimental, recognition of reality. In the dying process, this putting off of the truth prevents a person from being overwhelmed while promoting psychological survival. Denial plays an important stabilizing role, holding back more than could be otherwise managed while allowing the individual to marshall psychological resources and reserves. It enables patients to consider the possibility, even the inevitability, of death and then to put the consideration away so that they can pursue life in the ways that are still available. In this way, denial is truly a mechanism of defense.

Many other researchers, along with Kübler-Ross, report anger as the second stage of dying. The stage is also linked to rage, fury, envy, resentment, and loathing. When "This cannot be happening to me," becomes, "This is happening to me. There was no mistake," patients are beginning to replace denial with attempts to understand what is happening to and inside them. When they do, they often ask, "Why me?" Though logically an unanswerable, even illegitimate, question, the logic of the question is clear. People, to remain human, must try to make intelligible their experiences and reality. The asking of this question is an important feature of the way in which all dying persons adapt to and cope with the reality of death.

People react with anger when they lose something of value; they react with greater anger when something of value is taken away from them by someone or something. Rage and fury, in fact, are often more accurate descriptions of people's reactions to the loss of their own life than anger. Anger is a difficult stage for professionals and loved ones,

more so when the anger and rage are displaced and projected randomly into any corner and crevice of the patient's world. An unfortunate result is that caretakers often experience the anger as personal, and the caretakers' own feelings of guilt, shame, grief, and rejection can contribute to lessening contact with the dying person, which increases his or her sense of isolation.

Bargaining is Kübler-Ross' third stage, but it is also the one about which she wrote the least and the one that other thanatologists are most likely to leave unrepresented in their own models and stages of how people cope with dying. Nevertheless, it is a common phenomenon wherein dying people fall back on their faith, belief systems, or sense of the transcendent and the spiritual and try to make a deal—with God, life, fate, a higher power, or the composite of all the randomly colliding atoms in the universe. They ask for more time to help family members reconcile or to achieve something of importance. They may ask if they can simply attend their child's wedding or graduation or if they can see their first grandchild born. Then they will be ready to die; they will go willingly. Often, they mean that they will die without fighting death, if death can only be delayed or will delay itself. Some get what they want; others do not.

At some point, when terminally ill individuals are faced with decisions about more procedures, tests, surgeries, or medications or when their thinness, weakness, or deterioration becomes impossible to ignore, the anger, rage, numbness, stoicism, and even humor will likely give way to depression, Kübler-Ross' fourth stage and the one reaction that all thanatologists include in their models of how people cope with dying.

The depression can take many forms, for indeed there are always many losses, and each loss individually or several losses collectively might need to be experienced and worked through. For example, dying parents might ask themselves who will take care of the children, get them through school, walk them down the aisle, or guide them through life. Children, even adult children who are parents themselves, may ask whether they can cope without their own parents. They wonder who will support and anchor them in times of distress, who will (or could) love, nurture, and nourish them the way that their parents did. Depression accompanies the realization that each role, each function, will never be performed again. Both the dying and those who love them mourn.

Much of the depression takes the form of anticipatory grieving, which often occurs both in the dying and in those who will be affected most by their death. It is a part of the dying process experienced by the living, both terminal and nonterminal. Patients, family, and friends can psychologically anticipate what it will be like when the death does occur and what life will, and will not, be like afterward. The grieving begins while there is still life left to live.

Bereavement specialists generally agree that anticipatory grieving, when it occurs, seems to help people cope with what is a terrible and frightening loss. It is an adaptive psychological mechanism wherein emotional, mental, and existential stability is painfully maintained. When depression develops, not only in reaction to death but also in preparation for it, it seems to be a necessary part of how those who are left behind cope in order to survive the loss themselves. Those who advocate or advise cheering up or looking on the bright side are either unrealistic or unable to tolerate the sadness in themselves or others. The dying are in the process of losing everything and everyone they love. Cheering up does not help them; the advice to "be strong" only helps the "helpers" deny the truth of the dying experience.

Both preparatory and reactive depression are often accompanied by unrealistic self-recrimination, shame, and guilt in the dying person. Those who are dying may judge themselves harshly and criticize themselves for the wrongs that they committed and for the good that they did not accomplish. They may judge themselves to be unattractive, unappealing, and repulsive because of how the illness and its treatment have made them appear. These feelings and states of minds, which have nothing to do with the reality of the situation, are often amenable to the interventions of understanding and caring people. Disfigured breasts do not make a woman less a woman; the removal of the testes does not make a man less a man. Financial and other obligations can be restructured and reassigned. Being forgiven and forgiving can help finish what was left undone.

Kübler-Ross' fifth stage, acceptance, is an intellectual and emotional coming to terms with death's reality, permanence, and inevitability. Ironically, it is manifested by diminished emotionality and interests and increased fatigue and inner (many would say spiritual) self-focus. It is a time without depression or anger. Envy of the healthy, the fear of losing all, and bargaining for another day or week are also absent. This final stage is often misunderstood. Some see it either as resignation and giving up or as achieving a happy serenity. Some think that acceptance is the goal of dying well and that all people are supposed to go through this stage. None of these viewpoints is accurate. Acceptance, when it does occur, comes from within the dying person. It is marked more by an emotional void and psychological detachment from people and things once held important and necessary and by an interest in some transcendental value (for the atheist) or his or her God (for the theist). It has little to do with what others believe is important or "should" be done. It is when dying people become more intimate with themselves and appreciate their separateness from others more than at any other time.

Perspective and Prospects

All patients die—a fact that the actual practice of clinical Western medicine has too often discounted. Dealing with death is difficult in life, and it is difficult in medicine. As the ultimate outcome of all medical interventions, however, it is unavoidable. Dealing with the dying and those who care about them is also difficult. Patients ask questions that cannot be answered; families in despair and anger seek to find cause and sometimes lay blame. It takes courage to be with individuals as they face their deaths, struggling to find meaning in the time that they have left. It takes special courage simply to witness this struggle in a profession which prides itself on how well it intervenes. Working with death also reminds professionals of their own inevitable death. Facing that fact inwardly, spiritually, and existentially also requires courage.

Cure and treatment become care and management in the dying. They should live relatively pain-free, be supported in accomplishing their goals, be respected, be involved in decision making as appropriate, be encouraged to function as fully as their illness allows, and be provided with others to whom control can comfortably and confidently be passed. The lack of a cure and the certainty of the end can intimidate health care providers, family members, and close friends. They may dread genuine encounters with those whose days are knowingly numbered. Yet the dying have the same rights to be helped as any of the living, and how a society assists them bears directly on the meaning that its members are willing to attach to their own lives.

Today, largely in response to what dying patients have told researchers, medicine recognizes its role to assist these patients in working toward an appropriate death. Caretakers must determine the optimum treatments, interventions, and conditions which will enable such a death to occur. For each terminally ill person, these should be unique and specific. Caretakers should respond to the patient's needs and priorities, at the patient's own pace and as much as possible following the patient's lead. For some dying patients, the goal is to remain as pain-free as is feasible and to feel as well as possible. For others, finishing whatever unfinished business remains becomes the priority. Making amends, forgiving and being forgiven, resolving old conflicts, and reconciling with self and others may be the most therapeutic and healing of interventions. Those who are to be bereaved fear the death of those they love. The dying fear the separation from all they know and love, but they fear as well the loss of autonomy, letting family and friends down, the pain and invasion of further treatment, disfigurement, dementia, loneliness, the unknown, becoming a burden, and the loss of dignity.

The English writer C. S. Lewis said that bereavement is the universal and integral part of the experience of loss. It requires effort, authenticity, mental and emotional work, a willingness to be afraid, and an openness to what is happening and what is going to happen. It requires an attitude which accepts, tolerates suffering, takes respite from the reality, reinvests in whatever life remains, and moves on.

The only way to cope with dying or witnessing the dying of loved ones is by grieving through the pain, fear, loneliness, and loss of meaning. This process, which researcher Stephen Levine has likened to opening the heart in hell, is a viscous morass for most, and all people need to learn their own way through it and to have that learning respected. Healing begins with the first halting, unsteady, and frightening steps of genuine grief, which sometimes occur years before the "time of death" can be recorded as an historical event and which may never completely end.

—*Paul Moglia*

See also Aging; Depression; Grief and guilt; Midlife crisis; Phobias; Stress; Sudden infant death syndrome (SIDS); Suicide.

FOR FURTHER INFORMATION:

Becker, Ernest. *The Denial of Death*. New York: Free Press, 1973. Written by an anthropologist and philosopher, this is an erudite and insightful analysis and synthesis of the role that the fear of death plays in motivating human activity, society, and individual actions. A profound work.

Bluebond-Langer, Myra. *The Private Worlds of Dying Children*. Princeton, N.J.: Princeton University Press, 1978. Based on research that she conducted with hospitalized leukemic children, the anthropologist-author describes how children deal with their impending deaths in ways that give meaning and instruction to those who deal with the terminally ill. Filled with transcribed dialogue; at times a moving work.

Cook, Alicia Skinner, and Daniel S. Dworkin. *Helping the Bereaved: Therapeutic Interventions for Children, Adolescents, and Adults*. New York: BasicBooks, 1992. Though not a self-help book, this work is useful to professionals and nonprofessionals alike as a review of the state of the art in grief therapy. Practical and readable. Of special interest for those becoming involved in grief counseling.

Feifel, Herman, ed. *The Meaning of Death*. New York: McGraw-Hill, 1959. A classic of thanatological thinking before thanatology became a recognized specialty. Brings together systematized knowledge about death from multiple disciplines. An excellent resource of information fostering reflection.

Kübler-Ross, Elisabeth, ed. *Death: The Final Stage of Growth*. Englewood Cliffs, N.J.: Prentice Hall, 1975. A psychiatrist by training, Kübler-Ross brings together other researchers' views of how death provides the key to how human beings make meaning in their own personal worlds. The author, who is regarded as the pioneer in death and dying studies, addresses practical concerns over how people express grief and accept the death of those close to them, and how they might prepare for their own inevitable ends.

_____, ed. *Living with Death and Dying*. New York: Macmillan, 1981. Written in response to the concerns and questions of professionals and parents in dealing with dying generally and with children's understanding of death in particular, this is a conversational work based on the experience and insights of Kübler-Ross and two of her colleagues. Moving and genuine.

Kushner, Harold. *When Bad Things Happen to Good People*. New York: Summit, 1985. The first of Rabbi Kushner's works on finding meaning in one's life, it was originally his personal response to make intelligible the death of his own child. It has become a highly regarded reference for any who struggle with the meaning of pain, suffering, and death in their lives. Highly recommended.

Levine, Stephen. *Meetings at the Edge: Dialogues with the Grieving and the Dying, the Healing and the Healed*. Garden City, N.Y.: Anchor Press, 1984. An encouraging, realistic, and reassuring work by a nonphysician who addresses the suffering and pain of the dying and the bereaved. Advocates opening oneself to grief as a means of healing oneself with it. Though nonsectarian, this work has an Eastern, even Buddhist, slant. Clearly written with much practical application.

Linn, Matthew, Dennis Linn, and Sheila Fabricant. *Healing the Greatest Hurt*. New York: Paulist Press, 1985. A wonderful, reflective, and practical work written within the Christian tradition that would be of benefit to believers in other traditions as well. Grapples with the great unknown of what lies after death through the eschatological metaphor known as "the communion of saints."

DEMENTIA

SYSTEM AFFECTED: Brain

SPECIALISTS: Geriatric specialists, neurologists, psychiatrists

DEFINITION: A generally irreversible decline in intellectual ability resulting from a variety of causes; differs from mental retardation, in which the affected person never reaches an expected level of mental growth.

KEY TERMS:

basal ganglia: a collection of nerve cells deep inside the brain, below the cortex, that controls muscle tone and automatic actions such as walking

cortical dementia: dementia resulting from damage to the brain cortex, the outer layer of the brain that contains the bodies of the nerve cells

delirium: an acute condition characterized by confusion, a fluctuating level of consciousness, and visual, auditory, and even tactile hallucinations; often caused by acute disease, such as infection or intoxication

hydrocephalus: a condition resulting from the accumulation of fluid inside the brain in cavities known as ventricles; as fluid accumulates, it exerts pressure on the neighboring brain cells, which may be destroyed

subcortical dementia: dementia resulting from damage to the area of the brain below the cortex; this area contains nerve fibers that connect various parts of the brain with one another and with the basal ganglia

vascular dementia: dementia caused by repeated strokes, resulting in interference with the blood supply to parts of the brain

CAUSES AND SYMPTOMS

Dementia affects about four million people in the United States and is a major cause of disability in old age. Its prevalence increases with age. Dementia is characterized by a permanent memory deficit affecting recent memory in particular and of sufficient severity to interfere with the patient's ability to take part in professional and social activities. Although the aging process is associated with a gradual loss of brain cells, dementia is not part of the aging process. It also is not synonymous with benign senescent forgetfulness, which is very common in old age and affects recent memory. Although the latter is a source of frustration, it does not significantly interfere with the individual's professional and social activities because it tends to affect only trivial matters (or what the individual considers trivial). Furthermore, patients with benign forgetfulness usually can remember what was forgotten by utilizing a number of subterfuges, such as writing lists or notes to themselves and leaving them in conspicuous places. Individuals with benign forgetfulness also are acutely aware of their memory deficit, while those with dementia—except for in the early stages of the disease—have no insight into their memory deficit and often blame others for their problems.

In addition to the memory deficit interfering with the patient's daily activities, patients with dementia have evidence of impaired abstract thinking, impaired judgment, or other disturbances of higher cortical functions such as aphasia (the inability to use or comprehend language), apraxia (the inability to execute complex, coordinated movements), or agnosia (the inability to recognize familiar objects).

Dementia may result from damage to the cerebral cortex (the outer layer of the brain), as in Alzheimer's disease, or from damage to the subcortical structures (the structures below the cortex), such as white matter, the thalamus, or the basal ganglia. Although memory is impaired in both cortical and subcortical dementias, the associated features are different. In cortical dementias, for example, cognitive functions such as the ability to understand speech and to talk and the ability to perform mathematical calculations are severely impaired. In subcortical dementias, on the other hand, there is evidence of disturbances of arousal, motivation, and mood, in addition to a significant slowing of cognition and of information processing.

Alzheimer's disease, the most common cause of presenile dementia, is characterized by progressive disorientation, memory loss, speech disturbances, and personality disorders. Pick's disease is another cortical dementia, but unlike Alzheimer's disease, it is rare, tends to affect younger patients, and is more common in women. In the early stages of Pick's disease, changes in personality, disinhibition, inappropriate social and sexual conduct, and lack of foresight may be evident—features that are not common in Alzheimer's disease. Patients also may become euphoric or apathetic. Poverty of speech is often present and gradually progresses to mutism, although speech comprehension is usually spared. Pick's disease is characterized by cortical atrophy localized to the frontal and temporal lobes.

Vascular dementia is the second most common cause of dementia in patients over the age of sixty-five and is responsible for 8 percent to 20 percent of all dementia cases. It is caused by interference with the blood flow to the brain. Although the overall prevalence of vascular dementia is decreasing, there are some geographical variations, with the prevalence being higher in countries with a high incidence of cardiovascular and cerebrovascular diseases, such as Finland and Japan. About 20 percent of patients with dementia have both Alzheimer's disease and vascular dementia. Several types of vascular dementia have been identified.

Multiple infarct dementia (MID) is the most common type of vascular dementia. As its name implies, it is the result of multiple, discrete cerebral infarcts (strokes) that have destroyed enough brain tissue to interfere with the patient's higher mental functions. The onset of MID is usually sudden and is associated with neurological deficit, such as the paralysis or weakness of an arm or leg or the inability to speak. The disease characteristically progresses in steps: With each stroke experienced, the patient's condition suddenly deteriorates and then stabilizes or even improves slightly until another stroke occurs. In about 20 percent of patients with MID, however, the disease displays an insidious onset and causes gradual deterioration. Most patients also show evidence of arteriosclerosis and other factors predisposing them to the development of strokes, such as hypertension, cigarette smoking, high blood cholesterol, diabetes mellitus, narrowing of one or both carotid arteries, or cardiac disorders, especially atrial fibrillation (an irregular heartbeat). Somatic complaints, mood changes, depression, and nocturnal confusion tend to be more common in vascular dementias, although there is relative preservation of the patient's personality. In such cases, magnetic resonance imaging (MRI) or a computed tomography (CT) scan of the brain often shows evidence of multiple strokes.

Strokes are not always associated with clinical evidence of neurological deficits, since the stroke may affect a "silent" area of the brain or may be so small that its immediate impact is not noticeable. Nevertheless, when several of these small strokes have occurred, the resulting loss of brain tissue may interfere with the patient's cognitive functions. This is, in fact, the basis of the lacunar dementias. The infarcted tissue is absorbed into the rest of the brain, leaving a small cavity or lacuna. Brain-imaging techniques and especially MRI are useful in detecting these lacunae.

A number of neurological disorders are associated with dementia. The combination of dementia, urinary incontinence, and muscle rigidity causing difficulties in walking should raise the suspicion of hydrocephalus. In this condition, fluid accumulates inside the ventricles (cavities within the brain) and results in increased pressure on the brain cells. A CT scan demonstrates enlargement of the ventricles. Although some patients may respond well to surgical shunting of the cerebrospinal fluid, it is often difficult to identify those who will benefit from surgery. Postoperative complications are significant and include strokes and subdural hematomas.

Dementia has been linked to Parkinson's disease, a chronic, progressive neurological disorder that usually manifests itself in middle or late life. It has an insidious onset and a very slow progression rate. Although intellectual deterioration is not part of the classical features of Parkinson's disease, dementia is being recognized as a late manifestation of the disease, with as many as one-third of the patients eventually being afflicted. The dementing process also has an insidious onset and slow progression rate. Some of the medication used to treat Parkinson's disease also may induce confusion, particularly in older patients.

Subdural hematomas (collections of blood inside the brain) may lead to mental impairment and are usually precipitated by trauma to the head. Usually, the trauma is slight and the patient neither loses consciousness nor experiences any immediate significant effects. A few days or even weeks later, however, the patient may develop evidence of mental impairment. By that time, the patient and caregivers may have forgotten about the slight trauma that the patient had experienced. A subdural hematoma should be suspected in the presence of a fairly sudden onset and progressing course. Headaches are common. A CT scan can reveal the presence of a hematoma. The surgical removal of the hematoma is usually associated with a good prognosis if the surgery is done in a timely manner, before irreversible brain damage occurs.

Brain tumors may lead to dementia, particularly if they are slow growing. Most tumors of this type can be diagnosed by CT scanning or MRI. Occasionally, cancer may induce dementia through an inflammation of the brain.

Many chronic infections affecting the brain can lead to dementia; they include conditions that, when treated, may reverse or prevent the progression of dementia, such as syphilis, tuberculosis, slow viruses, and some fungal and protozoal infections. Human immunodeficiency virus (HIV) infection is also a cause of dementia, and it may be suspected if the rate of progress is rapid and the patient has risk factors for the development of HIV infection. Although the dementia is part of the acquired immunodeficiency syndrome (AIDS) complex, it may occasionally be the first manifestation of the disease.

It is often difficult to differentiate depression from dementia. Nevertheless, sudden onset—especially if preceded by an emotional event, the presence of sleep disturbances, and a history of previous psychiatric illness—is suggestive of depression. The level of mental functioning of patients with depression is often inconsistent. They may, for example, be able to give clear accounts of topics that are of personal interest to them but be very vague about, and at times may not even attempt to answer, questions on topics that are of no interest to them. Variability in performance during testing is suggestive of depression, especially if it improves with positive reinforcement.

TREATMENT AND THERAPY

It is estimated that dementia affects about 0.4 percent of the population aged sixty to sixty-four years and 0.9, 1.8, 3.6, 10.5, and 23.8 percent of the population aged sixty-five to sixty-nine, seventy to seventy-four, seventy-five to seventy-nine, eighty to eighty-four, and eighty-five to ninety-three years, respectively. Different surveys may yield different results, depending on the criteria used to define dementia.

For physicians, an important aspect of diagnosing patients with dementia is detecting potentially reversible causes which may be responsible for the impaired mental functions. A detailed history followed by a meticulous and thorough clinical examination and a few selected laboratory tests are usually sufficient to reach a diagnosis. Various investigators have estimated that reversible causes of dementia can be identified in 10 percent to 20 percent of patients with dementia. Recommended investigations include brain imaging (CT scanning or MRI), a complete blood count, and tests of erythrocyte sedimentation rate, blood glucose, serum electrolytes, serum calcium, liver function, thyroid function, and serum B_{12} and folate. Some investigators also recommend routine testing for syphilis. Other tests, such as those for the detection of HIV infection, cerebrospinal fluid examination, neuropsychological testing, drug and toxin screen, serum copper and ceruloplasmin analysis, carotid and cerebral angiography, and electroencephalography, are performed when appropriate.

It is of paramount importance for health care providers to adopt a positive attitude when managing patients with dementia. Although at present little can be done to treat and reverse dementia, it is important to identify the cause of the dementia. In some cases, it may be possible to prevent the disease from progressing. For example, if the dementia is the result of hypertension, adequate control of this condition may prevent further brain damage. Moreover, the prevalence of vascular dementia is decreasing in countries where efforts to reduce cardiovascular and cerebrovascular diseases have been successful. Similarly, if the dementia is the result of repeated emboli (blood clots reaching the brain) complicating atrial fibrillation, then anticoagulants or aspirin may be recommended.

Even after a diagnosis of dementia is made, it is important for the physician to detect the presence of other conditions that may worsen the patient's mental functions, such as the inadvertent intake of medications that may induce confusion and mental impairment. Medications with this potential are numerous and include not only those that act on the brain, such as sedatives and hypnotics, but also hypotensive agents (especially if given in large doses), diuretics, and antibiotics. Whenever the condition of a patient with dementia deteriorates, the physician meticulously reviews all the medications that the patient is taking, both medical prescriptions and medications that may have been purchased over the counter. Even if innocuous, some over-the-counter preparations may interact with other medications that the patient is taking and lead to a worsening of mental functions. Inquiries are also made into the patient's alcohol intake. The brain of an older person is much more sensitive to the effects of alcohol than that of a younger person, and some medications may interact with the alcohol to impair the patient's cognitive functions further.

Many other disease states also may worsen the patient's mental functions. For example, patients with diabetes mellitus are susceptible to developing a variety of metabolic abnormalities including a low or high blood glucose level, both of which may be associated with confusional states. Similarly, dehydration and acid-base or electrolyte disorders, which may result from prolonged vomiting or diarrhea, may also precipitate confusional states. Infections, particularly respiratory and urinary tract infections, often worsen the patient's cognitive deficit. Finally, patients with dementia may experience myocardial infarctions (heart attacks) that are not associated with any chest pain but that may manifest themselves with confusion.

The casual observer of the dementing process is often overwhelmed with concern for the patient, but it is the family that truly suffers. The patients themselves experience no physical pain or distress, and except for in the very early stages of the disease, they are oblivious to their plight as a result of their loss of insight. Health care professionals therefore are alert to the stress imposed on the caregivers by dealing with loved ones with dementia. Adequate support from agencies available in the community is essential.

When a diagnosis of dementia is made, the physician discusses a number of ethical, financial, and legal issues with the family, and also the patient if it is believed that he or she can understand the implications of this discussion. Families are encouraged to make a list of all the patient's assets, including insurance policies, and to discuss this information with an attorney in order to protect the patient's and the family's assets. If the patient is still competent, it is recommended that he or she select a trusted person to have durable power of attorney. Unlike the regular power of attorney, the former does not become invalidated when the patient becomes mentally incompetent and continues to be in effect regardless of the degree of mental impairment

of the person who executed it. Because durable power of attorney cannot be easily reversed once the person is incompetent, great care should be taken when selecting a person and the specific powers granted should be clearly specified. It is also important for the patient to make his or her desires known concerning advance directives and the use of life-support systems.

Courts may appoint a guardian or conservator to have charge and custody of the patient's property (including real estate and money) when no responsible family members or friends are willing or available to serve as guardian. Courts supervise the actions of the guardian, who is expected to report all the patient's income and expenditures to the court once a year. The court may also charge the guardian to ensure that the patient is adequately housed, fed, and clothed and receiving appropriate medical care.

PERSPECTIVE AND PROSPECTS

Dementia is a very serious and common condition, especially among the older population. Dementia permanently robs patients of their minds and prevents them from functioning adequately in their environment by impairing memory and interfering with the ability to make rational decisions. It therefore deprives patients of their dignity and independence.

Because dementia is mostly irreversible, cannot be adequately treated at present, and is associated with a fairly long survival period, it has a significant impact not only on the patient's life but also on the patient's family and caregivers and on society in general. The expense of long-term care for patients with dementia, whether at home or in institutions, is staggering. Every effort, therefore, is made to reach an accurate diagnosis and especially to detect any other condition that may worsen the patient's underlying dementia. Finally, health care professionals do not treat the patient in isolation but also concern themselves with the impact of the illness on the patient's caregivers and family.

Much progress has been made in defining dementia and determining its cause. Terms such as "senile dementia" are no longer in use, and even the use of the term "dementia" to diagnose a patient's condition is frowned upon because there are so many types of dementia. The recognition of the type of dementia affecting a particular patient is important because of its practical implications, both for the patient and for research into the prevention, management, and treatment of dementia. The prevalence of vascular dementia, for example, is decreasing in many countries where the prevention of cardiovascular diseases such as hypertension and arteriosclerosis has been successful.

Unfortunately, there is little that can be done to cure dementia and no effective means to regenerate nerve cells. Researchers, however, are feverishly trying to identify factors that control the growth and regeneration of nerve cells. Although no single medication is expected to be of benefit to all types of dementia, it is hoped that effective therapy for many dementias will be developed. —*Ronald C. Hamdy, Louis A. Cancellaro, and Larry Hudgins*

See also Aging; Alzheimer's disease; Amnesia and memory loss; Brain disorders; Hallucinations; Parkinsonism; Strokes and TIAs.

FOR FURTHER INFORMATION:

Coons, Dorothy H., ed. *Specialized Dementia Care Units.* Baltimore: The Johns Hopkins University Press, 1991. A collection of articles reviewing the benefits and disadvantages of caring for patients with dementia in specialized care units. Several problems encountered when running such units are addressed.

Hamdy, Ronald C., J. M. Turnbull, L. D. Norman, and M. M. Lancaster, eds. *Alzheimer's Disease: A Handbook for Caregivers.* St. Louis: C. V. Mosby, 1990. A comprehensive discussion of the symptoms and characteristic features of Alzheimer's disease and other dementias. Abnormal brain structure and function in these patients are discussed, and the normal effects of aging are reviewed. Gives caregivers practical advice concerning the encouragement of patients with dementia.

Howe, M. L., M. J. Stones, and C. J. Brainerd, eds. *Cognitive and Behavioral Performance Factors in Atypical Aging.* New York: Springer-Verlag, 1990. A review of the factors controlling behavior, test performance, and brain function in both young and older patients.

Terry, Robert D., ed. *Aging and the Brain.* New York: Raven Press, 1988. A review of the application of concepts in neurobiology and technology in the study of brain structure and function in normal elderly people and those with different types of dementia.

U.S. Congress. Office of Technology Assessment. *Confused Minds, Burdened Families: Finding Help for People with Alzheimer's and Other Dementias.* Washington, D.C.: Government Printing Office, 1990. A report from the Office of Technology Assessment analyzing the problems of locating and arranging services for people with dementia in the United States. Also presents a framework for an effective system to provide appropriate services and discusses congressional policy options for establishing such a system.

U.S. Congress. Office of Technology Assessment. *Losing a Million Minds: Confronting the Tragedy of Alzheimer's Disease and Other Dementias.* Washington, D.C.: Government Printing Office, 1987. A comprehensive report from the Office of Technology Assessment reviewing the nature and psychological, sociological, and economic implications of dementia in the United States. The various programs and services available are reviewed, and recommendations concerning future policies are made. The issues of personnel training and quality assurance are also addressed.

West, Robin L., and Jan D. Sinnott, eds. *Everyday Memory and Aging.* New York: Springer-Verlag, 1992. A review

of issues relating to memory research and methodology, especially as they apply to aging.

DENTAL DISEASES

SYSTEMS AFFECTED: Gums, teeth

SPECIALISTS: Dentists

DEFINITION: Diseases that affect the teeth, such as dental caries, and the gums, such as gingivitis, pyorrhea, or cancer.

KEY TERMS:

dental caries: tooth decay

dentin: a hard, bonelike tissue lying beneath the tooth enamel

enamel: the hard surface covering of teeth

gingivae: the soft tissue surrounding the teeth; the gums

gingivitis: an inflammation of the gums

periodontal diseases: diseases characterized by inflammation of the gingivae

pyorrhea: the second stage of gingivitis

tooth pulp: the tissue at the center of teeth, surrounded by dentin

Vincent's infection: a bacterial infection of the gingivae, also known as trench mouth

CAUSES AND SYMPTOMS

Dental diseases fall into four major categories: dental caries, or tooth decay; periodontal disease, including gingivitis and pyorrhea; Vincent's infection, or trench mouth; and oral cancer. The first of these diseases was the largest contributor to tooth loss among people under thirty-five in the United States before the widespread fluoridation of drinking water was begun; it remains a major cause of tooth loss in much of the world. Periodontal disease in its two stages, gingivitis and pyorrhea, is the most widespread dental problem for people over thirty-five. Most people who suffer the loss of all of their teeth are victims of this condition. Vincent's infection, which shares many characteristics with gingivitis, is a bacterial infection. The infection flares up, is treated, and disappears, whereas gingivitis is more often a continuing condition that requires both persistent home treatment and specialized treatment. The most serious but least frequently occurring dental disease is oral cancer. It is the only dental disease commonly considered life-threatening, and there is a risk that it may spread to other parts of the body.

Dental caries occur because the food that one eats becomes trapped in the irregularities of the teeth, creating lactic acids that penetrate the enamel through holes (often microscopic) in it. Once lodged between the teeth or below the gum line, carbohydrates and starches combine with saliva to form acids that, over time, can penetrate a tooth's enamel, enter the dentin directly below it, and progressively destroy the dentin while spreading toward the tooth's center, the pulp.

This process often is not confined to a single tooth. As decay spreads, adjoining teeth may be affected. Some people have much harder tooth enamel than others. Therefore, some individuals may experience little or no decay, whereas others who follow similar diets and practice similar methods of dental hygiene may develop substantial decay.

Toothache occurs when decay eats through the dentin and enters the nerve-filled dental pulp, causing inflammation, infection, and pain. A dull, continuous ache, either mild or severe and often pulsating, may indicate that the infection has entered the jawbone beneath the tooth. An aching or sensitivity in the back teeth during chewing is sometimes a side effect of sinusitis.

Periodontal disease. One of dentistry's nagging problems is periodontal disease, which results from a buildup of calculus, or tartar, formed by hardened plaque. Plaque is formed when food, particularly carbohydrates and starches, interact with the saliva that coats the teeth, creating a yellowish film. If this film is not removed, it inevitably lodges between the gums and the teeth, where, within twenty-four hours, it hardens into calculus. Dental hygienists can remove most of this calculus mechanically. If it is allowed to build up over extended periods, however, the calculus will irritate the gums, causing the soreness, swelling, and bleeding that signal gum infection. Eventually, this infection becomes entrenched and difficult to treat.

Periodontists can control but not cure most periodontal disease. In its early manifestations, periodontal disease results in gingivitis, marked by inflammation and bleeding. Untreated, it progresses to pyorrhea, which is characterized by gums that recede from the teeth and form pockets in which infections flourish. As pyorrhea advances, the bone that underlies the teeth and holds them in place is compromised and ultimately destroyed, causing looseness and eventual tooth loss.

Vincent's infection (trench mouth) is communicable through kissing or sharing eating utensils. Although it is sometimes mistaken for gingivitis, Vincent's infection has one distinguishing characteristic that gingivitis does not have: It is accompanied by a fever stemming from sustained bacterial infection, which also causes extremely foul breath. Vincent's infection is curable through proper treatment. It is unlikely to recur unless one is again exposed to the infection.

Oral cancer is the most serious of oral diseases. It often spreads quickly, destroying the tissues of the mouth during its ravaging advance. It not only threatens its original site but also can spread to other areas of the body and to vital organs. Fortunately, oral cancer is uncommon. Nevertheless, dentists look vigilantly for signs of it when they perform mouth examinations because early detection is vital to successful treatment, containment, and cure. People who have persistent mouth sores that do not heal may be experiencing the early manifestations of oral cancer and should see their dentists or physicians immediately.

Other conditions. Two other dental conditions afflict many people: malocclusion and toothache. Malocclusion

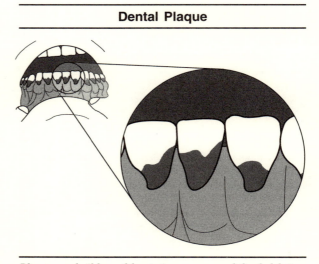

Dental Plaque

Plaque—a buildup of bacteria, mucus, and food debris— leads to dental caries (tooth decay) if not regularly removed by brushing, flossing, and professional tooth cleaning.

occurs when, for a variety of reasons, the teeth are out of alignment. People with malocclusion are prime candidates for dental caries and periodontal disease, largely because their teeth are difficult to reach and hard to clean. Malocclusion may also cause one or more teeth to strike the teeth above or below them, causing injury to teeth and possibly fracturing them.

TREATMENT AND THERAPY

Modern dentistry has succeeded in controlling most dental diseases. In the United States, dental caries have been almost eliminated in the young, for example, by the addition of fluoride to most water systems. Used over time, fluoride strengthens the teeth by increasing the hardness of the enamel, making it resistant to the acids that form in the mouth and cause decay.

Since the 1950's, many American children have been reared on fluoridated water. Those whose water supply is not fluoridated have usually had their teeth treated with fluoride by their dentists. Many have brushed their teeth regularly with fluoridated toothpaste, which offers considerable protection from dental caries. From the 1950's to the 1990's, fluoride reduced dental decay in Americans under the age of twenty-one by more than 70 percent.

Current research into ways of preventing dental decay centers on several projects of the National Institute of Dental Research. Researchers for this organization discovered in the mid-1960's that a substance found in the mouth's streptococcal bacteria creates dextran. Dextran enables bacteria to cling to the surface of the teeth and invade them with the lactic acid that they generate. Researchers ultimately discovered dextrase, an enzyme effective in dissolving dextran. Strides are being made to use dextrase in toothpaste or mouthwash in order to reduce or eliminate the effects of dextran.

Some people's teeth seem to be impervious to tooth decay. It has been determined that such people have a common substance in their blood that protects their teeth from dental caries. Attempts are being made to identify and isolate this substance and to make it generally available to the public and to dentists in an applicable form. Some dentists coat the teeth with a durable plastic substance to make them resistant to penetration by the acids that cause dental decay, creating a hard protective coating above the enamel and making it difficult for food to lodge between the teeth or in irregularities in the teeth.

Because malocclusion can lead to tooth decay, dentists have become increasingly aware of the need to replace lost teeth so that the alignment of the remaining teeth will not be disturbed. Tooth implantation, a process by which a tooth, either artificial or natural, is anchored directly and permanently in the gum, solves many dental problems that in the past were addressed by attaching artificial teeth to existing ones beside them. In situations where malocclusion is caused by malformations, the use of orthodontic braces results in a more regular alignment.

Nutrition has come to the forefront of recent research in dental health. A lack of calciferol, a form of vitamin D_2, may result in dental abnormalities, including malocclusion. Among substantial numbers of hospital patients who suffer from nutritional problems, the earliest symptoms occur in the soft tissue of the mouth.

Brushing the teeth after meals and before bed controls plaque, as does regular flossing. Such daily attention must be supplemented by twice-yearly cleaning, performed by a dentist or dental hygienist, and by annual or biennial wholemouth X rays to reveal incipient decay. Various mouthwashes also contain substances that control decay.

People who cannot brush after every meal should use a mouthwash or rinse the mouth out with water after eating, then brush as soon as they can. Special attention must be given to the back surfaces of the lower front teeth because the salivary glands are located there. This area is a breeding ground for the bacteria that cause the formation of lactic acid. Routine home care of this kind, particularly daily flossing, will help prevent both tooth decay and periodontal disease, and can also reverse some of the inroads that periodontal disease has made. When gingivitis advances to pyorrhea, however, dental surgery may be indicated.

The major villain in both gingivitis and pyorrhea is tartar, or calculus, which is produced when plaque hardens. When tartar accumulates beneath the gums, it causes an irritation that can lead to infection. Sometimes, this infection moves to other parts of the body, causing joint problems and other difficulties.

People can control plaque by practicing daily dental hygiene at home. They must also have accumulated tartar regularly scraped away or removed by ultrasound in the dentist's office. Malocclusions and defects in the production of saliva can be corrected by dentists and can greatly reduce the progress of periodontal disease.

When gum surgery is advised for the removal of the deep gum pockets that occur with pyorrhea, further surgery can usually be avoided by regular home care. Meanwhile, researchers are trying to develop a vaccine to immunize its recipients against the bacteria that cause tooth decay. Other decay-inhibiting agents are being studied closely with the expectation that they may in time be added to common foods and beverages.

Vincent's infection is successfully treated with antibiotics, accompanied by a prescribed course of dental hygiene that is begun in the dentist's office and continues at home on a daily basis. Some patients have found a peroxide mouthwash helpful in treating this disease.

Oral cancer, when it is discovered by a dentist, is usually referred immediately to the patient's family physician, who then refers the case to an oncologist. Laser treatment and radiation are used in controlling this sort of cancer, as are chemotherapy and surgery. The most important element in cancer treatment is time. It is essential, therefore, that specialized treatment be initiated as soon as oral cancer is discovered or suspected. In cases of oral cancer, a delay of even days can affect outcomes negatively.

The most immediate treatments for toothache range from the application of cold compresses to the taking of aspirin or some other analgesic every few hours. If the decayed part of the tooth is visible and reachable, sometimes applying a mixture of oil of cloves and benzocaine to the decayed area on a small swab soothes the pain. These treatments, however, offer only temporary relief.

Dentists resist treating toothache by removing the tooth, although removal offers an immediate solution to the problem. In some cases, dentists can drill out the decay and fill the tooth with silver amalgam, gold, or plastic. Quite often, by the time a tooth begins to ache, the pulp and dentin have been ravaged by decay and the best solution is endodontistry, or root canal, which will preserve the tooth but may necessitate the attachment of a crown.

PERSPECTIVE AND PROSPECTS

Great strides have been made in the United States in preventing and treating dental disease as researchers have reached deeper understandings of the root causes of such disease. Dentistry has become increasingly less painful through the use of anesthetics and high-speed, water-cooled drills. The public at large has grown aware of the close relationship between dental health and general health. People are unwilling to accept tooth loss as a natural consequence of aging. They have also begun to realize that orthodontistry is more than a cosmetic procedure. Rather, it is a necessary procedure for correcting misalignments of the teeth that can result in difficulty if uncorrected.

National attention has been given to preventing tooth decay through the fluoridation of water supplies and, although some groups still fight fluoridation, it is for most Americans an accepted fact of modern life. Fluoridation more than any other factor has changed the emphasis in dentistry from preventing and treating dental caries to more sophisticated pursuits such as orthodontistry, endodontistry, and periodontistry. The establishment of the National Institute for Dental Research by Congress in 1948 has, more than any other single factor, stimulated dental research in the United States.

Advances in preventing and treating dental disease are constantly being made. Through genetic engineering, it is almost inevitable that substances will soon be available to increase an individual's resistance to tooth decay. Nevertheless, controlling the buildup of calculus, the major factor in periodontal disease, will probably remain the responsibility of individuals through daily home care and twice yearly visits to their dentists. —*R. Baird Shuman*

See also Caries, dental; Endodontic disease; Gingivitis; Periodontitis; Toothache.

FOR FURTHER INFORMATION:

Anderson, Pauline C., and Martha R. Burkard. *The Dental Assistant.* 5th ed. Albany, N.Y.: Delmar, 1987. Designed as a textbook for dental hygienists, this popular volume is particularly clear in its discussion of periodontal disease and dental caries. Although it is not directed specifically to laypersons, the book is easily accessible to nonspecialized readers.

Foster, Malcolm S. *Protecting Our Children's Teeth: A Guide to Quality Dental Care from Infancy Through Age Twelve.* New York: Insight Books, 1992. This book, meant for parents, is clear and easy to understand. The illustrations are useful. A good starting point.

McGuire, Thomas. *The Tooth Trip: An Oral Experience.* New York: Random House, 1972. Although somewhat dated, this book provides accurate information about dental diseases. Its pen-and-ink drawings clarify some of the technical information that McGuire provides. Aimed at laypersons.

Renner, Robert. *An Introduction to Dental Anatomy and Esthetics.* Chicago: Quintessence, 1985. This standard work in the field is thorough and accurate. Presents extensive information about dental disease, its prevention and treatment. A fundamental resource.

Ring, Malvin E. *Dentistry: An Illustrated History.* New York: Harry N. Abrams, 1985. Ring's coverage of dentistry is broad and accurate. The illustrations are particularly useful in helping readers understand dental diseases. An excellent starting point for those unfamiliar with the topic.

Ward, Brian R. *Dental Care.* New York: Franklin Watts, 1986. Ward emphasizes the daily care of the teeth and the prevention of dental disease. Presents this informa-

tion lucidly and directly, using selective illustrations appropriately and well.

DEPRESSION

SYSTEMS AFFECTED: Psychic-emotional, heart, muscular

SPECIALISTS: Family physicians, psychiatrists, psychologists

DEFINITION: The single most common psychiatric disorder, caused by biological and/or psychological factors; approximately 15 percent of cases result in suicide.

KEY TERMS:

bipolar disorder: a mood disorder characterized by one or more manic and major depressive episodes occurring simultaneously or in cycles

cyclothymia: a mood disorder characterized as a less intense form of bipolar disorder

dysthymia: a mood disorder characterized as a less intense form of depressive disorder

electroconvulsive therapy: the use of electric shocks to induce seizure in depressed patients as a form of treatment

major depressive disorder: a pattern of major depressive episodes that form an identified psychiatric disorder

major depressive episode: a syndrome of symptoms characterized by depressed mood; required for the diagnosis of some mood disorders

manic episode: a syndrome of symptoms characterized by elevated, expansive, or irritable mood; required for the diagnosis of some mood disorders

psychopharmacology: the drug treatment of psychiatric disorders

psychosurgery: the surgical removal or destruction of part of the brain of depressed patients as a form of treatment

psychotherapy: the "talk" therapies that target the emotional and social contributors and consequences of depression

seasonal affective disorder: a mood disorder associated with the winter season, when the amount of daylight hours is reduced

CAUSES AND SYMPTOMS

The term "depression" is used to describe a fleeting mood, an outward physical appearance of sadness, or a diagnosable clinical disorder. It is estimated that 13 million Americans suffer from a clinically diagnosed depression, a mood disorder that often affects personal, vocational, social, and health functioning. The *Diagnostic and Statistical Manual of Mental Disorders* (rev. 3d ed., 1987, DSM-III-R) of the American Psychiatric Association delineates a number of mood disorders that subsume the various types of clinical depression.

A *major depressive episode* is a syndrome of symptoms, present during a two-week period and representing a change from previous functioning. The symptoms include at least five of the following: depressed or irritable mood, diminished interest in previously pleasurable activities, significant weight loss or weight gain, insomnia or hypersomnia, physical excitation or slowness, loss of energy, feelings of worthlessness or guilt, indecisiveness or a diminished ability to concentrate, and recurrent thoughts of death. The clinical depression cannot be initiated or maintained by another illness or condition, and it cannot be a normal reaction to the death of a loved one (some symptoms of depression are a normal part of the grief reaction).

In *major depressive disorder*, the patient experiences a major depressive episode and does not have a history of mania or hypomania. Major depressive disorder is often first recognized in the patient's late twenties, while a major depressive episode can occur at any age, including infancy. Women are twice as likely to suffer from the disorder than are men.

There are several potential causes of major depressive disorder. Genetic studies suggest a familial link with higher rates of clinical depression in first-degree relatives. There also appears to be a relationship between clinical depression and levels of the brain's neurochemicals, specifically serotonin and norepinephrine. Common causes of clinical depression include psychosocial stressors, such as the death of a loved one or the loss of a job, or any of a number of personal stressors; it is unclear why some people respond to a specific psychosocial stressor with a clinical depression and others do not. Finally, certain prescription medications have been noted to cause clinical depression. These drugs include muscle relaxants, heart medications, hypertensive medications, ulcer medications, oral contraceptives, and steroids. Thus there are many causes of clinical depression, and no single cause is sufficient to explain all clinical depressions.

Another category of clinical depression is *bipolar disorder*, which affects approximately 1 percent of the population. Bipolar disorder is characterized by one or more manic episodes along with one or more major depressive episodes. A *manic episode* is defined as a distinct period of abnormally and persistently elevated, expansive, or irritable mood. Three of the following symptoms must occur during the period of mood disturbance: inflated self-esteem, decreased need for sleep, unusual talkativeness or pressure to keep talking, racing thoughts, distractibility, excessive goal-oriented activities (especially in work, school, or social areas), and reckless activities with a high potential for negative consequences (such as buying sprees or risky business ventures). For a diagnosis of bipolar disorder, the symptoms must be sufficiently severe to cause impairment in functioning and/or concern regarding the person's danger to himself/herself or to others, must not be superimposed on another psychotic disorder, and must not be initiated or maintained by another illness or condition.

Patients with bipolar disorder will display cycles in which they experience a manic episode followed by a short episode of a major depressive episode, or vice versa. These cycles are often separated by a period of normal mood.

Occasionally, two or more cycles can occur in a year without a period of remission between them, in what is referred to as rapid cycling. The two mood disorders can also occur simultaneously in a single episode. Bipolar disorder is often first recognized in adolescence or in the patient's early twenties; it is not unusual, however, for the initial recognition to occur later in life. Bipolar disorder is equally common in both males and females.

Genetic patterns are strongly involved in bipolar disorder. Brain chemicals (particularly dopamine, acetylcholine, GABA, and serotonin), hormones, drug reactions, and life stressors have all been linked to its development. Of particular interest are findings which suggest that, for some patients with bipolar disorder, changes in the seasons affect the frequency and severity of the disorder. These meteorological effects, while not well understood, have been observed in relation to other disorders of mood.

Cyclothymia is another cyclic mood disorder related to depression; it has a reported lifetime prevalence of approximately 1 to 2 percent. This chronic mood disorder is characterized by manic episodes without marked social or occupational impairment ("hypomanic" episodes) and symptoms of major depressive episode that do not meet the clinical criteria (less than five of the nine symptoms described above). These symptoms must be present for at least two years, and if the patient has periods without symptoms, these periods cannot be longer than two months. Cyclothymia cannot be superimposed on another psychotic disorder and cannot be initiated or maintained by another illness or condition. This mood disorder has its onset in adolescence and early adulthood and is equally common in men and women. It is a particularly persistent and chronic disorder with an identified familial pattern. Cyclothymia often develops into bipolar disorder, and its causes are believed to be the same.

Dysthymia is a chronic mood disorder affecting approximately 2 to 4 percent of the population. Dysthymia is characterized by at least a two-year history of depressed mood and at least two of the following symptoms: poor appetite, insomnia or hypersomnia, low energy or fatigue, low self-esteem, poor concentration or decision making, or feelings of hopelessness. There cannot be evidence of a major depressive episode during the first two years of the dysthymia or a history of manic episodes or hypomanic episodes. The patient cannot be without the symptoms for more than two months at a time, the disorder cannot be superimposed on another psychotic disorder, and it cannot be initiated or maintained by another illness or condition. Dysthymia appears to begin at an earlier age, as young as childhood, with symptoms typically evident by young adulthood. Dysthymia is more common in adult females, equally common in both sexes of children, and with a greater prevalence in families. The causes of dysthymia are believed to be similar to those listed for major depressive disorder.

TREATMENT AND THERAPY

Crucial to the choice of treatment for clinical depression is determining the variant of depression being experienced. Each of the diagnostic categories has associated treatment approaches that are more effective for a particular diagnosis. Multiple assessment techniques are available to the health care professional to determine the type of clinical depression. The most valid and reliable is the clinical interview. The health care provider may conduct either an informal interview or a structured, formal clinical interview assessing the symptoms that would confirm the diagnosis of clinical depression. If the patient meets the criteria set forth in the DSM-III-R, then the patient is considered for depression treatments. Patients who meet many but not all diagnostic criteria are sometimes diagnosed with a "subclinical" depression. These patients might also be considered appropriate for the treatment of depression, at the discretion of their health care providers.

Another assessment technique is the "paper-and-pencil" measure, or depression questionnaire. A variety of questionnaires have proven useful in confirming the diagnosis of clinical depression. Questionnaires such as the Beck Depression Inventory, Hamilton Depression Rating Scale, Zung Self-Rating Depression Scale, and the Center for Epidemiologic Studies Depression Scale are used to identify persons with clinical depression and to document changes with treatment. This technique is often used as an adjunct to the clinical interview and rarely stands alone as the definitive assessment approach to diagnosing clinical depression.

Laboratory tests, most notably the dexamethasone suppression test, have also been used in the diagnosis of depression. The dexamethasone suppression test involves injecting a steroid (dexamethasone) into the patient and measuring the production levels of another steroid (cortisol) in response. Studies have demonstrated, however, that certain severely depressed patients do not reveal the suppression of cortisol production that would be expected following the administration of dexamethasone. The test has also failed to identify some patients who were depressed and has mistakenly identified others as depressed. Research continues to determine the efficacy of other laboratory measures of brain activity to include computed tomography (CT) scanning, positron emission tomography (PET) scanning, and magnetic resonance imaging (MRI). At this time, laboratory tests are not a reliable diagnostic strategy for depression.

Once a clinical depression (or a subclinical depression) is identified, there are at least four general classes of treatment options available. These options are dependent on the subtype and severity of the depression and include psychopharmacology (drug therapy), psychotherapy, electroconvulsive therapy (ECT), and other less traditional treatments. These treatment options can be provided to the patient as part of an outpatient program or, in certain severe cases of clinical depression in which the person is a danger to himself/herself or others, as part of a hospitalization.

Clinical depression often affects the patient physically, emotionally, and socially. Therefore, prior to beginning any treatment with a clinically depressed individual, the health care provider will attempt to develop an open and communicative relationship with the patient. This relationship will allow the health care provider to provide patient education on the illness and to solicit the collaboration of the patient in treatment. Supportiveness, understanding, and collaboration are all necessary components of any treatment approach.

Three primary types of medications are used in the treatment of clinical depression: cyclic antidepressants, monoamine oxidase inhibitors (MAOIs), and lithium salts. These medications are considered equally effective in decreasing the symptoms of depression, which begin to resolve in three to four weeks after initiating treatment. The health care professional will select an antidepressant based on side effects, dosing convenience (once daily versus three times a day), and cost.

The cyclic antidepressants are the largest class of antidepressant medications. As the name implies, the chemical makeup of the medication contains chemical rings, or "cycles." There are unicyclic (buproprion and fluoxetine, or Prozac), bicyclic (sertraline and trazodone), tricyclic (amitriptyline, desipramine, and nortriptyline), and tetracyclic (maprotiline) antidepressants. These antidepressants function to either block the reuptake of neurotransmitters by the neurons, allowing more of the neurotransmitter to be available at a receptor site, or increase the amount of neurotransmitter produced. The side effects associated with the cyclic antidepressants—dry mouth, blurred vision, constipation, urinary difficulties, palpitations, and sleep disturbance—vary and can be quite problematic. Some of these antidepressants have deadly toxic effects at high levels, so they are not prescribed to patients who are at risk of suicide.

Monoamine oxidase inhibitors (isocarboxazid, phenelzine, and tranylcypromine) are the second class of antidepressants. They function by slowing the production of the enzyme monoamine oxidase. This enzyme is responsible for breaking down the neurotransmitters norepinephrine and serotonin, which are believed to be responsible for depression. By slowing the decomposition of these transmitters, more of them are available to the receptors for a longer period of time. Restlessness, dizziness, weight gain, insomnia, and sexual dysfunction are common side effects of the MAOIs. MAOIs are most notable because of the dangerous adverse reaction (severely high blood pressure) that can occur if the patient consumes large quantities of foods high in tyramine (such as aged cheeses, fermented sausages, red wine, foods with a heavy yeast content, and pickled fish). Because of this potentially dangerous reaction, MAOIs are not usually the first choice of medication and are more commonly reserved for depressed patients who do not respond to the cyclic antidepressants.

A third class of medication used in the treatment of depressive disorders consists of the mood stabilizers, the most notable being lithium carbonate, which is used primarily for bipolar disorder. Lithium is a chemical salt that is believed to effect mood stabilization by influencing the production, storage, release, and reuptake of certain neurotransmitters. It is particularly useful in stabilizing and preventing manic episodes and preventing depressive episodes in patients with bipolar disorder.

Another drug occasionally used in the treatment of depression is alprazolam, a muscle-relaxant benzodiazepine commonly used in the treatment of anxiety. Alprazolam is believed to affect the nervous system by decreasing the sensitivity of neuronal receptors believed to be involved in depression. While this may in fact occur, the more likely explanation for its positive effect for some patients is that it reduces the anxiety or irritability often coexisting with depression in certain patients.

Psychotherapy refers to a number of different treatment techniques used to deal with the psychosocial contributors and consequences of clinical depression. Psychotherapy is a common supplement to drug therapy. In psychotherapy, the patients develop knowledge and insight into the causes and treatment for their clinical depression. In cognitive psychotherapy, cure comes from assisting patients in modifying maladaptive, irrational, or automatic beliefs that can lead to clinical depression. In behavioral psychotherapy, patients modify their environment such that social or personal rewards are more forthcoming. This process might involve being more assertive, reducing isolation by becoming more socially active, increasing physical activities or exercise, or learning relaxation techniques. Research on the effectiveness of these and other psychotherapy techniques indicates that psychotherapy is as effective as certain antidepressants for many patients and, in combination with certain medications, is more effective than either treatment alone.

Electroconvulsive (or "shock") therapy is the single most effective treatment for severe and persistent depression. If the clinically depressed patient fails to respond to medications or psychotherapy and the depression is life-threatening, electroconvulsive therapy is considered. This therapy involves inducing a seizure in the patient by administering an electrical current to specific parts of the brain. The therapy is quite sophisticated and safe, involving little risk to the patient. Patients undergo six to twelve treatments over a two-day to five-day period. Some temporary memory impairment is a common side effect of this treatment.

A variant of clinical depression is known as seasonal affective disorder. Patients with this illness demonstrate a pattern of clinical depression during the winter, when there is a reduction in the amount of daylight hours. For these pa-

tients, phototherapy has proven effective. Phototherapy involves exposing patients to bright light (greater than or equal to 2,500 lux) for two hours daily during the depression episode. The manner in which this treatment approach modifies the depression is unclear and awaits further research.

Psychosurgery, the final treatment option, is quite rare. It refers to surgical removal or destruction of certain portions of the brain believed to be responsible for causing severe depression. Psychosurgery is used only after all treatment options have failed and the clinical depression is life-threatening. Approximately 50 percent of patients who undergo psychosurgery benefit from the procedure.

PERSPECTIVE AND PROSPECTS

Depression, or the more historical term "melancholy," has had a history predating modern medicine. Writings from the time of the ancient Greek physician Hippocrates refer to patients with a symptom complex similar to the present-day definition of clinical depression.

Major depressive episodes and the various subtypes of depression are the leading psychiatric diagnoses treated by health care professionals. Prevalence rates from large-scale studies of depression suggest that approximately 1 in 20 adults will meet the criteria for a major depressive episode at some point in their lives; 1 in 100 for bipolar disorder; 1 in 33 for dysthymia; and 1 in 100 for cyclothymia.

The rates of clinical depression have increased since the early twentieth century, while the age of onset of clinical depression has decreased. Women appear to be at least twice as likely as men to suffer from clinical depression, and people who are happily married have a lower risk for clinical depression than those who are separated, divorced, or dissatisfied in their marital relationship. These data, along with recurrence rates of 50 to 70 percent, indicate the importance of this psychiatric disorder.

While most psychiatric disorders are nonfatal, clinical depression can lead to death. Of the approximately 30,000 suicide deaths per year in the United States, 40 to 80 percent are believed to be related to depression. Approximately 15 percent of patients with major depressive disorder will die by suicide. There are, however, other costs of clinical depression. In the United States, billions of dollars are spent on clinical depression, divided among the following areas: treatment, suicide, and absenteeism (the largest). Clinical depression obviously has a significant economic impact on a society.

The future of clinical depression lies in early identification and treatment. Identification will involve two areas. The first is improving the social awareness of mental health issues to include clinical depression. By eliminating the negative social stigma associated with mental illness and mental health treatment, there will be an increased level of the reporting of depression symptoms and thereby an improved opportunity for early intervention, preventing the progression of the disorder to the point of suicide. The sec-

ond approach to identification involves the development of reliable assessment strategies for clinical depression. Data suggest that the majority of those who commit suicide see a physician within thirty days of the suicide. The field will continue to strive to identify biological markers and other methods to predict and/or identify clinical depression more accurately. Treatment advances will focus on further development of pharmacological strategies and drugs with more specific actions and fewer side effects. Adjuncts to traditional drug therapies need continued development and refinement to maximize the success of integrated treatments.
—*Oliver Oyama*

See also Addiction; Alcoholism; Anxiety; Death and dying; Dementia; Eating disorders; Grief and guilt; Hypochondriasis; Manic-depressive disorder; Midlife crisis; Neurosis; Obsessive-compulsive disorder; Panic attacks; Paranoia; Phobias; Postpartum depression; Psychiatric disorders; Psychosomatic disorders; Stress; Suicide.

FOR FURTHER INFORMATION:

American Psychiatric Association. *Diagnostic and Statistical Manual of Mental Disorders*. Rev. 3d ed. Washington, D.C.: Author, 1987. This reference book lists the clinical criteria for psychiatric disorders, including the mood disorders that incorporate the depressions.

Beckham, E. Edward, and William R. Leber, eds. *Handbook of Depression: Treatment, Assessment, and Research*. Homewood, Ill.: Dorsey Press, 1985. This text reviews the field of depression from a scientific perspective. The twenty-seven chapters provide a thoroughly comprehensive review of depression assessment, treatment, and research.

Burns, David D. *Feeling Good: The New Mood Therapy*. New York: William Morrow, 1980. This well-written book is nontechnical and is designed for a general audience. The author describes depression—its assessment and treatment—from a self-help perspective. He introduces the principle of cognitive therapy, which focuses on treating depression by changing the way that people think.

DePaulo, J. Raymond, Jr., and Keith R. Ablow. *How to Cope with Depression: A Complete Guide for You and Your Family*. New York: McGraw-Hill, 1989. Written for patients diagnosed with depression and for their families and friends. The authors use case histories of patients seen at The Johns Hopkins University Hospital to highlight their clinical information. Includes a nice section on bipolar (manic-depressive) disorder.

Greist, John H., and James W. Jefferson. *Depression and Its Treatment*. Rev. ed. Washington, D.C.: American Psychiatric Press, 1992. A patient's guide to depression. The authors describe mood disorders and the identification of depression, and they review the various treatments that are available. The appendices offer a listing of national organizations concerned with depression and an excellent reading list.

Matson, Johnny L. *Treating Depression in Children and Adolescents*. New York: Pergamon Press, 1989. This book, written by one of the leaders in the scientific study of depression, presents a guide to the evaluation and treatment of depression in children and adolescents. The author describes the assessment and treatment approaches that are unique for this nonadult population.

Roesch, Roberta. *The Encyclopedia of Depression*. New York: Facts on File, 1991. This volume was written for both a lay and a professional audience. Covers all aspects of depression, including bereavement, grief, and mourning. The appendices are very up-to-date and include references, self-help groups, national associations, and institutes.

DERMATITIS

SYSTEM AFFECTED: Skin

SPECIALISTS: Dermatologists

DEFINITION: A wide range of skin disorders, some the result of allergy, some caused by contact with a skin irritant, and some attributable to other causes.

KEY TERMS:

allergen: a substance that excites an immunologic response; also called an antigen

crusting: the appearance of slightly elevated skin lesions made up of dried serum, blood, or pus; they can be brown, red, black, tan, or yellowish

immunoglobulin E (IgE): ordinarily, a relatively rare antibody; in patients with atopic dermatitis, levels can be significantly higher than in the general population

lesion: any pathologic change in tissue

scaling: a buildup of hard, horny skin cells

secondary infection: a bacterial, viral, or other infection that results from or follows another disease

wheal: a small swelling in the skin

CAUSES AND SYMPTOMS

The term "dermatitis" does not refer to a single skin disease, but rather to a wide range of disorders. "Dermatitis" is often used interchangeably with "eczema." The two most common dermatitides are atopic (allergic) dermatitis, in which the individual appears to inherit a predilection for the disease, and contact dermatitis, in which the individual's skin reacts immediately on contact with a substance, or develops sensitivity to it.

Atopic dermatitis often occurs in individuals with a personal or family history of allergy, such as hay fever or asthma. Thirty to 50 percent of children with atopic dermatitis develop asthma or hay fever, a rate that is three to five times higher than for the general population. These people often have high serum levels of a certain antibody, immunoglobulin E (IgE), which may be associated with their skin's tendency to break out, although a specific antigen-antibody reaction has not been demonstrated.

There are many distinct characteristics of atopic dermatitis, some of which depend on the age of the patient. The disease usually starts early in childhood. It is often first discovered in infants in the first months of life when redness and weeping, crusted lesions appear mostly on the face, although the scalp, arms, and legs may also be affected. There is intense itching. Papules (pimples), vesicles (small, blisterlike lesions filled with fluid), edema (swelling), serous exudation (discharge of fluid), and scaly crusts may be seen. At one year of age, oval, scaly lesions appear on the arms, legs, face, and torso. In older children and adults, the lesions are usually localized in the crook of the elbow and the back of the knees, and the face and neck may be involved. The course of the disease is variable. It usually subsides by the third or fourth year of life, but periodic remissions may occur throughout childhood, adolescence, and adulthood. In 75 percent of cases, atopic dermatitis improves between the ages of ten and fourteen. Cases persisting past the patient's middle twenties, or beginning then, are the most difficult to treat.

Dryness and itching are always present in atopic dermatitis. People with atopic dermatitis seem to lose skin moisture more readily than average people: Rather than soft, pliable skin, they develop dry, rough, sensitive skin that is particularly prone to chapping and splitting. The skin becomes itchy, and the individual's tendency to scratch significantly aggravates the condition in what is called the "itch-scratch-itch" cycle or the "scratch-rash-itch" cycle: The individual scratches to relieve the itching, which causes a rash, which in turn causes increased itching, which invites increased scratching and increased irritation. After years of itching and scratching, the skin of older children and adults with atopic dermatitis develops red, lichenified (rough, thickened) patches in the crook of the arm and behind the knees, as well as on the eyelids, neck, and wrists.

Constant chafing of the affected area invites bacterial infection and lymphadenitis (inflammation of lymph nodes). Furthermore, patients with atopic dermatitis seem to have altered immune systems. They appear to be more susceptible than others to skin infections, warts, and contagious skin diseases. *Staphylococcus aureus* and certain streptococci are common infecting bacteria in these patients. Pyoderma is often seen as a result of bacterial infection in atopic dermatitis. This condition features redness, oozing, scaling, and crusting, as well as the formation of small pustules (pus-filled pimples).

Patients with atopic dermatitis are also particularly sensitive to herpes simplex and vaccinia viruses. Exposure to either could cause a severe skin disease called Kaposi's varicelliform eruption. Vaccinia virus (the agent that causes cowpox) is used in the preparation of smallpox vaccine. Therefore, patients with atopic dermatitis must not be vaccinated against smallpox. Furthermore, they must be isolated from patients with active herpes simplex and those recently vaccinated against smallpox.

Patients with atopic dermatitis may also develop contact dermatitis, which can greatly exacerbate their condition.

They are also sensitive to a wide range of allergens, which can bring on outbreaks, as well as to low humidity (such as in centrally heated houses in winter), which would contribute to dry skin. They may not be able to tolerate woolen clothing.

A condition called keratosis pilaris often develops in the presence of atopic dermatitis. It is not seen in young infants, but it does appear in childhood. Hair follicles on the torso, buttocks, arms, and legs become plugged with horny matter and protrude above the skin, giving the appearance of goose bumps or "chicken skin." The palms of the hands of patients with atopic dermatitis have significantly more fine lines than those of average people. In many patients, there is a tiny "pleat" under the eyes. They are often prone to cold hands and may have pallor, seen as a blanching of the skin around the nose, mouth, and ears.

When ordinary skin is lightly rubbed with a pointed object, almost immediately there is a red line, followed by a red flare, and finally, a wheal or slight elevation of the skin along the line. In patients with atopic dermatitis, however, there is a completely different reaction: The red line appears, but almost instantly it becomes white. The flare and the wheal do not appear.

About 4 to 12 percent of patients with atopic dermatitis develop cataracts at an early age. Normally, cataracts do not appear until the fifties and sixties; those with atopic dermatitis may develop them in their twenties. These cataracts usually affect both eyes simultaneously and develop quickly.

Psychologically, children with atopic dermatitis often show distinct personality characteristics. They are reported to be bright, aggressive, energetic, and prone to fits of anger. Children with severe, unmanageable cases of atopic dermatitis may become selfish and domineering, and some go on to develop significant personality disorders.

It is not known exactly what happens to cause the itching and dry skin that are the fundamental signs of atopic dermatitis and the root of many of its complications. Various theories suggest various origins. It is by definition an allergic disorder, but the allergens that are specifically involved and how they produce the signs of atopic dermatitis are unknown. One of the most interesting theories involves the antibody IgE. Theoretically, the union of IgE with an antigen causes certain cells to release pharmacologic mediators, such as histamine, bradykinin, and slow-reacting substance (SRS-A), that cause itching and thus begin the cycle of scratching and irritation characteristic of atopic dermatitis. The fact that patients with atopic dermatitis have higher than normal levels of IgE, and that there is a relationship between IgE levels and the severity of atopic dermatitis, seems to lend support to this theory.

Contact dermatitis could resemble atopic dermatitis at certain stages, but the dry skin of atopic dermatitis may not be seen. Contact dermatitis is usually characterized by a rash consisting of small bumps, itchiness, blisters, and gen-

Contact dermatitis

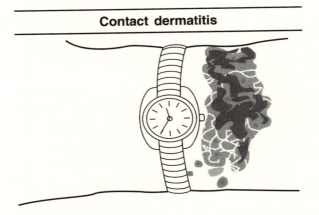

A person can be sensitive to a particular material, such as a nickel watch strap, and contract the itchy, blistering rash of contact dermatitis.

eral swelling. It occurs when the skin has been exposed to a substance to which the body is sensitive or allergic. If the contact dermatitis is caused by direct irritation by a caustic substance, it is called irritant contact dermatitis. The causative agents are primary irritants that cause inflammation at first contact. Some obvious irritants are acids, alkalis, and other harsh chemicals or substances. An example is fiberglass dermatitis, in which fine glass particles from fiberglass fabrics or insulation enter the skin and cause redness and inflammation.

If the dermatitis is caused by allergic sensitivity to a substance, it is called allergic contact dermatitis. In this case, it may take hours, days, weeks, or years for the patient to develop sensitivity to the point where exposure to these substances causes allergic contact dermatitis. These agents include soaps, acetone, skin creams, cosmetics, poison ivy, and poison sumac.

Allergic contact dermatitis comprises the largest variety of contact dermatitides, many of them named for the allergens that cause them. Hence, there is pollen dermatitis; plant and flower dermatitis, such as poison ivy or poison oak; clothing dermatitis; shoe, and even sandal strap, dermatitis; metal and metal salt dermatitis; cosmetic dermatitis; and adhesive tape dermatitis, among others. They all have one thing in common: The skin is exposed to an allergen from any of these sources and becomes so sensitive to it that further exposure causes a rash, itching, and blistering.

The development of sensitivity to an allergen is an immunological response to exposure to that substance. With many allergens, the first contact elicits no immediate immunological reaction. Sensitivity develops after the allergen has been presented to the T lymphocytes that mediate the immune response.

Because it often takes a long time to develop sensitivity, patients are surprised to discover that they have become allergic to substances that they have been using for years. For example, a patient who has been applying a topical medication to treat a skin condition may one day find that the medication causes an outbreak of dermatitis. Ironically, some of the ingredients in medications commonly used to treat skin conditions are among the major allergens that cause allergic contact dermatitis. These include antibiotics, antihistamines, topical anesthetics, antiseptics, as well as the inactive ingredients used in formulating the medication, such as stabilizers.

Other substances to which the patient may develop sensitivity include the chemicals used in making fabric for clothing, tanning chemicals used in making leather, dyes, and ingredients in cosmetics. Many patients develop sensitivity to allergens found in the workplace. The list of potential allergens in the industrial setting is virtually endless. It includes solvents, petroleum products, chemicals commonly used in manufacturing processes, and coal tar derivatives.

In some cases, the allergen requires sunlight or other forms of light to precipitate an outbreak of contact dermatitis. This is called photoallergic contact dermatitis, and it may be caused by such agents as aftershave lotions, sunscreens, topical sulfonamides, and other preparations applied to the skin. Another light reaction, termed phototoxic contact dermatitis, can be caused by exposure to sunlight after exposure to perfumes, coal tar, certain medications, and various chemicals.

A different form of dermatitis involves the sebaceous glands, which secrete sebum, a fatty substance that lubricates the skin and helps retain moisture. Sebaceous dermatitis is usually seen in areas of the body with high concentrations of sebaceous glands, such as on the scalp or face, behind the ears, on the chest, and in areas where skin rubs against skin, such as the buttocks and the groin. It is seen most often in infants and adolescents, although it may persist into adulthood or start at that time.

In infants, sebaceous dermatitis can begin within the first month of life and appears as a thick, yellow, crusted lesion on the scalp called cradle cap. There can be yellow scaling behind the ears and red pimples on the face. Diaper rash may be persistent in these infants. In older children, the lesion may appear as thick, yellow plaques in the scalp. When sebaceous dermatitis begins in adulthood, it starts slowly, and usually its only manifestation is scaling on the scalp (dandruff). In severe cases, yellowish-red scaling pimples develop along the hairline and on the face and chest. Its cause is unknown, but a yeast commonly found in the hair follicles, *Pityrosporum ovale*, may be involved.

There are many other kinds of dermatitis. Diaper dermatitis, or diaper rash, is a complex skin disorder that involves irritation of the skin by urine and feces, irritation by constant rubbing, and secondary infection by *Candida albicans*. Nummular dermatitis (from *nummus*, meaning coin) is characterized by crusting, scaly, disc-shaped papules and vesicles filled with fluid and often pus. Pityriasis alba is a common dermatitis with pale, scaly patches. In lichen simplex chronicus, there is intense itching, with lesions caused by, and perpetuated by, scratching and rubbing. Stasis dermatitis occurs at the ankles; brown discoloration, swelling, scaling, and varicose veins are common. Hyperimmunoglobulin E (Hyper IgE) syndrome is characterized by extremely high IgE levels, ten to one hundred times higher than normal, and a family history of allergy; the patient has frequent skin infections, suppurative (pus-forming) lymphadenitis, pustules, plaques, and abscesses. Pompholyx occurs on the hands and soles of the feet; there is excessive sweating, with eruptions of deep vesicles accompanied by burning or itching.

Friction can also cause dermatitis. In intertrigo, the friction of skin rubbing against skin causes inflammation that can become infected. In frictional lichenoid dermatitis, or sandbox dermatitis, it is thought that the abrasive action of sand or other gritty material on the skin causes the characteristic lesions. Winter eczema seems to be caused by the skin-drying effects of low humidity as well as by harsh soaps and overfrequent bathing; dry skin and itching are common. The acrodermatitis diseases (from *acro*, meaning the extremities) may be limited to the hands and feet, or, like acrodermatitis enteropathica, may erupt in other parts of the body, such as around the mouth and on the buttocks. In fixed-drug eruption, lesions appear in direct response to the administration of a drug; the lesions are generally in the same parts of the body, but they may spread. Swimmer's itch is a parasitic infection from an organism that lives in fresh water lakes and ponds, while seabather's eruption seems to be caused by a similar saltwater organism.

TREATMENT AND THERAPY

Many dermatitides resemble one another, and it is important for a physician to identify the patient's complaint precisely in order to treat it effectively. Therefore, the physician will confirm the identity of the condition through a process known as differential diagnosis. This method allows him or her to rule out all similar conditions, pinpoint the exact nature of the patient's problem, and develop a therapeutic regimen to treat it.

In treating atopic dermatitis, one of the first goals is to relieve dryness and itching. The patient is cautioned not to bathe excessively because this dries the skin. Lotions are used to lubricate the skin and retain moisture. The patient is advised not to scratch, because this could break the skin and invite infection. The patient is advised to avoid any known offending agents and not to apply any medication to the skin without the doctor's knowledge.

Wet compresses can bring relief to patients with atopic dermatitis. Topical corticosteroids are used to help resolve acute flare-ups, but only for short-term therapy, because their prolonged use might produce undesirable side effects. Oral antihistamines are often given to relieve itching and

to help the patient sleep. Diet may play a role in atopic dermatitis in infants: Some pediatric dermatologists and other physicians recommend elimination of milk, eggs, tomatoes, citrus fruits, wheat products, chocolate, spices, fish, and nuts from the diets of these patients. Soft cotton clothing is recommended, as is the avoidance of pets or fuzzy toys that might be allergenic. For secondary infections that arise from atopic dermatitis, the physician prescribes appropriate antibiotic therapy.

In primary irritant contact dermatitis, the offending agent is eliminated or avoided. In allergic contact dermatitis, one of the main goals is to discover the offending agent so that the patient can avoid contact with it. Sometimes this information can be elicited from the patient interview, and sometimes it is necessary to conduct a series of patch tests. In this procedure, known allergens are applied to the skin of the patient to find those that cause irritation. Avoidance of the offending agent can cause the patient some difficulty if the agent happens to be something that is found everywhere. An example is the metal nickel, which is in coins, jewelry, and hundreds of other objects. Patients who insist on wearing nickel-plated jewelry are advised to paint it with clear nail polish periodically to avoid contact of the metal with the skin. Similarly, many other allergens are in common use. Patients are advised to read cosmetic labels and food and medical ingredients lists in order to avoid contact with agents to which they are sensitive.

Because there is such a wide range of allergic contact dermatitides, treatment of the flare-ups varies considerably. Topical and oral steroids are used, as well as antihistamines. Sometimes the physician finds it necessary to drain large blisters and apply drying agents to weeping lesions. Sometimes the condition calls for wet compresses to relieve itching and soothe the patient. Specialized lotions, soaps, and shampoos are also used, some to treat dryness and others, as in the case of sebaceous dermatitis, to remove scales and to relieve oiliness.

Other treatments depend on the type of dermatitis from which the patient suffers. Patients with photoallergic or phototoxic dermatitis are advised to avoid light. Acrodermatitis enteropathica is caused by a zinc deficiency; in addition to palliative therapy to relieve the symptoms, these patients are given zinc sulfate, which results in complete remission of the disease. As with atopic dermatitis, bacterial infections occurring as a result of a flare-up of allergic contact dermatitis are treated with appropriate antibiotic therapy.

PERSPECTIVE AND PROSPECTS

The skin is the largest organ of the human body, and it is subject to an extraordinary range and number of diseases, with atopic dermatitis and contact dermatitis among the most common. They may afflict patients of all ages, but they are particularly prevalent in children. Many of the dermatitides start in the first weeks of life and continue through childhood. In many cases, the disease is resolved by the time that the child reaches adolescence, but in some it continues into adulthood.

In spite of the fact that disorders of the skin are readily apparent, an understanding of them has been imperfect throughout history. For example, the allergic nature of many of the dermatitides was not explained until the twentieth century. In addition, because their symptoms are similar to one another and to diseases that are not properly classified as dermatitides, there has been much confusion in identifying them. It has been suggested that many of the biblical lepers were in fact suffering only from a form of dermatitis. With prolonged exposure, however, they probably became lepers in time.

The dermatitides are often highly complex diseases, involving genetic, allergic, metabolic, and immune and infective factors, among many others. They are not usually life-threatening, but they take an enormous toll in pain, discomfort, and disfigurement, with an equal toll in psychological distress that can be suffered by patients.

Understanding of these disorders improves constantly, and with understanding comes new methods of treating them. Nevertheless, progress will probably be limited. There is the possibility that patients can be desensitized to allow them to tolerate the allergens that bring about their eruptions, as many hay fever sufferers have been desensitized against the pollens and dusts that trigger their allergy. It is unlikely, however, that there will ever be vaccines to immunize against this group of diseases, nor can many of them be cured, except in the sense that the discomfort that they bring can be treated and the agents that cause them can be avoided. —*C. Richard Falcon*

See also Acne; Allergies; Eczema; Keratoses; Pimples; Poisonous plants; Psoriasis; Rashes; Rosacea; Scabies; Skin cancer; Skin disorders; Warts.

FOR FURTHER INFORMATION:

Alexander, Dale. *Dry Skin and Common Sense*. West Hartford, Conn.: Witkower Press, 1978. Dry skin is a feature of atopic dermatitis. This book provides treatment tips for the layperson and suggests that dietary habits may improve the condition.

Dvorine, William. *A Dermatologist's Guide to Home Skin Treatment*. New York: Charles Scribner's Sons, 1983. This text features easy-to-understand descriptions of various skin diseases, including the dermatitides. Dvorine offers his recommendations on how to treat them at home.

Handbook of Nonprescription Drugs. 9th ed. Washington, D.C.: American Pharmaceutical Association, 1990. This drug reference work contains excellent background sections on the diseases treated by the thousands of drugs listed. It is well illustrated and particularly suited to teaching the lay reader about various disease conditions and how they can be treated. The section on skin diseases is clear, with excellent illustrations.

Larson, David E., ed. *Mayo Clinic Family Health Book*. New York: William Morrow, 1990. An excellent general reference for the lay reader, with good coverage of the dermatological diseases.

Walzer, Richard A. *Skintelligence*. New York: Appleton-Century-Crofts, 1981. This dermatologist offers advice on "how to be smart about your skin."

DIABETES MELLITUS

SYSTEMS AFFECTED: Endocrine, gastrointestinal, circulatory, visual, nervous

SPECIALISTS: Endocrinologists, family physicians, internists

DEFINITION: A hormonal disorder in which the pancreas is not able to produce sufficient insulin to process and maintain proper blood sugar levels; if left untreated, it leads to secondary complications such as blindness, dementia, and eventually death.

KEY TERMS:

beta cells: the insulin-producing cells located at the core of the islets of Langerhans in the pancreas; the alpha, or glucagon-producing, cells form an outer coat

cross-linking: a chemical reaction, triggered by the binding of glucose to tissue proteins, that results in the attachment of one protein to another and the loss of elasticity in aging tissues

glucosuria: a condition in which the concentration of blood glucose exceeds the ability of the kidney to reabsorb it; as a result, glucose spills into the urine, taking with it body water and electrolytes

insulin-dependent diabetes mellitus (IDDM): type 1 diabetes, a state of absolute insulin deficiency in which the body does not produce sufficient insulin to move glucose into the cells

insulin resistance: a lack of insulin action; a reduction in the effectiveness of insulin to lower blood glucose concentrations; characteristic of type 2 diabetes

insulitis: the selective destruction of the insulin-producing beta cells in type 1 diabetes

islets of Langerhans: clusters of cells scattered throughout the pancreas; they produce three hormones involved in sugar metabolism: insulin, glucagon, and somatostatin

non-insulin-dependent diabetes mellitus (NIDDM): type 2 diabetes, which is the state of a relative insulin deficiency; although insulin is released, its target cells do not adequately respond to it by taking up blood glucose

CAUSES AND SYMPTOMS

Diabetes mellitus is by far the most common of all endocrine (hormonal) disorders. The word "diabetes" is derived from the Greek word for "siphon" or "running through," a reference to the potentially large urine volume that can accompany the condition. *Mellitus*, the Latin word for "honey," was added when physicians began to make the diagnosis of diabetes mellitus based on the sweet taste of the patient's urine. The disease has been depicted as a state of starvation in the midst of plenty. Although there is plenty of sugar in the blood, without insulin it does not reach the cells that need it for energy. Glucose, the simplest form of sugar, is the primary source of energy for many vital functions. Deprived of glucose, cells starve and tissues begin to degenerate. The unused glucose builds up in the bloodstream, which leads to a series of secondary complications.

The acute symptoms of diabetes mellitus are all attributable to inadequate insulin action. The immediate consequence of an insulin insufficiency is a marked decrease in the ability of both muscle and adipose (fat) tissue to remove glucose from the blood. In the presence of inadequate insulin action, a second problem manifests itself. People with diabetes continue to make the hormone glucagon. Glucagon, which raises the level of blood sugar, can be considered insulin's biological opposite. Like insulin, glucagon is released from the pancreatic islets. The release of glucagon is normally inhibited by insulin; therefore, in the absence of insulin, glucagon action elevates concentrations of glucose. For this reason, diabetes may be considered a "two-hormone disease." With a reduction in the conversion of glucose into its storage forms of glycogen in liver and muscle and lipids in adipose cells, concentrations of glucose in the blood steadily increase (hyperglycemia). When the amount of glucose in the blood exceeds the capacity of the kidney to reabsorb this nutrient, glucose begins to spill into the urine (glucosuria). Glucose in the urine then drags additional body water along with it so that the volume of urine dramatically increases. In the absence of adequate fluid intake, the loss of body water and accompanying electrolytes (sodium) leads to dehydration and, ultimately, death caused by the failure of the peripheral circulatory system.

Insulin deficiency also results in a decrease in the synthesis of triglycerides (storage forms of fatty acids) and stimulates the breakdown of fats in adipose tissue. Although glucose cannot enter the cells and be used as an energy source, the body can use its supply of lipids from the fat cells as an alternate source of energy. Fatty acids increase in the blood, causing hyperlipidemia. With large amounts of circulating free fatty acids available for processing by the liver, the production and release of ketone bodies (breakdown products of fatty acids) into the circulation are accelerated, causing both ketonemia and an increase in the acidity of the blood. Since the ketone levels soon also exceed the capacity of the kidney to reabsorb them, ketone bodies soon appear in the urine (ketonuria).

Insulin deficiency and glucagon excess also cause pronounced effects on protein metabolism and result in an overall increase in the breakdown of proteins and a reduction in the uptake of amino acid precursors into muscle protein. This leads to the wasting and weakening of skeletal muscles and, in children who are diabetics, results in a reduction in overall growth. Unfortunately, the increased level

of amino acids in the blood provides an additional source of material for glucose production (gluconeogenesis) by the liver. All these acute metabolic changes in carbohydrates, lipids, and protein metabolism can be prevented or reversed by the administration of insulin.

There are two distinct types of diabetes mellitus. Type I, or insulin-dependent diabetes mellitus (IDDM), is an absolute deficiency of insulin that accounts for approximately 10 percent of all cases of diabetes. Until the discovery of insulin, people stricken with Type I diabetes faced certain death within about a year of diagnosis. In Type II or non-insulin-dependent diabetes mellitus (NIDDM), insulin secretion may be normal or even increased, but the target cells for insulin are less responsive than normal (insulin resistance); therefore, insulin is not as effective in lowering blood glucose concentrations. Although either type can be manifested at any age, Type I diabetes has a greater prevalence in children, whereas the incidence of Type II diabetes increases markedly after the age of forty and is the most common type of diabetes. Genetic and environmental factors are important in the expression of both types of diabetes mellitus.

Type I diabetes is an autoimmune process that involves the selective destruction of the insulin-producing beta cells in the islets of Langerhans (insulitis). The triggering event that initiates this process in genetically susceptible persons may be a virus or, more likely, the presence of toxins in the diet. The body's own T lymphocytes progressively attack the beta cells but leave the other hormone-producing

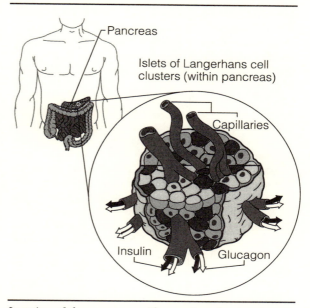

Pancreas

Islets of Langerhans cell clusters (within pancreas)

Capillaries

Insulin

Glucagon

Location of the pancreas, with a section showing the specialized cells (islets of Langerhans) that produce the sugar-metabolizing hormones.

Diabetes Mellitus

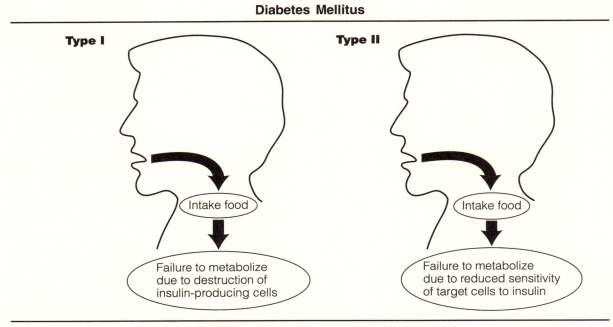

Type I

Intake food

Failure to metabolize
due to destruction of
insulin-producing cells

Type II

Intake food

Failure to metabolize
due to reduced sensitivity
of target cells to insulin

Diabetes mellitus results from the body's failure to metabolize sugar properly. Type I diabetes is an autoimmune process that destroys insulin-producing cells and is often found in children. Type II diabetes results from the reduced sensitivity of target cells to insulin, requiring increased secretion of insulin to maintain blood sugar levels; this type generally affects adults and is often caused by poor eating habits and lack of exercise over years.

cell types intact. T lymphocytes are white blood cells that normally attack virus-invaded cells and cancer cells. For up to ten years, there remains a sufficient number of insulin-producing cells to respond effectively to a glucose load, but when approximately 80 percent of the beta cells are destroyed, there is insufficient insulin release in response to a meal and the deadly spiral of the consequences of diabetes mellitus is triggered. Insulin injection can halt this lethal process and prevent it from recurring but cannot mimic the normal pattern of insulin release from the pancreas. It is interesting that not everyone who has insulitis actually progresses to experience overt symptoms of the disease, although it is known that the incidence of Type I diabetes around the world is on the increase.

Type II diabetes is normally associated with obesity and lack of exercise as well as with genetic predisposition. Family studies have shown that as many as 25 to 35 percent of persons with Type II diabetes have a sibling or parent with the disease. The risk of diabetes doubles if both parents are affected. Because there is a reduction in the sensitivity of the target cells to insulin, people with Type II diabetes must secrete more insulin to maintain blood glucose at normal levels. Because insulin is a storage, or anabolic, hormone, this increased secretion further contributes to obesity. In response to the elevated insulin concentrations, the number of insulin receptors on the target cell

gradually decreases, which triggers an even greater secretion of insulin. In this way, the excess glucose is stored despite the decreased availability of insulin binding sites on the cell. Over time, the demands for insulin eventually exceed even the reserve capacity of the "genetically weakened" beta cells, and symptoms of insulin deficiency develop as the plasma glucose concentrations remain high for increasingly larger periods of time. Because the symptoms of Type II diabetes are usually less severe than those of Type I diabetes, many persons have the disease but remain unaware of it. Unfortunately, once the diagnosis of diabetes is made in these individuals, they also exhibit symptoms of long-term complications that include atherosclerosis and nerve damage. Hence, Type II diabetes has been called the "silent killer."

TREATMENT AND THERAPY

Insulin is the only treatment available for Type I diabetes, and in many cases it is used to treat individuals with Type II diabetes. Insulin is available in many formulations, which differ in respect to the time of onset of action, activity, and duration of action. Insulin preparations are classified as fast-acting, intermediate-acting, and long-acting; the effects of fast-acting insulin last for thirty minutes to twenty-four hours, while those of long-acting preparations last from four to thirty-six hours. Some of the factors that affect the rate of insulin absorption include the site of injection, the patient's age and health status, and the patient's level of physical activity. For a person with diabetes, however, insulin is a reprieve, not a cure.

Because of the complications that arise from chronic exposure to glucose, it is recommended that glucose concentrations in the blood be maintained as close to physiologically normal levels as possible. For this reason, it is preferable to administer multiple doses of insulin during the day. By monitoring plasma glucose concentrations, the diabetic person can adjust the dosage of insulin administered and thus mimic normal concentrations of glucose relatively closely. Basal concentrations of plasma insulin can also be maintained throughout the day by means of electromechanical insulin-delivery systems. Whether internal or external, such insulin pumps can be programmed to deliver a constant infusion of insulin at a rate designed to meet minimum requirements. The infusion can then be supplemented by a bolus injection prior to a meal. Increasingly sophisticated systems automatically monitor blood glucose concentrations and adjust the delivery rate of insulin accordingly. These alternative delivery systems are intended to prevent the development of long-term tissue complications.

There are a number of chronic complications that account for the shorter life expectancy of diabetic persons. These include atherosclerotic changes throughout the entire vascular system. The thickening of basement membranes that surround the capillaries can affect their ability to exchange nutrients. Cardiovascular lesions are the most common cause of premature death in diabetic persons. Kidney disease, which is commonly found in longtime diabetics, can ultimately lead to kidney failure. For these persons, expensive medical care, including dialysis and the possibility of a kidney transplant, overshadows their lives. Diabetes is the leading cause of new blindness in the United States. In addition, diabetes leads to a gradual decline in the ability of nerves to conduct sensory information to the brain. For example, the feet of some diabetics feel more like stumps of wood than living tissue. Consequently, weight is not distributed properly; in concert with the reduction in blood flow, this problem can lead to pressure ulcers. If not properly cared for, areas of the foot can develop gangrene, which may then lead to amputation of the foot. Finally, in male patients, there are problems with reproductive function that generally result in impotence.

The mechanism responsible for the development of these long-term complications of diabetes is genetic in origin and dependent on the amount of time the tissues are exposed to the elevated plasma glucose concentrations. What, then, is the link between glucose concentrations and diabetic complications?

As an animal ages, most of its cells become less efficient in replacing damaged material, while its tissues lose their elasticity and gradually stiffen. For example, the lungs and heart muscle expand less successfully, blood vessels become increasingly rigid, and ligaments tighten. These apparently diverse age-related changes are accelerated in diabetes, and the causative agent is glucose. Glucose becomes chemically attached to proteins and deoxyribonucleic acid (DNA) in the body without the aid of enzymes to speed the reaction along. What is important is the duration of exposure to the elevated glucose concentrations. Once glucose is bound to tissue proteins, a series of chemical reactions is triggered that, over the passage of months and years, can result in the formation and eventual accumulation of cross-links between adjacent proteins. The higher glucose concentrations in diabetics accelerate this process, and the effects become evident in specific tissues throughout the body.

Understanding the chemical basis of protein cross-linking in diabetes has permitted the development and study of compounds that can intervene in this process. Certain compounds, when added to the diet, can limit the glucose-induced cross-linking of proteins by preventing their formation. One of the best-studied compounds, aminoguanidine, can help prevent the cross-linking of collagen; this fact is shown in a decrease in the accumulation of trapped lipoproteins on artery walls. Aminoguanidine also prevents thickening of the capillary basement membrane in the kidney. Aminoguanidine acts by blocking glucose's ability to react with neighboring proteins. Vitamins C and B_6 are also effective in reducing cross-linking. All these substances may be considered anti-aging compounds.

Alternatively, transplantation of the entire pancreas is an effective means of achieving an insulin-independent state in persons with Type I diabetes mellitus. Both the technical problems of pancreas transplantation and the possible rejection of the foreign tissue, however, have limited this procedure as a treatment for diabetes. Diabetes is usually manageable; therefore, a pancreas transplant is not necessarily life-saving. Some limited success in treating diabetes has been achieved by transplanting only the insulin-producing islet cells from the pancreas or grafts from fetal pancreas tissue. It may one day be possible to use genetic engineering to permit cells of the liver to self-regulate glucose concentrations by synthesizing and releasing their own insulin into the blood.

Some of the less severe forms of Type II diabetes mellitus can be controlled by the use of oral hypoglycemic agents that bring about a reduction in blood glucose. These drugs can be taken orally to drive the beta cells to release even more insulin than usual. These drugs also increase the ability of insulin to act on the target cells, which ultimately reduces the insulin requirement. The use of these agents remains controversial, because they overwork the already strained beta cells. If a diabetic person is reliant on these drugs for extended periods of time, the insulin cells could "burn out" and completely lose their ability to synthesize insulin. In this situation, the previously non-insulin-dependent person would have to be placed on insulin therapy for life.

If obesity is a factor in the expression of Type II diabetes, as it is in most cases, the best therapy is a combination of a reduction of calorie intake and an increase in activity. More than any other disease, Type II diabetes is related to lifestyle. It is often the case that people prefer having an injection or taking a pill to improving their quality of life by changing their diet and level of activity. Attention to diet and exercise results in a dramatic decrease in the need for drug therapy in nine out of ten diabetics. In some cases, the loss of only a small percentage of body weight results in an increased sensitivity to insulin. Exercise is particularly helpful in the management of both types of diabetes, because working muscle does not require insulin to metabolize glucose. Thus, exercising muscles take up and use some of the excess glucose in the blood, which reduces the overall need for insulin. Permanent weight reduction and exercise also help to prevent long-term complications and permit a healthier and more active lifestyle.

PERSPECTIVE AND PROSPECTS

Diabetes mellitus is a disease of ancient origin. The first written reference to diabetes, which was discovered in the tomb of Thebes in Egypt (1500 B.C.), described an illness associated with the passage of vast quantities of sweet urine and an excessive thirst.

The study of diabetes owes much to the Franco-Prussian War. In 1870, during the siege of Paris, it was noted by French physicians that the widespread famine in the besieged city had a curative influence on diabetic patients. Their glycosuria decreased or disappeared. These observations supported the view of clinicians at the time who had previously prescribed periods of fasting and increased muscular work for the treatment of the overweight diabetic individual.

It was Oscar Minkowski of Germany who, in 1889, accidentally traced the origin of diabetes to the pancreas. Following the complete removal of the pancreas from a dog, Minkowski's technician noted the animal's subsequent copious urine production. Acting on the basis of a hunch, Minkowski tested the urine and determined that its sugar content was greater than 10 percent.

In 1921, Frederick Banting and Charles Best, at the University of Toronto, successfully extracted the antidiabetic substance "insulin" using a cold alcohol-hydrochloric acid mixture to inactivate the harsh digestive enzymes of the pancreas. Using this substance, they first controlled the disease in a depancreatized dog and then, a few months later, successfully treated the first human diabetic patient. The clinical application of a discovery normally takes a long time, but in this case a mere twenty weeks had passed between the first injection of insulin into the diabetic dog and the first trial with a diabetic human. Three years later, in 1923, Banting and Best were awarded the Nobel Prize in Physiology or Medicine for their remarkable achievement.

Although insulin, when combined with an appropriate diet and exercise, alleviates the symptoms of diabetes to such an extent that a diabetic can lead an essentially normal life, insulin therapy is not a cure. The complications that arise in diabetics are typical of those found in the general population except that they happen much earlier in the diabetic. With regard to these glucose-induced complications, it was first postulated in 1908 that sugars could react with proteins. In 1912, Louis Camille Maillard further characterized this reaction at the Sorbonne and realized that the consequences of this reaction were relevant to diabetics. Maillard suggested that sugars were destroying the body's amino acids, which then led to increased excretion in diabetics. It was not until the mid-1970's, however, that Anthony Cerami in New York introduced the concept of the nonenzymatic attachment of glucose to protein and recognized its potential role in diabetic complications. A decade later, this development led to the discovery of aminoguanidine, the first compound to limit the cross-linking of tissue proteins and thus delay the development of certain diabetic complications.

In 1974, Josiah Brown published the first report showing that diabetes could be reversed by transplanting fetal pancreatic tissue. By the mid-1980's, procedures had been devised for the isolation of massive numbers of human islets that could then be transplanted into diabetics. For persons with diabetes, both procedures represent more than a treatment; they may offer a cure for the disease.

—*Hillar Klandorf*

See also Endocrine disorders; Gangrene; Hypoglycemia; Obesity; Pancreatitis.

FOR FURTHER INFORMATION:

Biermann, June, and Barbara Toohey. *The Peripatetic Diabetic*. Los Angeles: Jeremy P. Tarcher, 1984. Written for the diabetic patient and parents of the diabetic child, the book uses sound medical information and practical advice to help find solutions to problems in the real world. A popular and sometimes humorous book for people with diabetes.

Bliss, Michael. *The Discovery of Insulin*. Edinburgh: Paul Harris, 1987. An excellent historical perspective on the events leading to the discovery of insulin. The complete dedication of those individuals in their pursuit of what was hoped to be the "cure" for diabetes is well documented.

Cerami, Anthony, Helen Vlassara, and Michael Browlee. "Glucose and Aging." *Scientific American* 256 (May, 1987): 90-96. A pioneering article written by experts in the field of diabetic complications. This important work clearly explains the development of cross-linking in the tissues and challenges the reader with new approaches to treating a very old problem. Contains excellent figures and diagrams of the processes involved.

Krall, Leo P., and Richard S. Beaser. *Joslin Diabetes Manual*. 12th ed. Philadelphia: Lea & Febiger, 1989. First published in 1918, this book serves as an updated guide for people with diabetes. Its intent is to help diabetics understand the disease and permit them to take control of their lives.

Powers, Margaret A. *Handbook of Diabetic Nutritional Management*. Rockville, Md.: Aspen, 1987. A comprehensive book written by dietitians for persons interested in the nutritional management of diabetes; blends new scientific knowledge and thought with recent advances in clinical practice.

Diarrhea and dysentery

System affected: Gastrointestinal

Specialists: Family physicians, gastroenterologists, infectious disease physicians, internists, public health specialists, tropical medicine physicians

Definition: Intestinal disorders that may indicate minor emotional distress or a variety of diseases, some serious; diarrhea is loose, watery, copious bowel movements, whereas dysentery is an intestinal infection characterized by severe diarrhea.

Key terms:

electrolytes: inorganic ions dissolved in body water, including sodium, potassium, calcium, magnesium, chloride, phosphate, bicarbonate, and sulphate

functional disease: a derangement in the way that normal anatomy operates

gastroenterology: the medical subspecialty devoted to care of the digestive tract and related organs

intestines: the tube connecting the stomach and anus in which nutrients are absorbed from food; divided into the small intestine and the colon, or large intestine

mucosa: the semipermeable layers of cells lining the gut, through which fluid and nutrients are absorbed

organic disease: disease resulting from an identifiable cause, such as an enzyme deficiency, growth, hole, or organism

pathogen: an organism that causes disease

peristalsis: the wavelike muscular contractions that move food and waste products through the intestines; problems with peristalsis are called motility disorders

stool: the waste products expelled from the anus during defecation

Causes and Symptoms

A symptom of various diseases rather than a disease in itself, diarrhea is so difficult to define and can result from so many disparate causes that it is sometimes called the gastroenterologist's nightmare. Dysentery (bloody diarrhea), a more threatening symptom, presents even further complexity.

Uncontrolled, some forms of diarrhea result in dehydration, weakness, and malnutrition and quickly turn deadly. Diarrhea is implicated in more infant deaths worldwide than any other affliction. Even in mild forms, it produces so much distress in victims and has inspired so many remedies

that its psychological and economic toll is monumental. During the 1980's, diarrhea accounted for an estimated $23 billion annually in medical expenses and lost productivity in the United States alone, a figure that surpassed the government budgets of many states.

Common medical definitions of diarrhea seek to bring diagnostic precision to a nebulous complaint and to distinguish between acute and chronic forms and between organic and functional causes. For example, *The Merck Manual* (15th ed., 1987), a widely respected reference for physicians, associates diarrhea with increased amount and fluidity of fecal matter and frequent defecation relative to a person's usual pattern, emphasizing the importance of volume (more than three hundred grams of stool daily, of which 60 to 90 percent is water) in the definition. The key phrase here is "relative to a usual pattern": Because quantity, frequency, and firmness of bowel movements vary greatly among healthy people, a more precise generalization is difficult to make. Yet some specialists demand greater specificity from the definition. For example, W. Grant Thompson, a professor of medicine and popular author on the digestive tract, proposes the operational definition of "loose or watery stools more than 75 percent of the time" in *Gut Reactions* (1989). Acute diarrhea seldom lasts more than five days, although acute dysentery may continue up to ten days; most causes are infections, that is, resulting from the presence of microorganisms (viruses, bacteria, or parasites). Physicians differ over how long the symptoms must persist before a condition is identified as chronic diarrhea, proposing from two weeks to three months; impaired functioning of the intestinal tract (functional diarrhea) is usually responsible, although persistent malfunctions may originate from pathogens that in most cases provoke only acute diarrhea.

In a single day, water intake, saliva, gastric juice, bile, pancreatic juices, and electrolyte secretions in the upper small intestine produce about nine to ten liters of fluid in the average person. One to two liters of this amount empty into the colon, and 100 to 150 milligrams are excreted in the stool; the rest is absorbed through the intestinal mucosa. If for any reason more fluid enters the colon than it can absorb, diarrhea results. Schemes classifying diarrhea according to the biochemical mechanisms causing it vary considerably, although all authorities agree on three broad types of malfunction.

The first is secretory diarrhea. The intestines, especially the small intestine, normally add water and electrolytes—principally sodium, potassium, chloride, and bicarbonate—into the nutrient load during the biochemical reactions of digestion. In a healthy person, more fluid is absorbed than is secreted. Many agents and conditions can reverse this ratio and stimulate the mucosa to exude more water than can be absorbed: toxin-producing bacteria; various organic chemicals, including caffeine and some laxatives; acids;

hormones; some cancers; and inflammatory diseases of the bowel. Large stool volume (more than one liter a day), with little or no decrease during fasting and with normal sodium and potassium content in the body fluid, characterizes secretory diarrhea.

Second, the nutrient load in the gut may include substances that exert osmotic force but cannot be absorbed, causing osmotic diarrhea. Some laxatives (especially those containing magnesium), an inability to absorb the lactose in dairy products or the artificial sweeteners in diet foods, and enzyme deficiencies are the principal causes. Stool volume tends to be less than one liter a day and decreases during fasting; the sodium and potassium content of stool water is low.

Third, motility disorders occur when peristalsis, the natural wavelike contractions of the bowel wall that move waste matter toward the rectum for defecation, becomes deranged. Some drugs, irritable bowel syndrome (IBS), hyperthyroidism, and gut nerve damage (as from diabetes mellitus) may have this effect. Fluid passes through the intestines too quickly or in an uncoordinated fashion, and too little is removed from the waste matter.

These mechanisms do not conform exactly with popular names for diarrhea. For example, travelers' diarrhea, the most infamous, comprises a diverse group of microorganism infections that come from drinking polluted water or eating tainted foods. When a person is not a native to an area, and so has little or no resistance to locally abundant pathogens, these pathogens can radically alter the balance of intestinal flora or attack the mucosa, increasing secretion and disrupting absorption and motility. Similarly, terms such as "Montezuma's revenge," "the backdoor trots," and "beaver fever" can refer to a variety of organic diseases, although the last commonly refers to *Giardia lamblia* infection.

Dysentery occurs with infectious diarrhea, most commonly from bacteria and amoebas, such as shigella, salmonella, and *Escherichia coli* (*E. coli*), and with inflammatory diseases of the bowel, such as colitis and Crohn's disease. Any pathogen that injures and inflames the bowel wall, ulcerating the mucosa, may cause blood and pus to ooze into the feces. To the greatest threat from diarrhea—dehydration—dysentery often adds fever, chills, cramping, blood loss, and nausea, and in extreme cases delirium, convulsions, and coma.

Although most diarrheas result from physiological mechanisms, one relatively rare form of chronic diarrhea ultimately has a psychological origin: laxative abuse. Physicians consider this curious phenomenon a specialized manifestation of Münchausen's syndrome, named after the German soldier Baron Münchausen (1720-1797) who was famous for his wild tales of military exploits and injuries in battles. In order to be admitted to hospitals, patients mutilate themselves in such a way that the injuries mimic acute, dramatic, and convincing symptoms of serious physi-

ological diseases. Laxative abusers secretly dose themselves with nonprescription laxatives and suffer continual diarrhea, weight loss, and weakness. When they present themselves to physicians, they lie about taking laxatives, which makes a correct diagnosis extremely difficult; even when confronted with irrefutable evidence of the abuse, they deny it and persist in taking the laxatives.

TREATMENT AND THERAPY

Almost everyone, at one time or another, produces stools that seem somehow unusual; if the bowel movement comes swiftly and is preceded by intestinal cramps and if the stool has anything from a watery to an oatmeal-like consistency, victims are likely to believe that they have diarrhea. Such episodes seldom indicate anything except perhaps a dietary excess or a temporary motility disturbance. Normal bowel movement returns on its own, and no medical treatment is called for. When loose feces are uncontrollable, even explosive, however, and other symptoms coexist, such as nausea, bleeding, fever, bloating, and persistent intestinal pain, the distress may indicate serious illness.

Because so many organic and functional diseases can lead to diarrhea, physicians follow carefully designed algorithms when treating patients. Essentially, such an algorithm seeks to eliminate possibilities systematically. Step by step, physicians interview patients, conduct physical examinations, and, when called for, perform tests that gradually narrow the range of possible causes until one seems most likely. Only then can the physician decide upon an effective therapy. This painstaking approach is necessary because treatments for some mechanisms of diarrhea prove useless against or worsen other mechanisms. If the underlying disease is complex or uncommon, the process can be long and frustrating.

One treatment, however, always precedes a complete investigation. Because dehydration is the most immediately serious effect of diarrhea, the physician first tries to prevent or reduce dehydration in a patient through oral rehydration; that is, the patient is given fluids with electrolytes to drink. Often, mineral water or fruit juice with soda crackers is sufficient to restore fluid balance.

If the diarrhea lasts fewer than three days and no other serious symptoms accompany it, the physician is unlikely to recommend treatment other than oral rehydration because whatever caused the upset is already resolving itself. If the diarrhea is persistent, however, the physician queries the patient about his or her recent experience, which is called "taking a history." Fever, tenesmus (the urgent need to defecate without the ability to do so satisfactorily), blood in the stool, and abdominal pain will suggest that a pathogen has infected the patient. If the patient has recently eaten seafood, traveled abroad, suffered an immune system disorder, or engaged in sexual activity without the protection of condoms, the physician has reason to suspect that viruses, bacteria, or parasites are responsible.

At that point, a stool sample is taken. If few or no white cells turn up in the stool, then the diarrhea has not caused inflammation. Several common bacteria and parasites, usually contracted during travel, induce diarrhea without inflammation, most notably some types of *E. coli*, cryptosporidium, rotavirus, Norwalk virus, and *Giardia lamblia*. Further tests, such as the culturing and staining of stool samples and electron microscopy of stool or bowel wall tissue, will distinguish between bacterial and parasite infection. Most noninflammatory bacterial diarrheas are allowed to run their course without drug therapy; only the effects of the diarrhea (especially dehydration) are treated. If the agent responsible is a parasite, the patient is given specific antiparasite medications.

The presence of white cells in the stool is evidence of inflammatory diarrhea, and the physician considers a completely separate group of microorganisms, especially shigella, salmonella, amoebas, and various forms of *E. coli*. Because the inflammation may cause bleeding and pockets of pus, which in turn can lead to anemia and fever, inflammatory diarrhea often requires aggressive treatment. Cell cultures help identify the specific microorganism involved, and that identification enables the physician to select the proper antibiotic to kill the infecting agents.

If cell cultures, microscopic examination of stool samples, biopsies, or staining fails to identify a microorganism (and some, like the parasite *Giardia lamblia*, are difficult to spot), the physician suspects that the diarrhea derives from a source other than an infectious agent. Irritable bowel syndrome (IBS), a chronic and relapsing disorder, may be making its first appearance. Overuse of antibiotics, antacids, or laxatives is frequently the cause, in which case the cure is simple: Elimination of the drugs clears up the symptom.

When neither drugs nor IBS is responsible, the physician looks for other diseases, organic or functional; these can range from the readily identifiable to the obscure, and they are often chronic. Chemical tests, for example, can show that a patient has enzyme deficiencies that produce intolerance to types of food, such as dairy products, or conditions resulting from malfunctioning organs, such as hyperthyroidism and pancreatic insufficiency. Looking through an endoscope, a long flexible fiberoptic tube, the physician can locate diarrhea-causing tumors or the abrasions and inflammation typical of colitis and Crohn's disease. Yet neither tests nor direct examination may pin down the dysfunction. For example, diarrhea figures prominently among a group of symptoms, probably derived from assorted dysfunctions, that characterize IBS; this mild functional dis-

Cycle of Amebic Dysentery

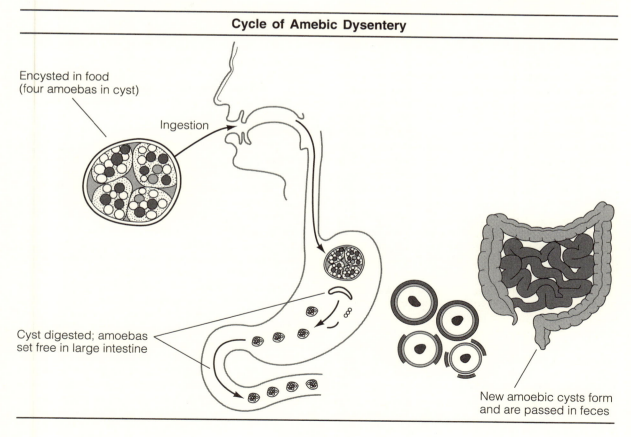

Encysted in food
(four amoebas in cyst)

Ingestion

Cyst digested; amoebas
set free in large intestine

New amoebic cysts form
and are passed in feces

Incidence of Amebic Dysentery

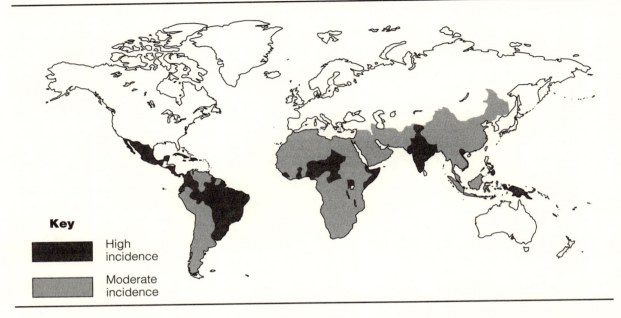

Key

■ High incidence

▩ Moderate incidence

ease is estimated to afflict between 10 and 20 percent of Americans.

Cancers, Crohn's disease, and some forms of colitis can be alleviated with surgery, although in the case of Crohn's disease the relief from diarrhea may be only temporary. The surgery itself, however, may impair bowel function, worsening diarrhea rather than stopping it. Food intolerances are managed by removing the offending food from the patient's diet; similarly, some types of colitis and IBS sometimes improve after the physician and patient experiment with altering the patient's diet. Medications are available that supplement or counteract the biochemical imbalances created by malfunctioning organs, such as treatment for hyperthyroidism. Yet, in many cases, the disease must simply be endured and the diarrhea can only be palliated with bulking agents, which often contain aluminum and bismuth, or opiates, such as morphine and codeine, which slow peristalsis.

The surest protection from diarrhea of all types is a balanced, moderate, pathogen-free diet, although diet alone seldom prevents organic diseases. When dietary control is difficult, such as when a person travels and especially when the itinerary includes underdeveloped countries, other measures may help. Bacterial infection accounts for 80 percent of cases of travelers' diarrhea, so some physicians recommend regular doses of antibiotics or a bismuth subsalicylate preparation (such as Pepto Bismol) to kill off the pathogens before they can cause trouble. Such prophylactic treatment is controversial because the drugs, taken over long periods, can have serious side effects, including rashes, tinnitus (ringing in the ear), sensitivity to sunlight, and shock. Also,

preventive doses of drugs may give travelers a false sense of security so that they fail to exercise caution in eating foreign foods. Also, widespread use of antibiotics for this purpose fosters the emergence of bacteria that are resistant to them, ultimately making the treatment of disease more difficult.

Perspective and Prospects

In effect, diarrhea is an urgent message from the body that something is wrong. Although it is often difficult for a physician to interpret, persistent diarrhea sends a signal that cannot be ignored without endangering the patient. Similarly, when significant numbers of people in an area suffer diarrhea, the disease is an urgent social and political message to local governments: Public health is endangered and steps must be taken to improve living conditions.

Although some endemic diarrheal diseases do exist in wealthy industrialized countries such as the United States, most severe, long-lasting plagues of diarrhea occur in impoverished nations that have inadequate sanitation systems and poor standards for food handling. Most viral, bacterial, and parasitic diarrheas are transmitted by food and water. Any food can harbor bacteria after being grown in or washed with infected water. Meat is especially vulnerable during slaughtering, but refrigerating, drying, salting, fermenting, freezing, or irradiating it prevents the bacteria from proliferating to numbers that cause illness. If the food is stored in a warm place, as is often the case in countries lacking the resources for refrigeration or other safe storage techniques, the diarrhea-causing organisms can spoil the food in hours. Spoiled food becomes a particular nuisance when served at restaurants or by street vendors, because great numbers and varieties of people are infected.

Organisms that cause many forms of diarrhea travel in human excrement. When an infected person defecates, the organism-rich stool enters the sewer system, and if that system is not well designed, the infected excrement may leak into the local water supply, spreading the infection when the water is drunk or used to wash food. Furthermore, infected persons, if they fail to wash themselves well, may have traces of excrement on their hands, and when they touch food during its preparation or touch other people directly, the organism can find a new host.

In 1989, the World Health Organization (WHO) issued ten rules for safe food preparation in an attempt to improve food handling practices worldwide and combat diarrheal diseases. The effort, it was hoped, would reduce infant mortality in developing countries, since diarrheal dehydration kills children younger than two years of age at rates disproportionate to other age groups. WHO advises food handlers to choose foods that are already processed, to cook foods thoroughly, to serve cooked foods immediately, to store foods carefully, to reheat foods thoroughly, to prevent raw and cooked foods from touching, to wash their hands repeatedly, to clean all kitchen surfaces meticulously, to protect foods from insects and rodents, and to use pure water.

Eliminating endemic infectious diarrheal diseases would improve general health significantly throughout the world, since diarrhea is one of the most incapacitating of afflictions even in its mild forms. International travel would also become safer; of the estimated 300 million people who cross national borders yearly, 20 to 50 percent contract diarrheal illnesses. Noninfectious diarrhea from chronic functional diseases will remain a knotty problem, but it is rare in comparison to acute infectious diarrhea, cannot be transmitted, and so has little or no effect on public health.

—*Roger Smith*

See also Abdominal disorders; Colitis; Colon cancer; Crohn's disease; Gastrointestinal disorders; Incontinence; Indigestion; Intestinal disorders.

FOR FURTHER INFORMATION:

DuPont, Herbert L., and Charles D. Ericsson. "Drug Therapy: Prevention and Treatment of Traveler's Diarrhea." *The New England Journal of Medicine* 328 (June 24, 1993): 1821-1826. This article, one of the Center for Infectious Diseases' periodic updates on the subject, is a review of existing knowledge. It should be basic reading for international travelers, or anyone who wants an accurate overview of travelers' diarrhea.

Gracey, Michael, ed. *Diarrhea*. Boca Raton, La.: CRC Press, 1991. The fourteen essays in this collection cover major types of acute and chronic diarrhea in depth. Although written by academic physicians, the essays are accessible to readers with a basic knowledge of physiol-

ogy, and the clarity and wealth of information make the book a valuable resource. Extensive bibliographies are included.

Greenberger, Norton J. *Gastrointestinal Disorders: A Pathophysiologic Approach*. 3d ed. Chicago: Year Book Medical Publishers, 1986. A medical text that requires college-level preparation in biochemistry and physiology to appreciate fully, yet its discussion of diseases is lucid and orderly. A solid introduction into the mechanisms involved in diarrhea and dysentery.

Janowitz, Henry D. *Your Gut Feelings: A Complete Guide to Living Better with Intestinal Problems*. New York: Oxford University Press, 1987. An eminent gastroenterologist and popular writer on intestinal subjects, Janowitz writes plainly and offers much helpful advice. His section on travelers' diarrhea is particularly valuable.

Sachar, David B., Jerome D. Waye, and Blair S. Lewis, eds. *Gastroenterology for the House Officer*. Baltimore: Williams & Wilkins, 1989. This handbook has two virtues: first, crisp definitions of disease types and mechanisms and, second, an easy-to-reference outline format. Readers must know medical and pharmaceutical terminology, however, to derive the full benefit of the text.

Scully, Robert E., Eugene J. Mark, and Betty U. McNeely. "Case Records of the Massachusetts General Hospital: Case 47-1985." *New England Journal of Medicine* 313 (November 21, 1985): 1341-1346. A moderately technical panel discussion, this report concerns a laxative abuser hospitalized with chronic diarrhea. The long battery of tests that were conducted, the patient's denials, and the detective work leading to the final diagnosis of this psychological aberration make fascinating reading and illustrate the complexity of the mental disease.

Thompson, W. Grant. *Gut Reactions: Understanding Symptoms of the Digestive Tract*. New York: Plenum Press, 1989. With much charm, Grant writes for the general reader, laying out the essential information that patients need in order to comprehend most gastrointestinal ailments. His chapter on diarrhea addresses only the functional diseases, and the book is perhaps best read as a thorough introduction to the gut and the medical specialties that care for it.

DIETARY DEFICIENCIES. *See* MALNUTRITION; VITAMIN AND MINERAL DEFICIENCIES.

DIPHTHERIA

SYSTEMS AFFECTED: Respiratory, heart, kidneys, nervous
SPECIALISTS: Emergency physicians, infectious disease physicians, public health specialists
DEFINITION: A major cause of death in children until effective immunization was developed, diphtheria is a highly contagious bacterial infection that usually affects

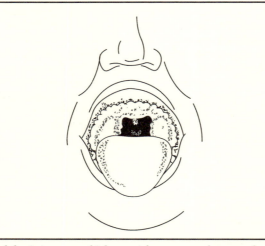

Diphtheria causes a thick, grayish green membrane to form over the larynx, tonsils, pharynx, and sinus cavities.

the respiratory system. When the bacteria, spread through the air or physical contact, cause a thick, grayish green membrane to form over the larynx, tonsils, pharynx, and sinus cavities, the result is hoarseness, a raspy cough, a sore throat, and a fever. Serious complications in the heart, kidneys, and nervous systems may occur when the bacteria release a dangerous toxin into the bloodstream. Treatment consists of the use of antitoxins and penicillin, which can destroy the diphtheria organisms. Although it has become rare in developed countries, diphtheria still has a mortality rate of 10 percent.

See also Bacterial infections; Childhood infectious diseases; Pulmonary diseases.

DISEASE

SYSTEMS AFFECTED: All

SPECIALISTS: All

DEFINITION: A morbid (pathological) process with a characteristic set of symptoms that may affect the entire body or any of its parts; the cause, pathology, and course of a disease may be known or unknown.

KEY TERMS:

diagnosis: the art of distinguishing one disease from another

lesion: any pathologic or traumatic discontinuity of tissue or loss of function of a body part

pathology: the study of the essential nature of disease, especially as it relates to the structural and functional changes that are caused by that disease

prognosis: a forecast regarding the probable cause and result of an attack of disease

syndrome: a congregation of a set of signs and symptoms that characterize a particular disease process, but without a specific etiology or a constant lesion

TYPES OF DISEASE

It is difficult to answer the question "What is disease?" To the patient, disease means discomfort and disharmony with the environment. To the treating physician or surgeon, it means a set of signs and symptoms. To the pathologist, it means one or more structural changes in body tissues, called lesions, which may be viewed with or without the aid of magnifying lenses.

The study of lesions, which are the essential expression of disease, forms part of the modern science of pathology. Pathology had its beginnings in the morgue and the autopsy room, where investigations into the cause of death lead to the appreciation of "morbid anatomy"—at first by gross (naked-eye) examination and later microscopically. Much later, the investigation of disease moved from the cold autopsy room to the patient's bedside, from the dead body to the living body, on which laboratory tests and biopsies are performed for the purpose of establishing a diagnosis and addressing proper treatment.

Diagnosis is the art of determining not only the character of the lesion but its etiology, or cause. Because so much of this diagnostic work is done in the laboratories, the term "laboratory medicine" has gained in popularity. The explosion in high technology has expanded the field of laboratory medicine tremendously. The diagnostic laboratory today is highly automated and sophisticated, containing a team of laboratory technologists and scientific researchers rather than a single pathologist.

The lesions laid bare by the pathologist usually bear an obvious relation to the symptoms, as in the gross lesions of acute appendicitis, the microscopic lesions in poliomyelitis, or even the chromosomal lesions in genetically inherited conditions such as Down syndrome. Yet there may be lesions without symptoms, as in early cancer or "silent" diseases such as tuberculosis. There may also be symptoms without obvious lesions, as in the so-called psychosomatic disease, functional disorders, and psychiatric illnesses. It is likely that future research will reveal the presence of "biochemical lesions" in these cases. The presence of lesions distinguishes organic disease, in which there are gross or microscopic pathologic changes in an organ, from functional disease, in which there is a disturbance of function without a corresponding obvious organic lesion. Although most diagnoses consist largely of naming the lesion (such as cancer of the lung or a tooth abscess), diseases should truly be considered in the light of disordered function rather than altered structure. Scientists are searching beyond the presence of obvious lesions in tissues and cells to the submicroscopic, molecular, and biochemical alterations affecting the chemistry of cells.

Not all diseases have a specific etiology. A syndrome is a complex of signs and symptoms with no specific etiology or constant lesion. It results from interference at some point with a chain of body processes, causing impairment of body function in one or more systems. With a syndrome, a specific biochemical molecular derangement caused by yet undiscovered agents is usually found. An example is acquired immunodeficiency syndrome (AIDS), for which a specific human immunodeficiency virus (HIV) agent is now accepted as its etiologic agent.

Some diseases have an acute (sudden) onset and run a relatively short course, as with acute tonsillitis (strep throat) or the common cold. Others run a long, protracted course, as with tuberculosis and rheumatoid arthritis; these are called chronic illnesses. The healthy body is in a natural state of readiness to combat disease, and thus there is a natural tendency to recover from disease. This is especially true in acute illness, in which inflammation tends to heal with full resolution of structure and function. Sometimes, however, healing does not occur and the disease overwhelms the body and leads to death. Therefore, a patient with acute pneumonia may have a full recovery, with complete healing and resolution of structure and function, or may die. The outcome of disease can vary between the extremes of full recovery or death and can run a chronic, protracted course eventually leading to severe loss of function. This outcome is the prognosis, a forecast of what may be expected to happen. The accurate diagnosis of disease is essential for its treatment and prognosis.

There are four aspects to the study of disease. The first is etiology or cause; for example, the common cold virus causes the common cold. The second is pathogenesis, or course; it refers to the sequence of events in the body that occurs in response to injury and the method of the lesion's production and development. The relation of an etiologic agent to disease, of cause to effect, is not always as simple a matter as it is in most acute illnesses; for example, a herpesvirus causes the development of fever blisters. In many illnesses, indeed in most chronic illnesses, the concept of one agent causing one disease is an oversimplification. In tuberculosis, for example, the causative agent is a characteristic slender microbe called tubercle bacillus (*Mycobacterium tuberculosis*). Many people may be exposed to and inhale the tuberculosis bacteria, but only a few will get the disease; also, the bacteria may lurk in the body for years and only become clinically active as a result of an unrelated, stressful situation that alters the body's immunity, such as prolonged strain, malnutrition, or another infection. In investigating the causation and pathogenesis of disease, several factors—such as heredity, sex, environment, nutrition, immunity, and age—must be considered. That is why there is no simple answer to the questions, "Does cigarette smoking cause cancer?" or "Does a cholesterol-rich diet cause hardening of the blood vessels (atherosclerosis)?" The third aspect to the study of disease relates to morphologic and structural changes associated with the functional alterations in cells and tissues that are characteristic of the disease. These are the gross and microscopic findings that allow the pathologist to establish a

diagnosis. The fourth aspect to disease study is the evaluation of functional abnormalities and their clinical significance; the nature of the morphologic changes and their distribution in different organs or tissues influence normal function and determine the clinical features, signs and symptoms, and course and outcome (prognosis) of disease.

All forms of tissue injury start with molecular and structural changes in cells. Cells are the smallest living units of tissues and organs. Along with their substructural components, they are the seat of disease. Cellular pathology is the study of disease as it relates to the origins, molecular mechanisms, and structural changes of cell injury.

The normal cell is similar to a factory. It is confined to a fairly narrow range of function and structure, dictated by its genetic code, the constraints of neighboring cells, the availability of and access to nutrition, and the disposal of its waste products. It is said to be in a "steady state," able to handle normal physiologic demands and to respond by adapting to other excessive or strenuous demands (such as the muscle enlargement seen in bodybuilders) to achieve a new equilibrium with a sustained workload. This type of adaptive response is called hypertrophy. Conversely, atrophy is an adaptive response to decreased demand, with a resulting diminished size and function.

If the limits of these adaptive responses are exceeded, or if no adaptive response is possible, a sequence of events follows which results in cell injury. Cell injury is reversible up to a certain point, but if the stimulus persists or is severe, then the cell suffers irreversible injury and eventual death. For example, if the blood supply to the heart muscle is cut off for only a few minutes and then restored, the heart muscle cells will experience injury but can recover and function normally. If the blood flow is not restored until one hour later, however, the cells will die.

Whether specific types of stress induce an adaptive response, a reversible injury, or cell death depends on the nature and severity of the stress and on other inherent, variable qualities of the cell itself. The causes of cell injury are many and range from obvious physical trauma, as in automobile accidents, to a subtle, genetic lack of enzymes or hormones, as in diabetes mellitus. Broadly speaking, the causes of cell injury and death can be grouped into the following categories: hypoxia, or a decrease in the delivery of available oxygen; physical agents, as with mechanical and thermal injuries; chemical poisons, such as carbon monoxide, alcohol, tobacco, and other addictive drugs; infectious agents, such as viruses and bacteria; immunological and allergic reactions, as in patients with certain sensitivities; genetic defects, as with sickle-cell anemia; and nutritional imbalances, such as severe malnutrition and vitamin deficiencies or nutritional excesses predisposing a patient to heart disease and atherosclerosis.

CAUSES OF DISEASE

By far the most common cause of disease is infection, especially by bacteria. Certain lowly forms of animal life known as animal parasites may also live in the body and produce disease; parasitic diseases are common in poor societies and countries. Finally, there are viruses, forms of living matter so minute that they cannot be seen with the most powerful light microscope; they are visible, however, with the electron microscope. Viruses, as agents of disease, have attracted much attention for their role in many diseases, including cancer.

Bacteria, or germs, can be divided into three morphologic groups: cocci, which are round; bacilli, which are rod-shaped; and spirilla or spirochetes, which are spiral-shaped, like a corkscrew. Bacteria produce disease either by their presence in tissues or by their production of toxins (poisons). They cause inflammation and either act on surrounding tissues, as in an abscess, or are carried by the bloodstream to other distant organs. Strep throat is an example of a local infection by cocci—in this case, streptococci. Some dysenteries and travelers' diarrheas are caused by coliform bacilli. Syphilis is an example of disease caused by a spirochete. The great epidemics of history, such as bubonic plague and cholera, are caused by bacteria, as are tuberculosis, leprosy, typhoid, gas gangrene, and many others. Bacterial infections are treatable with antibiotics, such as penicillin.

Viruses, on the other hand, are not affected by antibiotics; they infect the cell itself and live within it, and are therefore protected. Viruses cause a wide variety of diseases. Some are short-lived and run a few days' course, such as many childhood diseases, the measles, and the common cold. Others can cause serious body impairment, such as poliomyelitis and AIDS. Still others are probably involved in causing cancer and such diseases as multiple sclerosis.

Of the many physical agents causing injury, trauma is the most obvious; others relate to external temperatures, ones that are either too high or too low. A high temperature may produce local injury, such as a burn, or general disease, as in heat stroke. Heat stroke results from prolonged direct exposure to the sun (sunstroke) or from very high temperatures, so that the heat-regulating mechanism of the body becomes paralyzed. The internal, body temperature shoots up to alarming heights; collapse, coma, and even death may result. Low temperatures can cause local frostbite or general hypothermia, which can also lead to death.

Other forms of physical agents causing injury are radiation and atmospheric pressure. Increased atmospheric pressure is best illustrated by the "bends," a decompression sickness which can affect deep sea divers. The pressure of the water causes inert gases, such as nitrogen, to be dissolved in the blood plasma. If the diver passes too rapidly from a high to a normal atmospheric pressure, the excessive nitrogen is released, forming gas bubbles in the blood. These tiny bubbles can cause the blockage of small vessels of the brain and result in brain damage. The same problem can occur in high-altitude aviators unless the airplane is pressurized.

The study of chemical poisoning, or toxicology, as a cause of disease is a large and specialized field. Poisons may be introduced into the body by accident (especially in young children), because of suicide or homicide, and most important as industrial pollution. Lead poisoning is a danger because of its use in paints and soldering. Acids and carbon monoxide are emitted into the atmosphere by industry, and various chemicals are dumped into the ground and water. Such environmental damage will eventually affect plants, livestock, and humans.

Hypoxia (lack of oxygen) is probably the most common cause of cell injury, and it may also be the ultimate mechanism of cell death by a wide variety of physical, biological, and chemical agents. Loss of adequate blood and oxygen supply to a body part, such as a leg, is called ischemia. (This is a local loss of blood, in contrast to anemia, which is a general condition of poor oxygen-carrying capacity affecting the entire body.) If the blood loss is very severe, the result is hypoxia, or anoxia. This condition may also result from narrowing of the blood vessels, called atherosclerosis. If this narrowing occurs in the artery of the leg, as may be seen in patients with advanced diabetes, then the tissues of the foot will eventually die, a condition known as gangrene. An even more critical example of ischemia is blockage of the coronary arteries of the heart, resulting in a myocardial infarction (heart attack), with damage to the heart muscle. Similarly, severe blockage of arteries to the brain can cause a stroke.

Nutritional diseases can be caused either by an excessive intake and storage of foodstuffs, as in extreme obesity, or by a deficiency. Obesity is a complex condition, often associated with hereditary tendencies and hormonal imbalances. The deficiency conditions are many. Starvation and malnutrition can occur because of intestinal illnesses that prevent the delivery of food to the blood (malabsorption) or because of debilitating diseases such as advanced cancer. Even more important than general malnutrition as a cause of disease is a deficiency of essential nutrients such as minerals, vitamins, and other trace elements. Iron deficiency causes anemia, and calcium deficiency causes osteoporosis (bone fragility). Vitamin deficiencies are also numerous, and deficiency of the trace element iodine causes a thyroid condition called goiter.

Genetic defects as a cause of cellular injury and disease are of major interest to many biologists. The genetic injury may be as gross as the congenital malformations seen in patients with Down syndrome or as subtle as molecular alterations in the coding of the hemoglobin molecule that causes sickle-cell anemia.

Cellular injuries and diseases can be induced by immune mechanisms. The anaphylactic reaction to a foreign protein, such as a bee sting or drug, can actually cause death. In the so-called autoimmune diseases, such as lupus erythematosus, the immune system turns against the cellular components of the very body that it is supposed to protect.

Finally, neoplastic diseases, or cancer, are presently of unknown etiology. Some are innocuous growths, while others are highly lethal. Diagnosing cancer and determining its precise nature can be an elaborate, and elusive, process. The methods involve clinical observations and laboratory tests; a biopsy of the involved organ may be taken and analyzed.

PERSPECTIVE AND PROSPECTS

It is sometimes said that the nature of disease is changing, that one hears more often of people dying of heart failure and cancer than was once the case. This does not mean that these diseases have actually become more common, although more people do die from them. This increase is attributable to a longer life span and vastly improved diagnostic methods.

For primitive humans, there were no diseases, only patients stricken by evil; therefore, magic was the plausible recourse. Magic entails recognition of the principle of causality—that, given the same predisposing conditions, the same results will follow. In a profound sense, magic is early science. In ancient Egypt, the priests assumed the role of healers. Unlike magic, however, religion springs from a different source. Here the system is based on the achievement of results against, or in spite of, a regular sequence. Religion heals with miracles and antinaturals that require the violation of causality. The purely religious concept of disease, as an expression of the wrath of gods, became embodied in many religious traditions.

The ancient Greeks are credited with attempts at introducing reason to the study of disease by asking questions about the nature of things and considering the notion of health as a harmony, as the adjustment of such opposites as high and low, hot and cold, dry and moist. Disease, therefore, was a disharmony of the four elements that make up life: earth, air, fire, and water. This concept was refined by Galen in the second century and became dogma throughout the Dark Ages until the Renaissance, when the seat of disease was finally assigned to organs within the body itself through autopsy studies. Much later, in the nineteenth century, the principles espoused by French physiologist Claude Bernard were introduced, whereby disease was considered not a thing but a process that distorts normal physiologic and anatomic features. The nineteenth century German pathologist Rudolf Virchow emphasized the same principle—that disease is an alteration of life's processes—by championing the concept of cellular pathology, identifying the cell as the smallest unit of life and as the seat of disease.

As new diseases are discovered and old medical mysteries are deciphered, as promising new medicinal drugs and vaccines are tested and public health programs implemented, the age-old goal of medicine as a healing art seems to be closer at hand. —*Victor H. Nassar*

See also Arthropod-borne diseases; Childhood infectious diseases; Environmental diseases; Infection; Parasitic diseases; Zoonoses; *specific diseases.*

FOR FURTHER INFORMATION:

Boyd, William. *Boyd's Introduction to the Study of Disease.* 11th ed. Philadelphia: Lea & Febiger, 1992. A textbook for students in the medical and allied health sciences. The text and illustrations emphasize the view of disease as a disturbed functional alteration.

Grist, Norman R., et al. *Diseases of Infection: An Illustrated Textbook.* 2d ed. Oxford, England: Oxford University Press, 1992. An informative survey of communicable diseases. Contains copious illustrations.

Jones, Kenneth L., Louis W. Shainberg, and Curtis O. Byer. *Disease.* 2d ed. San Francisco: Canfield Press, 1975. A popular work designed to educate the general reader about both communicable and noncommunicable diseases. Examines the causes of these diseases, as well as general theories of causation.

Perez-Tamayo, Ruy. *Mechanisms of Disease: An Introduction to Pathology.* 2d ed. Chicago: Yearbook Medical Publishers, 1985. A fascinating examination of the nature and mechanism of disease. Written for the advanced student.

Robbins, Stanley L., Ramzi S. Cotran, and Vinay Kumar. *Robbins' Pathologic Basis of Disease.* 4th ed. Philadelphia: W. B. Saunders, 1989. The standard textbook on disease for medical students. This work is a revision of the third edition.

DISLOCATION. *See* FRACTURE AND DISLOCATION.

DIVERTICULITIS AND DIVERTICULOSIS

SYSTEM AFFECTED: Gastrointestinal

SPECIALISTS: Colorectal surgeons, gastroenterologists, general surgeons, internists

DEFINITION: Diverticulosis is a disease involving multiple outpouchings, or diverticuli, of the wall of the colon; these diverticuli may become inflamed, leading to the painful condition called diverticulitis.

KEY TERMS:

colon: the portion of the large intestine excluding the cecum and rectum; it includes the ascending, transverse, descending, and sigmoid colon

dietary fiber: indigestible plant substances that humans eat; fiber may be soluble, meaning that it dissolves in water, or insoluble, meaning that it does not dissolve in water

hernia: the bulging out of part or all of an organ through the wall of the cavity that usually contains it

infection: multiplication of disease-causing microorganisms in the body; the body normally also contains microorganisms that do not cause disease

inflammation: a tissue response to injury involving local reactions that attempt to destroy the injurious material and begin healing

lumen: the channel within a hollow or tubular organ

mucosa: the inner lining of the digestive tract; in the colon, the major function of the mucosal cells is to reabsorb liquid from feces, creating a semisolid material

perforation: an abnormal opening, such as a hole in the wall of the colon

peritoneal cavity: the cavity in the abdomen and pelvis that contains the internal organs

prevalence: the frequency of disease cases in a population, often expressed as a fraction (such as cases per 100,000)

CAUSES AND SYMPTOMS

Diverticulosis is an acquired condition of the colon that involves a few to hundreds of blueberry-sized outpouchings of its wall called diverticuli. Diverticular disease is usually manifested by the presence of multiple diverticuli that are at risk of causing abdominal pain, inflammation, or bleeding.

Although the wall of the colon is thin, microscopically it has four layers. The innermost layer is called the mucosa. Its main function is to absorb fluids from the substance entering the colon, turning it into a semisolid material called feces. Outside the mucosa is the submucosa, a layer which contains blood vessels as well as nerve cells that control the functions of mucosal cells. Outside the submucosa is the muscularis, which contains muscle cells that are able to contract, pushing feces along the colon and eventually out through the rectum. Outside the muscularis is the serosa, which forms a wrap around the colon and helps prevent infections in this organ from spreading beyond its walls.

The definition of a diverticulum, taken from *Stedman's Medical Dictionary* (25th ed., 1990), is "a pouch or sac opening from a tubular or saccular organ, such as the gut or bladder." The diverticuli that form in the colon are not true diverticuli, in that the entire wall is not present in the outpouching. If examined microscopically, only the mucosal and submucosal layers pouch out through weakened areas in the muscularis layer. If examined by the naked eye, however, it appears as if the entire wall of the colon is involved in the tiny outpouching. The mucosa bulges out in the part of the colonic wall that is weakened: This is where arteries penetrate through clefts in the muscularis.

The large intestine begins with the cecum, which is connected to the small intestine. The cecum is a pouch leading to the colon, whose components are the ascending, transverse, descending, and sigmoid colon. The sigmoid colon leads to the rectum, which is connected to the outside of the body by the anal canal. Although diverticuli can appear at a variety of locations in the gastrointestinal (GI) tract, they are usually located in the colon, most commonly in the sigmoid colon.

The most common form of diverticulosis is called spastic colon diverticulosis, which is a condition involving diverticuli in the sigmoid colon whose lumen is abnormally narrowed. Since the circumference of the colon normally alternately narrows and widens along its length, muscle contractions may result in local occlusions of the lumen at the narrowed sections. Occlusion may cause the lumen of the colon to become multiple, separate chambers. When this happens, the pressure within the chambers can increase to the point where the mucosa herniates out through small clefts in the muscularis, creating diverticuli.

Most people with diverticulosis never notice it. When abdominal pain related to painful diverticular disease develops, it is felt in the lower abdomen and may last for hours or days. Eating usually makes it worse, whereas passing gas or having a bowel movement may relieve it.

Besides causing abdominal pain, diverticuli may cause rectal bleeding, which may vary from mild to life-threatening. Usually, there is a sudden urge to defecate followed by passagen of red blood, clots, or maroon-colored stool. If the stool is black, the bleeding is probably from the upper GI tract.

Since the colon may be studded with multiple diverticuli, and the bleeding may stop by the time of evaluation, it is

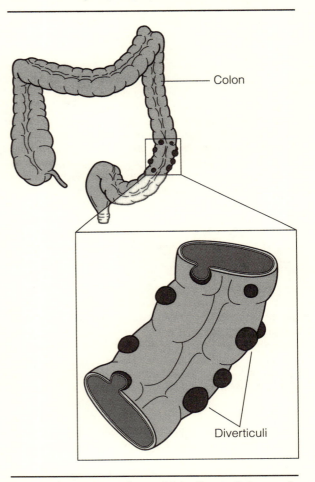

Diverticulosis occurs when multiple diverticuli (outpouchings) appear on the colon wall.

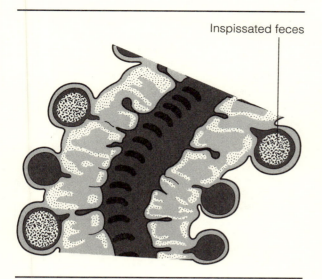

Inspissated feces

Diverticulitis begins when fecal material invades diverticuli and thickens (inspissated feces); when a diverticulum perforates, bacteria travel outside the colon into other regions and cause serious symptoms, including lower abdominal pain, fever, chills, and abscesses.

often difficult to tell which one bled. Diverticulosis is most common in elderly people, who may have other conditions of the colon that are associated with bleeding. Therefore, it is often impossible to confirm that the cause of bleeding was from diverticular disease—even if the colon is lined with hundreds of diverticuli.

What is most important is to establish what part of the GI tract is bleeding. To find out if the bleeding could have come from the upper GI tract, a tube is passed through the nose into the stomach and the contents are aspirated. If blood is not present, this suggests lower GI bleeding. In addition, the esophagus, stomach, and upper small intestine can be visualized with a flexible, snakelike instrument called an endoscope to exclude a source such as a bleeding ulcer.

It is more difficult to examine the lower GI tract. The simplest procedure is anoscopy, by which the physician can examine the inside of the anal canal for hemorrhoids. Proctosigmoidoscopy, a procedure similar to endoscopy, offers a view of the rectum and part of the sigmoid colon. It may reveal diverticuli or other lesions such as a bleeding growth called a polyp.

Angiography is a test done in the radiology department; it involves injecting dye into the vessels that lead to the colon. If there is active bleeding, it can help localize the source. Even if the bleeding has stopped, this procedure can sometimes identify abnormal blood vessel formations suggestive of cancer or a blood vessel abnormality called angiodysplasia. Colonoscopy is most easily performed after bleeding has stopped. It requires cleaning out the contents

of the colon and then inserting a long, flexible instrument called a colonoscope all the way to the cecum. The entire lining of the colon can be visualized while withdrawing the colonoscope.

About 15 percent of people with diverticulosis suffer from one or more episodes of diverticulitis, which is an inflammatory condition that may progress to an infection. Initially, feces may become trapped and inspissated (thickened) in a diverticulum, irritating it and leading to inflammation. Inflammation is a tissue response to injury which involves local reactions that attempt to destroy the injurious material and begin the healing process. It is usually the first step in the body's attempt to prevent infection and involves the migration of white blood cells out of blood vessels and into tissues, where they begin to fight off bacteria. The white blood cells release enzymes that cause tissue destruction. Because it is thin, the wall of the diverticulum may develop a tiny perforation.

Feces are made up of waste material and bacteria that normally do not cause problems when confined within the lumen of the colon. When a diverticulum perforates, however, they travel outside the colon and into other regions such as the peritoneal cavity, causing an infection. This infection along the outside of the colon is often limited, because many adjacent structures are able to wall off the bacteria, limiting their ability to extend through the peritoneal cavity. Although they become sealed off, they often form a pus-filled lesion called an abscess.

Fever and abdominal pain are the most common symptoms of diverticulitis. The fever may be high and associated with shaking chills. The pain is often sudden in onset, continuous, and may radiate from the left lower abdomen to the back. Laboratory findings usually include an elevated white blood cell count, a nonspecific finding that occurs with a variety of infections.

Radiographic studies are helpful for diagnosing and assessing the severity of diverticulitis. For example, a computed tomography (CT) scan can detect diverticuli or a thickening of the bowel wall associated with diverticulitis and can help assess whether abscesses are present.

TREATMENT AND THERAPY

There are two treatment goals in treating uncomplicated, painful diverticular disease: prevention of further development of diverticuli and pain relief. It is important to understand that the pressure that is able to develop inside the lumen of the colon is inversely related to the radius of the lumen. Therefore, if the lumen's radius can be increased, the pressures within the lumen will lessen, theoretically decreasing the chance of diverticuli formation. One key to increasing the radius of the lumen of the colon is to increase the bulk of the stool by the addition of dietary fiber.

A Western diet tends to be high in fiber-free animal foods and to lose much of its fiber during processing. This low-fiber diet may contribute to the cause of diverticulosis, which is prevalent in countries that have low-fiber diets. The typical American diet contains an average of 12 grams of fiber per day, whereas diets from Africa and India contain from 40 to 150 grams of fiber per day. A high-fiber diet can increase stool bulk by 40 to 100 percent. Fiber adds bulk to the stool because it acts like a sponge, retaining water that would normally be reabsorbed by the colonic mucosa. Fiber also increases stool bulk because 50 to 70 percent of the fiber is degraded by the bacteria in the colon and the products of degradation attract water by a process called osmosis.

The main fibers that increase stool bulk are the water-insoluble fibers, such as cellulose, hemicellulose, and lignin; they are derived from plants such as vegetables and whole grain cereals. Diets high in these fibers have been shown to decrease the intraluminal pressure in the sigmoid colon, as well as to relieve the pain associated with uncomplicated diverticular disease. The best results have been with the addition of 10 to 25 grams per day of coarse, unprocessed wheat bran to various liquid and semisolid foods. The sudden addition of large amounts of bran to one's diet, however, may cause bloating. Commercial preparations such as methylcellulose may be better tolerated during the first few weeks of therapy; their use may then be tapered off as bran is added to the diet. There are also various antispasmodic drugs available for inhibiting the muscle spasms of the colon, but many of those used in the United States are not very effective for decreasing symptoms.

For diverticular bleeding, the most effective therapy is patience. Most episodes stop on their own, and conservative treatments such as maintaining the patient's blood volume with intravenous fluids and possibly performing blood transfusions are all that is necessary. In those patients with continued active bleeding and in whom the source of the bleeding can be identified with angiography, a drug called vasopressin may be administered into the artery over several hours. This causes constriction of the vessel and stops bleeding most of the time. Once the vasopressin is stopped, however, patients may resume bleeding.

If vasopressin fails, surgery may be necessary. Surgery is most often successful if the bleeding site has been well localized before the operation. In that case, only the involved segment of the colon needs to be removed. If the bleeding site cannot be identified, it may be necessary to remove a majority of the colon; this procedure is associated with a higher rate of postoperative complications.

Diverticulitis that warrants hospitalization is initially treated with intravenous antibiotics for seven to ten days. Antibiotics help prevent 70 to 85 percent of patients from needing surgery. Most of those who respond to antibiotics will not have future attacks severe enough to warrant hospitalization.

Other measures may be necessary for the care of someone with diverticulitis, because the inflammation around the colon may be associated with problems such as narrowing of the bowel lumen to the point where it causes a partial or complete colonic obstruction. In this case, nothing should be given by mouth, and a tube should be passed through the nose into the stomach in order to suck out air and the stomach contents. This suction helps to reduce the amount of material that can pass through the colon and worsen the dilation of the colon that occurs proximal to the obstruction.

If the fever persists for more than a few days, the diverticulitis may be associated with complications. One complication is the formation of a large abscess outside the colon, which may be detected by a CT scan. An abscess has a rim around it that makes it difficult for antibiotics to penetrate the liquid center. If it does not go away despite antibiotic therapy, surgery may be necessary. If the abscess is small, it is possible to remove the involved segment of bowel and reattach the two free ends. If the abscess is very large, it may be necessary first to drain the abscess and then to cut across the colon proximal to the diseased segment, attaching the free end of the proximal segment to the abdominal wall, a procedure called a diverting colostomy. Later, the diseased segment of colon can be removed, and the remaining two free ends of colon can be joined. Another option is to drain the abscess with the aid of visual guidance by the CT scan and then operate on the colon. Draining the abscess in this manner helps get the infection under control before surgery is performed. Other indications for surgery in diverticulitis include complications such as a persistent bowel obstruction. In this case, it is often necessary to use a two-stage approach rather than to cure the problem in one operation.

Another complication of diverticulitis is a generalized infection of the peritoneal cavity, called peritonitis. Surgery for peritonitis involves removing the leaking segment of bowel and attaching the remaining two free ends of the colon to the abdominal wall. In addition, the peritoneal cavity is rinsed with a sterile solution in an attempt to clean out the contaminating materials.

Diverticulitis may also be complicated by the presence of a perforation of a diverticulum leading to a fistula, an abnormally existing channel connecting two hollow organs. When there is a fistula between the colon and the bladder, stool can travel into the bladder. The bacteria in the stool can cause severe, recurrent urinary tract infections. Another symptom is that bowel gas gets into the bladder; when the patient urinates, there is an intermittent stream because of colonic gas being passed along with the urine. When a fistula exists, it is necessary to remove the diseased segment of colon, the fistula tract, and a small portion of the bladder where the tract entered it.

Even if a patient with diverticulitis seems to improve and is able to return home from the hospital without needing surgery, there is still a chance that surgery will be necessary in the future. Surgery may be needed if the patient continues to have repeated, severe attacks of diverticulitis, or when a fistula between the colon and bladder causes recurring urinary tract infections. Another reason for surgery is when there is persistent partial colonic obstruction and it is impossible to inspect the narrowed region of colon to exclude a constricting cancerous lesion as the cause of the obstruction.

PERSPECTIVE AND PROSPECTS

Diverticuli are quite common in the United States and other developed countries that tend to eat processed, low-fiber foods. In the United States, for example, diverticulosis is uncommon before the age of forty but is seen in 30 to 50 percent of elderly people at autopsy. Of those with diverticuli, only about one-fifth suffer any symptoms. Although members of ethnic groups who live in underdeveloped countries and eat a high-fiber diet tend to have a low prevalence of diverticulosis, their risk of developing this disease increases within ten years of moving to more developed countries.

Before 1900, the presence of colonic diverticuli in the United States was considered a curiosity, whereas now it is found in one-third to one-half of all autopsies of people over the age of sixty. There are a few possible explanations for why this increasing prevalence is seen.

First, the change in the American diet probably plays a large part in the pathogenesis of diverticular disease. Fiber consumption may have fallen off by as much as 30 percent during the twentieth century. Many people in the United States eat foods such as quick-cooking rice, highly processed cereals, and processed flour, all which contains less fiber than their unprocessed counterparts. In addition, the population tends to eat more fats and proteins and less carbohydrates. Many fibers are from food sources rich in carbohydrates and are carbohydrates themselves.

The increasing prevalence of diverticular disease may also be attributable to the changing survival pattern. In 1900, the average life expectancy in the United States was forty-nine; in 1983, it was seventy-one years for men and seventy-eight years for women. The proportion of people over sixty-five has risen: It was 4.1 percent in 1900 and increased to 11.6 percent in 1986. Thus, the American population is not only growing but also getting older. Since diverticulosis is seen in increasing frequencies with aging, it is understandable that more of it was seen in the late twentieth century than during the early 1900's.

Most poor people in the world live largely on plant foods rich in fiber, being largely dependent on cereal grains such as wheat, rice, and corn for both their calorie and their protein sources. Although one can look at the amount of fiber in the diet of rural Africans and compare it to that in the United States, there may be other differences in lifestyles that contribute to the higher prevalence of diverticular disease in the United States. Living in rural Africa, without traffic jams and the fast pace of developed countries, may cause people to have less stressful lives, and the lower stress is associated with fewer muscle spasms in the colon. Since it has been documented that stress can increase colonic contractions, and stress may worsen another disorder of the colon involving muscle spasm called irritable bowel syndrome (IBS), one might postulate that the stress of Western society contributes to the spasms in the sigmoid colon that may lead to diverticular disease.

Another reason for the increase in the prevalence of diverticular disease could be improvements in detection. Now it is detected not only at autopsy but also by barium enema, during sigmoidoscopy, and during surgery. Thus, there are more opportunities for discovering diverticulosis.

—*Marc H. Walters*

See also Colon cancer; Constipation; Gastrointestinal disorders; Intestinal disorders; Peritonitis.

FOR FURTHER INFORMATION:

Achkar, Edgar, et al. *Clinical Gastroenterology*. 2d ed. Philadelphia: Lea & Febiger, 1992. This book is written by gastroenterologists from the Cleveland Clinic. Contains excellent chapters on abdominal pain, gastrointestinal bleeding, and diverticular disease. Less detailed but more readable than Marvin Sleisenger and John Fordtran's textbook (below).

Ganong, William F. *Review of Medical Physiology*. 16th ed. Norwalk, Conn.: Appleton and Lange, 1993. This classic paperback has a nice section emphasizing normal gastrointestinal physiology which would provide a solid background for understanding diverticulosis.

Hackford, Alan W., and Malcolm C. Veidenheimer. "Diverticular Disease of the Colon: Current Concepts and Management." *Surgical Clinics of North America* 65 (April, 1985): 347-363. This article emphasizes the medical and surgical options for treating diverticulitis.

Kumar, Vinay, Ramzi S. Cotran, and Stanley L. Robbins. *Basic Pathology*. 5th ed. Philadelphia: W. B. Saunders, 1992. An introductory pathology textbook. Less detailed than texts used by physicians, but still contains useful information on diverticular disease.

Segal, I. A. Solomon, and J. A. Hunt. "Emergence of Diverticular Disease in the Urban South African Black." *Gastroenterology* 72 (February, 1977): 215-219. This article discusses the emergence of diverticulosis in urban South African blacks, coincident with decreasing dietary fiber intake.

Sleisenger, Marvin H., and John S. Fordtran, eds. *Gastrointestinal Disease: Pathophysiology/Diagnosis/Management*. 5th ed. 2 vols. Philadelphia: W. B. Saunders, 1993. This text is the best comprehensive textbook of gastrointestinal diseases and physiology. Contains excellent information on diverticular disease.

Tortora, Gerard J., and Sandra R. Grabowski. *Principles of Anatomy and Physiology*. 7th ed. New York: HarperCollins, 1993. An outstanding textbook of human anatomy and physiology, and a good first text to consult before reading more advanced gastroenterology and journal articles. Many supplements are available, including an anatomy and physiology laserdisc.

Dizziness and fainting

Systems affected: Circulatory, brain

Specialists: Cardiologists, emergency physicians, family physicians, internists, neurologists

Definition: Dizziness is a feeling of light-headedness and unsteadiness, sometimes accompanied by a feeling of spinning or other spatial motion; fainting is a loss of consciousness as a result of insufficient amounts of blood reaching the brain. Both are symptoms of many conditions, which may be harmless or serious.

Key terms:

cardiac output: the amount of blood that the heart can pump per unit time (usually per minute); if the brain does not receive enough of the cardiac output, the person becomes dizzy and may faint

dizziness: a sensation of whirling with difficulty balancing

fainting: a weak feeling followed by a loss of consciousness, usually due to a lack of blood flow to the brain; also called syncope

hypertension: a condition in which the patient's blood pressure is higher than what the body demands

hypotension: decrease in blood pressure to the point that insufficient blood flow causes symptoms

vasoconstriction: a reduction in the diameter of arteries, which increases the amount of work required for the heart to move blood

vasodilation: an increase in the diameter of arteries, which decreases the amount of work required for the heart to move blood

venous return: the amount of blood returning to the heart; one factor that determines the amount of blood the heart can pump out

vertigo: a sensation of moving in space or having objects move about when the patient is stationary, the most common symptom of which is dizziness; vertigo results from a disturbance in the organs of equilibrium

Causes and Symptoms

Humans have evolved several mechanisms by which adequate blood flow to organs is maintained. Without a constant blood supply, the body's tissues would die from a lack of essential nutrients and oxygen. In particular, the brain and heart are very sensitive to changes in their blood supply as they, more than any other organs, must receive oxygen and nutrients at all times. If they do not, their cells will die and cannot be replaced.

While the heart supplies most of the force needed to propel the blood throughout the body, tissues rely on changes in the size of arteries to redirect blood flow to where it is needed most. For example, after a large meal the blood vessels that lead to the gastrointestinal tract enlarge (vasodilate) so that more blood can be present to collect the nutrients from the meal. At the same time, the blood vessels that supply muscles decrease in diameter (vasoconstrict) and effectively shunt the blood toward the stomach and intestines. On the other hand, during exercise, the blood vessels that supply the muscles dilate and the ones leading to the intestinal tract vasoconstrict. This mechanism allows the cardiovascular system to supply the most blood to the most active tissues.

The brain is somewhat special in that the body tries to maintain a nearly constant blood flow to it. Located in the walls of the carotid arteries, which carry blood to the brain, are specialized sensory cells that have the ability to detect changes in blood pressure. These cells are known as baroreceptors. If the blood pressure going to the brain is too low, the baroreceptors send an impulse to the brain which in turn speeds up the heart rate and causes a generalized vasoconstriction. This reflex response raises the body's blood pressure, reestablishing adequate blood flow to the brain. If the baroreceptors detect too high a blood pressure, they send a signal to the brain which in turn slows the heart rate and causes the arteries of the body to dilate. These reflexes prevent large fluctuations in blood flow to the brain and other tissues.

Most people have experienced a dizzy feeling or maybe even a fainting response when they have stood up too quickly from a prone position. The ability of the baroreceptors to maintain relatively constant arterial pressure is extremely important when a person stands after having been lying down. Immediate upon standing, the pressure in the carotid arteries falls and a reduction of this pressure can cause dizziness or even fainting. Fortunately, the falling pressure at the baroreceptors elicits an immediate reflex, resulting in a more rapid heart rate and vasoconstriction and minimizing the decrease in blood flow to the brain.

Blood pressure is not the only factor that is essential in maintaining tissue viability. The accumulation of waste products and a lack of essential nutrients and gases can also have a profound effect on how much blood flows through a particular tissue and how quickly. In a region of the carotid arteries near the baroreceptors are chemoreceptors. Chemoreceptors detect the concentration of the essential gas, oxygen, and the concentration of the gaseous waste product, carbon dioxide. When carbon dioxide concentrations increase and oxygen concentrations decrease, the chemoreceptors stimulate regions in the brain to increase the heart rate and blood pressure in an attempt to supply the tissues with more oxygen and flush away the excess carbon dioxide. If the chemoreceptors detect high levels of oxygen and low levels of carbon dioxide, an impulse is transmitted to the brain which in turn slows the heart rate and decreases the blood pressure.

Normally, most of the control of blood flow to the brain is accomplished by the baroreceptor and chemoreceptor reflexes. However, the brain has a backup system. If blood flow decreases enough to cause a deficiency of nutrients and oxygen and an accumulation of waste products, special nerve cells respond directly to the lack of adequate energy sources and become strongly excited. When this occurs, the heart is stimulated and blood pressure rises.

Dizziness is a sensation of light-headedness often accompanied by a sensation of spinning (vertigo). Occasionally, a person experiencing dizziness will feel nauseous and may even vomit. Most attacks of dizziness are harmless, resulting from a brief reduction in blood flow to the brain. There are several causes of dizziness, and each alters blood flow to the brain for a slightly different reason.

A person rising rapidly from a sitting or lying position may become dizzy. This is known as postural hypotension, which is caused by a relatively slow reflexive response to the reduced blood pressure in the arteries providing blood to the brain. Rising requires increased blood pressure to supply the brain with adequate amounts of blood. Postural hypotension is more common in the elderly and in individuals prescribed antihypertensive medicines (drugs used to lower high blood pressure).

If the patient experiences vertigo with dizziness, the condition is usually caused by a disorder of the inner ear equilibrium system. Two disorders of the inner ear that can cause dizziness are labyrinthitis and Ménière's disease. Labyrinthitis, inflammation of the fluid-filled canals of the inner ear, is usually caused by a virus. Since these canals are involved in maintaining equilibrium, when they become infected and inflamed one experiences the symptom of dizziness. Ménière's disease is a degenerative disorder of the ear in which the patient experiences not only dizziness but also progressive hearing loss.

Some brain-stem disorders also cause dizziness. The brain stem houses the vestibulocochlear nerve, which transmits messages from the ear to several other parts of the nervous system. Any disorder that alters the functions of this nerve will result in dizziness and vertigo. Meningitis (inflammation of the coverings of the brain and spinal cord), brain tumors, and blood-flow deficiency disorders such as atherosclerosis may affect the function of the vestibulocochlear nerve.

Syncope (fainting) is often preceded by dizziness. Syncope is the temporary loss of consciousness as a result of an inadequate blood flow to the brain. In addition to losing consciousness, the patient may be pale and sweaty. The most common cause of syncope is a vasovasal attack, in which an overstimulation of the vagus nerve slows the heart down. Often vasovagal syncope results from severe pain, stress, or fear. For example, people may faint when hearing bad news or at the sight of blood. More commonly, individuals who have received a painful injury will faint. Rarely, vasovagal syncope may be caused by prolonged coughing, straining to defecate or urinate, pregnancy, or forcing expiration. Standing still for long periods of time or standing up rapidly after lying or sitting can cause fainting. With the exception of vasovagal syncope, all the other causes of syncope are attributable to inadequate blood returning to the heart. If blood pools in the lower extremities, there is a reduced amount available for the heart to pump to the brain. In vasovagal syncope and some disorders of heart rhythm such as Adams-Stokes syndrome, it is the heart itself that does not force enough blood toward the brain.

TREATMENT AND THERAPY

Short periods of dizziness usually subside after a few minutes. Deep breathing and rest will usually help relieve the symptom. Prolonged episodes of dizziness and vertigo should be brought to the attention of a physician.

Recovery from fainting likewise will occur when adequate blood flow to the brain is reestablished. This happens within minutes because falling to the ground places the head at the same level as the heart and helps return the blood from the legs. If a person does not regain consciousness within a few minutes, a physician or emergency medical team should be notified.

The most common cause of syncope is decreased cerebral blood flow resulting from limitation of cardiac output. When the heart rate falls below its normal seventy-five beats per minute to approximately thirty-five beats per minute, the patient usually becomes dizzy and faints. Although slow heart rates can occur in any age group, it is most often found in elderly people who have other heart conditions. Drug-induced syncope can also occur. Drugs for congestive heart failure (digoxin) or antihypertensive medications that slow the heart rate (propranolol, metoprolol) may reduce blood flow to the brain sufficiently to cause dizziness and fainting.

Exertional syncope occurs when individuals perform some physical activity to which they are not accustomed. These physical efforts demand more work from the cardiovascular system, and in patients with some obstruction of the arteries which leave the heart, the cardiovascular system is overstressed. This defect, combined with the vasodilation in the blood vessels that provide blood to the working muscles, reduces the amount of blood available for use by the brain. If the person also hyperventilates during exercise, he or she will effectively reduce the amount of carbon dioxide in the blood and rid the cardiovascular system of this normal stimulus for increasing heart rate and blood flow to the brain. Some persons also hold their breath during periods of high exertion. For example, people attempting to lift something very heavy often take a deep breath just prior to exerting and then hold their breath when they lift the object. This practice, known as the Valsalva maneuver, increases the pressure within the chest cavity, which in turn reduces the amount of blood returning to the heart. A decrease in blood returning to the heart (venous return) causes a decrease in the availability of blood to be pumped out of the heart and reduces cardiac output. The reduction in cardiac output decreases the amount of blood flowing to the brain and initiates a fainting response. It is interesting to note that humans also use the Valsalva maneuver when defecating or urinating, particularly when they strain. These acts can also lead to exertional syncope.

In order for a physician to diagnose and treat dizziness and fainting accurately, he or she must take an accurate medical history, paying particular attention to cardiovascular and neurological problems. In addition to experiencing episodes of dizziness and fainting, patients often have a weak pulse, low blood pressure (hypotension), sweating, and shallow breathing. Heart rate and blood pressure are monitored while the patient assumes different positions. The clinician also listens to the heart and carotid arteries to determine whether there are any problems with these tissues, such as a heart valve problem or atherosclerosis of the carotid arteries. An electrocardiogram (ECG or EKG) can detect abnormal heart rates and rhythms that may reduce cardiac output. Laboratory tests are used to determine whether the patient has low blood sugar (hypoglycemia), too little blood volume (hypovolemia), too few red blood cells (anemia), or abnormal blood gases suggesting a lung disorder. Finally, if the physician suspects a neurological problem such as a seizure disorder, he or she may run an electroencephalogram (EEG) to record brain activity.

Treatment for any of these underlying disorders may cure the dizziness and fainting episodes. In patients with postural hypotension, merely being aware of the condition will allow them to change their behavior to lessen the chances of becoming dizzy and fainting. These patients should not make any sudden changes in posture that could precipitate an attack. Often, this means simply slowing down their movements and learning to assume a horizontal position if they feel dizzy. Patients also can learn to contract their leg muscles and not hold their breath when rising. This increases the amount of blood available for the heart to pump toward the brain. If these techniques do not provide an adequate solution for postural hypotension, then a physician can prescribe drugs such as ephedrine, which increase blood pressure.

Heart rhythm disturbances that cause an abnormally fast or slow heart rate can be corrected with drug therapy such as quinidine or disopyramide (if the rate is too rapid) or a pacemaker (if the rate is too slow). It is interesting to note that even too fast a heart rate can cause dizziness and fainting. In patients with this type of arrhythmia, the heart beats at such a rapid rate that it cannot efficiently fill with blood before the next contraction. Therefore, less blood is pumped with each beat.

Other treatments for dizziness and fainting may include correcting the levels of certain blood elements. Patients with hypoglycemia often feel dizzy. The brain and spinal cord require glucose as their energy source. In fact, the brain and spinal cord have a very limited ability to utilize other substrates such as fat or protein for energy. Because of this, patients often feel light-headed when there are inadequate levels of glucose in the blood. Patients can correct this condition by eating more frequent meals, and if necessary, physicians can administer drugs such as epinephrine or glucagon. These agents liberate glucose from storage sites in the liver.

Individuals with a low blood volume are often dehydrated and upon becoming rehydrated no longer have dizziness or fainting episodes. If dehydration is not corrected and becomes worse, the patient can go into shock, a state of inadequate blood flow to tissues that will result in death if left untreated. In addition to being dizzy or fainting, the patient is often cold to the touch and has a rapid heart rate, low blood pressure, bluish skin, and rapid breathing. These patients are treated by emergency medical personnel, who keep the individual warm, elevate the legs, and infuse fluid into a vein. Drugs may be used to help bring blood pressure back to normal. The cause of the shock should be identified and corrected.

PERSPECTIVE AND PROSPECTS

As humans evolved, they assumed an upright posture. This was advantageous because it allows for the use of the front limbs for other things besides locomotion. Unlike most four-legged animals, however, humans have their brains above their hearts and must continually force blood uphill to reach this vital tissue. This adaptation to the upright posture is a continuing physiological problem because the cardiovascular system must counteract the forces of gravity to provide the brain with blood. If this does not occur, the individual becomes dizzy and faints.

Another significant problem that humans face is adaptation to brain blood flow during exercise. The amount of blood flowing to a tissue is usually proportional to the metabolic demand of the tissue. At rest, various organs throughout the body receive a certain amount of the cardiac output. For example, blood flow to abdominal organs such as the spleen and the kidneys requires about 43 percent of the total blood volume. The total flow to the brain is estimated to be only 13 percent, and the skin and skeletal muscles require 21 percent and 9 percent, respectively. Other areas such as the gastrointestinal tract and heart receive the remaining 14 percent. During exercise, the skeletal muscles may receive up to 80 percent of the cardiac output while the rest of the organs are perfused at a much-reduced rate.

Most data indicate that the brain receives only 3 percent of the total cardiac output during heavy exercise. Even though there is a large change in the redistribution of cardiac output, physiologists do not know the absolute amount of blood reaching the brain or the mechanism for the change in the perfusion rate.

With strenuous aerobic exercise such as jogging, there is an increase in cardiac output. During strenuous anaerobic exercise such as weight lifting, however, there may be a decrease in cardiac output attributable to the Valsalva maneuver. Therefore, it has been difficult to predict accurately, using available techniques, the volume of blood reaching this critical tissue. —*Matthew Berria*

See also Anxiety; Brain disorders; Meningitis; Neuralgia, neuritis, and neuropathy; Palpitations; Unconsciousness.

FOR FURTHER INFORMATION:

Astrand, Per-Olof, and Kaare Rodahl. *Textbook of Work Physiology: Physiological Bases of Exercise.* 3d ed. New York: McGraw-Hill, 1986. This text can be used by individuals who want a basic understanding of how the cardiovascular system responds to physical stresses. It can also be used by readers with an extensive background in physiology. For these professionals, some of the text includes highly detailed explanations of physiological adaptations to exercise.

Babakian, Viken K., and Lawrence R. Wechsler, eds. *Transcranial Doppler Ultrasonography.* St. Louis: Mosby Year Book, 1993. Describes a noninvasive way to measure blood flow to the brain using ultrasound techniques. The authors provide information on how drugs such as anesthetics alter blood flow to the brain. They also discuss the importance of monitoring cerebral blood flow during surgeries.

Clayman, Charles B., ed. *The American Medical Association Encyclopedia of Medicine.* New York: Random House, 1989. This encyclopedia lists in alphabetical order medical terms, diseases, and medical procedures. It does an excellent job of explaining rather complex medical subjects for the nonprofessional audience. In the sections on dizziness and fainting, flow charts detail the appropriate first aid treatments.

Geelen, G., and J. E. Greenleaf. "Orthostasis: Exercise and Exercise Training." *Exercise and Sport Sciences Reviews* 21 (1993): 201-230. Provides an excellent, complete discussion of the relationship between exercise and dizziness and fainting. These authors describe the current theories on blood flow regulation to the brain in athletes.

Guyton, Arthur C. *Human Physiology and Mechanisms of Disease.* 5th ed. Philadelphia: W. B. Saunders, 1991. This textbook introduces human physiology and basic pathology for individuals without an extensive background in medicine. Guyton offers several chapters on blood pressure regulation in humans and gives brief explanations as to what happens when blood pressure is not adequately regulated.

DOMESTIC VIOLENCE

SYSTEMS AFFECTED: Psychic-emotional, skin, all bodily systems

SPECIALISTS: Emergency physicians, family physicians, geriatric specialists, internists, pediatricians, psychiatrists, psychologists, public health specialists

DEFINITION: Assaultive behavior intended to punish, dominate, or control another in an intimate family relationship; physicians are often best able to identify situations of domestic violence and assist victims to implement preventive interventions.

KEY TERMS:

cycle of violence: a repeating pattern of violence characterized by increasing tension, culminating in violent action, and followed by remorse

family violence: violence against an intimate partner, typically to assert domination, control actions, or punish, which occurs as a pattern of behavior, not as a single, isolated act; also called battering, marital violence, domestic violence, relationship violence, child abuse, or elder abuse

funneling: an interviewing technique for assessing violence in a patient's relationship, beginning with broad questions of relationship conflict and gradually narrowing to focus on specific violent actions

hands-off violence: indirect attacks meant to terrorize or control a victim; may include property or pet destruction, threats, intimidating behavior, verbal abuse, stalking, and monitoring

hands-on violence: direct attacks upon the victim's body, including physical and sexual violence; comprises a continuum of acts ranging from seemingly minor to obviously severe

lethality: the potential, given the particular dynamics of violence in a relationship, for one or both partners to be killed

safety planning: the development of a specific set of actions and strategies to enable a victim either to avoid violence altogether or, once violence has begun, to escape and minimize damage and injury

CAUSES AND SYMPTOMS

Domestic or family violence is the intentional use of violence against an intimate partner. The purpose of the violence is to assert domination, to control the victim's actions, or to punish the victim for some actions. Family violence generally occurs as a pattern of behavior over time rather than as a single, isolated act.

Forms of family violence include child physical abuse, child sexual abuse, spousal or partner abuse, and elder abuse. These forms of violence are related, in that they occur within the context of the family unit. Therefore, the victims and perpetrators know one another, are related to one another, may live together, and may love one another. These various forms of violence also differ insofar as victims may be children, adults, or frail, elderly adults. The needs of victims differ with age and independence, but there are also many similarities between the different types of violence. One such similarity is the relationship between the offender and the victim. Specifically, victims of abuse are always less powerful than abusers. Power includes the ability to exert physical and psychological control over situations. For example, a child abuser has the ability to lock a child in a bathroom or to abandon him or her in a remote area in order to control access to authorities. A spouse abuser has the ability to physically injure a spouse, disconnect the phone, and keep the victim from leaving for help. An elder abuser can exert similar control. Such differences in power between victims and offenders are seen as a primary cause of abuse; that is, people batter others because they can.

Families that are violent are often isolated. The members usually keep to themselves and have few or no friends or relatives with whom they are involved, even if they live in a city. This social isolation prevents victims from seeking help from others and allows the abuser to establish rules for the relationship without answering to anyone for these actions. Abuse continues and worsens because the violence occurs in private, with few consequences for the abuser.

Victims of all forms of family violence share common experiences. In addition to physical violence, victims are also attacked psychologically, being told they are worthless and responsible for the abuse that they receive. Because they are socially isolated, victims do not have an opportunity to take social roles where they can experience success, recognition, or love. As a result, victims often have low self-esteem and truly believe that they cause the violence. Without the experience of being worthwhile, victims often become severely depressed and anxious, and they experience more stress-related illnesses such as headaches, fatigue, or gastrointestinal problems.

Child and partner abuse are linked in several ways. About half of the men who batter their wives also batter their children. Further, women who are battered are more likely to abuse their children than are nonbattered women. Even if a child of a spouse-abusing father is not battered, living in a violent home and observing the father's violence has negative effects. Such children often experience low self-esteem, aggression toward other children, and school problems. Moreover, abused children are more likely to commit violent offenses as adults. Children, especially males, who have observed violence between parents are at increased risk of assaulting their partners as adults. Adult sexual offenders have an increased likelihood of having been sexually abused as children. Yet, while these and other problems are reported more frequently by adults who were abused as children than by adults who were not, many former victims do not become violent. The most common outcomes of childhood abuse in adults are emotional problems. Although much less is known about the relationship between child abuse and future elder abuse, many elder abusers did suffer abuse as children. While most people who have been abused do not themselves become abusers, this intergenerational effect remains a cause for concern.

In its various forms, family violence is a public health epidemic in the United States. Once thought to be rare, family violence occurs with high frequency in the general population. Although exact figures are lacking and domestic violence tends to be underreported, it is estimated that each year 1.9 million children are physically abused; 250,000 children are sexually molested; 1.6 million women are assaulted by their male partners; and between 500,000 and 2.5 million elders are abused. Rates of violence directed toward unmarried heterosexual women, married heterosexual women, and members of homosexual male and female couples tend to be similar. No one is immune: Victims come from all social classes, races, and religions. Partner violence directed toward heterosexual men, however, is rare and usually occurs in relationships in which the male hits first.

Because family violence is so pervasive, physicians encounter many victims. One out of every three to five women visiting emergency rooms is seeking medical care for injuries related to partner violence. In primary care clinics, including family medicine, internal medicine, and obstetrics and gynecology, one out of every four female patients reports violence in the past year, and two out of five report violence at some time in their lives. It is therefore reasonable to expect all physicians and other health care professionals working in primary care and emergency rooms to provide services for victims of family violence.

Family violence typically consists of a pattern of behavior occurring over time and involving both hands-on and hands-off violence. Hands-on violence consists of direct attacks against the victim's body. Such acts range from pushing, shoving, and restraining to slapping, punching, kicking, clubbing, choking, burning, stabbing, or shooting. Hands-on violence also includes sexual assault, ranging from forced fondling of breasts, buttocks, and genitals; to forced touching of the abuser; to forced intercourse with the abuser or with other people.

Hands-off violence includes physical violence that is not directed at the victim's body but is intended to display destructive power and assert domination and control. Examples include breaking through windows or locked doors, punching holes through walls, smashing objects, destroying personal property, and harming or killing pet animals. The victim is often blamed for this destruction and forced to clean up the mess. Hands-off violence also includes psychological control, coercion, and terror. This includes name calling, threats of violence or abandonment, gestures suggesting the possibility of violence, monitoring of the victim's whereabouts, controlling of resources (such as money, transportation, and property), forced viewing of pornography, sexual exposure, or threatening to contest child custody. These psychological tactics may occur simultaneously with physical assaults or may occur separately. Whatever the pattern of psychological and physical tactics, abusers exert extreme control over their partners.

Neglect—the failure of one person to provide for the basic needs of another dependent person—is another form of hands-off abuse. Neglect may involve failure to provide food, clothing, health care, and shelter. Children, older adults, and developmentally delayed or physically handicapped people are particularly vulnerable to neglect.

Family violence differs in two respects from violence directed at strangers. First, the offender and victim are related and may love each other, live together, share property, have children, and share friends and relatives. Hence, unlike victims of stranger violence, victims of family violence cannot quickly or easily sever ties with or avoid seeing their assailants. Second, family violence often increases slowly in intensity, progressing until victims feel immobilized, unworthy, and responsible for the violence that is directed toward them. Victims may also feel substantial and well-grounded fear about leaving their abusers or seeking legal help, because they have been threatened or assaulted in the past and may encounter significant difficulty obtaining help to escape. In the case of children, the frail and elderly, or people with disabilities, dependency upon the caregiver and cognitive limitations make escape from an abuser difficult. Remaining in the relationship increases the risk of continued victimization. Understanding this unique context of the violent family can help physicians and other health care providers understand why battered victims often have difficulty admitting abuse or leaving the abuser.

Family violence follows a characteristic cycle. This cycle of violence begins with escalating tension and anger in the abuser. Victims describe a feeling of "walking on eggs." Next comes an outburst of violence. Outbursts of violence sometimes coincide with episodes of alcohol and drug abuse. Following the outburst, the abuser may feel remorse and expect forgiveness. The abuser often demands reconciliation, including sexual interaction. After a period of calm, the abuser again becomes increasingly tense and angry. This cycle generally repeats, with violence becoming increasingly severe. In partner abuse, victims are at greatest risk when there is a transition in the relationship such as pregnancy, divorce, or separation. In the case of elder abuse, risk increases as the elder becomes increasingly dependent on the primary caregiver, who may be inexperienced or unwilling to provide needed assistance. Without active intervention, the abuser rarely stops spontaneously and often becomes more violent.

TREATMENT AND THERAPY

Physicians play an important role in stopping family violence by first identifying people who are victims of violence, then taking steps to intervene and help. Physicians use different techniques with each age group because children, adults, and older adults each have special needs and varying abilities to help themselves. This section will first consider the physician's role with children and then will examine the physician's role with adults and older adults.

Because children do not usually tell a physician directly if they are being abused physically or sexually, physicians use several strategies to identify child and adolescent victims. Physicians screen for abuse during regular checkups by asking children if anyone has hurt them, touched them in private places, or scared them. To accomplish this screening with five-year-old patients having a routine checkup, physicians may teach their young patients about private areas of the body; let them know that they can tell a parent, teacher, or doctor if anyone ever touches them in private places; and ask the patients if anyone has ever touched them in a way that they did not like. For fifteen-year-old patients, physicians may screen potential victims by providing information on sexual abuse and date rape, then ask the patients if they have ever experienced either.

A second strategy that physicians use to identify children who are victims of family violence is to remain alert for general signs of distress that may indicate a child or youth lives in a violent situation. General signs of distress in children, which may be caused by family violence or by other stressors, include depression, anxiety, low self-esteem, hyperactivity, disruptive behaviors, aggressiveness toward other children, and lack of friends.

In addition to general signs of distress, there are certain specific signs and symptoms of physical and sexual abuse in children which indicate that the child has probably been exposed to violence. For example, bruises that look like a handprint, belt mark, or rope burn would indicate abuse. X rays can show a history of broken bones that are suspicious. Intentional burns from hot water, fire, or cigarettes often have a characteristic pattern. Sexually transmitted diseases in the genital, anal, or oral cavity of a child who is aged fourteen or under would suggest sexual abuse.

A physician observing specific signs of abuse or violence in a child, or even suspecting physical or sexual abuse, has an ethical and legal obligation to provide this information to state child protective services. Every state has laws that require physicians to report suspected child abuse. Physicians do not need to find proof of abuse before filing a report. In fact, the physician should never attempt to prove abuse or interview the child in detail because this can interfere with interviews conducted by experts in law, psychology, and the medicine of child abuse. When children are in immediate danger, they may be hospitalized so that they may receive a thorough medical and psychological evaluation while also being removed from the dangerous situation. In addition to filing a report, the physician records all observations in the child's medical chart. This record includes anything that the child or parents said, drawings or photographs of the injury, the physician's professional opinion regarding exposure to violence, and a description of the child abuse report.

The physician's final step is to offer support to the child's family. Families of child victims often have multiple problems, including violence between adults, drug and alcohol abuse, economic problems, and social isolation. Appropriate interventions for promoting safety include foster care for children, court-ordered counseling for one or both parents, and in-home education in parenting skills. The physician's goal, however, is to maintain a nonjudgmental manner while encouraging parental involvement.

Physicians also play a key role in helping victims of partner violence. Like children and adolescents, adult victims will usually not disclose violence. Therefore physicians should screen for partner violence and ask about partner violence whenever they notice specific signs of abuse or general signs of distress. Physicians screen for current and past violence during routine patient visits, such as during initial appointments; school, athletic, and work physicals; premarital exams; obstetrical visits; and regular checkups. General signs of distress include depression, anxiety disorders, low self-esteem, suicidal ideation, drug and alcohol abuse, stress illnesses (headache, stomach problems, chronic pain), or patient comments about a partner being jealous, angry, controlling, or irritable. Specific signs of violence include physical injury consistent with assault, including those requiring emergency treatment.

When a victim reports partner violence, there are five steps that a physician can take to help. Communicating belief and support is the first step. Sometimes abuse is extreme and patient reports may seem incredible. The physician validates the victim's experience by expressing belief in the story and exonerating the patient of blame. The physician can begin this process by making eye contact and telling the victim, "You have a right to be safe and respected" and "No one should be treated this way."

The second step is helping the patient assess danger. This is done by asking about types and severity of violent acts, duration and frequency of violence, and injuries received. Specific factors that seem to increase the risk of death in violent relationships include the abuser's use of drugs and alcohol, threats to kill the victim, and the victim's suicidal ideation or attempts. Finally, the physician should ask if the victim feels safe returning home. With this information, the physician can help the patient assess lethal potential and begin to make appropriate safety plans.

The third step is helping the patient identify resources and make a safety plan. The physician begins this process by simply expressing concern for the victim's safety and providing information about local resources such as mandatory arrest laws, legal advocacy services, and shelters. For patients planning to return to an abusive relationship, the physician should encourage a detailed safety plan by helping the patient identify safe havens with family members, friends, or a shelter; assess escape routes from the residence; make specific plans for dangerous situations or when violence recurs; and gather copies of important papers, money, and extra clothing in a safe place in or out of the home in the event of a quick exit. Before the patient leaves, the physician should give the patient a follow-up appointment within two weeks. This provides the victim with a specific, known resource. Follow-up visits should continue until the victim has developed other supportive resources.

The physician's final step is documentation in the patient's medical chart. This written note includes the victim's report of violence, the physician's own observations of injuries and behavior, assessment of danger, safety planning, and follow-up. This record can be helpful in the event of criminal or civil action taken by the victim against the offender. The medical chart, and all communications with the patient, is kept strictly confidential. Confronting the offender about the abuse can place the victim at risk of further, more severe violence. Improper disclosure can also result in loss of the patient's trust, precluding further opportunities for help.

There are several things that a physician should never do when working with a patient-victim. The physician should not encourage a patient to leave a violent relationship as a first or primary choice. Leaving an abuser is the most dangerous time for victims and should be attempted only with adequate planning and resources. The physician should not recommend couples counseling. Couples counseling endangers victims by raising the victim's expectation that issues can be discussed safely. The abuser often batters the victim after disclosure of sensitive information. Finally, the physician should not overlook violence if the violence appears to be "minor." Seemingly minor acts of aggression can be highly injurious.

Physicians also play an important role in helping adults who are older, developmentally delayed, or physically disabled. People in all three groups experience a high rate of family violence. Each group presents unique challenges for the physician. One common element among all three groups is that the victims may be somewhat dependent upon other adults to meet their basic needs. Because of this dependence, abuse may sometimes take the form of failing to provide basic needs such as adequate food or medical care. In many states, adults who are developmentally delayed are covered by mandatory child abuse reporting laws.

The signs and symptoms of the abuse of elders are similar to the other forms of family violence. These include physical injuries consistent with assault, signs of distress, and neglect, including self-neglect. Elder abuse victims are often reluctant to reveal abuse because of fear of retaliation, abandonment, or institutionalization. Therefore, a key to intervention is coordinating with appropriate social service and allied health agencies to support an elder adequately, either at home or in a care center. Such agencies include aging councils, visiting nurses, home health aids, and respite or adult day care centers. Counseling and assistance for caregivers is also an important part of intervention.

Many states require physicians to report suspected elder abuse. Because many elder abuse victims are mentally competent, however, it is important that they be made part of the decision-making and reporting process. Such collaboration puts needed control in the elder's hands and therefore facilitates healing. Many other aspects of intervention described for partner abuse apply to working with elders, including providing emotional support, assessing danger, safety planning, and documentation.

In addition to helping the victims of acute, ongoing family violence, physicians have an important role to play in helping survivors of past family violence. People who have survived family violence may continue to experience negative effects similar to those experienced by acute victims. Physicians can identify survivors of family violence by screening for past violence during routine exams. A careful history can determine whether the patient has been suffering medical or psychological problems related to the violence. Finally, the physician should identify local resources for the patient, including a mutual help group and a therapist.

Physicians can also help prevent family violence. One avenue of prevention is through education of patients by discussing partner violence with patients at key life transitions, such as during adolescence when youths begin dating, prior to marriage, during pregnancy, and during divorce or separation. A second avenue of prevention is making medical clinic waiting rooms and examination rooms into education centers by displaying educational posters and providing pamphlets.

PERSPECTIVE AND PROSPECTS

Despite its frequency, family violence has not always been viewed as a problem. In the 1800's, it was legal in the United States for a man to beat his wife, or for parents to use brutal physical punishment with children. Although the formation of the New York Society for the Prevention of Cruelty to Children in 1874 signaled rising concern about child maltreatment, the extent of the problem was underestimated. As recently as 1960, family violence was viewed as a rare, aberrant phenomenon and women who were victims of violence were often seen as partially responsible because of "masochistic tendencies." Several factors combined to turn the tide during the next thirty years. Medical research published in the early 1960's began documenting the severity of the problem of child abuse. By 1968, every state in the United States had passed a law requiring that physicians report suspected child abuse, and many states established child protective services to investigate and protect vulnerable children.

Progress in the battle against partner violence was slower. The battered women's movement brought new attention and a feminist understanding to the widespread and serious nature of partner violence. This growing awareness provided the impetus, during the 1970's and 1980's, for reform in the criminal justice system, scientific research, continued growth of women's shelters, and the development of treatment programs for offenders.

The medical profession's response to partner abuse followed these changes. In 1986, Surgeon General C. Everett Koop declared family violence to be a public health problem and called upon physicians to learn to identify and intervene with victims. In 1992, the American Medical Association (AMA) echoed the Surgeon General and stated that physicians have an ethical obligation to identify and assist victims of partner violence, and it established standards and protocols for identifying and helping victims of family violence. Because partner and elder abuse have been recognized only recently by the medical community, many physicians are just beginning to learn about their essential role.

Family violence has at various times been considered as a social problem, a legal problem, a political problem, and a medical problem. Because of this shifting understanding and because of the grassroots political origins of the child and partner violence movements, some may question why physicians should be involved. There are three compelling reasons.

First, there is a medical need: Family violence is one of the most common causes of injury, illness, and death for women and children. Victims seeking treatment for acute injuries make up a sizable portion of emergency room visits. Even in outpatient clinics, women report high rates of recent and ongoing violence and injury from partners. In addition to physical injuries, many victims experience stress-related medical problems for which they seek medical care. Among obstetrical patients who are battered, there is a risk of injury to both the woman and her unborn child. Hence, physicians working in clinics and emergency rooms will see many people who are victims.

Second, physicians have a stake in breaking the cycle of violence because they are interested in injury prevention and health promotion. When a physician treats a child or adult victim for physical or psychological injury but does not identify root causes, the victim will return to a dangerous situation. Prevention of future injury requires proper diagnosis of root causes, rather than mere treatment of symptoms.

Third, physicians have a stake in treatment of partner violence because it is a professional and ethical obligation. Two principles of medical ethics apply. First, a physician's actions should benefit the patient. Physicians can benefit patients who are suffering the effects of family violence only if they correctly recognize the root cause and intervene in a sensitive and professional manner. Physicians should also "do no harm." A physician who fails to recognize and treat partner violence will harm the patient by providing inappropriate advice and treatment.

—*L. Kevin Hamberger and Bruce Ambuel*

See also Addiction; Depression; Intoxication; Manic-depressive disorder; Paranoia; Psychiatric disorders; Psychosis; Schizophrenia; Stress.

FOR FURTHER INFORMATION:

Bass, Ellen, and Laura Davis. *The Courage to Heal: A Guide for Women Survivors of Child Sexual Abuse.* Rev. ed. New York: Harper-Perennial, 1992. A practical guide to understanding child sexual abuse for women survivors. Informative, but not intended as a substitute for professional therapy.

Island, David, and Patrick Letellier. *Men Who Beat the Men Who Love Them.* New York: Haworth Press, 1991. The first published book that tackles the issue of gay male partner violence. The authors write in a lively, straightforward manner which is easy to understand. Proposes novel ways of thinking about partner violence.

Jones, Ann, and Susan Schechter. *When Love Goes Wrong: What to Do When You Can't Do Anything Right.* New York: HarperCollins, 1992. Contains practical and useful information for women caught in controlling and abusive relationships, such as how to leave an abusive relationship.

Levine, Murray, and Adeline Levine. *Helping Children: A Social History.* New York: Oxford University Press, 1992. The Levines provide an excellent history of child maltreatment in the United States, as well as the various legal, social, and medical strategies that have been used to help abused children.

Pagelow, Mildred. *Family Violence.* New York: Praeger, 1984. One of the most comprehensive texts on family violence available. Though an academic text, it is easy to read and provides a balanced discussion of the major definitions, issues, and controversies in the field of family violence.

Straus, Murray A., Richard J. Gelles, and Suzanne K. Steinmetz. *Behind Closed Doors: Violence in the American Family.* Garden City, N.Y.: Anchor Press/Doubleday, 1980. A report of the first national survey on violence in the American family. Though many statistics are presented, they are explained in layperson's terms.

DOWN SYNDROME

SYSTEMS AFFECTED: Brain, nervous, heart

SPECIALISTS: Embryologists, geneticists, obstetricians, pediatricians

DEFINITION: A congenital abnormality characterized by moderate to severe mental retardation and a distinctive physical appearance caused by a chromosomal aberration, the result of either an error during embryonic cell division or the inheritance of defective chromosomal material.

KEY TERMS:

chromosomes: small, threadlike bodies containing the genes that are microscopically visible during cell division

gametes: the egg and sperm cells that unite to form the fertilized egg (zygote) in reproduction

gene: a segment of the DNA strand containing instructions for the production of a protein

homologous chromosomes: chromosome pairs of the same size and centromere position that possess genes for the same traits; one homologous chromosome is inherited from the father and the other from the mother

meiosis: the type of cell division that produces the cells of reproduction, which contain one-half of the chromosome number found in the original cell before division

mitosis: the type of cell division that occurs in nonsex cells, which conserves chromosome number by equal allocation to each of the newly formed cells

translocation: an aberration in chromosome structure resulting from the attachment of chromosomal material to a nonhomologous chromosome

CAUSES AND SYMPTOMS

Down syndrome is an example of a genetic disorder, that is, a disorder arising from an abnormality in an individual's genetic material. Down syndrome results from an incorrect transfer of genetic material in the formation of cells. Genetic information is contained in large "library" molecules of deoxyribonucleic acid (DNA). DNA molecules are formed by joining together units called nucleotides which come in four different varieties: adenosine, thymine, cytosine, and guanine (identified by their initials A, T, C, and G). These nucleotides store hereditary information by forming "words" with this four-letter alphabet. In a gene, a section of DNA which contains the chemical message controlling an inherited trait, three consecutive nucleotides combine to specify a particular amino acid. This word order forms the "sentences" of a recipe telling cells how to construct proteins, such as those coloring the hair and eyes, from amino acids.

In living systems, tissue growth occurs through cell-division processes in which an original cell divides to form two cells containing duplicate genetic material. Just before a cell divides, the DNA organizes itself into distinct, compact bundles called chromosomes. Normal human cells, diploid cells, contain twenty-three pairs (or a total of forty-six) of these chromosomes. Each pair is a set of homologues containing genes for the same traits. These chromosomes are composed of two DNA strands, chromatids, joined at a constricted region known as the centromere. The bundle is similar in shape to the letter *X*. The arms are the parts above and below the constriction, which may be centered or offset toward one end (giving arms of equal or different lengths, respectively). During mitosis, the division of nonsex cells, the chromatids separate at the centromere, forming two sets of single-stranded chromosomes, which migrate to opposite ends of the cell. The cell then splits into two genetically equivalent cells, each containing twenty-three single-stranded chromosomes that will duplicate to form the original number of forty-six chromosomes.

In sexual reproduction, haploid egg and sperm cells, each containing twenty-three single-stranded chromosomes, unite in fertilization to produce a zygote cell with forty-six chromosomes. Haploid cells are created through a different, two-step cell-division process termed meiosis. Meiosis begins when the homologues in a diploid cell pair up at the equator of the cell. The attractions between the members of each pair then break, allowing the homologues to migrate to opposite ends of the cell, each twin to a different pole, without splitting at the centromere. The parent cell then divides once to give two cells containing twenty-three double-stranded chromosomes, and then divides again through the process of mitosis to form cells that contain only twenty-three single-stranded chromosomes. Thus, each cell contains half of the original chromosomes.

Although cell division is normally a precise process, occasionally an error called nondisjunction occurs when a chromosome either fails to separate or fails to migrate to the proper pole. In meiosis, the failure to move to the proper pole results in the formation of one gamete having twenty-four chromosomes and one having twenty-two chromosomes. Upon fertilization, zygotes of forty-seven or forty-five chromosomes are produced, and the developing embryo must function with either extra or missing genes. Since every chromosome contains a multitude of genes, problems result from the absence or excess of proteins produced. In fact, the embryos formed from most nondisjunctional fertilizations die at an early stage in development and are spontaneously aborted. Occasionally, nondisjunction occurs in mitosis, when a chromosome migrates before the chromatids separate, yielding one cell with an extra copy of the chromosome and no copy in the other cell.

Down syndrome is also termed trisomy 21 because it most commonly results from the presence of an extra copy of the smallest human chromosome, chromosome 21. Actually, it is not the entire extra chromosome 21 that is responsible, but rather a small segment of the long arm of this chromosome. Only two other trisomies occur with any significant frequency: trisomy 13 (Patau's syndrome) and trisomy 18 (Edwards' syndrome). Both of these disorders are accompanied by multiple severe malformations, resulting in death within a few months of birth. Most incidences of Down syndrome are a consequence of a nondisjunction during meiosis. In about 75 percent of these cases, the extra chromosome is present in the egg. About 1 percent of Down syndrome cases occur after the fertilization of normal gametes from a mitosis nondisjunction, producing a mosaic in which some of the embryo's cells are normal and some exhibit trisomy. The degree of mosaicism and its location will determine the physiological consequences of the nondisjunction. Although mosaic individuals range from apparent normality to completely affected, typically the disorder is less severe.

In about 4 percent of all Down syndrome cases, the individual possesses not an entire third copy of chromosome 21 but rather extra chromosome 21 material, which has been incorporated via a translocation into a nonhomologous chromosome. In translocation, pieces of arms are swapped between two nonrelated chromosomes, forming "hybrid" chromosomes. The most common translocation associated with Down syndrome is that between the long arm (Down gene area) of chromosome 21 and an end of chromosome 14. The individual in whom the translocation has occurred shows no evidence of the aberration, since the normal complement of genetic material is still present, only at different chromosomal locations. The difficulty arises when this individual forms gametes. A mother who possesses the 21/14 translocation, for example, has one normal 21, one normal 14, and the hybrid chromosomes. She is a genetic carrier for the disorder, because she can pass it on to her offspring even though she is clinically normal. This mother could produce three types of viable gametes: one containing the normal 14 and 21; one containing both translocations, which would result in clinical normality; and one containing the normal 21 and the translocated 14 having the long arm of 21. If each gamete were fertilized by normal sperm, two apparently normal embryos and one partial trisomy 21 Down syndrome embryo would result. Down syndrome that results from the passing on of translocations is termed familial Down syndrome and is an inherited disorder.

The presence of an extra copy of the long arm of chromosome 21 causes defects in many tissues and organs. One major effect of Down syndrome is mental retardation. The intelligence quotients (IQs) of affected individuals are typically in the range of 40-50. The IQ varies with age, being higher in childhood than in adolescence or adult life. The disorder is often accompanied by physical traits such as short stature, stubby fingers and toes, protruding tongue, and an unusual pattern of hand creases. Perhaps the most recognized physical feature is the distinctive slanting of the eyes, caused by a vertical fold (epicanthal fold) of skin near the nasal bridge which pulls and tilts the eyes slightly toward the nostrils. For normal Caucasians, the eye runs parallel to the skin fold below the eyebrow; for Asians, this skin fold covers a major portion of the upper eyelid. In contrast, the epicanthal fold in trisomy 21 does not cover a major part of the upper eyelid.

It should be noted that not all defects associated with Down syndrome are found in every affected individual. About 40 percent of Down syndrome patients have congenital heart defects, while about 10 percent have intestinal blockages. Affected individuals are prone to respiratory infections and contract leukemia at a rate twenty times that of the general population. Although Down syndrome children develop the same types of leukemia in the same proportions as other children, the survival rate of the two groups is markedly different. While the survival rate for non-Down-syndrome patients after ten years is about 30 percent, survival beyond five years is negligible in Down

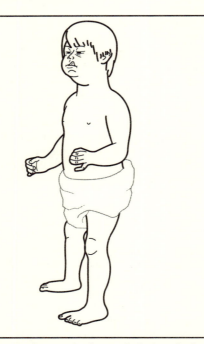

Down syndrome is characterized not only by impaired mental ability but also by a complex of physical traits that may include short stature, stubby fingers and toes, protruding tongue, a single transverse palm crease, slanting of the eyes, small nose and ears, abnormal finger orientation, congenital heart defects, and other defects that vary from individual to individual.

syndrome patients. It appears that the extra copy of chromosome 21 not only increases the risk of contracting the cancer but also exerts a decisive influence on the disease's outcome. Reproductively, males are sterile while some females are fertile. Although many Down syndrome infants die in the first year of life, the mean life expectancy is about thirty years. This reduced life expectancy results from defects in the immune system, causing a high susceptibility to infectious disease. Most older Down syndrome individuals develop an Alzheimer's-like condition, and less than 3 percent live beyond fifty years of age.

TREATMENT AND THERAPY

Trisomy 21 is one of the most common human chromosomal aberrations, occurring in about 0.5 percent of all conceptions and in one out of every seven hundred to eight hundred live births. About 15 percent of the patients institutionalized for mental deficiency suffer from Down syndrome.

Even before the chromosomal basis for the disorder was determined, the frequency of Down syndrome births was correlated with increased maternal age. For mothers at age twenty, the incidence of Down syndrome is about 0.05 percent, which increases to 0.9 percent by age thirty-five and

3 percent for age forty-five. Studies comparing the chromosomes of the affected offspring with both parents have shown that the nondisjunction event is maternal about 75 percent of the time. This maternal age effect is thought to result from the different manner in which the male and female gametes are produced. Gamete production in the male is a continual, lifelong process, while it is a one-time event in females. Formation of the female's gametes begins early in embryonic life, somewhere between the eighth and twentieth weeks. During this time, cells in the developing ovary divide rapidly by mitosis, forming cells called primary oocytes. These cells then begin meiosis by pairing up the homologues. The process is interrupted at this point, and the cells are held in a state of suspended animation until needed in reproduction, when they are triggered to complete their division and form eggs. It appears that the frequency of nondisjunction events increases with the length of the storage period. Studies have demonstrated that cells in a state of meiosis are particularly sensitive to environmental influences such as viruses, X rays, and cytotoxic chemicals. It is possible that environmental influences may play a role in nondisjunction events. Up to age thirty-two, males contribute an extra chromosome 21 as often as do females. Beyond this age, there is a rapid increase in nondisjunctional eggs, while the number of nondisjunctional sperm remains constant. Where the maternal age effect is minimal, mosaicism may be an important source of the trisomy. An apparently normal mother who possesses undetected mosaicism can produce trisomy offspring if gametes with an extra chromosome are produced. In some instances, characteristics such as abnormal fingerprint patterns have been observed in the mothers and their Down-syndrome offspring.

Techniques such as amniocentesis, chorionic villus sampling, and alpha-fetoprotein screening are available for prenatal diagnosis of Down syndrome in fetuses. Amniocentesis, the most widely used technique for prenatal diagnosis, is generally performed between the fourteenth and sixteenth weeks of pregnancy. In this technique, about one ounce of fluid is removed from the amniotic cavity surrounding the fetus by a needle inserted through the mother's abdomen. Although some testing can be done directly on the fluid (such as the assay for spina bifida), more information is obtained from the cells shed from the fetus that accompany the fluid. The mixture obtained in the amniocentesis is spun in a centrifuge to separate the fluid from the fetal cells. Unfortunately, the chromosome analysis for Down syndrome cannot be conducted directly on the amount of cellular material obtained. Although the majority of the cells collected are nonviable, some will grow in culture. These cells are allowed to grow and multiply in culture for two to four weeks, and then the chromosomes undergo karyotyping, which will detect both trisomy 21 and translocational aberration.

In karyotyping, the chromosomes are spread on a microscope slide, stained, and photographed. Each type of chromosome gives a unique, observable banding pattern when stained which allows it to be identified. The chromosomes are then cut out of the photograph and arranged in homologous pairs, in numerical order. Trisomy 21 is easily observed, since three copies of chromosome 21 are present, while the translocation shows up as an abnormal banding pattern. Termination of the pregnancy in the wake of an unfavorable amniocentesis diagnosis is complicated, because the fetus at this point is usually about eighteen to twenty weeks old, and elective abortions are normally performed between the sixth and twelfth weeks of pregnancy. Earlier sampling of the amniotic fluid is not possible because of the small amount of fluid present.

An alternate testing procedure called chorionic villus sampling became available in the mid-1980's. In this procedure, a chromosomal analysis is conducted on a piece of placental tissue that is obtained either vaginally or through the abdomen during the eighth to eleventh week of pregnancy. The advantages of this procedure are that it can be done much earlier in the pregnancy and that enough tissue can be collected to conduct the chromosome analysis immediately, without the cell culture step. Consequently, diagnosis can be completed during the first trimester of the pregnancy, making therapeutic abortion an option for the parents. Chorionic villus sampling does have some negative aspects. One disadvantage is the slightly higher incidence of test-induced miscarriage as compared to amniocentesis—around 1 percent (versus less than 0.5 percent). Also, because tissue of both the mother and the fetus are obtained in the sampling process, they must be carefully separated, complicating the analysis. Occasionally, chromosomal abnormalities are observed in the tested tissue that are not present in the fetus itself.

Prenatal maternal alpha-fetoprotein testing has also been used to diagnose Down syndrome. Abnormal levels of a substance called maternal alpha-fetoprotein are often associated with chromosomal disorders. Several research studies have described a high correlation between low levels of maternal alpha-fetoprotein and the occurrence of trisomy 21 in the fetus. By correlating alpha-fetoprotein levels, the age of the mother, and specific female hormone levels, between 60 percent and 80 percent of fetuses with Down syndrome can be detected. Although techniques allow Down syndrome to be detected readily in a fetus, there is no effective intrauterine therapy available to correct the abnormality.

The care of a Down syndrome child presents many challenges for the family unit. Until the 1970's, most of these children spent their lives in institutions. With the increased support services available, however, it is now common for such children to remain in the family environment. Although many Down syndrome children have happy dispositions, a significant number have behavioral problems that can consume the energies of the parents, to the detriment of the other children. Rearing a Down syndrome child often places a large financial burden on the family: Such children are, for example, susceptible to illness; they also have special educational needs. Since Down syndrome children are often conceived late in the parents' reproductive period, the parents may not be able to continue to care for these children throughout their offspring's adult years. This is problematic because many Down syndrome individuals do not possess sufficient mental skills to earn a living or to manage their affairs without supervision.

All women in their mid-thirties have an increased risk of producing a Down syndrome infant. Since the resultant trisomy 21 is not of a hereditary nature, the abnormality can be detected only by the prenatal screening, which is recommended for all pregnancies of women older than age thirty-four.

For parents who have produced a Down syndrome child, genetic counseling can be beneficial in determining their risk factor for future pregnancies. The genetic counselor determines the specific chromosomal aberration that occurred utilizing chromosome studies of the parents and affected child, along with additional information provided by the family history. If the cause was nondisjunction and the mother is young, the recurrence risk is much less than 1 percent; for mothers over the age of thirty-four, it is about 5 percent. If the cause was translocational, the Down syndrome is hereditary and risk is much greater—statistically, a one-in-three chance. In addition, there is a one-in-three chance that clinically normal offspring will be carriers of the syndrome, producing it in the next generation. For couples who come from families having a history of spontaneous abortions, which often result from lethal chromosomal aberrations and/or incidence of Down syndrome, it is suggested that they undergo chromosomal screening to detect the presence of a Down syndrome translocation.

PERSPECTIVE AND PROSPECTS

English physician John L. H. Down is credited with the first clinical description of Down syndrome, in 1886. Since the distinctive epicanthic fold gave Down children an appearance that John Down associated with Asians, he termed the condition "mongolism"—an unfortunate term showing a certain racism on Down's part, since it implies that those affected with the condition are throwbacks to a more "primitive" racial group. Today, the inappropriate term has been replaced with the term "Down syndrome."

A French physician, Jérôme Lejeune, suspected that Down syndrome had a genetic basis and began to study the condition in 1953. A comparison of the fingerprints and palm prints of affected individuals with those of unaffected individuals showed a high frequency of abnormalities in the prints of those with Down syndrome. These prints are developed very early in development and serve as a record of events that take place early in embryogenesis. The extent of the changes in print patterns led Lejeune to the conclusion that the condition was not a result of the action of one or two genes but rather of many genes or even an entire chromosome. Upon microscopic examination, he observed that Down syndrome children possess forty-seven chromosomes instead of the forty-six chromosomes found in normal children. In 1959, Lejeune published his findings, showing that Down syndrome is caused by the presence of an extra chromosome which was later identified as an extra copy of chromosome 21. This first observation of a human chromosomal abnormality marked a turning point in the study of human genetics. It demonstrated that genetic defects not only were caused by mutations of single genes but also could be associated with changes in chromosome number. Although the presence of an extra chromosome allows varying degrees of development to occur, most of these abnormalities result in fetal death, with only a few resulting in live birth. Down syndrome is unusual in that the affected individual often survives into adulthood.

—*Arlene R. Courtney*

See also Genetic diseases; Mental retardation.

FOR FURTHER INFORMATION:

Blatt, Robin J. R. *Prenatal Tests.* New York: Vintage Books, 1988. Discusses tests available for prenatal screening, their benefits, the risk factors of the tests, and how to decide whether to have prenatal testing.

Ford, E. H. R. *Human Chromosomes.* New York: Academic Press, 1973. A complete treatise discussing all aspects of human chromosomes, including what they look like, their composition, how they are studied, how they function, and the effects of chromosomal abnormalities.

Holtzman, Neil A. *Proceed with Caution: Predicting Genetic Risks in the Recombinant DNA Era.* Baltimore: The Johns Hopkins University Press, 1989. Discusses genetic counseling, how genetic disorders are diagnosed, and social implications.

Nyhan, William L. *The Heredity Factor: Genes, Chromosomes, and You.* New York: Grosset & Dunlap, 1976. Provides a good introduction to the field of medical genetics. Discusses chromosomal disease and how chromosomes are analyzed.

Pueschel, Siegfried. *A Parent's Guide to Down Syndrome.* Baltimore: Paul H. Brookes, 1990. An informative guide highlighting the important developmental stages in the life of a child with Down syndrome.

Tingey, Carol, ed. *Down Syndrome: A Resource Handbook.* Boston: Little, Brown, 1988. A practical resource for rearing a Down syndrome child, including guidelines on daily life, developmental expectations, and health and medical needs.

DRUG ADDICTION. *See* ADDICTION.

DWARFISM

SYSTEMS AFFECTED: Endocrine, muscular, skeletal, brain

SPECIALISTS: Endocrinologists, geneticists, orthopedists

DEFINITION: Underdevelopment of the body, most often caused by a variety of genetic or endocrinological dysfunctions and resulting in either proportionate or disproportionate development, sometimes accompanied by other physical abnormalities and/or mental deficiencies.

KEY TERMS:

amino acid: the building blocks of protein

autosomal: refers to all chromosomes except the X and Y chromosomes (sex chromosomes) that determine body traits

cleft palate: a gap in the roof of the mouth, sometimes present at birth and frequently combined with harelip

collagen: protein material of which the white fibers of the connective tissue of the body are composed

hypoglycemia: low blood sugar

laminae: arches of the vertebral bones

spondylosis: a condition characterized by restriction of movement of the vertebral bones; occurs naturally as a child grows

stenosis: any narrowing of a passage or orifice of the body

CAUSES AND SYMPTOMS

A person of unusually small stature is generally termed a "dwarf." Dwarfism in humans may be caused by a number of conditions that occur either before birth or in early childhood. When short stature is the only observable feature, growth—though abnormal relative to height—is proportionate. Short stature is nearly always blamed on endocrinological dysfunction, but few cases are actually the result of endocrinopathy. If shortness is caused by endocrinopathy, it is often attributable to a deficiency in one or two glands: the pituitary gland (which produces growth hormone) and the thyroid gland. Those who are unusually short but have no other obvious disease are divided into two categories: those who were afflicted prenatally and those who were afflicted postnatally. Many of those born "growth-retarded" are actually the result of chromosomal aberrations and skeletal abnormalities; other events that may cause prenatal growth retardation might include magnesium deficiency (which would prohibit ribosome synthesis and, in turn, halt protein synthesis) or a uterus that is too small. Postnatal growth retardation may be caused by heredity if both parents are short; there is no skeletal abnormality at fault. Other short-statured children may simply mature at a much slower rate, yet grow normally. Typically, one of the parents may have had a late onset of puberty; such children may reach normal height in their late teens.

Unusually short-statured males are those who are shorter than five feet tall; in females, fifty-eight inches and below is short-statured. Children are classified as dwarfs if their height is below the third percentile for their age. When this is the case, doctors will look primarily to four major causes of dwarfism: an underactive or inactive pituitary gland, achondroplasia (failure of normal development in cartilage), emotional or nutritional deprivation, or Turner's syndrome (the possession of a single, X chromosome). If the answer is not found in one of these alternatives, then it may be found in rarer causes, either genetically based or disease-induced.

Growth hormone, also called somatotropin, determines a person's height. Growth hormone does not affect brain growth but may influence the brain's functions. In addition, it may enhance the growth of nerves radiating from the brain so that they can reach their targets. Growth hormone elevates the appetite, increases metabolic rate, maintains the immune system, and works in coordination with other hormones to regulate carbohydrate, protein, lipid, nucleic acid, water, and electrolyte metabolism. Target areas for growth hormone include cell membranes, as well as other cell organelles, in bone, cartilage, bone marrow, adipose tissue, and the liver, kidney, heart, pancreas, mammary glands, ovaries, testes, thymus gland, and hypothalamus. Fetuses not producing growth hormone still grow normally until birth; they may even weigh more than average at birth. The baby may thrive at first, but if no growth hormone is administered, they will be "miniature" adults with a maximum height of two and one-half feet. Other telltale physical attributes include higher-than-average body fat, a high forehead, wrinkled skin, and a high-pitched voice. During childhood, there may be episodic hypoglycemia attacks. If the endocrine system is functioning properly, puberty may be delayed but still will occur. Complete reproductive maturity will be reached, and there is great likelihood that the afflicted person will develop his or her complete intellectual potential. When it is inherited, growth hormone deficiency occurs as an autosomal recessive trait. Yet the genetic basis for growth hormone deficiency may not simply be caused by a gene. The condition could, in theory, be the result of a structural defect in the pituitary gland or the hypothalamus, or in the secretory mechanisms of growth hormone itself.

Prenatal thyroid dysfunction that goes untreated results in cretinism. Cretins do not undergo nervous, skeletal, or reproductive maturation; they may not grow over thirty inches tall. Before two months of age, treatment can cause a complete reversal of symptoms. Delayed treatment, however, cannot reverse brain damage, although growth and reproductive organs can be dramatically affected.

Achondroplasia is inherited as an autosomal dominant form of short-limb dwarfism. Only when one dominant gene is inherited is achondroplasia expressed; when an offspring inherits the dominant gene from both parents, the condition is lethal. Incidence of achondroplasia increases with parental age and is more closely related to the father's age. Mutations may account for a majority of cases of achondroplasia, since in only 15 to 20 percent of cases is there an afflicted parent. Achondroplasia results from abnormal embryonic

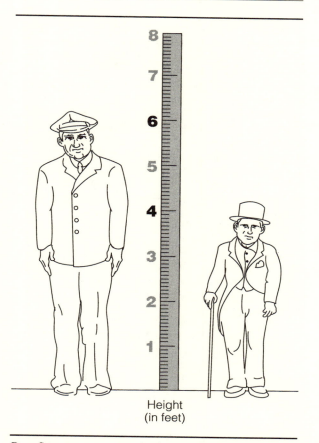

Height
(in feet)

Dwarfism occurs as a result of endocrine dysfunction; generally, adult males are classified as dwarfs if less than five feet tall, females if less than fifty-eight inches tall. Dwarfism may result simply in short stature or in a complex of other physical features such as skeletal abnormalities and reproductive difficulties.

development that affects bone growth; metaphyseal development is prevented, which means that cartilaginous bone growth is impaired. This impairment is accompanied by unusually small laminae of the spine, resulting in spinal stenosis. The spinal cord may become compressed during the normal process of spondylosis. These individuals may experience slowly progressing spastic weakness of the legs as a result of the spinal cord compression. The torso may be normal, but the head will be disproportionately large and the limbs may be dwarfed and curved. In addition, there will be a prominent forehead and a depressed nasal bridge. A shallow thoracic cage and pelvic tilt may cause a protuberant abdomen. Bowlegs are caused by overly long fibulae. Many infants so affected are stillborn. Those surviving to adulthood are typically three feet to five feet tall and have unusual muscular strength; reproductive and mental development are not affected, and neither is longevity.

Marasmus, severe emaciation resulting form malnutrition prenatally or in early infancy, may be considered a form of dwarfism. It is caused by extremely low caloric and protein intake, which causes a wasting of body tissues. Usually marasmus is found in babies either weaned very early or never breastfed. All growth is retarded, including head circumference. If the area housing the brain fails to grow, then it cannot house a normal-sized brain, and some degree of retardation will occur. Not only is growth stunted, but such infants will be apathetic and hyperirritable as well. As they lie in bed, they are completely unresponsive to their environment and are irritable when moved or handled. Although the symptoms are treatable and may disappear, the growth failure is permanent.

Occasionally, dwarfism may be induced by emotional starvation. This type of child abuse causes extreme growth retardation, inhibition of skeletal growth, and delayed psychomotor development. Fortunately, it can be reversed by social and dietary changes. These children are extremely small but perfectly proportioned; however, they have a distended abdomen.

The height achieved in females with Turner's syndrome is typically between four and one-half and five feet. Turner's syndrome results when an egg has no X chromosome and is fertilized by an X-bearing sperm. The offspring are females with only one X; their ovaries never develop and are unable to function. These individuals cannot undergo puberty; physical manifestations of Turner's syndrome include short stature, stocky build, and a webbed neck.

Another cause of short stature may be as a consequence of chronic disease. Children suffering from chronic renal (kidney) failure nearly always experience growth retardation because of hormonal, metabolic, and nutritional abnormalities, effects seen in 35 to 65 percent of children with renal failure. The failure to grow occurs more often in children with congenital renal disease than in those with acquired renal disease.

With congenital heart disease, several factors may prohibit growth. Growth failure may be a direct result of the disease or an indirect result of other problems associated with heart disease. These babies experience stress, with periods of cardiac failure, and either caloric or protein deficiency. These inadequacies grossly slow the multiplication of cells and hence growth. If surgery corrects the condition, some catching up can be expected, but normal growth is dependent on how much time has elapsed without treatment.

TREATMENT AND THERAPY

In the United States population in 1992, there were roughly five million people of short stature, with 40 percent of this number under the age of twenty-one. The more a child is below the average stature, the greater is the likelihood of determining the cause. A child who is short-statured should be evaluated so that, if an endocrine disorder is the root, the child can be treated. Time is an important consideration with hypothyroidism especially, since the longer it goes untreated, the more likely it is that mental development will be arrested.

Children born with congenital growth-hormone deficiency are sometimes small for their gestational age; however, the majority of growth-hormone-deficient children acquire the disorder after birth. The first year or two, the children grow normally; then growth dramatically decreases. Diagnosis of growth-hormone deficiency requires numerous tests and sampling. If bone age appears the same as the child's age, then growth-hormone deficiency can be eliminated. A test for normal growth-hormone secretion is done by measuring a blood sample for growth hormone twenty minutes after exercise in a fasting child. If this test shows a hormone deficiency, then growth-hormone therapy may help the child overcome the obstacles of being labeled "short."

At first, growth hormone was harvested from human pituitary glands after a person's death. This process was so expensive, however, that few children with hormone deficiency could be treated. Even worse, some of those who did get this treatment were inadvertently infected with a slow-acting, virus that proved fatal. In the mid-1980's, it was found that some men who had received human growth hormone died at an early age of a neurological disorder called Creutzfeldt-Jakob disease (CJD). These men were found to have been given the disease via a growth hormone that had been obtained from pituitary glands during autopsies. Once the relationship was determined, more victims were traced. CJD is a nervous disorder caused by a slow-acting, viruslike particle. Its symptoms include difficulty in balance while walking, loss of muscular control, slurred speech, impairment of vision, and other muscular disorders including spasticity and rigidity. Behavioral changes and mental incapacities may also occur (memory loss, confusion, dementia). The symptoms appear, progress rapidly over the next months, and usually cause death in less than a year. There is no treatment or cure.

These unfortunate circumstances led to the development of a synthetic growth hormone. It is made by encoding bacterial deoxyribonucleic acid (DNA) with the sequence of human growth hormone; the bacteria used are those that grow normally in the human intestinal tract. The bacteria synthesize human growth hormone using the preprogrammed human sequence of DNA; it is then purified so that no bacteria remain in the hormone that is used for treatment. The Food and Drug Administration (FDA) approved the biosynthetic hormone in 1985. The sole difference in the synthetic and the naturally produced growth hormone was one amino acid; in 1987, a new synthetic form without the extra amino acid became available. This synthetic hormone works exactly as natural growth hormone does. Moreover, it does not carry the danger of contamination attributed to human growth hormone. In most cases, the patient's immune system fails to interfere with the synthetic growth hormone's effectiveness. In fact, no major health-threatening side effects have surfaced in using artificial growth hormone. In 1992, there were more than 150,000 growth-hormone-deficient children in the United States receiving growth-hormone therapy.

Those children suffering from various forms of chondrodystrophies (cartilage disorders), such as achondroplasia, are diagnosed by using skeletal measurements, clinical manifestations, X rays, laboratory study and analysis of cartilage, and observed abnormalities of the body's proteins, such as collagen and cell membranes. In chondrodystrophies, skeletal growth is disproportionate, with shortened limbs more common than a shortened trunk. If visual examination is not confirmation enough, the diagnosis may be assured through X rays. Although histological studies do not necessarily enhance diagnosis, making an analysis of the patient's cartilage may lead to a better understanding of the disease. Biochemical studies of abnormal proteins in chondrodystrophies actually have little diagnostic value, but they too may lead to better understanding. Because achondroplasia is genetically inherited, prevention of the affliction involves genetic counseling before conception.

A child so affected may be treated symptomatically; surgery on the fibulae to correct bowlegs may be desirable, either for cosmetic reasons or for functional reasons. Laminectomies or skull surgery may be indicated for neurological problems. If hearing loss occurs because of recurrent ear infections, then corrective surgery may be necessary. Achondroplasiacs generally enjoy a normal life span, barring complications to symptoms.

Other chondrodystrophies that cause dwarfism may have more severe symptoms than achondroplasia. Cockayne syndrome, a type of progeria, is the sudden onset of premature old age in extremely young children. It is the result of inheritance of an autosomal recessive gene. Physical signs of the disease begin after a normal first year of life. In the second year, growth begins to falter, and psychomotor development becomes abnormal. As time passes, dwarfism, and sometimes mental retardation, becomes evident. Other observable characteristics that develop are a shrunken face with sunken eyes and a thin nose, optic degeneration, cavities of the teeth, a photosensitive skin rash that produces scarring, disproportionately long limbs with large hands and feet, and hair loss. The life span for children with this disease is very short.

Another chondrodystrophy inherited through autosomal recessive genes is thanotophoric dwarfism. All known cases have died during the first four weeks of life as a result of respiratory distress; most are stillborn. Postnatal death occurs as a result of an extremely small thoracic cage with only eleven pairs of ribs present. Other physical characteristics of the disease are that the infant has a large skull relative to its face, which is often elongated with a prominent forehead. The eyes are widely spaced, and there is a broad, flat nasal bridge. Frequently, cleft palate is present. The ears are low-set and poorly formed, and the neck is short and fleshy. The limbs, particularly the legs, are bowed; clubfoot is common, as are dislocated hip joints.

A small percentage of short-statured individuals may be unusually short because of social and psychological factors. This condition is called psychosocial dwarfism. This type of nongrowth is secondary to emotional deprivation and is representative of a type of child abuse. The behavior of such children is characterized by apathy and inadequate interpersonal relationships, with retarded motor and language development. They generally do not gain weight in spite of their extraordinary appetite and excessive thirst; they may steal and hoard food yet have the distended abdomen of a starving child. Diagnosis generally identifies a growth-hormone deficiency, and when these children are moved to stimulating and accepting environments, their behavior becomes more normal. Their caloric intake decreases as their growth-hormone secretion becomes normal and their growth undergoes a dramatic catch-up.

PERSPECTIVE AND PROSPECTS

Dwarfism is certainly not a new phenomenon. Two well-known Egyptian deities, Bes and Ptah, are represented as dwarfs. At one time, short-statured individuals were an attraction in the royal courts. Jeffery Hudson, a favorite of Charles I of England, is said to have been only eighteen inches high at the age of thirty; and Bébé, the celebrated dwarf in the court of Stanisław I of Poland, was thirty-three inches tall. More recently, perfectly proportioned dwarfs have made a living by working in circuses and sideshows. It is likely that the best known of these individuals was P. T. Barnum's General Tom Thumb (Charles Stratton), who at twenty-five was thirty-one inches tall.

Today, because of the negative consequences afforded the short-statured, counseling should begin early if treatment is not feasible. Counseling would begin with a physical examination to determine the nature of the affliction. If it is ascertained that the short stature cannot be treated, both patient and parents should be informed of the nature of the disease. The patient should be assured that intelligence will not be affected, even if the head is somewhat large. Ear infections are common, and the child should be closely watched to avoid hearing loss. Normal fertility is the rule, but giving birth will necessitate a cesarean section. These characteristics of a majority of dwarfism cases should assure families that, as the child matures, he or she will not be limited physically or mentally. The problems that the patients may face usually deal with social and emotional consequences. Short-statured children will usually be thought younger than their age; finding appropriate clothes and shoes may be difficult. Children are often cruel, and as afflicted individuals are highly noticeable, they may be the butt of jokes and teasing and will experience discrimination on many fronts. Seeking affiliation with support groups may aid in coping with the difficulties that a short-statured person will undoubtedly meet.

The rate at which those diagnosed with dwarfism develop psychologically is directly related to two components: if their parents treat them according to their age rather than their size, and if they can cope with the notoriety that their size brings them. It is common for such children to lag in development; personality traits often exhibited with delayed maturation are withdrawal, inhibition, dissociation, and learning problems. There have been no observed tendencies toward aggression or acting out. Inhibition and withdrawal are likely if affected children are appalled by their notoriety; if they use it to measure popularity, they may act the clown to minimize their size difference.

—*Iona C. Baldridge*

See also Congenital heart disease; Endocrine disorders; Gigantism; Growth.

FOR FURTHER INFORMATION:

Bergsma, Daniel, ed. *Birth Defects: Atlas and Compendium*. Baltimore: Williams & Wilkins, 1973. This large volume includes a section of photographs of birth defects, followed by alphabetical descriptions of hundreds of such defects. Such important information as genetic likelihood, complications, treatment, and prognosis is included by Bergsma, an authority on types of dwarfism.

Cheek, Donald B. *Human Growth*. Philadelphia: Lea & Febiger, 1968. Every aspect of growth, including physiology, biochemistry, and psychology, is covered in this volume. More information is accorded growth-retarded children than those undergoing normal growth or overgrowth. Each chapter ends with an extensive bibliography.

Kelly, Thaddeus E. *Clinical Genetics and Genetic Counseling*. 2d ed. Chicago: Year Book Medical Publishers, 1986. This text of genetic disorders and their treatment was written to aid medical students and physicians. Aside from the sometimes difficult medical terminology, the case illustrations and discussions of genetic counseling are interesting.

Martin, Constance R. *Endocrine Physiology*. New York: Oxford University Press, 1985. This textbook covers virtually every aspect of endocrinology, gland by gland. Human physiology is emphasized, and the topics should be comprehensible to students with a basic background in animal physiology. Some knowledge in biochemistry is useful.

Morgan, Brian L. G., and Roberta Morgan. *Hormones*. Los Angeles: Body Press, 1989. A book written for use by the general reader as a resource for hormones and their roles in the human body. Very readable, it also contains sections about hormonal diseases and includes a bibliography.

DYSENTERY. *See* DIARRHEA AND DYSENTERY.

DYSLEXIA

SYSTEMS AFFECTED: Auditory, brain, psychic-emotional, visual

SPECIALISTS: Child psychiatrists, neurologists, psychologists, speech pathologists

DEFINITION: Severe reading disability in children with average to above-average intelligence.

KEY TERMS:

auditory dyslexia: the inability to perceive individual sounds that are associated with written language

cognitive: relating to the mental process by which knowledge is acquired

computed tomography (CT) scan: a detailed X-ray picture that identifies abnormalities of fine tissue structure

dysgraphia: illegible handwriting resulting from impaired hand-eye coordination

electroencephalogram: a graphic record of the brain's electrical activity

imprinting: training that overcomes reading problems by use of repeated, exaggerated language drills

kinesthetic: related to sensation of body position, presence, or movement, resulting mostly from the stimulation of sensory nerves in muscles, tendons, and joints

phonetics: the science of speech sounds; also called phonology

visual dyslexia: the inability to translate observed written or printed language into meaningful terms

CAUSES AND SYMPTOMS

Nearly 25 percent of the individuals in the United States and of many other industrialized societies who otherwise possess at least average intelligence cannot read well. Many such people are viewed as suffering from a neurological disorder called dyslexia. This term was first introduced by the German ophthalmologist Rudolf Berlin in the nineteenth century. Berlin defined it as designating all those individuals who possessed average or above-average intelligence quotients (IQs) but who could not read adequately because of their inability to process language symbols. At the same time as Berlin and later, others reported on dyslexic children. These children saw everything perfectly well but acted as if they were blind to all written language. For example, they could see a bird flying but were unable to identify the written word "bird" seen in a sentence.

The problem involved in dyslexia has been defined and redefined many times, since its introduction. The modern definition of the disorder, which is close to Berlin's definition, is based on long-term, extensive studies of dyslexic children. These studies have identified dyslexia as a complex syndrome composed of a large number of associated behavioral dysfunctions that are related to visual-motor brain immaturity and/or brain dysfunction. These problems include a poor memory for details, easy distractibility, poor motor skills, visual letter and word reversal, and the inability to distinguish between important elements of the spoken language.

Understanding dyslexia in order to correct this reading disability is crucial and difficult. To learn to read well, an individual must acquire many basic cognitive and linguistic skills. First, it is necessary to pay close attention, to concentrate, to follow directions, and to understand the language spoken in daily life. Next, one must develop an auditory and visual memory, strong sequencing ability, solid word decoding skills, the ability to carry out structural-contextual language analysis, the capability to interpret the written language, a solid vocabulary which expands as quickly as is needed, and speed in scanning and interpreting written language. These skills are taught in good developmental reading programs, but some or all are found to be deficient in dyslexic individuals.

Two basic explanations have evolved for dyslexia. Many physicians propose that it is caused by brain damage or brain dysfunction. Evolution of the problem is attributed to accident, disease, and/or hereditary faults in body biochemistry. Here, the diagnosis of dyslexia is made by the use of electroencephalograms (EEGs), computed tomography (CT) scans, and related neurological technology. After such evaluation is complete, medication is often used to diminish hyperactivity and nervousness, and a group of physical training procedures called patterning is used to counter the neurological defects in the dyslexic individual.

In contrast, many special educators and other researchers believe that the problem of dyslexia is one of dormant, immature, or undeveloped learning centers in the brain. Many proponents of this concept strongly encourage the correction of dyslexic problems by the teaching of specific reading skills. While such experts agree that the use of medication can be of great value, they attempt to cure dyslexia mostly through a process called imprinting. This technique essentially trains dyslexic individuals and corrects their problems via the use of exaggerated, repeated language drills.

Another interesting point of view, expressed by some experts, is the idea that dyslexia may be the fault of the written languages of the Western world. For example, Rudolf F. Wagner notes that Japanese children exhibit an incidence of dyslexia that is less than 1 percent. The explanation for this, say Wagner and others, is that unlike Japanese, the languages of Western countries require both reading from right to left and phonetic word attack. These characteristics—absent in Japanese—may make the Western languages either much harder to learn or much less suitable for learning.

A number of experts propose three types of dyslexia. The most common type and the one most often identified as dyslexia is called visual dyslexia, the lack of ability to translate the observed written or printed language into meaningful terms. The major difficulty is that afflicted people see certain words or letters backward or upside down. The resultant problem is that—to the visual dyslexic—any written

b   d

p   q

on   no

Dyslexia may make it difficult to distinguish letters and words that are mirror images of each other, thus making it difficult for an otherwise intelligent child to learn to read.

sentence is a jumble of many letters whose accurate translation may require five or more times as much effort as is needed by an unafflicted person. The other two problems viewed as dyslexia are auditory dyslexia and dysgraphia. Auditory dyslexia is the inability to perceive individual sounds of spoken language. Despite having normal hearing, auditory dyslexics are deaf to the differences between certain vowel and/or consonant sounds, and what they cannot hear they cannot write. Dysgraphia is the inability to write legibly. The basis for this problem is a lack of the hand-eye coordination that is required to write clearly.

Many children who suffer from visual dyslexia also exhibit elements of auditory dyslexia. This complicates the issue of teaching many dyslexic students because only one type of dyslexic symptom can be treated at a time. Also, dyslexia appears to be a sex-linked disorder, being much more common in boys than in girls. Estimates vary between three and seven times as many boys having dyslexia as girls.

TREATMENT AND THERAPY

The early diagnosis and treatment of dyslexia is essential to its eventual correction. Many experts agree that if a treatment begins before the third grade, there is an 80 percent probability that the dyslexia can be corrected. If the disorder remains undetected until the fifth grade, however, success at treating dyslexia is cut in half. If treatment does not begin until the seventh grade, the probability of successful treatment drops below 5 percent.

The preliminary identification of a dyslexic child can be made from symptoms that include poor written schoolwork, easy distractibility, clumsiness, poor coordination, poor spatial orientation, confused writing and/or spelling, and poor left-right orientation. Because numerous nondyslexic children also show many of these symptoms, a second step is required for such identification: the use of written tests designed to identify dyslexics. These tests include the Peabody Individual Achievement Test, the Halstead-Reitan Neuropsychological Test Battery, and the SOYBAR Criterion Tests.

Electroencephalograms and CT scans are often performed in the hope of pinning down concrete brain abnormalities in dyslexic patients. There is considerable disagreement, however, over the value of these techniques, beyond finding evidence of tumors or severe brain damage—both of which may indicate that the condition observed is not dyslexia. Most researchers agree that children who seem to be dyslexic but who lack tumors or damage are no more likely to have EEG or CT scan abnormalities than nondyslexics. An interesting adjunct to EEG use is a technique called brain electrical activity mapping (BEAM). BEAM converts an EEG into a brain map. Viewed by some workers in the area as a valuable technique, BEAM is contested by many others.

Once conclusive identification of a dyslexic child has been made, it becomes possible to begin corrective treatment. Such treatment is usually the preserve of special education programs. These programs are carried out by the special education teacher in school resource rooms. They also involve special classes limited to children with reading disabilities and schools that specialize in treating learning disabilities.

An often-cited method used is that of Grace Fernald, which utilizes kinesthetic imprinting, based on combined language experience and tactile stimulation. In this popular method or adaptations of it, a dyslexic child learns to read in the following way. First, the child tells a spontaneous story to the teacher, who transcribes it. Next, each word that is unknown to the child is written down by the teacher, and the child traces its letters repeatedly until he or she can write the word without using the model. Each word learned becomes part of the child's word file. A large number of stories are handled this way. Though the method is quite slow, many reports praise its results. Nevertheless, no formal studies of its effectiveness have been made.

A second common teaching technique that is utilized by special educators is the Orton-Gillingham-Stillman method, which was developed in a collaboration between two teachers and a pediatric neurologist, Samuel T. Orton. The method evolved from Orton's conceptualization of language as developing from a sequence of processes in the nervous system that ends in its unilateral control by the left cerebral hemisphere. He proposed that dyslexia arises from conflicts between this cerebral hemisphere and the right cerebral hemisphere, which is usually involved in the handling of nonverbal, pictorial, and spatial stimuli.

Consequently, the corrective method that is used is a multisensory and kinesthetic approach, like that of Fernald. It begins, however, with the teaching of individual letters and phonemes. Then, it progresses to dealing with syllables, words, and sentences. Children taught by this method are drilled systematically, to imprint them with a mastery of phonics and the sounding out of unknown written words. They are encouraged to learn how the elements of written language look, how they sound, how it feels to pronounce them, and how it feels to write them down. Although the Orton-Gillingham-Stillman method is as laborious as that of Fernald, it is widely used and appears to be successful.

Another treatment aspect that merits discussion is the use of therapeutic drugs in the handling of dyslexia. Most physicians and educators propose the use of these drugs as a useful adjunct to the special education training of those dyslexic children who are restless and easily distracted and who have low morale because of continued embarrassment in school in front of their peers. The drugs that are utilized most often are amphetamine, dexidrine, and methylphenidate (Ritalin).

These stimulants, given at appropriate dose levels, will lengthen the time period during which certain dyslexic children function well in the classroom and can also produce feelings of self-confidence. Side effects of their overuse, however, include loss of appetite, nausea, nervousness, and sleeplessness. Furthermore, there is also the potential problem of drug abuse. When they are administered carefully and under close medical supervision, however, the benefits of these drugs far outweigh any possible risks.

A proponent of an entirely medical treatment of dyslexia is psychiatrist Harold N. Levinson. He proposes that the root of dyslexia is in inner ear dysfunction and that it can be treated with the judicious application of proper medications. Levinson's treatment includes amphetamines, antihistamines, drugs used against motion sickness, vitamins, health food components, and nutrients mixed in the proper combination for each patient. He asserts that he has cured more than ten thousand dyslexics and documents many cases. Critics of Levinson's work pose several questions, including whether the studies reported were well controlled and whether the patients treated were actually dyslexics. A major basis for the latter criticism is Levinson's statement that many of his cured patients were described to him as outstanding students. The contention is that dyslexic students are never outstanding students and cannot work at expected age levels.

An important aspect of dyslexia treatment is parental support of these children. Such emotional support helps dyslexics to cope with their problems and with the judgment of their peers. Useful aspects of this support include a positive attitude toward an afflicted child, appropriate home help that complements efforts at school, encouragement and praise for achievements, lack of recrimination when repeated mistakes are made, and positive interaction with special education teachers.

PERSPECTIVE AND PROSPECTS

The identification of dyslexia by German physician Rudolf Berlin and England's W. A. Morgan began the efforts to solve this unfortunate disorder. In 1917, Scottish eye surgeon James Hinshelwood published a book on dyslexia, which he viewed as being a hereditary problem, and the phenomenon became much better known to many physicians.

Attempts at educating dyslexics were highly individualized until the endeavors of Orton and his coworkers and of Fernald led to more standardized and widely used methods. These procedures, their adaptations, and several others not mentioned here became the standard treatments for dyslexia by the late twentieth century.

Interestingly, many famous people—including Hans Christian Andersen, Winston Churchill, Albert Einstein, General George Patton, and Woodrow Wilson—had symptoms of dyslexia, which they subsequently overcame. This was fortunate for them, because adults who remain dyslexic are very often at a great disadvantage. In many cases in modern society, such people are among the functionally illiterate and the poor. Job opportunities open to dyslexics of otherwise adequate intelligence are quite limited.

Furthermore, with the development of a more complete understanding of the brain and its many functions, better counseling facilities, and the conceptualization and actualization of both parent-child and parent-counselor interactions, the probability of successful dyslexic training has improved greatly. Moreover, while environmental and socio-economic factors contribute relatively little to the occurrence of dyslexia, they strongly affect the outcome of its treatment.

The endeavors of special education have so far made the greatest inroads in the treatment of dyslexia. It is hoped that many more advances in the area will be made as the science of the mind grows and diversifies, and the contributions of psychologists, physicians, physiologists, and special educators mesh even more effectively. Perhaps BEAM or the therapeutic methodology suggested by Levinson may provide or contribute to definitive understanding of and treatment of dyslexia. —*Sanford S. Singer*

See also Learning disabilities.

FOR FURTHER INFORMATION:

Hartstein, Jack. *Current Concepts in Dyslexia.* St. Louis: C. V. Mosby, 1971. Introduces readers to terms, specialists, and some available dyslexia treatments. Topical coverage includes dyslexia diagnosis and treatment, the role of teachers, the dimensions of reading disability, the use of medications, and the functions of neurologists.

Huston, Anne Marshall. *Common Sense About Dyslexia.* Lanham, Md.: Madison Books, 1987. Explains dyslexia, describes its three main types, identifies causes and treatments, and covers useful teaching techniques. A bibliography, a useful glossary, appendices of publishers on dyslexia, and special teaching materials are valuable additions.

Jordan, Dale R. *Dyslexia in the Classroom.* 2d ed. Columbus, Ohio: Charles E. Merrill, 1977. Seeks to provide information to "grass-roots" professionals who work with group problems seen as comprising dyslexia. Included are definitions of the three types of dyslexia, their classroom characteristics, correction methods, methods for distinguishing dyslexia from other learning disabilities, and useful screening tests.

Klasen, Edith. *The Syndrome of Specific Dyslexia: With Special Consideration of Its Physiological, Psychological, Testpsychological, and Social Correlates.* Baltimore: University Park Press, 1972. A study of five hundred dyslexics that provides much useful information on aspects of dyslexia origin, speech disorders, organic-sensory and neuropsychological symptoms, psychopathology, therapy, psychologic test results, socioeconomic and family background, and parental attitudes.

Levinson, Harold N. *Smart but Feeling Dumb.* New York: Warner Books, 1984. Based on "thousands of cases cured," this book explains the basis and treatment of dyslexia as inner ear dysfunction that can be cured with judicious application of the correct medications. Included are an overview, case studies, a summary, useful appendices, and a bibliography.

Routh, Donald K. "Disorders of Learning." In *The Practical Assessment and Management of Children with Disorders of Development and Learning,* edited by Mark L. Wolraich. Chicago: Year Book Medical Publishers, 1987. This succinct article summarizes salient facts about learning disorders, including etiology, assessment, management, and outcome. Interested readers will also find many useful references.

Snowling, Margaret. *Dyslexia: A Cognitive Developmental Perspective.* New York: Basil Blackwell, 1989. Covers aspects of dyslexia, including its identification, associated cognitive defects, the basis for language skill development, and the importance of phonetics. Also contains many references.

Valett, Robert E. *Dyslexia: A Neuropsychological Approach to Educating Children with Severe Reading Disorders.* Belmont, Calif.: David S. Lake, 1980. This text, containing hundreds of references, is of interest to readers wishing detailed information on dyslexia and on educating dyslexics. Its two main sections are the neuropsychological foundations of reading (including neuropsychological factors, language acquisition, and diagnosis) and a wide variety of special education topics.

Wagner, Rudolf F. *Dyslexia and Your Child: A Guide for Teachers and Parents.* Rev. ed. New York: Harper & Row, 1979. This clear, useful book is "for teachers and parents concerned with children referred to as dyslexic."

Includes a careful exposition of dyslexic symptoms, commentary on the problem, ways to treat dyslexia and associated problems, recommended reading, and a glossary.

DYSMENORRHEA

SYSTEM AFFECTED: Reproductive (female)

SPECIALISTS: Gynecologists

DEFINITION: Dysmenorrhea is cramplike abdominal pain generally occurring just before or during a menstrual period. Primary dysmenorrhea, which is not related to an identifiable cause, has been linked to excessive levels of prostaglandin, the hormone that triggers uterine contractions; it may be treated with mild painkillers, heat, and prostaglandin inhibitors, and it usually occurs in teenage girls and young women. The source of painful menstruation in women who are over twenty-five or who have given birth is usually secondary dysmenorrhea, which is attributable to an underlying condition such as endometriosis, pelvic inflammatory disease, or tumors; treatment consists of addressing this condition, perhaps with surgery.

See also Endometriosis; Menstruation; Pelvic inflammatory disease (PID).

DYSPHASIA. *See* APHASIA AND DYSPHASIA.

DYSTROPHY

SYSTEMS AFFECTED: All

SPECIALISTS: Neurologists, ophthalmologists

DEFINITION: Dystrophy is a progressive condition that occurs when required nutrients do not reach tissues or organs, causing an inability of these structures to carry out their proper functions; such defective nutrition can result from poor circulation or nerve damage, and many dystrophies are inherited. Muscular dystrophies, in which the muscles degenerate, are the most common example. Dystrophy can also occur in the eyes, resulting in blindness, and in the nerve fibers of the brain, causing severe neurological problems.

See also Muscular dystrophy.

EAR INFECTIONS AND DISORDERS

SYSTEM AFFECTED: Auditory

SPECIALISTS: Audiologists, neurologists, otolaryngologists

DEFINITION: Infections or disorders of the outer, middle, or inner ear, which may result in hearing impairment or loss.

KEY TERMS:

conductive loss: a hearing loss caused by an outer-ear or middle-ear problem which results in reduced transmission of sound

frequency: the number of vibrations per second of a source of sound, measured in hertz; correlates with perceived pitch

intensity of sound: the physical phenomenon that correlates approximately with perceived loudness; measured in decibels

otitis: any inflammation of the outer or middle ear

sensory-neural loss: a hearing loss caused by a problem in the inner ear; this impairment is caused by a hair cell or nerve problem and is usually not amenable to surgical correction

CAUSES AND SYMPTOMS

The hearing mechanism, one of the most intricate and delicate structures of the human body, consists of three sections: the outer ear, the middle ear, and the inner ear. The outer ear converts sound waves into the mechanical motion of the eardrum (tympanic membrane), and the middle ear transmits this mechanical motion to the inner ear, where it is transformed into nerve impulses sent to the brain.

The outer ear consists of the visible portion, the ear canal, and the eardrum. The middle ear is a small chamber containing three tiny bones—the auditory ossicles, termed malleus (hammer), incus (anvil), and stapes (stirrup)—which transmit the vibrations of the eardrum (attached to the hammer) into the inner ear. The chamber is connected to the back of the throat by the Eustachian tube, which allows equalization with the external air pressure. The inner ear, or cochlea, is a fluid-filled cavity containing the complex structure necessary to convert the mechanical vibrations of the cochlear fluid into nerve pulses. The cochlea, shaped something like a snail's shell, is divided lengthwise by a slightly flexible partition into upper and lower chambers. The upper chamber begins at the oval window, to which the stirrup is attached. When the oval window is pushed or pulled by the stirrup, vibrations of the eardrum are transformed into cochlear fluid vibrations.

The lower surface of the cochlear partition, the basilar membrane, is set into vibration by the pressure difference

Anatomy of the Ear

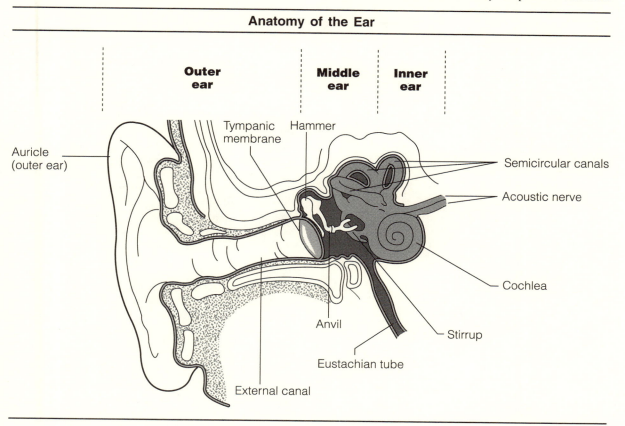

Outer ear

Middle ear

Inner ear

Auricle (outer ear)

Tympanic membrane

Hammer

Semicircular canals

Acoustic nerve

Cochlea

Anvil

Stirrup

Eustachian tube

External canal

between the fluids of the upper and lower ducts. Lying on the basilar membrane is the organ of Corti, containing tens of thousands of hair cells attached to the nerve transmission lines leading to the brain. When the basilar membrane vibrates, the cilia of these cells are bent, stimulating them to produce electrochemical impulses. These impulses travel along the auditory nerve to the brain, where they are interpreted as sound.

Although well protected against normal environmental exposure, the ear, because of its delicate nature, is subject to various infections and disorders. These disorders, which usually lead to some hearing loss, can occur in any of the three parts of the ear.

The ear canal can be blocked by a buildup of waxy secretions or by infection. Although earwax serves the useful purpose of trapping foreign particles that might otherwise be deposited on the eardrum, if the canal becomes clogged with an excess of wax, less sound will reach the eardrum and hearing will be impaired.

Swimmer's ear, or otitis externa, is an inflammation caused by contaminated water which has not been completely drained from the ear canal. A moist condition in a region with little light favors fungal growth. Symptoms of swimmer's ear include an itchy and tender ear canal and a small amount of foul-smelling drainage. If the canal is allowed to become clogged by the concomitant swelling, hearing will be noticeably impaired.

Otitis Externa

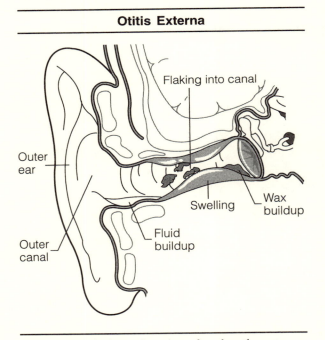

Otitis externa (swimmer's ear) results when the outer ear is inflamed by contaminated water that has not been completely drained from the ear canal.

A perforated eardrum may result from a sharp blow to the side of the head, an infection, the insertion of objects into the ear, or a sudden change in air pressure (such as a nearby explosion). Small perforations are usually self-healing, but larger tears require medical treatment.

Inflammation of the middle ear, acute otitis media, is one of the most common ear infections, especially among children. Infection usually spreads from the throat to the middle ear through the Eustachian tube. Children are particularly susceptible to this problem because their short Eustachian tubes afford bacteria in the throat easy access to the middle ear. When the middle ear becomes infected, pus begins to accumulate, forcing the eardrum outward. This pressure stretches the auditory ossicles to their limit and tenses the ligaments so that vibration conduction is severely impaired. Untreated, this condition may eventually rupture the eardrum or permanently damage the ossicular chain. Furthermore, the pus from the infection may invade nearby structures, including the facial nerve, mastoid bones, the inner ear, or even the brain. The most common symptom of otitis is a sudden severe pain and an impairment of hearing resulting from the reduced mobility of the eardrum and the ossicles.

Secretory otitis media is caused by occlusion of the Eustachian tube as a result of conditions such as a head cold, diseased tonsils and adenoids, sinusitis, improper blowing of the nose, or riding in unpressurized airplanes. People with allergic nasal blockage are particularly prone to this condition. The blocked Eustachian tube causes the middle-ear cavity to fill with a pale yellow, noninfected discharge which exerts pressure on the eardrum, causing pain and impairment of hearing. Eventually, the middle-ear cavity is completely filled with fluid instead of air, impeding the movement of the ossicles and causing hearing impairment.

A mild, temporary hearing impairment resulting from airplane flights is termed aero-otitis media. This disorder results when a head cold or allergic reaction does not permit the Eustachian tube to equalize the air pressure in the middle ear with atmospheric pressure when a rapid change in altitude occurs. As the pressure outside the eardrum becomes greater than the pressure within, the membrane is forced inward, while the opening of the tube into the upper part of the throat is closed by the increased pressure. Symptoms are a severe sense of pressure in the ear, pain, and hearing impairment. Although the pressure difference may cause the eardrum to rupture, more often the pain continues until the middle ear fills with fluid or the tube opens to equalize pressure.

Chronic otitis media may result from inadequate drainage of pus during the acute form of this disease or from a permanent eardrum perforation that allows dust, water, and bacteria easy access to the middle-ear cavity. The main symptoms of this disease are fluids discharging from the

Otitis Media

Otitis media occurs when infection spreads from the throat to the middle ear via the Eustachian tube; it is a serious condition which, left untreated, may lead to permanent ear damage and even infection of the brain.

outer ear and hearing loss. Perforations of the eardrum result in hearing loss because of the reduced vibrating surface and a buildup of fibrous tissue which further induces conductive losses. In some cases, an infection may heal but still cause hearing loss by immobilizing the ossicles. There are two distinct types of chronic otitis, one relatively harmless and the other quite dangerous. An odorless, stringy discharge from the mucous membrane lining the middle ear characterizes the harmless type. The dangerous type is characterized by a foul-smelling discharge coming from a bone-invading process beneath the mucous lining. If neglected, this process can lead to serious complications, such as meningitis, paralysis of the facial nerve, or complete sensory-neural deafness.

The ossicles may be disrupted by infection or by a jarring blow to the head. Most often, a separation of the linkage occurs at the weakest point, where the anvil joins the stirrup. A partial separation results in a mild hearing loss, while complete separation causes severe hearing impairment.

Disablement of the mechanical linkage of the middle ear may also occur if the stirrup becomes calcified, a condition termed otosclerosis. The normal bone is resorbed and replaced by very irregular, often richly vascularized bone. The increased stiffness of the stirrup produces conductive hearing loss. In extreme cases, the stirrup becomes completely immobile and must be surgically removed. Although

the exact cause of this disease is unknown, it seems to be hereditary. About half of the cases occur in families in which one or more relatives have the same condition, and it occurs more frequently in females than in males. There is also some evidence that the condition may be triggered by a lack of fluoride in drinking water and that increasing the intake of fluoride may retard the calcification process.

Tinnitus is characterized by ringing, hissing, or clicking noises in the ear that seem to come and go spontaneously without any sound stimulus. While technically tinnitus is not a disease of the ear, it is a common symptom of various ear problems. Possible causes of tinnitus are earwax lodged against the eardrum, a perforated or inflamed eardrum, otosclerosis, high aspirin dosage, or excessive use of the telephone. Tinnitus is most serious when caused by an inner-ear problem or by exposure to very intense sounds, and it often accompanies hearing loss at high frequencies.

Ménière's disease is caused by an excess production of cochlear fluid which increases the pressure in the cochlea. This condition may be precipitated by allergy, infection, kidney disease, or any number of other causes, including severe stress. The increased pressure is exerted on the walls of the semicircular canals, as well as on the cochlear partition. The excess pressure in the semicircular canals (the organs of balance) is interpreted by the brain as a rapid spinning motion, and the victim experiences abrupt attacks of vertigo and nausea. The excess pressure in the cochlear partition has the same effect as a very loud sound and rapidly destroys hair cells. A single attack causes a noticeable hearing loss and could result in total deafness without prompt treatment.

Of all ear diseases, damage to the hair cells in the cochlea causes the most serious impairment. Cilia may be destroyed by high fevers or from a sudden or prolonged exposure to intensely loud sounds. Problems include destroyed or missing hair cells, hair cells which fire spontaneously, and damaged hair cells that require unusually strong stimuli to excite them. At the present time, there is no means of repairing damaged cilia or of replacing those which have been lost.

Viral nerve deafness is a result of a viral infection in one or both ears. The mumps virus is one of the most common causes of severe nerve damage, with the measles and influenza viruses as secondary causes.

Ototoxic (ear-poisoning) drugs can cause temporary or permanent hearing impairment by damaging auditory nerve tissues, although susceptibility is highly individualistic. A temporary decrease of hearing (in addition to tinnitus) accompanies the ingestion of large quantities of aspirin or quinine. Certain antibiotics, such as those of the mycin family, may also create permanent damage to the auditory nerves.

Repeated exposure to loud noise (in excess of 90 decibels) will cause a gradual deterioration of hearing by destroying cilia. The extent of damage, however, depends on the loudness and the duration of the sound. Rock bands often exceed 110 decibels; farm machinery averages 100 decibels.

Presbycusis (hearing loss with age) is the inability to hear high-frequency sounds because of the increasing deterioration of the hair cells. By age thirty, a perceptible high-frequency hearing loss is present. This deterioration progresses into old age, often resulting in severe impairment. The problem is accelerated by frequent unprotected exposure to noisy environments. The extent of damage depends on the frequency, intensity, and duration of exposure, as well as on the individual's predisposition to hearing loss.

Treatment and Therapy

The simplest ear problems to treat are a buildup of earwax, swimmer's ear, and a perforated eardrum. A large accumulation of wax in the ear canal is best removed by having a medical professional flush the ear with a warm solution under pressure. One should never attempt to remove wax plugs with a sharp instrument. A small accumulation of earwax may be softened by a few drops of baby oil left in the ear overnight, then washed out with warm water and a soft rubber ear syringe. Swimmer's ear can usually be prevented by thoroughly draining the ears after swimming. The disease can be treated by an application of antibiotic eardrops after the ear canal has been thoroughly cleaned. A small perforation of the eardrum will usually heal itself. Larger tears, however, require an operation, tympanoplasty, that grafts a piece of skin over the perforation.

Fortunately, the bacteria that usually cause acute otitis respond quickly to antibiotics. Although antibiotics may relieve the symptoms, complications can arise unless the pus is thoroughly drained. The two-part treatment—draining the fluid from the middle ear and antibiotic therapy—resolves the acute otitis infection within a week. Secretory otitis is cured by finding and removing the cause of the occluded Eustachian tube. The serous fluid is then removed by means of an aspirating needle or by an incision in the eardrum so as to inflate the tube by forcing air through it. In some cases, a tiny polyethylene tube is inserted through the eardrum to aid in reestablishing normal ventilation. If the Eustachian tube remains inadequate, a small plastic grommet may be inserted. The improvement in hearing is often immediate and dramatic. The pain and hearing loss of aero-otitis is usually temporary and disappears of its own accord. If, during or immediately after flight, yawning or swallowing does not allow the Eustachian tube to open and equalize the pressure, medicine or surgical puncture of the eardrum may be required. The harmless form of chronic otitis is treated with applied medications to kill the bacteria and to dry the chronic drainage. The eardrum perforation may then be closed to restore the functioning of the ear and to recover hearing. The more dangerous chronic form of this disease does not respond well to antibacterial agents, but careful

X-ray examination allows diagnosis and surgical removal of the bone-eroding cyst.

Ossicular interruption can be surgically treated to restore the conductive link by repositioning the separated bones. This relatively simple operation has a very high success rate. Otosclerosis is treated by operating on the stirrup in one of several ways. The stirrup can be mechanically freed by fracturing the calcified foot plate, or by fracturing the foot plate and one of the arms. Although this operation is usually successful, recalcification often occurs. Alternatively, the stirrup can be completely removed and replaced by a prosthesis of wire or silicon, yielding excellent and permanent results.

Since tinnitus has many possible, and often not readily identifiable, causes, only about 10 percent of the cases are treated successfully. The tinnitus masker has been invented to help sufferers live with this annoyance. The masker, a noise generator similar in appearance to a hearing aid, produces a constant, gentle humming sound which masks the tinnitus.

Ménière's disease, usually treated by drugs and a restricted diet, may also require surgical correction to relieve the excess pressure in the inner ear. If this procedure is unsuccessful, the nerves of the inner ear may be cut. In drastic cases, the entire inner ear may be removed.

Presently there is no cure for damaged hair cells; the only treatment is to use a hearing aid. It is more advantageous to take preventive measures, such as reducing noise at the source, replacing noisy equipment with quieter models, or using ear protection devices. Recreational exposure to loud music should be severely curtailed, if not completely eliminated.

Perspective and Prospects

For many centuries, treatment of the ear was associated with that of the eye. In the nineteenth century, the development of the laryngoscope (to examine the larynx) and the otoscope (to examine the ears) enabled doctors to examine and treat disorders such as croup, sore throat, and draining ears, which eventually led to the control of these diseases. As an offshoot of the medical advances made possible by these technological devices, the connection between the ear and throat became known, and otologists became associated with laryngologists.

The study of ear diseases did not develop scientifically until the early nineteenth century, when Jean-Marc-Gaspard Itard and Prosper Ménière made systematic investigations of ear physiology and disease. In 1853, William R. Wilde of Dublin published the first scientific treatise on ear diseases and treatments, setting the field on a firm scientific foundation. Meanwhile, the scientific investigation of the diseased larynx was aided by the laryngoscope, invented in 1855 by Manuel Garcia, a Spanish singing teacher who used his invention as a teaching aid. During the late nineteenth century, this instrument was adopted for detailed studies of larynx pathology by Ludwig Türck and Jan

Czermak, who also adapted this instrument to investigate the nasal cavity, which established the link between laryngology and rhinology. Friedrich Voltolini, one of Czermak's assistants, further modified the instrument so that it could be used in conjunction with the otoscope. In 1921, Carl Nylen pioneered the use of a high-powered binocular microscope to perform ear surgery. The operating microscope opened the way for delicate operations on the tiny bones of the middle ear. With the founding of the American Board of Otology in 1924, otology (later otolaryngology) became the second medical specialty to be formally established in North America.

Prior to World War II, the leading cause of deafness was the various forms of ear infection. Advances in technology and medicine have now brought ear infections under control. Today the leading type of hearing loss in industrialized countries is conductive loss, which occurs in those who are genetically predisposed to such loss and who have had lifetime exposure to noise and excessively loud sounds. In the future, ear protection devices and reasonable precautions against extensive exposure to loud sounds should reduce the incidence of hearing loss to even lower levels.

—*George R. Plitnik*

See also Altitude sickness; Hearing loss; Ménière's disease; Motion sickness; Nasopharyngeal disorders; Sinusitis; Speech disorders; Tonsillitis.

FOR FURTHER INFORMATION:

Davis, Hallowell, and S. R. Silverman. *Hearing and Deafness*. 4th ed. New York: Holt, Rinehart and Winston, 1978. Although somewhat technical, this text is written for the nonspecialist.

Jerger, James, ed. *Hearing Disorders in Adults: Current Trends*. San Diego: College-Hill Press, 1984. A reliable and readable introductory treatise on common hearing disorders.

Lutman, M. E., and M. P. Haggard, eds. *Hearing Science and Hearing Disorders*. New York: Academic Press, 1983. A monograph on acoustic perception and impairments.

Pender, Daniel J. *Practical Otology*. Philadelphia: J. B. Lippincott, 1992. A well-illustrated text on diseases of the ear and their surgical correction.

Strong, W. J., and G. R. Plitnik. *Music, Speech, Audio*. Provo, Utah: Soundprint, 1992. Comprehensive treatment for the layperson covering many aspects of hearing, including chapters on the ear, hearing impairments, noise, and controlling environmental sound.

EATING DISORDERS

SYSTEMS AFFECTED: Psychic-emotional, gastrointestinal, endocrine, reproductive

SPECIALISTS: Psychiatrists, psychologists

DEFINITION: A set of emotional disorders centering on body image that lead to misuse of food in a variety of ways—through overeating, overeating and purging, or undereating—that severely threaten the physical and mental well-being of the individual.

KEY TERMS:

amenorrhea: the cessation of menstruation

anorexia nervosa: a disorder characterized by the phobic avoidance of eating, the relentless pursuit of thinness, and fear of gaining weight

arrythmia: irregularity or loss of rhythm, especially of the heartbeat

bulimia: a disorder characterized by binge eating followed by self-induced vomiting

electrolytes: ionized salts in blood, tissue fluid, and cells, including salts of potassium, sodium, and chloride

CAUSES AND SYMPTOMS

The presence of an eating disorder in a patient is defined by an abnormal mental and physical relationship between body image and eating. While obesity is considered an eating disorder, the most prominent conditions are anorexia nervosa and bulimia nervosa. Anorexia nervosa (the word "anorexia" comes from the Greek for "loss of appetite") is an illness characterized by the relentless pursuit of thinness and fear of gaining weight. Bulimia nervosa (the word "bulimia" comes from the Greek for "ox appetite") refers to binge eating followed by self-induced vomiting. These conditions are related in intimate, yet ill-defined ways.

Anorexia nervosa affects more women than men by the overwhelming ratio of nineteen to one. It most often begins in adolescence and is more common among the upper and middle classes of the Western world. According to most studies, its incidence increased severalfold from the 1970's to the 1990's. Prevalence figures vary from 0.5 to 0.8 cases per one hundred adolescent girls. A familiar pattern of anorexia nervosa is often present, and studies indicate that 16 percent of the mothers and 23 percent of the fathers of anorectic patients had a history of significantly low adolescent weight or weight phobia.

The criteria for anorexia nervosa include intense fear of becoming obese, which does not diminish with the progression of weight loss; disturbance of body image, or feeling "fat" even when emaciated; refusal to maintain body weight over a minimal weight for age and height; the loss of 25 percent of original body weight or being 25 percent below expected weight based on standard growth charts; and no known physical illness that would account for the weight loss. Anorexia nervosa is also classified into primary and secondary forms. The primary condition is the distinct constellation of behaviors described above. In secondary anorexia nervosa, the weight loss results from another emotional or organic disorder.

The most prominent symptom of anorexia nervosa is a phobic avoidance of eating that goes beyond any reasonable level of dieting in the presence of striking thinness. Attending this symptom is the characteristic distorted body image and faulty perceptions of hunger and satiety, as well as a pervasive sense of inadequacy.

The distortion of body image renders patients unable to evaluate their body weight accurately, so that they react to weight loss by intensifying their desire for thinness. Patients characteristically describe themselves as "fat" and "gross" even when totally emaciated. The degree of disturbance in body image is a useful prognostic index. Faulty perception of inner, visceral sensations, such as hunger and satiety, extends also to emotional states. The problem of nonrecognition of feelings is usually intensified with starvation.

Other cognitive distortions are also common in anorectic patients. Dichotomous reasoning—the assessment of self or others—is either idealized or degraded. Personalization of situations and a tendency to overgeneralize are common. Anorectics display an extraordinary amount of energy, directed to exercise and schoolwork in the face of starvation, but may curtail or avoid social relationships. Crying spells and complaints of depression are common findings and may persist in some anorectic patients even after weight is gained.

Sleep disturbances have also been reported in anorectics. Obsessive and/or compulsive behaviors, usually developing after the onset of the eating symptoms, abound with anorexia. Obsession with cleanliness and house cleaning, frequent handwashing, compulsive studying habits, and ritualistic behaviors are common.

As expected, the most striking compulsions involve food and eating. Anorectics' intense involvement with food belies their apparent lack of interest in it. The term "anorexia" is, in fact, a misnomer because lack of appetite is rare until late in the illness. Anorectics often carry large quantities of sweets in their purses and hide candies or cookies in various places. They frequently collect recipes and engage in elaborate meal preparation for others. Anorectics' behavior also includes refusal to eat with their families and in public places. When unable to reduce food intake openly, they may resort to such subterfuge as hiding food or disposing of it in toilets. If the restriction of food intake does not suffice for losing weight, the patient may resort to vomiting, usually at night and in secret. Self-induced vomiting then becomes associated with bulimia. Some patients also abuse laxatives and diuretics.

Commonly reported physical symptoms include constipation, abdominal pain, and cold intolerance. With severe weight loss, feelings of weakness and lethargy replace the drive to exercise. Amenorrhea (cessation of menstruation) occurs in virtually all cases, although it is not essential for a diagnosis of anorexia. Weight loss generally precedes the loss of the menstrual cycle. Other physical symptoms reveal the effects of starvation. Potassium depletion is the most frequent serious problem occurring with both anorexia and bulimia. Gastrointestinal disturbances are common, and death may occur from either infection or electrolyte imbalance.

Bulimia usually occurs between the ages of twelve and forty, with greatest frequency between the ages of fifteen and thirty. Unlike anorectics, bulimics usually are of normal weight, although some have a history of anorexia or obesity. Like anorectics, however, they are not satisfied by normal food intake. The characteristic symptom of bulimia is episodic, uncontrollable binge eating followed by vomiting or purging. The binge eating, usually preceded by a period of dieting lasting a few months or more, occurs when patients are alone at home and lasts about one hour. In the early stages of the illness, patients may need to stimulate their throat with a finger or spoon to induce vomiting, but later they can vomit at will. At times, abrasions and bruises on the back of the hand are produced during vomiting. The binge-purge cycle is usually followed by sadness, self-deprecation, and regret. Bulimic patients have troubled interpersonal relationships, poor self-concept, a high level of anxiety and depression, and poor impulse control. Alcohol and drug abuse are not uncommon with bulimia, in contrast to their infrequency with anorexia.

From the medical perspective, bulimia is nearly as damaging to its practitioners as anorexia. Dental problems, including discoloration and erosion of tooth enamel and irritation of gums by highly acidic gastric juice, are frequent. Electrolyte imbalance, such as metabolic alkalosis or hypokalemia (low potassium levels) caused by the self-induced vomiting, is a constant threat. Parotid gland enlargement, esophageal lacerations, and acute gastric dilatation may occur. Cardiac irregularities may also result. The chronic use of emetics such as ipecac to induce vomiting after eating may result in cardiomyopathy (disease of the middle layer of the walls of the heart, the myocardium), occasionally with a fatal outcome. While their menstrual periods are irregular, these patients are seldom amenorrheic.

Another eating disorder, obesity, is the most prevalent nutritional disorder of the Western world. Using the most commonly accepted definition of obesity—a body weight greater than 20 percent above an individual's normal or desirable weight—approximately 35 percent of adults in the United States were considered obese in the early 1990's. This figure represents twice the proportion of the population that was obese in 1900. Evidently, more sedentary lifestyles strongly contributed to this increase, since the average caloric intake of the population decreased by 5 percent since 1910. Although the problem affects both sexes, obesity is found in a larger portion of women than men. In the forty- to forty-nine-year-old age group, 40 percent of women, while only 30 percent of men, were found to meet the criterion for obesity. Prevalence of obesity increases with both age and lower socioeconomic status.

While results of both animal and human studies suggest that obesity is genetically influenced to some degree, most human obesity is reflective of numerous influences and conditions. Evidence indicates that the relationship between caloric intake and adipose tissue is not as straightforward as had been assumed. In the light of this evidence, the failure to lose unwanted pounds and the failure to maintain hard-won weight loss experienced by many dieters seem much more understandable. In the past, obese individuals often were viewed pejoratively by others and by themselves. They were seen as having insufficient willpower and self-discipline. It was incorrectly assumed that it is no more difficult for most obese individuals to lose fat by decreasing caloric intake than it is for individuals in a normal weight range and that it would be just as easy for the obese to maintain normal weight as it is for those who have never been obese.

TREATMENT AND THERAPY

The management of anorectic patients, in either hospital or outpatient settings, may include individual psychotherapy, family therapy, behavior modification, and pharmacotherapy. Many anorectic patients are quite physically ill when they first consult a physician, and medical evaluation and management in a hospital may be necessary at this stage. A gastroenterologist or other medical specialist familiar with this condition may be required to evaluate electrolyte disturbance, emaciation, hypothermia, skin problems, hair loss, sensitivity to cold, fatigue, and cardiac arrhythmias. Starvation may cause cognitive and psychological disturbances that limit the patient's cooperation with treatment.

Indications for hospitalization are weight loss exceeding 30 percent of ideal body weight or the presence of serious medical complications. Most clinicians continue the hospitalization until 80 percent to 85 percent of the ideal body weight is reached. The hospitalization makes possible hyperalimentation (intravenous infusion of nutrients) when medically necessary. Furthermore, individual and family psychiatric evaluations can be performed and a therapeutic alliance established more rapidly with the patient hospitalized.

Most programs utilize behavior modification during the course of hospitalization, making increased privileges such as physical and social activities and visiting contingent on weight gain. A medically safe rate of weight gain is approximately one-quarter of a pound a day. Patients are weighed daily, after the bladder is emptied, and daily fluid intake and output are recorded. Patients with bulimic characteristics may be required to stay in the room two hours after each meal without access to the bathroom to prevent vomiting. Some behavior modification programs emphasize formal contracting, negative contingencies, the practice of avoidance behavior, relaxation techniques, role-playing, and systematic desensitization.

The goal of dynamic psychotherapy is to achieve patient autonomy and independence. The female anorectic patient often uses her body as a battleground for the separation or individuation struggle with her mother. The cognitive therapeutic approach begins with helping the patient to articulate beliefs, change her view of herself as the center of the universe, and render her expectations of the consequences of food intake less catastrophic. The therapist acknowledges the patient's beliefs as genuine, particularly the belief that her self-worth is dependent on achieving and maintaining a low weight. Through a gradual modification of self-assessment, the deficits in the patient's self-esteem are remedied. The therapist also challenges the cultural values surrounding body shape and addresses behavioral and family issues such as setting weight goals and living conditions.

The behavioral management of bulimia includes an examination of the patient's thinking and behavior toward eating and life challenges in general. The patient is made fully aware of the extent of her binging by being asked to keep a daily record of her eating and vomiting practices. A contract is then established with the patient to help her restrict her eating to three or four planned meals per day. The second stage of treatment emphasizes self-control in eating as well as in other areas of the patient's life. In the final stage of treatment, the patient is assisted in maintaining her new, more constructive eating behaviors.

Almost all clinicians work intensively with the family of anorectic patients, particularly in the initial stage of treatment. Family treatment begins with the current family structure and later addresses the early family functioning that can influence family dynamics dramatically. Multigenerational sources of conflict are also examined.

Family therapy with bulimics explores the sources of family conflicts and helps the family to resolve them. Particular attention is directed toward gender roles in the family, as well as the anxiety of the parents in allowing their children autonomy and self-sufficiency. The roots of impulsive and depressive behaviors and the role of parental satisfaction with the patients' lives and circumstances are often explored and addressed.

In the treatment of obesity, the use of a reduced-calorie diet regimen alone does not appear to be an effective treatment approach for many patients, and it is believed that clinicians may do more harm than good by prescribing it. In addition to the high number of therapeutic failures and possible exacerbation of the problem, negative emotional responses are common side effects. Depression, anxiety, irritability, and preoccupation with food appear to be associated with dieting. Such responses have been found to occur in as many as half of the general obese population while on weight-loss diets and are seen with even greater frequency in the severely obese. Some researchers conclude that some cases are better off with no treatment. Their reasoning is based not only on the ineffectiveness of past treatments and the evidence of biological bases for differences in body size but also on the fact that mild to moderate obesity does not appear to put women (or men) at significant health risk. Moreover, an increase in the incidence of serious eating disorders in women has accompanied the increasingly stringent cultural standards of thinness for women. Given the present level of knowledge, it may be that some individuals would benefit most by adjusting to a weight that is higher than the culturally determined ideal.

When an individual of twenty-five to thirty-four years of age is more than 100 percent above normal weight level, however, there is a twelve-fold increase in mortality, and the need for treatment is clear. Although much of the increased risk is related to the effects of extreme overweight on other diseases (such as diabetes, hypertension, and arthritis), these risks can decrease with weight loss. Conservative treatments have had very poor success rates with this group, both in achieving weight reduction and in maintaining any reductions accomplished. Inpatient starvation therapy has had some success in reducing weight in the severely obese but is a disruptive, expensive, and risky procedure requiring very careful medical monitoring to avoid fatality. Furthermore, for those patients who successfully reduce their weight by this method, only about half will maintain the reduction.

Severe obesity seems to be treated most effectively by surgical measures, which include wiring the jaws to make oral intake nearly impossible, reducing the size of the stomach by suturing methods, or short-circuiting a portion of the intestine so as to reduce the area available for uptake of nutrients. None of these methods, however, are without risk.

Perspective and Prospects

The apparent increase in the incidence of anorexia and bulimia in the 1980's and the interest that they have generated both within the scientific community and among the general public have created the impression that these are new diseases. Although scientific writings on the two disorders were uncommon before the early 1960's, eating disorders are by no means recent developments.

Many early accounts of what might have been the condition of anorexia nervosa exist. The clearest and most detailed account is probably the treatise by Richard Morton, a London physician, in his *Phthisiologica: Or, A Treatise of Consumptions* (1964), first published in Latin. In the book, he described several conditions of consumption, devoting one section to the condition of "nervous consumption" in which the emaciation occurred without any remarkable fever, cough, or shortness of breath. He believed the illness to be the result of violent "passions of the mind," the intemperate drinking of alcohol, and an "unwholesome air." He then described two cases, an eighteen-year-old woman who subsequently died following a "fainting fit" and a sixteen-year-old boy who made a partial recovery.

The term "anorexia nervosa" was first used by Sir William Gull (1816-1890), a physician at Guy's Hospital in London, in a paper published in 1874 in which he described the case histories of four women, including one for whom the illness was fatal. He had first mentioned the illness, briefly calling it "apepsia hysterica," in a lengthy address on diagnosis in medicine that he delivered in Oxford, England, in 1868. By 1874, however, he believed that the term "anorexia" would be more correct, and he preferred the more general term "nervosa," since the disease occurs in males as well as females. As part of the clinical picture of the illness, he emphasized the presence of amenorrhea, constipation, bradycardia, loss of appetite, emaciation, and in some cases low body temperature, edema in the legs, and cyanotic peripheries. He commented particularly on the remarkable restlessness and "mental perversity" of the patients and was convinced that the loss of appetite was central in origin. He found the illness to occur mainly in young females between the ages of sixteen and twenty-three.

Ernest Charles Laseque (1816-1883), a professor of clinical medicine in Paris, published an article in 1873 in which he reported on eight patients. He found the illness to occur mostly in young women between the ages of fifteen and twenty, with the onset precipitated by some emotional upset. He also described the occurrence of diminished food intake, constipation, increased activity, amenorrhea, and the patient's contentment with her condition despite the entreaties and threats of family members.

Despite these promising beginnings, the concept of anorexia nervosa was not clearly established until modern times. The main reason for the conceptual confusion was the overgeneralized interpretation of the nature of the patient's refusal to eat. A second source of confusion was the erroneous view that severe emaciation was a frequent, if not primary, feature of hypopituitarism, a condition first described in 1914. That anorexia nervosa was not related to hypopituitarism was finally clarified by researchers in 1949, but the overgeneralized interpretation of the nature of the food refusal persisted into the early 1960's.

If anorexia is taken to mean a loss of the desire to eat, then there is no doubt that the term "anorexia nervosa" is a misnomer. Anorectic patients refuse to eat not because they have no appetite, but because they are afraid to eat; the food refusal or aversion to eating is the result of an implacable and distorted attitude toward weight, shape, and fatness. The idea that this characteristic attitude is the primary feature of the disorder was not clearly formulated until the early 1960's. Once the concept took hold, the illness of anorexia nervosa became distinguishable from other illnesses that led to similar malnutrition. Thus, for example, a person with hysteria may refuse to eat because of a genuine loss of appetite but does demonstrate the characteristic pursuit of thinness. In the 1980's, there was a revival of the idea that the eating disorders are merely variants of an affective illness.

After occurrences of vomiting and binge eating in a context of anorexia nervosa were described, other investigators proposed two subgroups of anorectic patients: the restrictors and the vomiters. This idea was taken further in 1980 by researchers who divided anorexia nervosa into the restrictor and the bulimic subgroups. The occurrence of binge eating in the context of obesity was described as early as 1959, and in 1970, one investigator described the condition as the "stuffing syndrome." Meanwhile, in 1977, several researchers in Japan proposed that *kibarashigui* (binge eating with an orgiastic quality) be delineated as a separate syndrome from anorexia nervosa. The confusion produced by using a symptom (bulimia) to describe a syndrome (also bulimia) is considerable, and in the English-speaking world the terms "bulimarexia," "dietary chaos syndrome," and "abnormal normal weight control syndrome" have been proposed for the binge-eating syndrome in patients with a normal or near-normal weight.

In 1980, the American Psychiatric Association (APA) distinguished bulimia as a syndrome from anorexia nervosa, and in 1987, the APA replaced the term with "bulimia nervosa." Doubts still persisted, however, regarding the identification of the eating disorders. On the one hand, the boundary between the disorders and "normal" dieting behavior seems blurred. On the other hand, the eating disorders are sometimes considered to be variants of other psychiatric illnesses, previously schizophrenia, obsessive-compulsive disorder, and in the 1980's, the mood disorders. A discussion of the eating disorders is necessary if researchers are to agree on definitions so that the disorders are distinguishable from a major depression or from each other. —*Genevieve Slomski*

See also Addiction; Anorexia nervosa; Bulimia; Malnutrition; Obesity; Obsessive-compulsive disorder; Vitamin and mineral deficiencies.

FOR FURTHER INFORMATION:

Bruch, Hilde. *Eating Disorders: Obesity, Anorexia Nervosa, and the Person Within*. New York: Basic Books, 1973. Intended for the general audience, this work provides useful information on eating disorders, their detection, and treatment alternatives. Contains a bibliography.

Field, Howard L., and Barbara B. Domangue, eds. *Eating Disorders Throughout the Life Span*. New York: Praeger, 1987. This collection of essays, intended for the layperson as well as the professional, offers insight into eating disorders of infancy and childhood, adolescent and adult eating disorders, and eating disturbances in the elderly. Includes a bibliography.

Harkaway, Jill Elka, ed. *Eating Disorders*. Rockville, Md.: Aspen, 1987. This edited volume discusses anorexia nervosa and obesity. The authors recognize the complexity of eating disorders and present several models for treatment. These excellent essays present case illustrations, descriptions of techniques, and ideas for family and therapists alike.

Hsu, L. K. George. *Eating Disorders*. New York: Guilford Press, 1990. The work provides a summary of the knowledge about the eating disorders of anorexia and bulimia, a historical development of the concepts, their clinical features, methods of diagnostic evaluation, and various treatment options.

Stunkard, Albert J., and Eliot Stellar, eds. *Eating and Its Disorders*. New York: Raven Press, 1984. This scholarly volume begins with an in-depth analysis of the brain mechanisms underlying appetite control and the signals in the brain that activate these mechanisms. The second section presents a synthesis of scientific thinking on body weight regulation. The concluding section features clinical approaches to obesity, anorexia, and bulimia.

ECLAMPSIA

SYSTEMS AFFECTED: Circulatory, nervous

SPECIALISTS: Obstetricians

DEFINITION: Hypertension induced by pregnancy is known in its convulsive form as eclampsia and in its nonconvulsive form as preeclampsia; the cause of this dangerous rise in blood pressure has not been identified. Preeclampsia may appear in the second or third trimesters and may be associated with edema (especially of the face) and sudden excessive weight gains; treatment may range from bed rest and sedatives to the induction of labor if the pregnancy is near term. If the preeclampsia worsens, life-threatening eclampsia may develop, resulting in seizures and possibly stillbirth, premature labor, renal failure, liver damage, and coma. If the seizures can be controlled, a cesarean section is usually performed.

See also Hypertension; Pregnancy and gestation; Seizures.

ECTOPIC PREGNANCY

SYSTEM AFFECTED: Reproductive (female)

SPECIALISTS: General surgeons, obstetricians

DEFINITION: An ectopic pregnancy is one in which the fertilized egg implants itself in a location other than in the uterus; these other sites may include the Fallopian tubes, the ovaries, or the internal cervical os (near the cervix). Symptoms may range from those normally associated with intrauterine pregnancy to mild abdominal pain. In rare cases, the fetus may survive if the ovum implants in the abdominal viscera, but otherwise surgical intervention may be required to save the mother, if possible leaving the Fallopian tubes and ovaries intact for future pregnancies. Ectopic pregnancy may be caused by congenital defects, sexually transmitted diseases, or the use of an intrauterine contraceptive device (IUD).

Ectopic pregnancy

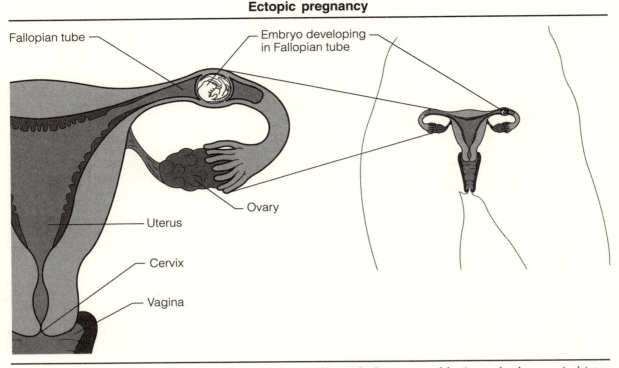

Fallopian tube

Embryo developing in Fallopian tube

Ovary

Uterus

Cervix

Vagina

Ectopic pregnancy results when the fertilized egg implants itself outside the uterus and begins to develop; surgical intervention is usually required.

See also Conception; Female genital disorders; Miscarriage; Pregnancy and gestation.

ECZEMA

SYSTEM AFFECTED: Skin

SPECIALISTS: Allergists, dermatologists, toxicologists

DEFINITION: Eczema, usually called dermatitis, is a skin disorder characterized by a general pattern of reddening, swelling, blistering, crusting, and scabbing. Chronic cases result in thickening of the skin, peeling, and changes in skin color. Both phases feature itching that may be intense. Dermatitis is associated with allergic reactions, infections, toxic reactions, and skin irritations. For example, atopic dermatitis is a genetic condition in which the patient has widespread sensitivities to certain substances and environmental factors, while contact dermatitis is caused by a reaction to a mild irritant over a long period of time or to a specific substance after sensitization to it. Treatment depends on the cause and may include corticosteroid creams.

See also Allergies; Dermatitis; Rashes; Skin disorders.

EDEMA

SYSTEMS AFFECTED: Skin, circulatory, lymphatic, liver

SPECIALISTS: Internists, nephrologists

Common Sites of Eczema

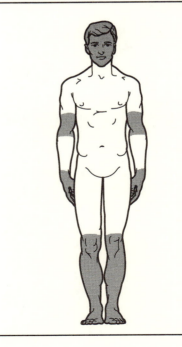

DEFINITION: Accumulation of fluid in body tissues that may indicate a variety of diseases, including cardiovascular, kidney, liver, and medication problems.

KEY TERMS:

extracellular fluid: the fluid outside cells; includes the fluid within the vascular system and the lymphatic system and the fluid surrounding individual cells

hydrostatic pressure: the physical pressure on a fluid, such as blood; it tends to push fluids across membranes toward areas of lower pressure

interstitial fluid: the fluid between the vascular system and cells; nutrients from the vascular compartment must diffuse across the interstitial compartment to enter the cells

intracellular fluid: the fluid within cells

intravascular fluid: the fluid carried within the blood vessels; it is in a constant state of motion because of the pumping action of the heart

osmotic pressure: the ability of a concentrated fluid on one side of a membrane to draw water away from a less concentrated fluid on the other side

PROCESS AND EFFECTS

Edema is not a disease, but a condition that may be caused by a number of diseases. It signals a breakdown in the body's fluid-regulating mechanisms. The body's water can be envisioned as divided into three compartments: the intracellular compartment, the interstitial compartment, and the vascular compartment. The intracellular compartment consists of the fluid contained within the individual cells. The vascular compartment consists of all the water that is contained within the heart, the arteries, the capillaries, and the veins. The last compartment, and in many ways the most important for a discussion of edema, is called the interstitial compartment. This compartment includes all the water not contained in either the cells or the blood vessels. The interstitial compartment contains all the fluids between the intracellular compartment and the vascular compartment and the fluid in the lymphatic system. The sizes of these compartments are approximately as follows: intracellular fluid at 66 percent, interstitial fluid at 25 percent, and the vascular fluid at only 8 percent of the total body water.

When the interstitial compartment becomes overloaded with fluid, edema develops. To understand the physiology of edema formation, it may be helpful to follow a molecule of water as it travels through the various compartments, beginning when the molecule enters the aorta soon after leaving the heart. The blood has just been ejected from the heart under high pressure, and it speedily begins its trip through the body. It passes from the great vessel, the aorta, into smaller and smaller arteries that divide and spread throughout the body. At each branching, the pressure and speed of the water molecule decreases. Finally, the molecule enters a capillary, a vessel so small that red blood cells must flow in a single file. The wall of this vessel is composed only of the membrane of a single capillary cell. There

Edema

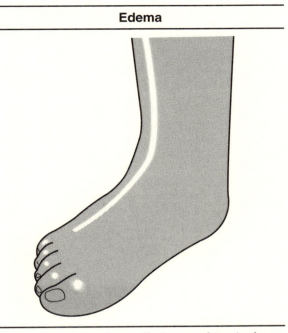

Edema may appear chronically (as seen here, in the ankles), with characteristic swelling and stretched, shiny skin; it can be a symptom of many diseases.

are small passages between adjacent capillary cells leading to the interstitial compartment, but they are normally closed.

The hydrostatic pressure on the water molecule is much lower than when it was racing through the aorta, but it is still higher than the surrounding interstitial compartment. At the arterial end of the capillary, the blood pressure is sufficient to overcome the barrier of the capillary cell's membrane. A fair number of water and other molecules are pushed through the membrane into the interstitial compartment.

In the interstitial compartment, the water molecule is essentially under no pressure, and it floats amid glucose molecules, oxygen molecules, and many other compounds. Glucose and oxygen molecules enter the cells, and when the water molecule is close to a glucose molecule it is taken inside a cell with that molecule. The water molecule is eventually expelled by the cell, which has produced extra water from the metabolic process.

Back in the interstitial compartment, the molecule floats with a very subtle flow toward the venous end of the capillary. This occurs because, as the arterial end of the capillary pushes out water molecules, it loses hydrostatic pressure, eventually equaling the pressure of the interstitial compartment. Once the pressure equalizes, another phenomenon that has been thus far overshadowed by the hydrostatic pressure takes over—osmotic pressure. Osmotic pressure is the force exercised by a concentrated fluid that is separated by a membrane from a less concentrated fluid. It draws water molecules across the membrane from the less concentrated side. The more concentrated is the fluid, the greater is the drawing power. The ratio of nonwater molecules to that of water molecules determines concentration.

The fluid that stays within the capillary remains more concentrated than the interstitial fluid for two reasons. First, the plasma proteins in the vascular compartment are too large to be forced across the capillary membrane; albumin is one such protein. These proteins stay within the vascular compartment and maintain a relatively concentrated state, compared to the interstitial compartment. At the same time, the concentration of the fluid in the interstitial compartment is being lowered constantly by the cellular compartment's actions. Cells remove molecules of substances such as glucose to metabolize, and afterward they release water—a by-product of the metabolic process. Both processes conspire to lower the total concentration of the interstitial compartment. The net result of this process is that water molecules return to the capillaries at the venous end because of osmotic pressure.

The water molecule is caught by this force and is returned to the vascular compartment. Back in the capillary, the molecule's journey is not yet complete. Now in a tiny vein, it moves along with blood. On the venous side of the circulatory system, the process of branching is reversed, and small veins join to form increasingly larger ones. The water molecule rides along in these progressively larger veins. The pressure surrounding the molecule is still low, but it is now higher than the pressure at the venous end of the capillary. One may wonder how this is possible if the venous pressure at the beginning of the venous system is essentially zero, and there is only one pump, the heart, in the body. As the molecule flows through the various veins, it occasionally passes one-way valves that allow blood to flow only toward the heart. The action of these valves, combined with muscular contractions from activities such as walking or tapping the foot, force blood toward the heart. Without these valves, it would be impossible for the venous blood to flow against gravity and return to the heart; the blood would simply sit at the lowest point in the body. Fortunately, these valves and contractions move the molecule against gravity, returning it to the heart to begin a new cycle.

In certain disease states, there is marked capillary dilation and excessive capillary permeability, and excessive amounts of fluid are allowed to leave the intravascular compartment. The fluid accumulates in the interstitial space. When capillary permeability is increased, plasma proteins also tend to leave the vascular space, reducing the intravascular compartment's osmotic pressure while increasing the interstitial compartment's osmotic pressure. As a result, the rate of return of fluid from the interstitial compartment to the vascular compartment is lowered, thus increasing the interstitial fluid levels.

Another route of return of interstitial fluid to the circulation is via the lymphatic system. The lymphatic system is similar to the venous system, but it carries no red blood cells. It runs through the lymph nodes, carrying some of the interstitial fluid that has not been able to return to the vascular compartment at the capillary level. If lymphatic vessels become obstructed, water in the interstitial compartment accumulates and edema may result.

CAUSES AND SYMPTOMS

Heart failure is a major cause of edema. When the right ventricle of the heart fails, it cannot cope with all the venous blood returning to the heart. As a consequence, the veins become distended, the interstitial compartment is overloaded, and edema occurs. If the patient with heart failure is mostly upright, the edema collects in the legs; if the patient has been lying in bed for some time, the edema tends to accumulate in the lower back. Other clinical signs of right heart failure include distended neck veins, an enlarged and tender liver, and a "galloping" sound on listening to the heart with a stethoscope.

When the left ventricle of the heart fails, the congestion affects the pulmonary veins instead of the neck and leg veins. Fluid accumulates in the same fashion within the interstitial compartment of the lungs; this condition is termed pulmonary edema. Patients develop shortness of breath with minimal activity, upon lying down, and periodically through the night. They may need to sleep on several pillows to minimize this symptom. This condition can usually be diagnosed by listening to the lungs and heart through a stethoscope and by taking an X ray of the chest.

Deep vein thrombosis is another common cause of edema of the lower limbs. When a thrombus (a blood clot inside a blood vessel) develops in a large vein of the legs, the patient usually complains of pain and tenderness of the affected leg. There is usually redness and edema as well. If the thrombus affects a small vein, it may not be noticed. The diagnosis can be made by several specialized tests, such as ultrasound testing and/or impedance plethysmography. Other tests may be needed to make the diagnosis, such as injecting radiographic dye in a vein in the foot and then taking X rays to determine whether the flow in the veins is obstructed, or using radioactive agents that bind to the clot. Risks for developing venous thrombosis include immobility (even for relatively short periods of time such as a long car or plane ride), injury, a personal or family history of venous thrombosis, the use of birth control pills, and certain types of cancer. Elderly patients are at particular risk because of relative immobility and an increased frequency of minor trauma to the legs.

When repeated or large thrombi develop, the veins deep inside the thigh (the deep venous system) become blocked, and blood flow shifts toward the superficial veins. The deep veins are surrounded by muscular tissue, and venous flow is assisted by muscular contractions of the leg (the muscular pump), but the superficial veins are surrounded only by skin and subcutaneous tissue and cannot take advantage of the muscular pump. As a consequence, the superficial veins become distended and visible as varicose veins.

When vein blockage occurs, the valves inside become damaged. Hydrostatic pressure of the venous system below the blockage then rises. The venous end of the capillary is normally where the osmotic pressure of the vascular compartment pulls water from the interstitial compartment back into the vascular compartment. In a situation of increased hydrostatic pressure, however, this process is slowed or stopped. As a result, fluid accumulates in the interstitial space, leading to the formation of edema.

A dangerous complication of deep vein thrombosis occurs when part of a thrombus breaks off, enters the circulation, and reaches the lung; this is called a pulmonary embolus. It blocks the flow of blood to the lung, impairing oxygenation. Small emboli may have little or no effect on the patient, while larger emboli may cause severe shortness of breath, chest pain, or even death.

Another potential cause of edema is the presence of a mass in the pelvis or abdomen compressing the large veins passing through the area and interfering with the venous return from the lower limbs to the heart. The resulting venous congestion leads to edema of the lower limbs. The edema may affect either one or both legs, depending on the size and location of the mass. This diagnosis can usually be established by a thorough clinical examination, including rectal and vaginal examinations and X-ray studies.

Postural (or gravitational) edema of the lower limbs is the most common type of edema affecting older people; it is more pronounced toward the end of the day. It can be differentiated from the edema resulting from heart failure by the lack of signs associated with heart failure and by the presence of diseases restricting the patients' degree of mobility. These diseases include Parkinson's disease, osteoarthritis, strokes, and muscle weakness. Postural edema of the lower limbs results from a combination of factors, the most important being diminished mobility. If a person stands or sits for prolonged periods of time without moving, the muscular pump becomes ineffective. Venous compression also plays an important role in the development of this type of edema. It will occur when the veins in the thigh are compressed between the weight of the body and the surface on which the patient sits, or when the edge of a reclining chair compresses the veins in the calves. Other factors that aggravate postural edema include varicose veins, venous thrombi, heart failure, some types of medication, and low blood albumin levels.

Albumin is formed in the liver from dietary protein. It is essential to maintaining adequate osmotic pressure inside the blood vessels and ensuring the return of fluid from the interstitial space to the vascular compartment. When edema is caused by inadequate blood levels of albumin, it tends to be quite extensive. The patient's entire body and even face are often affected. There are several reasons that the liver may be unable to produce the necessary amount of albumin, including malnutrition, liver impairment, the aging process, and excessive protein loss.

In cases of malnutrition, the liver does not receive a sufficient quantity of raw material from the diet to produce albumin; this occurs when the patient does not ingest enough protein. Healthy adults need at least 0.5 gram of protein for each pound of their body weight. Two groups of people are particularly susceptible to becoming malnourished: the poor and the elderly. Infants and children of poor families who cannot afford to prepare nutritious meals often suffer from malnutrition. The elderly, especially men living on their own, are also vulnerable, regardless of their income.

A liver damaged by excessive and prolonged consumption of alcohol, diseases, or the intake of some type of medication or other chemical toxins will be unable to manufacture albumin at the necessary rate to maintain a normal concentration in the blood. Clinically, the patient shows other evidence of liver impairment in addition to edema. For example, fluid may also accumulate in the abdominal cavity, a condition known as ascites. The diagnosis of liver damage is made by clinical examination and supporting laboratory investigations. The livers of older people, even in the absence of disease, are often less efficient at producing albumin.

The albumin also can be deficient if an excessive amount of albumin is lost from the body. This condition may occur in certain types of diseases affecting the kidneys or the gastrointestinal tract. An excessive amount of protein also may be lost if a patient has large, oozing pressure ulcers, extensive burns, or chronic lung conditions that produce large amounts of sputum.

Patients with strokes and paralysis sometimes develop edema of the paralyzed limb. The mechanism of edema formation in these patients is not entirely understood. It probably results from a combination of an impairment of the nerves controlling the dilation and a constriction of the affected limb blood vessels, along with postural and gravitational factors.

Severe allergic states, toxic states, or local inflammation are associated with increased capillary permeability that results in edema. The amount of fluid flowing out to the capillaries far exceeds the amount that can be returned to the capillaries at the venous end. A number of medications can induce edema by promoting the retention of fluid, including steroids, estrogens, some arthritis medications, a few blood pressure medications, and certain antibiotics. Salt intake tends to cause a retention of fluid as well. Obstruction of the lymphatic system often leads to accumulation of fluid in the interstitial compartment. Obstruction can occur in certain types of cancer, after radiation treatment, and in certain parasitic infestations.

TREATMENT AND THERAPY

The management of edema depends on the specific reason for its presence. To determine the cause of edema, a thorough history, including current medications, dietary habits, and activity level, is of prime importance. Performing a detailed physical examination is also a vital step. It is frequently necessary to obtain laboratory, ultrasound, and/or X-ray studies before a final diagnosis is made. Once a treatable cause is found, then therapy aimed at the cause should be instituted.

If no treatable, specific disease is responsible for the edema, conservative treatment aimed at reducing the edema to manageable levels without inducing side effects should be initiated. Frequent elevation of the feet to the level of the heart, support stockings, and an avoidance of prolonged standing or sitting are the first steps. If support stockings are ineffective or are too uncomfortable, then custom-made, fitted stockings are available. A low-salt diet is important in the management of edema because a high salt intake worsens the fluid retention. If all these measures fail, then diuretics in small doses may be useful.

Diuretics work by increasing the amount of urine produced. Urine is made of fluids removed from the vascular compartment by the kidneys. The vascular compartment then replenishes itself by drawing water from the interstitial compartment. This reduction in the amount of interstitial fluid improves the edema. There are various types of diuretics, which differ in their potency, duration of action, and side effects. Potential side effects include dizziness, fatigue, sodium and potassium deficiency, excessively low blood pressure, dehydration, sexual dysfunction, the worsening of a diabetic's blood sugar control, increased uric acid levels, and increased blood cholesterol levels. Although diuretics are a convenient and effective means of treating simple edema, it is important to keep in mind that the cure should not be worse than the disease. When the potential side effects of diuretic therapy are compared to the almost total lack of complications of conservative treatment, one can see that mild edema which is not secondary to significant disease is best managed conservatively. Edema caused by more serious diseases, however, calls for more intensive measures.

PERSPECTIVE AND PROSPECTS

The prevalence of edema could decrease as people become more health-conscious and medical progress is made. Nutritious diets, avoidance of excessive salt, and an increased awareness of the dangers of excessive alcohol intake and of the benefits of regular physical exercise all contribute to decreasing the incidence of edema. Improved methods for the early detection, prevention, and management of diseases that may ultimately result in edema could also significantly reduce the scope of the problem. It is also

expected that safer and more convenient methods of treating edema will become available. —*Ronald C. Hamdy, Mark R. Doman, and Katherine Hoffman Doman*

See also Atherosclerotic disease; Elephantiasis; Heart disease; Heart failure; Kidney disorders; Kwashiorkor; Liver disorders; Malnutrition; Phlebitis; Thrombosis and thrombus; Varicosis; Venous insufficiency.

FOR FURTHER INFORMATION:

Andreoli, Thomas, et al., eds. *Cecil Essentials of Medicine.* 2d ed. Philadelphia: W. B. Saunders, 1990. A good introductory text to internal medicine that can also be easily understood by nonscientists.

Bergan, John J., and James S. T. Yao, eds. *Venous Problems.* Chicago: Yearbook Medical Publishers, 1978. Contains the most thorough treatment of human venous problems. Causality, diagnosis (including the tests used to make a diagnosis), and the surgical treatment of venous abnormalities are discussed.

Guyton, Arthur C. *Human Physiology and Mechanisms of Disease.* 5th ed. Philadelphia: W. B. Saunders, 1992. The standard reference text in human physiology. A background in basic physiology is helpful in understanding this work.

Michaelson, Cydney, ed. *Congestive Heart Failure.* St. Louis: C. V. Mosby, 1983. An excellent basic, yet thorough, treatise on the subject of heart failure. The authors discuss the circulatory system in states of both health and disease, low-salt diets, and the drug treatment for heart failure.

Physician's Desk Reference. 47th ed. Oradell, N.J.: Medical Economics Data, 1993. The most up-to-date listing of drugs and drug side effects that is regularly available. The information contained is required by the Food and Drug Administration to allow the marketing of medications. Includes all reported drug side effects, although it can be difficult to sort out the more frequent side effects and adverse reactions from the rare ones.

Spence, Alexander, and Elliott Mason. *Human Anatomy and Physiology.* 2d ed. Menlo Park, Calif.: Benjamin/ Cummings, 1983. This text is a basic introduction to physiology and anatomy.

Staub, Norman, and Aubrey Taylor, eds. *Edema.* New York: Raven Press, 1984. A thorough and advanced treatment of edema—its many forms and causes.

ELECTRICAL SHOCK

SYSTEMS AFFECTED: Heart, nervous, skin

SPECIALISTS: Burn specialists, emergency physicians, neurologists

DEFINITION: The physical effect of an electrical current entering the body and the resulting damage.

CAUSES AND SYMPTOMS

Electric shock ranges from a harmless jolt of static electricity to a power line's lethal discharge. The severity of the shock depends on the current flowing through the body, and the current is determined by the skin's electrical resistance. Dry skin has a very high resistance; thus 110 volts produces a small, harmless current. The resistance for perspiring hands, however, is lower by a factor of 100, resulting in potentially fatal currents. Because of their proximity to the heart, currents traveling between bodily extremities are particularly dangerous.

Electric shock causes injury or death in one of three ways: paralysis of the breathing center in the brain, paralysis of the heart, or ventricular fibrillation (extremely rapid and uncontrolled twitching of the heart muscle).

The threshold of feeling (the minimum current detectable) ranges from 0.5 to 1.0 milliamperes. Currents up to 5.0 milliamperes, the maximum harmless current, are not hazardous, unless they trigger an accident by involuntary reaction. Currents in this range create a tingling sensation. The minimum current that causes muscular paralysis occurs between 10 and 15 milliamperes. Currents of this magnitude cause a painful jolt. Above 18 milliamperes, the current contracts chest muscles and breathing ceases. Unconsciousness and death follow within minutes unless the current is interrupted and respiration resumed. A short exposure to currents of 50 milliamperes causes severe pain, possible fainting, and complete exhaustion, while currents in the 100 to 300 milliampere range produce ventricular fibrillation, which is fatal unless quickly corrected. During ventricular fibrillation, the heart stops its rhythmic pumping and flutters uselessly. Since blood stops flowing, the victim dies from oxygen deprivation to the brain in a matter of minutes. This is the most common cause of death for victims of electric shock.

Relatively high currents (above 300 milliamperes) may produce ventricular paralysis, deep burns in the body's tissue, or irreversible damage to the central nervous system. Victims are more likely to survive a large but brief current, even through smaller, sustained currents are usually lethal. Burning or charring of the skin at the point of contact may be a contributing factor to the delayed death that often follows severe electric shock. Very high voltage discharges of short duration, such as a lightning strike, tend to disrupt the body's nervous impulses, but victims may survive. On the other hand, any electric current large enough to raise body temperature significantly produces immediate death.

TREATMENT AND THERAPY

Before medical treatment can be applied, the current must be stopped or the shock victim must be separated from the current source without being touched. Nonconducting materials such as dry, heavy blankets or pieces of wood can be used for this purpose. If the victim is not breathing, artificial respiration immediately applied provides adequate short-term life support, though the victim may become stiff or rigid in reaction to the shock. Victims of electric shock may suffer from severe burns and perma-

nent aftereffects, including eye cataracts, angina, or disorders of the nervous system.

Electric shock can usually be prevented by strictly adhering to safety guidelines and using commonsensical precautions. Careful inspection of appliances and tools, compliance with manufacturers' safety standards, and the avoidance of unnecessary risks greatly reduce the chance of an electric shock. Electrical appliances or tools should never be used when standing in water or on damp ground, and dry gloves, shoes, and floors provide considerable protection against dangerous shocks from 110 volt circuits.

Electrical safety is also provided by isolation, guarding, insulation, grounding, and ground fault interrupters. Isolation means that high-voltage wires strung overhead are not within reach, while guarding provides a barrier around high voltage devices, such as are found in television sets.

Old wire insulation may become brittle with age and develop small cracks. Defective wires are hazardous and should be replaced immediately. Most modern power tools are double-insulated; the motor is insulated from the plastic insulating frame. These devices do not require grounding, as no exposed metal parts become electrically live if the wire insulation fails.

In a home, grounding is accomplished by a third wire in outlets, connected through a grounding circuit to a water pipe. If an appliance plug has a third prong, it will ground the frame to the grounding circuit. In the event of a short circuit, the grounding circuit provides a low resistance path, resulting in a current surge which trips the circuit breaker.

In some instances, however, the current may be inadequate to trip a circuit breaker (which usually requires 15 or 20 amperes), but current in excess of 10 milliamperes could still be lethal to humans. A ground-fault interrupter ensures nearly complete protection by detecting leakage currents as small as 5 milliamperes and breaking the circuit. This relatively inexpensive device operates very rapidly and provides an extremely high degree of safety against electrocution in the household. Many localities now have codes which require the installation of ground-fault interrupters in bathrooms, kitchens, and other areas where water is used.

—*George R. Plitnik*

See also Burns and scalds; Shock; Unconsciousness.

FOR FURTHER INFORMATION:

Beausoliel, Robert W., and W. J. Meese. *Survey of Ground Fault Circuit Interrupter Usage for Protection Against Hazardous Shock.* Washington, D.C.: Government Printing Office, 1976. A monograph on ground-fault interrupters and their use.

Bridges, J. E., et al., eds. *International Symposium on Electrical Shock Safety Criteria.* New York: Pergamon Press, 1985. The summary of a symposium covering the physiological effects of shock, bioelectrical conditions, and safety measures.

Hewitt, Paul G. *Conceptual Physics*. 7th ed. New York: HarperCollins College Publishers, 1993. Comprehensive coverage of physics for the layperson that includes detailed discussions of the laws of electricity and electrical devices.

U.S. Department of Labor. Occupational Safety and Health Administration. *Controlling Electrical Hazards*. Washington, D.C.: Government Printing Office, 1991. A report which identifies common electrical hazards and discusses their prevention.

ELEPHANTIASIS

SYSTEM AFFECTED: Lymphatic

SPECIALISTS: Epidemiologists, tropical medicine physicians

DEFINITION: A grossly disfiguring disease caused by a roundworm parasite; it is the advanced stage of the disease Bancroft's filariasis, contracted through roundworms.

KEY TERMS:

acute disease: a disease in which symptoms develop rapidly and which runs its course quickly

chronic disease: a disease that develops more slowly than an acute disease and persists for a long time

host: any organism on or in which another organism (called a parasite) lives, usually for the purpose of nourishment or protection

inflammation: a response of the body to tissue damage caused by injury or infection and characterized by redness, pain, heat, and swelling

lymph nodes: globular structures located along the routes of the lymphatic vessels that filter microorganisms from the lymph

lymphatic system: a body system consisting of lymphatic vessels and lymph nodes that transports lymph through body tissues and organs; closely associated with the cardiovascular system

lymphatic vessels: vessels that form a system for returning lymph to the bloodstream

parasite: an organism that lives on or within another organism, called the host, from which it derives sustenance or protection at the host's expense

CAUSES AND SYMPTOMS

Elephantiasis is found worldwide, mostly in the tropics and subtropics. Most cases of elephantiasis are a result of infection with a parasitic worm called *Wuchereria bancrofti* (*W. bancrofti*). *W. bancrofti* belongs to a group of worms called filaria, or roundworms, and infection with a filarial worm is called filariasis. Filariasis caused by *W. bancrofti* is the most common and widespread type of human filarial infection and is often called Bancroft's filariasis. Elephantiasis is the advanced, chronic stage of Bancroft's filariasis, and only a small percentage of persons with Bancroft's filariasis will develop elephantiasis. During Bancroft's filariasis, adult forms of *W. bancrofti* live inside the human lymphatic system, and it is the person's reaction to the presence of the worm that causes the symptoms of the disease. The worm's life cycle is important in understanding how the disease is transmitted from one person to another, how the symptoms develop, and how to prevent and reduce the incidence of the disease.

The adult worms live in human lymphatic vessels and lymph nodes and measure about four centimeters in length for the male and nine centimeters in length for the female. Both are threadlike and about 0.3 millimeter in diameter. After mating, the female releases large numbers of embryos or microfilariae (microscopic roundworms), which are more than one hundred times smaller in length and ten times thinner than their parents. They make their way from the lymphatic system into the bloodstream, where they can circulate for two years or longer. Interestingly, most strains of microfilariae (all except those found in the South Pacific Islands) exhibit a nocturnal periodicity, in which they appear in the peripheral blood system (the outer blood vessels, such as those in the arms, legs, and skin) only at night, mostly between the hours of 10 P.M. and 2 A.M., and the remainder of the time they spend in the blood vessels of the lungs and other internal organs. This nighttime cycling into the peripheral blood is somehow related to the patient's sleeping habits, and although it is unknown exactly how or why the microfilariae do this, it is necessary for the survival of the worms. The microfilariae must develop through at least three different stages (called the first, second, and third larval stages) before they are ready to mature in adults; these stages take place not within humans, but within certain types of mosquitoes, which bite at night. Thus, the microfilariae appear in the peripheral blood just in time for the mosquitoes to bite an infected human and extract them so that they can continue their life cycle. It is important to note, therefore, that both humans and the proper type of mosquito are needed to keep a filariasis infection going in a particular area.

Female night-feeding mosquitoes of the genera *Culex*, *Aedes*, and *Anopheles* serve as intermediate hosts for *Wuchereria bancrofti*. The mosquitoes bite an infected person and ingest microfilariae from the peripheral blood. The microfilariae pass into the intestines of the mosquito, invade the intestinal wall, and within a day find their way to the thoracic muscles (the muscles in the middle part of the mosquito's body). There they develop from first-stage to third-stage larvae in about two weeks, and the new third-stage larvae move from the thoracic muscles to the head and mouth of the mosquito. Only the third-stage larvae are able to infect humans successfully, and the third stage can mature only inside humans. When the mosquito takes a blood meal, infective larvae make their way through the proboscis (the tubular sucking organ with which a mosquito bites a person) and enters the skin through the puncture wound. After they enter the skin, the larvae move by an unknown route to the lymphatic system, where they develop into adult worms. It takes about one year or longer for the larvae to grow into adults, mate, and produce more microfilariae.

A person contracts Bancroft's filariasis by being bitten by an infected mosquito. Various forms of the disease can occur, depending on the person's immune response and the number of times the person is bitten. The period of time from when a person is first infected with larvae to the time microfilariae appear in the blood can be between one and two years. Even after this time some persons, especially young people, show no symptoms at all, yet they may have numerous microfilariae in their blood. This period of being a carrier of microfilariae without showing any signs of disease may last several years, and such carriers act as reservoirs for infecting the mosquito population.

In those patients showing symptoms from the infection, there are two stages of the disease: acute and chronic. In acute disease, the most common symptoms are a recurrent fever and lymphangitis and/or lymphadenitis in the arms, legs, or genitals. These symptoms are caused by an inflammatory response to the adult worms trapped inside the lymphatic system. Lymphangitis, an inflammation of the lymph vessels, is characterized by a hard, cord-like swelling or a

Elephantiasis

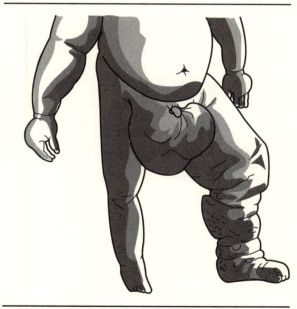

The common symptoms of acute elephantiasis are a recurrent fever and lymphangitis and/or lymphadenitis in the arms, legs, or genitals; if the conditions develop into chronic elephantiasis, the result can be layers of scar tissue that block the lymphatic vessels, leading to a buildup of fluid in the tissues. Grotesque swellings and tissue growth may result.

red superficial streak that is tender and painful. Lymphadenitis is characterized by swollen and painful lymph nodes. The attacks of fever and lymphangitis or lymphadenitis recur at irregular intervals and may last from three weeks up to three months. The attacks usually become less frequent as the disease becomes more chronic. In the absence of reinfection, there is usually a steady improvement in the victim, each relapse being milder. Thus, without specific therapy, this condition is self-limiting and presumably will not become chronic in those acquiring the infection during a brief visit to an area where the disease is endemic.

The most obvious symptoms caused as a result of *W. bancrofti* infection, such as elephantiasis, are noted in the chronic stage. Chronic disease occurs only after years of repeated infection with the worms. It is seen only in areas where the disease is endemic and only occurs in a small percentage of the infected population. The symptoms are the result of an accumulation of damage caused by inflammatory reactions to the adult worms. The inflammation causes tissue death and a buildup of scar tissue that eventually results in the blockage of the lymphatic vessels in which the worms live. One of the functions of lymphatic vessels is to carry excess fluid away from tissues and bring it back to the blood, where it enters the circulation again as the fluid portion of the blood. If the lymphatic vessels are blocked, the excess fluid stays in the tissues, and swelling occurs. When this swelling is extensive, grotesque enlargement of that part of the body occurs. Elephantiasis is characterized by gross enlargement of a body part caused by the accumulation of fluid and connective tissue. It most frequently affects the legs, but may also occur in the arms, breasts, scrotum, vulva, or any other body part. The disease starts with the slight enlargement of one leg or arm (or other body part). The limb increases in size with recurrent attacks of fever. Gradually, the affected part swells, and the swelling, which is soft at first, becomes hard following the growth of connective tissue in the area. In addition, the skin over the swollen area changes so that it becomes coarse and thickened, looking almost like elephant hide. The elephant-like skin, along with the enlarged body parts, gave the disease the name "elephantiasis."

TREATMENT AND THERAPY

One way in which doctors can tell whether a person has Bancroft's filariasis is by taking a sample of peripheral blood between 10 P.M. and 2 A.M. and looking at the blood under a microscope to try to find microfilariae. Sometimes, the ability to find microfilariae is enhanced by filtering the blood to concentrate the possible microfilariae in a smaller volume of liquid. Many persons infected with *W. bancrofti* have no detectable microfilariae in their blood, so other methods are available. In the absence of microfilariae, a diagnosis can be made on the basis of a history of exposure, symptoms of the disease, positive antibody or skin tests, or the presence of worms in a sample of lymph tissue. It is important to note that occasionally a few other filarial worms and at least one bacteria can also cause elephantiasis; therefore, if symptoms of elephantiasis are observed, it is important to discover the correct cause so that the proper treatment can be given. Since chronic infection occurs after prolonged residence in areas where the disease occurs, patients with acute disease should be removed from those areas. They also should be reassured that elephantiasis is a rare complication that is limited to persons who have had constant exposure to infected mosquitoes for years.

The best way to avoid contracting filariasis when traveling to an affected area is to avoid being bitten by mosquitoes. Insect repellent, mosquito netting, and other methods are helpful in this regard. No drugs or vaccines are available to prevent infection once a person is bitten.

A problem in the treatment of all parasitic diseases is finding a drug that will kill the parasite without harming the human host. The drug diethylcarbamazine (DEC) is the drug of choice in treating Bancroft's filariasis. Its advantages are that it can be taken orally, patients have a relatively high tolerance to the drug, and it has relatively rapid, beneficial, clinical effects. Generally, in the treatment of acute disease, excellent results are obtained when the proper dosage of the drug is given. There are only two relatively mild side effects of DEC. The first is nausea or vomiting. This symptom depends on the amount of the drug given; therefore, lower doses help alleviate this side effect. The second is fever and dizziness, the severity of which depends on the number of microfilariae a person has in his or her blood; the more microfilariae, the more severe the reaction. It is important to warn patients ahead of time about the fever reaction and encourage them to continue taking their doses anyway. The fever reaction is a sign that the patient is being cured, but the cure will not completely work if the patient does not finish the whole regimen of drug doses. Other drugs have been used in the treatment of filariasis (suramin, metrifonate, levamisole) but are generally less effective or more toxic than DEC. Additional treatment measures include bed rest and supportive measures, such as using hot and cold compresses to reduce swelling. The administration of antibiotics for patients with secondary bacterial infections and painkillers as well as anti-inflammatory agents during the painful, acute stage is helpful. Sometimes, swollen limbs can be wrapped in pressure bandages to force the lymph from them. If the distortion is not too great, this method is successful. It should also be noted that, although drugs such as DEC might be effective in killing *W. bancrofti*, the chronic lesions resulting from the infection are mostly incurable. Signs of chronic filariasis, such as elephantiasis of the limbs or the scrotum, are usually unaffected or only incompletely cured by medication, and it sometimes becomes necessary to apply surgical or other symptomatic treatments to relieve the suffering of the patients. Chronic obstruction in less advanced stages is some-

times improved by surgery. The surgical removal of an elephantoid breast, vulva, or scrotum is sometimes necessary.

Theoretically, it should be possible first to control and eventually to eliminate Bancroft's filariasis. Conditions that are highly favorable for continued propagation of the infection include a pool of microfilariae carriers in the human population and the right species of mosquitoes breeding near human habitations. Thus, control can be effected by treating all microfilariae carriers in an affected area and eliminating the necessary mosquitoes. Microfilariae carriers can be effectively treated with DEC. The decision usually is between giving mass drug treatment to the entire population in an affected area or only treating those persons who are microfilariae positive. Usually, if the infection is at a high rate and very widespread in an area, it is best to treat the entire population, since it would be very time consuming, difficult, and expensive to find all the microfilariae carriers. In other areas that are smaller or in which the pockets of infection are well defined, it is better to identify all the microfilariae-positive persons and treat only those persons until they are cured. The second control measure is to eliminate the mosquito population. It is important to note that eliminating the mosquitoes alone will not control the disease, especially in tropical areas, since the breeding period and season in which the disease can be transmitted is so extensive. In some temperate areas, where Bancroft's filariasis used to be endemic, measures that removed the mosquitoes alone aided in the elimination of the disease from that area, since in temperate areas the breeding period and thus the season for transmission is so short. In tropical areas, both DEC therapy and mosquito control must be applied in order to control the disease. The mosquito population can be controlled in four ways. First, general sanitation measures can be carried out in order to reduce the areas where the mosquitoes are breeding; for example, draining swamps. Second, insecticides can be used to kill the adult mosquitoes. Third, larvacides can be applied to sources of water where mosquitoes breed in order to kill the mosquito larvae. Finally, natural mosquito predators, such as certain species of fish, can be introduced into waters where mosquitoes breed to eat the mosquito larvae. Numerous problems stand in the way of eradication, such as poor sanitation, persons who do not cooperate with medical intervention, mosquitoes that become resistant to all known insecticides, increasing technology that yields increasing water supplies and therefore places for mosquitoes to breed, large populations, ignorance of the cause of the disease, and lack of medicine and a way of distributing that medicine.

PERSPECTIVE AND PROSPECTS

Dramatic symptoms of elephantiasis, especially the enormous swelling of legs or scrotum, were recorded in much of the ancient medical literature of India, Persia, and the Far East. The embryonic form of microfilariae was first discovered and described by a Frenchman in Paris in 1863.

The organism was named for O. Wucherer, who also discovered microfilariae in 1866, and Joseph Bancroft, who discovered the adult worm in 1876. Two important facts about *W. bancrofti*—namely, its development in mosquitoes and the nocturnal periodicity of the microfilariae—were discovered by Patrick Manson between 1877 and 1879. This was the first example of a disease being transmitted by a mosquito, and its discovery earned for Manson the title of Father of Tropical Medicine. These and most of the other essential facts of the disease were discovered before the end of the nineteenth century. Progress in the epidemiology and control of filariasis came after World War II. In 1947, DEC was shown to kill filariae in animals, and this result was followed by the successful use of DEC in the treatment of humans. The first promising results in the control of Bancroft's filariasis by mass administration of DEC were reported in 1957 on a small island in the South Pacific. Through subsequent studies, it has become clear that effective control of the infection can be achieved if sufficient dosages of DEC are administered to infected populations.

Filariasis is a serious health hazard and public health problem in many tropical countries. Infection with *Wuchereria bancrofti* has been recorded in nearly all countries or territories in the tropical and subtropical zones of the world. The infection occurs primarily in coastal areas and islands that experience long periods of high humidity and heat. Infections have also been noted from some temperate zone districts, such as mainland Japan, central China, and some European countries. There is more Bancroft's filariasis now than there was a hundred years ago, principally because of increases in population in affected areas and in increased resistance of mosquitoes to insecticides. In 1947, it was estimated that 189 million people were infected with *W. bancrofti*. More recently, the World Health Organization estimated that 250 million people are infected and 400 million are at risk.

Bancroft's filariasis was introduced into and became endemic to Charleston, South Carolina, until 1920. It disappeared in the United States before World War II, presumably because of a reduction of mosquitoes resulting from improved sanitation. Servicemen in the Pacific in World War II were concerned about contracting elephantiasis; although several thousand showed signs of acute filariasis, only twenty had microfilariae in their blood, and no one developed elephantiasis. In the United States today, the infection is most frequently seen in immigrants, military veterans, and missionaries. It is important for physicians to be aware of this and other tropical diseases so that they can treat the occasional patient who is suffering from one of them, since most of these diseases are more successfully treated in the early stages of the disease. —*Vicki J. Isola*

See also Edema; Inflammation; Lymphadenopathy and lymphoma; Parasitic diseases; Worms.

FOR FURTHER INFORMATION:

Beaver, Paul C., and Rodney C. Jung. *Animal Agents and Vectors of Human Disease*. 5th ed. Philadelphia, Pa.: Lea & Febiger, 1985. Discusses all major parasitic diseases. Chapter 12, "Filariae," which describes those diseases caused by filarial worms, contains helpful photographs and diagrams.

Foster, William D. *A History of Parasitology*. Edinburgh: E. & S. Livingstone, 1965. Describes the history of the discovery of the causes of parasitic diseases. Chapter 7, "*Wuchereria Bancrofti*," gives a detailed and interesting account of the history behind the discovery of the causes and nature of Bancroft's filariasis.

Ransford, Oliver. '*Bid the Sickness Cease.*' London: John Murray, 1983. Discusses the effect of disease on the development of Africa. Chapter 6, "The Father of Tropical Medicine," describes how Patrick Manson made the original discoveries of the cause of elephantiasis.

Sasa, Manabu. *Human Filariasis*. Baltimore: University Park Press, 1976. This book, though written as a field guide for the person working in some aspect of filariasis, is extremely well organized and easy to read. It describes in detail every filarial disease, including infections with *Wuchereria bancrofti*. It gives comprehensive details of the geographic distribution of the disease in every country in the world and describes the current methodology in studying filariasis and trying to control the disease.

Schmidt, G. D., and L. S. Roberts. *Foundations of Parasitology*. 4th ed. St. Louis, Mo.: Times Mirror/Mosby College, 1989. Gives a good general description of all parasitic diseases, their causes, effects, and treatments. Chapter 31, "Filarial Worms," deals specifically with diseases caused by filariae, including *Wuchereria bancrofti*.

Zinsser, Hans. *Zinsser Microbiology*. Edited by W. K. Joklik et al. 19th ed. Norwalk, Conn.: Appleton and Lange, 1988. The information presented in this textbook is thorough, logical, and supplemented by interesting diagrams, photographs, and charts. Chapter 90, "Medical Helminthology," contains a thorough description of Bancroft's filariasis.

EMBOLISM

SYSTEMS AFFECTED: Circulatory, heart, brain, respiratory
SPECIALISTS: Internists, vascular surgeons
DEFINITION: Embolism is the obstruction of circulation through a blood vessel by an embolus, such as a blood clot, a piece of tissue, cholesterol, fat, bone marrow, or an air bubble. Pulmonary embolism, the presence of an obstruction in the lung, is the most common site because all the blood in the body must pass through the lungs with every circuit made. Emboli can form after an operation or prolonged inactivity because of illness or injury: Blood clots may form in the deep veins of the legs, and pieces of these clots break away to travel through

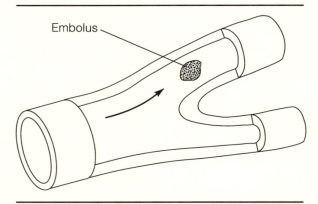

Embolus

An embolus is any material that is flowing in the bloodstream that obstructs a blood vessel; it may, for example, be a piece of a fatty plaque that has broken off an arterial wall.

the bloodstream. Emboli can be removed surgically, or drugs to dissolve blood clots and to prevent their formation may be administered.

See also Atherosclerotic disease; Cholesterol; Claudication; Phlebitis; Thrombosis and thrombus.

EMPHYSEMA

SYSTEM AFFECTED: Respiratory

SPECIALISTS: Internists, pulmonologists

DEFINITION: A disease of the lung characterized by enlargement of the small bronchioles or lung alveoli, the destruction of alveoli, decreased elastic recoil of these structures, and the trapping of air in the lungs, resulting in shortness of breath, reduced oxygen to the body, and a variety of serious and eventually fatal complications.

KEY TERMS:

alveoli: tiny, delicate, balloonlike air sacs composed of blood vessels that are supported by connecting tissue and enclosed in a very thin membrane; these sacs are found at the ends of the bronchioles

bronchioles: small branches of the bronchi, which are extensions of the trachea (the central duct that conducts air from the environment to the pulmonary system)

bullous emphysema: localized areas of emphysema within the lung substance

centrilobular (centriacinar) emphysema: a type of emphysema that destroys single alveoli, entering directly into the walls of terminal and respiratory bronchioles

diffusion: the passage of oxygen into the bloodstream from the alveoli and the return or exchange of carbon dioxide across the membrane between the blood vessels and the alveoli

panlobular (panacinar) emphysema: a type of emphysema that involves weakening and enlargement of the air sacs, which are clustered at the end of respiratory bronchioles

perfusion: the flow of blood through the lungs or other vessels in the body

ventilation: the transport of air from the mouth through the bronchial tree to the air sacs and back through the nose or mouth to the outside; ventilation includes both inspiration (breathing in) and expiration (breathing out)

CAUSES AND SYMPTOMS

Emphysema is a lung disease in which damage to these organs causes shortness of breath and can lead to heart or respiratory failure. A discussion of the structure and function of the normal lung can illuminate the nature and effects of this damage.

Gases, smoke, germs, allergens, and environmental pollutants pass from the nose and mouth into a large duct called the trachea. The trachea branches into smaller ducts, the bronchi and bronchioles (small branches of the bronchi), which lead to tiny air sacs called alveoli. The respiratory system is like a tree: The trachea is the trunk, the bronchi and bronchioles are similar to the branches, and the alveoli are similar to the leaves. The blood vessels of the alveoli carry red blood cells, which pick up oxygen and transport it to the rest of the body. The cellular waste product, carbon dioxide, is released to the alveoli from the bloodstream and then exhaled. The alveoli are supported by a framework of delicate elastic fibers and give the lung a very distensible quality and the ability to "snap back," or recoil.

The lungs and bronchial tubes are surrounded by the chest wall, composed of bone and muscle and functioning like a bellows. The lung is elastic and passively increases in size to fill the chest space during inspiration and decreases in size during expiration. As the lung (including the alveoli) enlarges, air from the environment flows in to fill this space. During exhalation, the muscles relax, the elasticity of the lung returns it to a normal size, and the air is pushed out. Air must pass through the bronchial tree to the alveoli before oxygen can get into the bloodstream and carbon dioxide can get out, because it is the alveoli that are in contact with blood vessels. The bronchial tree has two kinds of special lining cells. The first type can secrete mucus as a sticky protection against injury and irritation. The second type of cell is covered with fine, hairlike structures called cilia. These cells are supported by smooth muscle cells and elastic and collagen fibers. The cilia wave in the direction of the mouth and act as a defense system by physically removing germs and irritating substances. The cilia are covered with mucus, which helps to trap irritants and germs.

When alveoli are exposed to irritants such as cigarette smoke, they produce a defensive cell called an alveolar macrophage. These cells engulf irritants and bacteria and call for white blood cells, which aid in the defense against foreign bodies, to come into the lungs. The lung tissue also becomes a target for the enzymes or chemical substances produced by the alveolar macrophages and leukocytes (white blood cells). In a healthy body, natural defense systems inhibit the enzymes released by the alveolar macrophages and leukocytes, but it seems that this inhibiting function is impaired in smokers. In some cases, an individual may inherit a deficiency in an enzyme inhibitor. The enzymes vigorously attack the elastin and collagen of the lungs, the lung loses its elastic recoil, and air is trapped.

Emphysema, and a related disease, bronchitis, often work in concert. They are often lumped under the term "chronic obstructive pulmonary disease." Chronic bronchitis weakens and narrows the bronchi. Often, bronchial walls collapse, choking off the vital flow of air. Air is also trapped within the bronchial walls. Weakened by enzymes, the walls of the alveoli rupture and blood vessels die. Lung tissue is replaced with scar tissue, leaving areas of destroyed alveoli that appear as "holes" on an X ray. Small areas of destroyed alveoli are called blebs, and larger ones are called bullae.

As emphysema progresses, a patient has a set of large, overexpanded lungs with a weakened and partially plugged bronchial tree subject to airway collapse and air trapping with blebs and bullae. Breathing, especially exhalation, becomes a slow and difficult process. The patient often develops a "barrel chest" and is known, in medical circles, as a "blue bloater." The scientific world calls the mismatching of breathing to blood distribution a ventilation-to-perfusion imbalance; that is, when air arrives in the alveolus, there are no blood vessels there to transport their vital gaseous cargo to the cells (as a result of enzymatic damage). A person with chronic obstructive pulmonary disease has a bronchial tree with a narrow, defective trunk and sparse leaves.

The loss of elasticity of the lung and alveoli is a critical problem in the emphysemic patient. About one-half of the lungs' elastic recoil force comes from surface tension. The other half comes from the elastic nature of certain fibers throughout the lungs' structure. Emphysema weakens both of these forces because it destroys the elastic fibers and interferes with the surface tension. Fluid, a saline solution, bathes all the body's cells and surfaces. In the lung, this fluid contains surfactant, a substance that interferes with water's tendency to form a spherical drop with a pull into its center (and ultimate collapse). The tissue that gives shape to the lungs is composed of specialized fibers which contain a protein called elastin. These elastic fibers are also found in the alveolar walls and in the elastic connective tissue of the airways and air sacs. The amount of elastin in lung tissue determines its behavior. Healthy lungs maintain a proper balance between destruction of elastin and renewal. (Other parts of the body, such as bones, do this as well.) If too little elastin is destroyed, the lungs have difficulty expanding. If too much is destroyed, the lungs overexpand and cannot recoil properly.

The process of elastin destruction and renewal involves complex regulation. Specialized lung cells produce new elastin protein. Others produce elastase, an enzyme that destroys elastin. The liver plays a role in the production of a special enzyme known as alpha-1-antitrypsin, which controls the amount of elastase so that too much elastin is not digested. In emphysema, these regulatory systems fail: Too much elastin is destroyed because elastase is no longer controlled, apparently because alpha-1-antitrypsin production has been reduced to a trickle.

The loss of elastin (and thus elastic recoil) means that the lungs expand beyond the normal range during inspira-

Emphysema

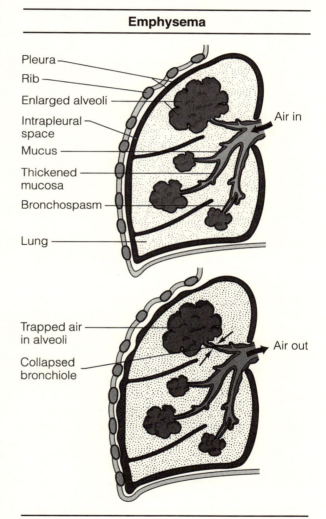

In emphysema, the body releases enzymes in response to inhaling irritants in the air, such as cigarette smoke; these enzymes reduce the lung's elasticity, compromising the bronchioles' ability to expand and contract normally. Air becomes trapped in the alveoli upon inhalation (top) and cannot escape upon exhalation (bottom). Over time, breathing becomes extremely difficult.

tion and cannot resume their resting size during expiration. Thus, alveoli overinflate and rupture. This further reduces elasticity because the loss of each alveolus further impairs the surface tension contribution to the lungs' ability to recoil. Thus, a state of hyperinflation is assumed in the emphysemic patient. This leads to stretched and narrowed alveolar capillaries, loss of elastic tissue, and dissolution of alveolar walls. The lungs increase in size, the thoracic (chest) cage assumes the inspiratory position, and the diaphragm becomes low and flat instead of convex. The patient becomes short of breath with any type of exertion. As the disease worsens, the patient's skin takes on a cyanotic color, as a result of poor oxygenation and perfusion. Wheezing is often present, and coughing is difficult and tiring. In the worst cases, even talking is enough exertion to produce a spasmodic cough. The hyperinflated chest causes inspiration to become a major effort, and the entire chest cage lifts up, resulting in considerable strain. The head moves with each inspiration while the chest remains relatively fixed.

Emphysema may be diagnosed by the early symptom of dyspnea (shortness of breath) on exertion. In advanced cases, the distended chest, depressed diaphragm, increased blood carbon dioxide content, and severe dyspnea clearly point to the disease.

TREATMENT AND THERAPY

The initial step in treating emphysema is to open the airways by eliminating the causes of irritation: smoke, dry air, infection, and allergies. The second treatment is to clean out the airways. There are several techniques and medicines for loosening airway mucus and expelling it. In most chronic obstructive lung diseases, including emphysema, the mucus becomes thick and purulent; coughing up mucus of this type is difficult. In addition, in emphysema the natural cleansing action of the cilia and lung elasticity are impaired. Thus, treatment is aimed at the patient consciously taking over the function of cleaning out the lungs. Coughing is nature's way of bringing up mucus (phlegm), and the emphysemic patient is urged to cough. Since the mucus is thick, one needs to do whatever is necessary to thin it out and to lubricate the airways so that the mucus slips up easily with coughing. The cough must come from deep within the chest in order to be "productive" (to raise mucus).

Moisture is helpful in loosening up thick mucus; hence, drinking large amounts of fluid is encouraged. Adding a humidifier or a vaporizer to a home is often helpful to the emphysemic patient. There are also machines known as nebulizers and intermittent positive pressure breathing (IPPB) machines that can help to add moisture to the airway of the patient with emphysema. Nebulizers are more effective in getting moisture beyond the throat and major airways than cold vaporizers. Nebulizers, which get their name from the Latin word for cloud or mist, create a mist that is a profusion of tiny droplets that keep themselves apart, even as they bump into one another. Nebulizers release only the smallest droplets—those which can penetrate far down into air passages, where thick mucus is likely to be. (Atomizers produce small droplets as well, but they also spray large droplets.) IPPBs have a special kind of valve that opens when one begins to breathe and allows the air to move into the lungs under mild pressure. As soon as the patient has come to the end of the inhalation, the valve closes and allows the patient to exhale freely.

When phlegm cannot be brought up by breathing mist, a technique called postural drainage is often combined with chest wall percussion or vibration. The idea is to move one's body to a position such that airways are perpendicular to the floor, or at least tilted down, so that gravity can help pull the mucus toward the larger airways, from which the phlegm can be coughed up. Percussion, or clapping the chest, is another way to loosen the mucus in the airways so that it can be coughed up.

A number of medications are useful in the treatment of emphysema. The bronchodilator drugs are xanthines, such as theophylline (Theo-Dur), that relieve bronchospasms; reduce wheezing and dyspnea, and improve respiratory muscle function. Theophylline is a drug that is similar chemically to caffeine. Whereas caffeine stimulates the skeletal muscles and the central nervous system, however, theophylline is potent as a cardiac stimulant and a smooth muscle relaxer. It has also been learned that theophylline stimulates mucociliary clearance of the airways, strengthens the diaphragm, and suppresses edema. Theophylline holds two benefits for the chronic obstructive pulmonary diseased patient: It helps get rid of mucus, and it strengthens the diaphragm, the main respiratory muscle. Common side effects are nausea, stomach pain, vomiting, insomnia, rapid heartbeat, loss of appetite, and restlessness. Another category of bronchodilator are the beta adrenergic-stimulants such as metaproterenol (Alupent). Their side effects include nervousness, headache, nausea, and muscle cramps.

The antibiotics sometimes prescribed for emphysemic patients are used to combat bacterial infection. Common antibiotics include tetracycline, penicillin, cephalosporin, erythromycin, and sulfa drugs. Their side effects include a burning sensation in the stomach, vomiting, diarrhea, increased sensitivity to sunlight, rashes, itching, hives, fever, and weakness.

The steroid hormones, such as prednisone, decrease swelling, inflammation, and bronchospasms; they also relieve wheezing. Side effects include blurred vision, frequent urination, thirst, black stools, bone pain, mood changes, weight gain, swelling of the feet, muscle weakness, hoarseness, and a sore mouth.

Other drugs given for emphysema include digitalis, cardiac glycosides, diuretics, mast cell inhibitors, expectorants, and parasympatholytics. Digitalis and cardiac glycosides, such as digoxin, improve the strength of heart contractions and treat disturbances in heart rhythm. Side effects are loss of appetite, abdominal pain, nausea, slow uneven pulse, blurred vision, diarrhea, mood changes, and weakness. Diuretics, such as furosemide (Lasix), are often given to prevent excessive fluid retention. Such drugs cause loss of hearing, skin rashes, hives, bleeding, bruising, jaundice, an irregular or fast heartbeat, muscle cramps, light-headedness, dizziness, and weakness. Mast cell inhibitors are a unique category of drugs that inhibit the release of body chemicals that cause wheezing and bronchospasm; however, they also cause weakness, nosebleeds, and nasal congestion. Expectorants, such as Robitussin, are used to thin secretions and have no known side effects. The parasympatholytics are a type of bronchodilator drug that inhibits the nerves that cause bronchospasm. They are apparently free from the many side effects associated with other bronchodilator drugs.

The emphysemic patient should avoid both excessive heat and excessive cold. If body temperature rises above normal, the heart works faster, as do the lungs. Excessive cold stresses the body to maintain its normal temperature. Smog, air pollution, dusts, powders, and hairspray should be avoided. Finally, a healthy diet consisting of foods high in calcium, vitamins, complex carbohydrates, proteins, and fiber is advised for the lung-diseased patient.

A healthy core diet is high in complex carbohydrates; is low in sugars, fats, and cholesterol; and has adequate protein for moderate stress. It should be high in fiber and contain approximately 1,000 milligrams of calcium, 15,000 milligrams of Vitamin A, and 250 milligrams of Vitamin C. Snack foods can include skim milk, fruit, popcorn, and fresh salads. The respiratory distress of the emphysemic patient uses vast amounts of energy, and the patient should eat several small meals a day so as not to distend the stomach and limit movement of the diaphragm. Liquids are important in keeping airways clear. Good nutrition is helpful in maintaining strength and improving the quality of life for the lung-diseased patient.

PERSPECTIVE AND PROSPECTS

Chronic bronchitis and emphysema are responsible for at least fifty thousand deaths a year in the United States alone. An increase in air pollution and cigarette consumption are apparent causes for this rise. In males over forty, chronic obstructive pulmonary disease (COPD) is second to heart disease as a cause of disability. With more females and young people smoking, the incidence of lung disease is likely to increase. Aside from death, a disease such as emphysema can cause long years of disability, joblessness, loss of income, depression, hospitalization, and an inability to perform normal activities.

Smoking is, by far, the single most important risk factor for emphysema. In the United States especially, social acceptance of women smokers began after World War II and has increased the number of women being diagnosed with COPD. Socioeconomic status also influences smoking habits. In many countries in Europe, the mortality rate from lung disease for the lowest socioeconomic class has been six times higher than for the highest. In the United States, the COPD mortality rate among unskilled and semiskilled laborers is twice as high as among professionals. Families with lower incomes usually live in small, often overcrowded apartments; such overcrowding makes respiratory infections more frequent. Often, family members of the COPD patient also smoke, increasing the surrounding air pollution.

In the United States, COPD causes 3 percent of all deaths. In some cases, it causes another 100,000 Americans to be too weak to survive other, unrelated medical conditions. Therefore, an annual figure of 150,000 deaths from COPD-related diseases is more realistic. The expanding COPD population is a growing market for pharmaceutical firms. For example, greater amounts of bronchodilator medications will be needed; hence, pharmaceutical firms are anxious to find longer-acting and more effective drugs for these patients to buy.

A number of economic pressures are likely to move COPD treatment from the hospital to the home. When effectively carried out by a well-trained health team, home care can lower medical costs. The COPD patient who finds a knowledgeable doctor and who begins a comprehensive rehabilitation program is the one who can look forward to a life that is more productive and more comfortable.

—Jane A. Slezak

See also Environmental diseases; Pulmonary diseases.

FOR FURTHER INFORMATION:

Bates, David V. *Respiratory Function in Disease*. 3d ed. Philadelphia: W. B. Saunders, 1989. Summarizes the effects of disease on pulmonary function. Also discussed are some of the more sophisticated pulmonary-function tests. Exercise testing, obesity, and the effects of drugs are other topics reviewed in this work.

Berland, Theodore, and Gordon L. Snider. *Living with Your Bronchitis and Emphysema*. New York: St. Martin's Press, 1972. A book for persons suffering from respiratory disease and making adjustments, both emotionally and physically, because of the disease. An invaluable source of information on healthy and unhealthy breathing in the modern world.

Haas, François, and Sheila Sperber Haas. *The Chronic Bronchitis and Emphysema Handbook*. New York: John Wiley & Sons, 1990. Helps patients with COPD learn to lead full and productive lives. Provides information pertinent to their disease and describes the treatments and medications available to them in order to improve their quality of life.

Shayevitz, Myra, and Berton Shayevitz. *Living Well with Emphysema and Bronchitis*. Garden City, N.Y.: Doubleday, 1985. Provides suggestions for living a full life in spite of lung disease. It clearly explains the causes and complications of emphysema, treatment modalities, and the medications available to alleviate discomfort.

Wolff, Ronald K. "Effects of Airborne Pollutants on Mucociliary Clearance." *Environmental Health Perspectives* 66 (April, 1986): 223-237. The role of mucociliary clearance as a lung defense mechanism is described in this article. The abnormal elimination of bronchial mucus is considered a possible factor in the pathogenesis of COPD. The role of certain pollutants, which pose a challenge to the mucociliary system, are detailed.

ENCEPHALITIS

SYSTEMS AFFECTED: Brain, nervous

SPECIALISTS: Infectious disease physicians, neurologists

DEFINITION: A family of diseases resulting from viral infection or complications from another disease; inflammation of the brain resulting in a variety of usually serious symptoms and sometimes death.

KEY TERMS:

athetosis: involuntary writhing movements of limbs and/or body, face, and tongue

dementia: loss of mental ability as a result of brain deterioration

diabetes insipidus: production of copious amounts of urine

hemiplegia: paralysis of one side of the body

nuchal: having to do with the nape of the neck

pleocytosis: an increase in the number of white blood cells in the cerebrospinal fluid

postencephalitic symptoms: symptoms commencing immediately after or years after an attack of encephalitis lethargica as a direct or indirect consequence of the infection

viremia: invasion of cells by viruses

CAUSES AND SYMPTOMS

Encephalitis, a noncontagious disease, is an inflammation of the brain. It most often results from viral infection, but it may also arise as a complication of measles, chickenpox, herpes simplex virus 1, or several other diseases. A nonviral form, encephalitis lethargica (sometimes referred to as "sleeping sickness") is implicated in parkinsonism. Between one thousand and five thousand cases are reported annually to the Centers for Disease Control in Atlanta, Georgia; the highest incidence is in the summer and early fall months, and worldwide, most cases are reported in the tropics. The disease affects the sexes equally, and no age group is unaffected.

The viruses that cause most cases of encephalitis are called arboviruses, animal viruses carried by arthropods and transmitted to vertebrate hosts. In a vertebrate, one of these viruses undergoes viremia, then multiplies in an arthropod when it feeds on the vertebrate host. The arthropod then passes the virus to another vertebrate, also while feeding. Arthropods implicated in passing on the virus to humans are mosquitoes, and rarely, ticks. Mosquitoes (and ticks)

pick up the virus as they feed on an infected host. There are several variables, however, that determine whether the virus will be passed on to the next host. First, each different virus has a "preferred" arthropod carrier. Second, the concentration of the virus in the vertebrate host is crucial; more than 100,000 infectious doses per millimeter may be required for infection. Third, the incubation period for replication of the virus in the arthropod must be met; four days to two weeks generally must pass before the carrier can infect a vertebrate, but the virus may remain infective for several weeks after that. The incubation period is often influenced by environmental temperature; high temperature often accelerates incubation times and frequently results in epidemics.

Symptoms of encephalitis develop one to two weeks after the bite of the mosquito and may come on gradually or quite suddenly and forcefully. Acute viral infection of the central nervous system varies from disease to disease because each virus may affect different parts of the nervous system and/or nerve cells. For example, if the meninges (outer covering of the brain and cord) are infected, symptoms may include headache, fever, stiff neck, and pleocytosis. If the fundamental tissues of the brain (parenchymal cells) are involved, loss of consciousness, seizures, focal neurological deficits, and an increased pressure within the brain (such is the case with encephalitis) may also occur. In addition to all other symptoms, if the hypothalamic-pituitary region becomes involved, sudden increases or decreases in body temperature may occur, and diabetes insipidus may result from a lack of antidiuretic hormone secretion. Swelling of the brain may lead to coma and is often followed by cardiac and respiratory arrest. In these cases, the disease may be deemed fatal. If the spinal cord becomes infected, symptoms manifested include paralysis of bowel and bladder.

The three most common symptoms of the acute state (with sudden, forceful onset) are headache, disturbances of sleep rhythm, and visual abnormalities (blurred vision or double vision). Headaches, though common, are not often severe but may accompany vomiting and other body aches. Sleep disturbances generally include lethargy during the day and insomnia at night. More severe cases suffer fever and delirium. Other common symptoms might include drowsiness, stupor, and eye muscle weakness. Because of the infrequency with which encephalitis strikes and the complete change in symptoms in the latter half of the twentieth century, the acute stage may never be observed. Still, in a study of two thousand cases, 38 percent of the patients died, and whose who did died during the acute phase. These deaths occurred during the first month, most frequently on the fourteenth day. Those most likely to succumb were children under one year of age and adults over the age of seventy. Young adults between the ages of twenty and thirty were most likely to survive. Complete recovery, however, occurred in only about one-fourth of the cases. The remainder of the survivors suffered some degree of dementia.

Symptoms of the chronic stage include sleep disturbances (lethargy and/or insomnia), some dementia, depression, irritability, and anxiety in adults. Children often experience such behavior disorders as stealing, animal cruelty, and other criminal mischief. Respiratory disorders are common in chronic cases, but visual disturbances persist in only a few cases. Since the epidemic during and after World War I that brought so much attention to the disease, the symptoms have undergone remarkable changes. With the epidemic form, the symptoms came on suddenly and with force. Years later, the onset became less terrifying but the chronic stage was often more severe. The most noted symptom in current cases is not during the course of the disease but later. Such is the case with those suffering postencephalitic parkinsonism. The long-range effects may be delayed as long as forty years before onset. Other lingering aftereffects may be deterioration of mental faculties. In children who have contracted the disease, behavioral disorders may result.

Very infrequently, encephalitis has been implicated in epilepsy. This link would be likely only if the disease caused lesions in the brain. Injuries to or inflammation of a child's nervous system may be the basis for hyperactivity in as many of 80 percent of those children suffering from hyperactivity. Although there are many ways these events can happen, it is not unreasonable to expect that some children who have recovered from encephalitis will experience hyperactivity. In fact, their hyperactivity may be the only real neurological aftermath of the disease.

The encephalitis that was prevalent during World War I was usually accompanied by sleep lasting days or even weeks. (Sometimes called "sleeping sickness" or "sleepy sickness," this type of encephalitis is not to be confused with African sleeping sickness, which is caused by the parasite trypanosoma, borne by the tsetse fly.) Its scientific name is encephalitis lethargica, and it is sometimes referred to as von Economo's disease. This sleep results from lesions in the midbrain as well as the hypothalamic and subthalamic regions of the brain. The lesions also induce continual drowsiness as well as motor deficiencies. Encephalitis lethargica is a type of coma, but the patient can be easily roused with stimulation although he or she lies inert, making no sound. The patient's eyes can follow movement or watch the observer carefully. Rarely, encephalitis lethargica may produce symptoms suggestive of chorea (characterized by involuntary movements).

Postinfection encephalitis may occur during, or as a result of, infectious diseases such as influenza or measles. It may also appear after vaccination against rabies, smallpox, or measles. Postinfection encephalitis does not occur as frequently as the other types, but neither is it affected by the sufferer's age. Because children are most often vaccinated, however, they are more susceptible to postinfection encephalitis.

In the United States, four types are commonly recognized. St. Louis encephalitis is geographically the most widespread as well as the most common type of arbovirus-induced encephalitis. It is found primarily in the South and Midwest and mostly victimizes the elderly. Affected areas of the nervous system include the basal ganglia, brainstem, and white matter of the brain and occasionally the spinal cord. The usual symptoms are fever, reduced heart rate, drowsiness, stupor, nuchal rigidity, athetoses and tremors of the hands, and sometimes seizures. Unusual symptoms may include urinary dysfunction (painful urination and pus in the urine), uncoordinated muscular movements, diabetes insipidus as a result of a lack of antidiuretic hormone, and oculomotor paralysis. Even so, recovery rates are considered to be good for St. Louis encephalitis.

Eastern equine encephalitis is very rare, but the most deadly, with 20 to 40 percent mortality. It is mostly found all along the East Coast where there are horses and pheasants. Eastern equine encephalitis produces numerous large lesions in the brain and is accompanied by high fever, drowsiness, cyanosis (lack of oxygen because of respiratory distress), twitching, seizures, and nuchal rigidity. Not only are mortality rates high, but there is likelihood of severe disabilities including speech difficulties, paralyses, and mental retardation as well.

California encephalitis, sometimes called Western encephalitis, is also rare. Found west of the Mississippi, it is not often fatal or serious. It comes on strong with headache, fever, vomiting, confusion, stupor with perhaps coma, seizures, and respiratory failure. The respiratory failure may cause death in 5 percent of the cases. Aftereffects are rare but might include parkinsonism or learning difficulties. A fourth type of encephalitis found in the United States is LaCrosse, which occurs in the north-central states and West Virginia. Its victims are most often young children.

Encephalitis may occur sporadically as a result of other viral infections such as herpes simplex virus 1, measles (it rarely follows German measles), mumps, rabies, and even during the course of human immunodeficiency virus (HIV) infection. The most common form of fatal sporadic encephalitis is caused by herpes simplex virus 1. It accounts for 5 to 10 percent of the total number of encephalitis cases in the United States each year. If untreated, it is fatal in as many as 70 percent of the cases. Herpes simplex-induced encephalitis produces fever, headache, seizures, and coma and is sometimes preceded by a span of bizarre behavior. These personality changes are likely the result of lesions in the temporal lobes and may include terror and hallucinations. The patient may suffer some paralysis, particularly of the face and arm. Deep coma with respiratory arrest may occur. Of those surviving herpes-induced encephalitis, about half continue to suffer major motor and sensory deficits, speech problems, and frequently, an amnestic syndrome (Korsakoff's psychosis). Two antiviral agents are used to combat the disease with moderate success: acyclovir (often the drug of choice) and adenosine arabinoside. Acyclovir is active only in the cells invaded by the herpes simplex virus and inhibits deoxyribonucleic acid (DNA) replication (effectively halting cell division and numerical growth). HIV-infected patients often experience herpes simplex virus 1, which means that acquired immunodeficiency syndrome (AIDS) patients with this herpes virus may develop encephalitis.

Occasionally, a child under two years of age apparently fights off a bout of measles, only to succumb to a slow invasion of encephalitis that may be fatal. The encephalitis may appear before the rash, with the rash, or after the rash. It may not make an appearance until the child is between ages four and eighteen. In these rare cases (one in every 200,000 cases), known as subacute sclerosing panencephalitis (SSPE), the initial symptoms may be mild. The child may experience poor concentration at first; then symptoms might progress through stages of erratic jerking of the limbs, blindness, severe mental retardation, and then death. There may be a sudden onset with symptoms of fever, lethargy, delirium, catatonia, or excitement. Seizures are common, and mortality rates are high. SSPE results when the measles virus persists in the brain, killing some nerve cells and destroying the myelin sheath surrounding others. SSPE is rare because of the widespread use of anti-measles vaccines.

Another disease of the nervous system that most frequently affects children is acute toxic encephalitis. The difference occurs in the changes it induces in the nervous system. There is not only brain cell degeneration but also edema of the brain and small hemorrhages. Acute toxic encephalitis may also occur in children suffering from burns because of the toxemic effects that burns have on nerve cells.

Several theories have been proposed to answer why other diseases lead to encephalitis. One of these is that the central nervous system reacts to the virus that caused the original disease. Another theory suggests that there may be poisonous substances that develop during the course of the original disease that induce encephalitis. The least popular theory is that enzymes already in the patient or enzymes produced by the original disease are activated. These enzymes destroy the myelin around the nerve cells. Still others believe that postinfection encephalitis is an autoimmune disease. Because of the rarity of postinfection encephalitis, it may be years before the answer is found.

TREATMENT AND THERAPY

Generally, in order to diagnose a patient with encephalitis (which is often indistinguishable from viral meningitis), a physician must review the patient's medical history in the light of the presence or absence of an epidemic, as well as the presence of signs and symptoms. If they indeed are indicative of the possibility, a lumbar puncture and examination of spinal fluid are performed. The amount of pressure the fluid exerts is checked; if pleocytosis and an elevated protein level are found, they too, indicate the likelihood of encephalitis. In some cases, the blood is found to contain increased numbers of neutralizing antibodies. Because the onset of fever, the aches and pains, and other symptoms characterize many infections and diseases as well as encephalitis, specific diagnosis can be made only by isolating the virus or sometimes through a blood workup. Because it is extremely difficult to isolate the virus in the blood, successful diagnosis may be made when two specific antibodies increase in the blood. Although sometimes misdiagnosed as poliomyelitis or multiple sclerosis, encephalitis can be distinguished from these diseases by the sleep disturbances it causes and by the visual disturbances that it may induce. It is unlikely to cause paralysis and only infrequently results in convulsions, unlike the other diseases. Encephalitis is also occasionally misdiagnosed as meningitis but differs from it in that the spinal fluid does not contain an excess of cells as in meningitis. An electroencephalogram (EEG) can be useful because it might show the appropriate disturbance of cerebral activity.

At one time, as many as seventy-five methods of treatment for encephalitis were reported. Yet none of these actually influences how the disease progresses. The only thing that can be treated, therefore, is the symptoms. Placement in intensive care as early as possible is desirable because of the rapid progression of the illness. Relieving the headache and reducing the fever so the sufferer can be as comfortable as possible would likely be the first course taken. Seizures can be treated with anticonvulsant drugs such as phenytoin. Intracranial pressure should be monitored, and if the pressure does rise, nasotracheal intubation (a tube placed in the nose) with hyperventilation from a ventilator might aid in decreasing pressure. During convalescence, speech and physical therapy may be necessary. The length of convalescence depends on how severe the illness has been, but it may take several months for recovery. The prognosis for those with viral encephalitis depends on the causative agent. In order to control the spread of the mosquito-borne encephalitis virus, a thorough knowledge and understanding of the mosquito population is necessary. Breeding sites must be located, and the distribution and density of the adult mosquito population must be determined, especially those in areas near human populations. This information can be used to contain the mosquito population by using larvivorous fish or chemical insecticides. If one is in an area that is experiencing an outbreak, the best prevention is to remain indoors after dark, thereby avoiding the time that mosquitoes are feeding. If one must go out, one should spray exposed areas with insect repellent and/or wear long sleeves and pants of tightly woven material. The use of window screens, residual insecticide application on and around screen doors, and mosquito netting over cribs offers other ways to retard the number of mosquitoes that can enter the house or to prevent mosquito bites.

PERSPECTIVE AND PROSPECTS

A look at history reveals numerous cases and minor epidemics of encephalitis. In 1580, Europe was inundated with a fever-causing lethargic disease resulting in parkinsonism and other long-lasting neurological effects. Other serious epidemics occurred in London between 1672 and 1673 and again between 1673 and 1675. The most common (and highly unusual) symptom of this epidemic was hiccuping. Epidemics also occurred in the German city of Tübingen from 1712 to 1713, in France and Germany in the latter half of the eighteenth century, and in Italy following a deadly influenza outbreak in 1889 and 1890. None of these epidemics, however, was nearly as widespread as the pandemic that began in the winter of 1916-1917. This major outbreak began in the European city of Vienna, and within three years it had spread worldwide. It seemed each case was different; no two patients experienced the same signs and symptoms the same way. Because of such variations, diagnosis such as epidemic delirium, epidemic schizophrenia, epidemic parkinsonism, rabies, and polio were erroneously made. Seemingly, thousands of new diseases were instantly pervading the globe. It was Constantin von Economo who, through his pathological studies on the brain tissues of many of those who died, not only found a unique pattern of damage but also isolated the virus common to all. Von Economo named this "new" disease encephalitis lethargica.

As this epidemic seized the world, more than five million people were either killed or severely affected. It lasted ten years, leaving as suddenly as it had come. Of those who died, one-third succumbed during the acute stages of the sleeping sickness (in such a deep comatose state as to preclude arousal, or in such a state of sleeplessness as to invalidate sedation). Even those who survived the coma/wakefulness attacks were so affected that they failed to recover to their predisease alertness. Many were simply conscious, unaware, speechless, motionless, and without energy, motivation, appetite, or desire. They knew what was occurring around them but were totally apathetic to the events, showing no behavior at all.

Sixty years after the epidemic of World War I, many survivors were still alive. Some had active lives despite parkinsonism, tics, and other problems. They were the lucky few; most postencephalitic patients suffered gross debilitating neurological damage, never to function independently again. Many of the survivors were bedridden and robbed of movement, speech, and perhaps memory. Most of them were banished to asylums, nursing homes, or other "special" places where they were untreated and forgotten.
—*Iona C. Baldridge*

See also Bites and stings; Brain disorders; Dementia; Hemiplegia; Parasitic diseases; Sleeping sickness; Viral infections.

FOR FURTHER INFORMATION:

Aminoff, Michael J., ed. *Neurology and General Medicine.* New York: Churchill Livingstone, 1989. This compilation by numerous contributors relates neurological disorders that may occur as a result of or in conjunction with general medical disorders. The intended audience is medical professionals.

Bowsher, David, ed. *Neurological Emergencies in Medical Practice: A Handbook for the Non-Specialist.* London: Croom Helm, 1988. A brief book delineating the recognition and treatment of neurological emergencies written by doctors for doctors. Therefore, it is filled with medical language and is not easily read by the layperson.

Horsfall, Frank L., Jr., and Igor Tamm, eds. *Viral and Rickettsial Infections of Man.* 4th ed. Philadelphia: J. B. Lippincott, 1965. A somewhat dated but well-organized, comprehensive look at many infections caused by viruses and rickettsias. Written as an aid to medical students and graduate students, but still fairly readable.

Johnson, Richard T. *Viral Infections of the Nervous System.* New York: Raven Press, 1982. A readable volume, with a clinical audience in mind; punctuated with pictures and tables. Emphasizes the biology of nervous system infections, and references to laboratory diagnoses, prevention, and therapy are also included.

Sacks, Oliver. *Awakenings.* New York: Summit Books, 1987. An insightful and intriguing look into twenty case histories of patients suffering from postencephalitic symptoms. Traces the history of the first drug treatment of these patients and their reentry into "life."

Taylor, Joyce W., and Sally Ballenger. *Neurological Dysfunctions and Nursing Intervention.* New York: McGraw-Hill, 1980. This text is filled with medical terminology regarding the brain and its related diseases. Written for nursing students, but most readers can achieve a basic understanding of neurological diseases with this work.

Walton, John N., and W. Russell Brain. *Diseases of the Nervous System.* 8th ed. Oxford, England: Oxford University Press, 1977. A lengthy, complex volume written to educate and inform medical professionals on all aspects of neurological dysfunctions. Its completeness provides a wide range of material, but it is intended for diagnostic usage.

ENDOCARDITIS

SYSTEM AFFECTED: Heart

SPECIALISTS: Cardiologists, internists, vascular surgeons

DEFINITION: Inflammatory lesions of the endocardium, the lining of the heart.

CAUSES AND SYMPTOMS

The lesions of endocarditis may be noninfective, as in rheumatic fever, or infective. The latter are characterized

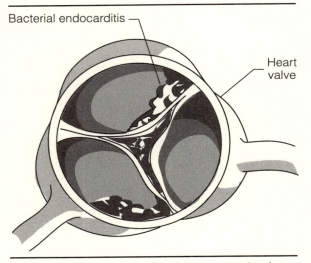

Bacterial endocarditis

Heart valve

Bacterial endocarditis of a heart valve occurs when bacteria invade and cause inflammatory lesions; untreated, the condition is usually fatal.

by direct invasion of the endocardium by microorganisms, most often bacteria. Bacterial endocarditis may occur on normal or previously damaged heart valves and also on artificial (prosthetic) heart valves. Rarely, endocarditis may occur on the wall (mural surface) of the heart or at the site of an abnormal hole between the pumping chambers of the heart, called a ventricular septal defect.

In areas of turbulent blood flow, platelet-fibrin deposition can occur, providing a nidus for subsequent bacterial colonization. Transient bacteremia may accompany infection elsewhere in the body or some medical and dental procedures, and these circulating bacteria can adhere to the endocardium, especially at platelet-fibrin deposition sites, and produce endocarditis. Intravenous drug abusers using unsterile equipment and drugs often inject bacteria along with the drugs, which can result in endocarditis. The lesions produced by these depositions plus bacteria are called vegetations. Clinical symptoms and signs usually begin about two weeks later.

Bacterial endocarditis usually involves either the mitral or the aortic heart valve. In intravenous drug abusers, the tricuspid heart valve is more commonly affected because it is the first valve to be reached by the endocardium-damaging drugs and contaminating bacteria. The pulmonic valve is only rarely the site of endocarditis. Occasionally, more than one heart valve is infected; this occurs most often in intravenous drug abusers or patients with multiple prosthetic heart valves.

Gram-positive cocci are the most common cause of bacterial endocarditis. Different species predominate in various conditions or situations: *Streptococcus viridans* in native valves, *Staphylococcus aureus* in the valves of intravenous drug abusers, and *Staphylococcus epidermidis* in prosthetic heart valves. Gram-negative bacilli are found in association with prosthetic heart valves or intravenous drug addiction.

The clinical manifestations of endocarditis are varied and often nonspecific. Early symptoms are similar to those encountered in most infections: fever, malaise, and fatigue. As the disease progresses, more cardiovascular and renal-related symptoms may appear: dyspnea, chest pain, and stroke. Fever and heart murmurs are found in most patients. Enlargement of the spleen, skin lesions, and evidence of emboli are commonly present.

The key to the diagnosis of bacterial endocarditis is to suspect the presence of the illness and obtain blood cultures. Febrile patients who have a heart murmur, cardiac failure, a prosthetic heart valve, history of intravenous drug abuse, preexisting valvular disease, stroke (especially in young adults), multiple pulmonary emboli, sudden arterial occlusion, unexplained prolonged fever, or multiple positive blood cultures are likely to have endocarditis. The hallmark of bacterial endocarditis is continuous bacteremia; thus, nearly all blood cultures will be positive. Other nonspecific blood tests, such as an erythrocyte sedimentation rate, or specific blood tests, such as tests for teichoic acid antibodies, may be helpful in establishing a diagnosis.

TREATMENT AND THERAPY

Endocarditis may be prevented by administering prophylactic antibiotics to patients with preexisting heart abnormalities that predispose them to endocarditis when they are likely to have transient bacteremia. An example would be a patient with an artificial heart valve scheduled to have a dental cleaning.

Endocarditis is one of the few infections that is nearly always fatal if mistreated. Antibacterial therapy with agents capable of killing the offending bacteria, along with supportive medical care and cardiac surgery when indicated, cures most patients.

PERSPECTIVE AND PROSPECTS

The first demonstration of bacteria in vegetations associated with endocarditis was by Emmanuel Winge of Oslo, Norway, in 1869. Fifty years later, a fresh section was cut from the preserved heart valve described by Winge, and staining by modern methods revealed a chain of streptococci verifying his discovery. It was not until 1943, when Leo Loewe successfully treated seven cases of bacterial endocarditis with penicillin, that the era of modern therapy of this serious illness began.

Endocarditis accounts for approximately one case in every 1,000 hospital admissions in the United States. The incidence remained fairly constant between the 1960's and the 1990's, but the type of patient has changed: Heroin addicts, the elderly, and patients with prosthetic heart valves constitute an increasing percentage of endocarditis cases.
—*H. Bradford Hawley*

See also Heart disease; Mitral insufficiency; Rheumatic fever.

FOR FURTHER INFORMATION:

Kaye, Donald, ed. *Infective Endocarditis*. Baltimore: University Park Press, 1976. An excellent text covering all the features of endocarditis in the modern era.

Kerr, Andrew. *Subacute Bacterial Endocarditis*. Springfield, Ill.: Charles C Thomas, 1955. The classic monograph describing the history and natural course of the disease.

Magilligan, Donald J., Jr., and Edward L. Quinn, eds. *Endocarditis: Medical and Surgical Management*. New York: Marcel Dekker, 1986. Discusses the treatment of endocarditis and its complications.

ENDOCRINE DISORDERS

SYSTEM AFFECTED: Endocrine

SPECIALISTS: Endocrinologists

DEFINITION: Breakdowns in the normal functioning of the endocrine system, which controls the metabolic processes of the body.

KEY TERMS:

cyclic AMP: a chemical that acts as a second messenger to bring about a response by the cell to the presence of some hormones at their receptors

endocrine: a secretion into the bloodstream rather than by way of a duct, such as hormones

feedback: the mechanism whereby a hormone inhibits its own production; often involves the inhibition of the hypothalamus and tropic hormones

hypothalamohypophysial: relating to the hypothalamus and the hypophysis (pituitary gland)

target cell or organ: a cell or organ possessing the specific hormone receptors needed to respond to a given hormone

tropic: hormones that feed a particular physiological state

tropin: hormones that cause a "turning toward" a particular physiological state

PROCESS AND EFFECTS

In order to understand endocrine disorders, it is necessary to review briefly the location of the principal endocrine glands, the hormones secreted, and the normal functions of the hormones. The hormones are released into the bloodstream and are carried throughout the body, where they affect target cells or organs that have receptors for the given hormone.

The pituitary gland, or hypophysis, is sometimes called the master gland because of its widespread influences on many other endocrine glands and the body as a whole. It is located in the midline on the lower part of the brain just above the posterior part of the roof of the mouth. The pituitary has three lobes: the posterior lobe, the intermediate lobe, and the anterior lobe.

The posterior lobe does not synthesize hormones, but it does have nerve fibers coming into it from the hypothalamus of the brain. The ends of these axons release two hormones that are synthesized in the hypothalamus, oxytocin and antidiuretic hormone (ADH). Oxytocin causes the contraction of the smooth muscles of the uterus during childbirth and the contraction of tissues in the mammary glands to release milk during nursing. ADH causes the kidneys to reabsorb water and thereby reduce the volume of urine to normal levels when necessary.

The intermediate lobe of the pituitary secretes melanocyte-stimulating hormone (MSH), a hormone with an uncertain role in humans but known to cause the darkening of melanocytes in animals. Sometimes, the intermediate lobe is considered to be a part of the anterior lobe.

The anterior lobe of the pituitary is under the control of releasing hormones produced by the hypothalamus and carried to the anterior lobe by special blood vessels. In response to these releasing hormones, some stimulatory and some inhibitory, the anterior lobe produces thyroid-stimulating hormone (TSH), adrenocorticotropic hormone (ACTH), follicle-stimulating hormone (FSH), luteinizing hormone (LH), prolactin, and somatotropin or growth hormone (GH). TSH stimulates the thyroid to produce thyroxine, ACTH stimulates the adrenal cortex to produce some of its hormones, FSH stimulates the growth of the cells surrounding eggs in the ovary and causes the ovary to produce estrogen, LH induces ovulation (the release of an egg from the ovary) and stimulates the secretion of progesterone by the ovary, prolactin is essential for milk production and various metabolic functions, and GH is needed for normal growth.

The pineal gland, or epiphysis, is a neuroendocrine gland attached to the roof of the diencephalon in the brain. It produces melatonin, which is released into the bloodstream during the night and has important functions related to an individual's biological clock.

The thyroid gland is located below the larynx in the front of the throat. It produces the hormones thyroxine (T_3) and triiodothyronine (T_4), which are essential for maintaining a normal level of metabolism and heat production, as well as enabling normal development of the brain in young children. C-cells in the thyroid produce calcitonin, which is involved in blood calcium regulation. This is also true for parathyroid hormone, a product of the nearby parathyroid glands. The thymus, located under the breast bone or sternum, produces the hormone thymosin that stimulates the immune system. Even the heart is an endocrine gland: It produces atrial natriuretic factor, which stimulates sodium excretion by the kidneys. The pancreas, located near the stomach and small intestine, produces digestive enzymes that pass to the duodenum, but also it produces insulin and glucagon in special cells called pancreatic islets. Insulin causes blood sugar (glucose) to be taken up from the blood into the tissues of the body, and glucagon causes stored starch (glycogen) to be broken down in the liver and thereby increases blood glucose levels.

Glands of the Endocrine System

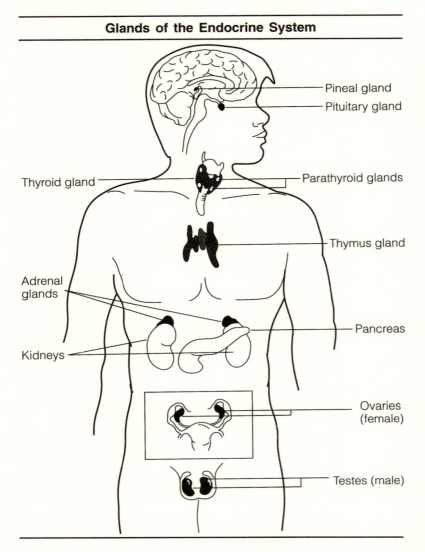

techniques for showing the existence of hypothesized hormones.

The posterior pituitary releases both oxytocin and ADH. Chemicals similar to oxytocin are sometimes given to induce contractions in pregnant women so that birth will occur at a predetermined time. The other hormone released from the posterior pituitary, ADH, normally causes the reabsorption of water within the tubules of the kidney. A deficiency of ADH leads to diabetes insipidus, a condition in which many liters of water a day are excreted by the urinary system; this necessitates that the patient drink huge quantities of water simply to stay alive. A synthetic form of ADH, desmopressin acetate, can be given in the form of a nasal spray that diffuses into the bloodstream and thus restores the reabsorption of water by the kidneys.

The anterior lobe of the pituitary produces six known hormones. The production of these hormones is stimulated and/or inhibited by special releasing hormones secreted by the hypothalamus and carried to the anterior lobe by the hypothalamohypophysial portal system of blood vessels. Thus, the source of some anterior pituitary disorders can reside in the hypothalamus. Tumors of anterior pituitary cells can result in the overproduction of a hormone, or if the tumor is destructive, the underproduction of a hormone. Radiation or surgery can be used to destroy tumors and thereby restore normal pituitary functioning.

The pair of adrenal glands, located on the kidneys, are made up of two components: first, a cortex that produces glucocorticoids, mineralocorticoids, and sex steroids or androgens; and second, a medulla, or inner part, that secretes adrenaline and noradrenaline. The gonads, testes or ovaries, are located in the pelvic region and produce several hormones, including the estrogen and progesterone that are essential for reproduction in females and the testosterone that is essential for reproduction in males. The kidneys and digestive tract also produce hormones that regulate red blood cell formation and the functioning of the digestive tract, respectively.

COMPLICATIONS AND DISORDERS

A wide variety of endocrine disorders can be treated successfully. In fact, the ability to restore normal endocrine function with replacement therapy has long been one of the

Anterior pituitary hormones can be the basis of a variety of disorders. As with other hormones, there may be below-normal production of the hormone (hyposecretion) or over-production of the hormone (hypersecretion). Because the pituitary hormones are often supportive of hormone secretion by the target organ or tissue, hyposecretion or hypersecretion of the tropic or supportive hormone leads to a similar change in the production of hormones by the target organ or tissue.

For example, hyperthyroidism, or Graves' disease, can be caused by excessive secretion of TSH by the pituitary, leading to hypersecretion of thyroxine or by nodules within the thyroid that produce excessive thyroxine. In the diagnosis process, blood levels of both TSH and thyroxine are usually measured to determine the specific cause of the disorder. Similarly, hypothyroidism can be induced by deficits at several levels. The lack of iodine in the diet can prevent the production of thyroxine, which requires iodide as part of its molecular composition. The production of thyroxine usually has a negative feedback effect on the hypothalamus and pituitary, reducing TSH production. The failure to produce thyroxine causes high blood levels of TSH and an abnormal growth of the thyroid that results in a greatly enlarged thyroid, called a goiter. The addition of iodine to salt has eliminated the incidence of goiter in developed countries. Even with an adequate supply of iodine in the diet, however, hypothyroidism can still develop from other sources. The usual treatment is to ingest a dose of thyroxine daily.

Other examples of anterior pituitary disorders include those involving changes in GH secretion. Undersecretion of GH can lead to short stature or even dwarfism, in which an individual has normal body proportions but is smaller than normal. Now it is possible to obtain human GH from bacteria genetically engineered to produce it. Replacement GH can be given during the normal growth years to enhance growth. A tumor sometimes develops in the pituitary cells that produce GH, and this can cause abnormally increased growth or gigantism. If the tumor develops during the adult years, only a few areas of abnormal growth can occur, such as in the facial bones and the bones of the hands and feet. This condition is called acromegaly. Abraham Lincoln is thought to have had abnormal levels of GH that caused gigantism in his youth and then acromegaly in his later years. Acromegaly can be treated by radiation or surgery of the anterior pituitary.

Pineal gland tumors have been associated with precocious puberty, in which children become sexually developed in early childhood. It is thought that melatonin normally inhibits sexual development during this period. The pineal gland is influenced by changes in the daily photoperiod, so that the highest levels of melatonin appear in the blood during the night, especially during the long nights of winter. Seasonal affective disorder (SAD), a mental depression that occurs during the late fall and winter, has been linked to seasonally high melatonin levels. Daily exposure to bright lights to mimic summer has been used to treat SAD. The pineal gland and melatonin are also being studied with regard to jet lag and disorders associated with shift work. The pineal gland thus seems to be involved in the functioning of the body's biological clock.

The pancreatic islets, also called the islets of Langerhans, produce insulin and glucagon. Diabetes mellitus is caused by insufficient insulin production (type 1 or juvenile-onset diabetes) or by the lack of functional insulin receptors on body cells (type 2 or maturity-onset diabetes). Type 1 diabetes can be treated with insulin injections, an implanted insulin pump, or even a transplant of fetal pancreatic tissue. Type 2 diabetes is treated with diet and weight loss. Weight loss induces an increase in insulin receptors. In addition to the symptoms of high blood sugar levels in the diabetic, long-term damage to the kidneys, blood vessels to the retina, and blood vessels in the legs and feet are important concerns.

The adrenal cortex produces glucocorticoids, mineralocorticoids, and androgens, any of which can be the basis of hyposecretion or hypersecretion. Addison's disease is caused by hyposecretion, whereas Cushing's syndrome is caused by hypersecretion or more-than-sufficient replacement therapy. Similar to those of the thyroid, the adrenal cortex secretions have a negative feedback on the hypothalamus and the anterior pituitary. Addison's disease is characterized by low blood pressure and a poor physiological response to stress. The high levels of ACTH—high because of inadequate feedback of corticoids on the hypothalamus and anterior pituitary—cause a bronzing of the skin because ACTH is similar in its molecular composition to MSH. During an adrenal crisis, exogenous adrenal corticoids are essential to avoid death. Corticoids can be given to prevent inflammation, but their overuse can lead to adrenal cortex suppression by the negative feedback mechanism. The abuse of androgens by athletes wanting to buildup their muscles can also result in adrenal suppression, sterility, and damage to the heart. Tumors of androgen-producing cells in women can cause beard growth, increased muscle development, and other changes associated with sex hormones.

PERSPECTIVE AND PROSPECTS

The early history of endocrinology noted that boys who were castrated failed to undergo the changes associated with puberty. A. A. Berthold in 1849 described the effects of castration in cockerels. The birds failed to develop large combs and waddles and failed to show male behavior. He noted that these effects could be reversed if testes were transplanted back into the cockerels. W. M. Bayliss and E. H. Starling in 1902 first introduced the term "hormone" to refer to secretin. They found that secretin is produced by the small intestine in response to acid in the chyme and that secretin causes the pancreas to release digestive enzymes into the small intestine. Most important, F. G. Banting and G. H. Best in 1922 reported their extraction of insulin from the pancreas of dogs and their success in alleviating diabetes in dogs by means of injections of the insulin. Fredrick Sanger in 1953 established the amino acid sequence for insulin and later won a Nobel Prize for this achievement.

Another Nobel Prize was awarded to Earl W. Sutherland, Jr., in 1971 for his demonstration in 1962 of the role of cyclic AMP as a second messenger in the sequence involved in the stimulation of cells by many hormones. Andrew V. Schally and Roger C. L. Guillemin in 1977 received a Nobel Prize for their work in isolating and determining the structures of hypothalamic regulatory peptides.

More recent achievements in endocrinological research have centered on the identification of receptors that bind with the hormone when the hormone stimulates a cell and on the genetic engineering of bacteria to produce hormones such as human growth hormone. The use of fetal tissues in endocrinological research and therapy—the host usually does not reject fetal implants—continue to be areas for future research. —*John T. Burns*

See also Addison's disease; Amenorrhea; Cushing's syndrome; Diabetes mellitus; Dwarfism; Dysmenorrhea; Endometriosis; Female genital disorders; Gigantism; Goiter; Growth; Hyperparathyroidism and hypoparathyroidism; Hypoglycemia; Infertility in females; Infertility in males; Male genital disorders; Menopause; Menorrhagia; Ovarian cysts; Pancreatitis; Pregnancy and gestation; Puberty and adolescence; Thyroid disorders.

FOR FURTHER INFORMATION:

Griffin, James E., and Sergio R. Ojeda, eds. *Textbook of Endocrine Physiology.* 2d ed. New York: Oxford University Press, 1992. A detailed account of normal and abnormal functioning of the endocrine system written by specialists. Intended for first year medical students.

Hadley, Mac E. *Endocrinology.* 3d ed. Englewood Cliffs, N.J.: Prentice Hall, 1992. A college-level text covering the endocrine system, primarily in humans and mammals. Recommended for a technical but understandable coverage of the field.

Jubiz, William. *Endocrinology: A Logical Approach for Clinicians.* 2d ed. New York: McGraw-Hill, 1985. An excellent source of information on specific endocrine disorders, symptoms and current treatment. Not recommended for the unmotivated reader.

Martini, Frederic. *Fundamentals of Anatomy and Physiology.* 2d ed. Englewood Cliffs, N.J.: Prentice Hall, 1992. A good place to start for a solid overview of the anatomy and physiology of the endocrine system before considering the details of disease states.

Thibodeau, Gary A., and Kevin T. Patton. *Anatomy and Physiology.* 2d ed. St. Louis: Mosby Year Book, 1993. An elementary examination of the endocrine system is provided.

ENDODONTIC DISEASE

SYSTEMS AFFECTED: Gums, teeth

SPECIALISTS: Dentists

DEFINITION: Endodontics is the field of dentistry concerned with diseases of the dental pulp found within teeth and diseases of the surrounding tissues, the gums. Endodontic disease can be caused by damage to the nerves in the teeth and gums and resulting infection by microorganisms. Dental caries, commonly known as cavities, are one example of pulp decay that must be removed. If the entire pulp has died or becomes untreatable, root canal treatment may be required, in which the pulp is

completely replaced with filling paste and the surface of the tooth is sealed with a cement crown.

See also Caries, dental; Dental diseases; Gingivitis; Periodontitis; Toothache.

ENDOMETRIOSIS

SYSTEM AFFECTED: Reproductive (female)

SPECIALISTS: Gynecologists

DEFINITION: Growth of cells of the uterine lining at sites outside the uterus, causing severe pain and infertility.

KEY TERMS:

cervix: an oval-shaped organ that separates the uterus and the vagina

dysmenorrhea: painful menstruation

dyspareunia: painful sexual intercourse

endometrium: the tissue that lines the uterus, builds up, and sheds at the end of each menstrual cycle; when it grows outside the uterus, endometriosis occurs

Fallopian tubes: two tubes extending from the ovaries to the uterus; during ovulation, an egg travels down one of these tubes to the uterus

hysterectomy: surgery that removes part or all of the uterus

implant: an abnormal endometrial growth outside the uterus

laparoscopy: a surgical procedure in which a small incision made near the navel is used to view the uterus and other abdominal organs with a lighted tube called a laparoscope

laparotomy: a surgical procedure, often exploratory in nature, carried out through the abdominal wall; it may be used to correct endometriosis

laser: a concentrated, high-energy light beam often used to destroy abnormal tissue

oophorectomy (or *ovariectomy*): removal of the ovaries, which is often necessary in cases of severe endometriosis

prostaglandins: fatlike hormones that control the contraction and relaxation of the uterus and other smooth muscle tissue

CAUSES AND SYMPTOMS

Endometriosis, the presence of endometrial tissue outside its normal location as the lining of the uterus, is a disabling disease in women that causes severe pain and in many cases infertility. The classic symptoms of endometriosis are very painful menstruation (dysmenorrhea), painful intercourse (dyspareunia), and infertility. Some other common endometriosis symptoms include nausea, vomiting, diarrhea, and fatigue.

It has been estimated that endometriosis affects between five million and twenty-five million American women. Often, it is incorrectly stereotyped as being a disease of upwardly mobile, professional women. According to many experts, the incidence of endometriosis worldwide and across most racial groups is probably very similar. They propose that the reported occurrence rate difference for some racial groups, such as a lower incidence in African

Americans, has been a socioeconomic phenomenon attributable to the social class of women who seek medical treatment for the symptoms of endometriosis and to the highly stratified responses of many health care professionals who have dealt with the disease.

The symptoms of endometriosis arise from abnormalities in the effects of the menstrual cycle on the endometrial tissue lining the uterus. The endometrium normally thickens and becomes swollen with blood (engorged) during the cycle, a process controlled by female hormones called estrogens and progestins. This engorgement is designed to prepare the uterus for conception by optimizing conditions for implantation in the endometrium of a fertilized egg, which enters the uterus via one of the Fallopian tubes leading from the ovaries.

By the middle of the menstrual cycle, the endometrial lining is normally about ten times thicker than that at its beginning. If the egg that is released into the uterus is not fertilized, pregnancy does not occur and decreases in production of the female sex hormones result in the breakdown of the endometrium. Endometrial tissue mixed with blood leaves the uterus as the menstrual flow and a new menstrual cycle begins. This series of uterine changes occurs repeatedly, as a monthly cycle, from puberty (which usually occurs between the ages of twelve and fourteen) to the menopause (which usually occurs between the ages of forty-five and fifty-five).

In women who develop endometriosis, some endometrial tissue begins to grow ectopically (in an abnormal position) at sites outside the uterus. The ectopic endometrial growths may be found attached to the ovaries, the Fallopian tubes, the urinary bladder, the rectum, other abdominal organs, and even the lungs. Regardless of body location, these implants behave as if they were still in the uterus, thickening and bleeding each month as the menstrual cycle proceeds. Like the endometrium at its normal uterine site, the ectopic tissue responds to the hormones that circulate through the body in the blood. Its inappropriate position in the body prevents this ectopic endometrial tissue from leaving the body as menstrual flow; as a result, some implants grow to be quite large.

In many cases, the endometrial growths that form between two organs become fibrous bands called adhesions. The fibrous nature of adhesions is attributable to the alternating swelling and breakdown of the ectopic tissue, which yields fibrous scar tissue. The alterations in size of living portions of the adhesions and other endometrial implants during the monthly menstrual cycle cause many afflicted women considerable pain. Because the body location of implants varies, the site of the pain may be almost anywhere, such as the back, the chest, the rectum, or the abdomen. For example, dyspareunia occurs when adhesions hold a uterus tightly to the abdominal wall, making its movement during intercourse painful.

Common Sites of Endometriosis

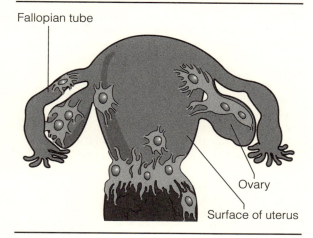

Fallopian tube

Ovary

Surface of uterus

The presence of endometriosis is usually confirmed by laparoscopy, viewed as being the most reliable method for its diagnosis. Laparoscopy is carried out after a physician makes an initial diagnosis of probable endometriosis from a combined study including an examination of the patient's medical history and careful exploration of the patient's physical problems over a period of at least six months. During prelaparoscopy treatment, the patient is very often maintained on pain medication and other therapeutic drugs that will produce symptomatic relief.

For laparoscopy, the patient is anesthetized with a general anesthetic, a small incision is made near the navel, and a flexible lighted tube—a laparoscope—is inserted into this incision. The laparoscope, equipped with fiber optics, enables the examining physician to search the patient's abdominal organs for endometrial implants. Visibility of the abdominal organs in laparoscopic examination can be enhanced by pumping harmless carbon dioxide gas into the abdomen, causing it to distend. Women who undergo laparoscopy usually require a day of postoperative bed rest, followed by seven to ten days of curtailed physical activity. After a laparoscopic diagnosis of endometriosis is made, a variety of surgical and therapeutic drug treatments can be employed to manage the disease.

About 40 percent of all women who have endometriosis are infertile; contemporary wisdom evaluates this relationship as one of cause and effect, which should make this disease the second most common cause of fertility problems. The actual basis for this infertility is not always clear, but it is often the result of damage to the ovaries and Fallopian tubes, scar tissue produced by implants on these and other abdominal organs, and hormone imbalances.

Because the incidence of infertility accompanying endometriosis increases with the severity of the disease, all potentially afflicted women are encouraged to seek early diagnosis. Many experts advise all women with abnormal menstrual cycles, dysmenorrhea, severe menstrual bleeding, abnormal vaginal bleeding, and repeated dyspareunia to seek the advice of a physician trained in identifying and dealing with endometriosis. Because the disease can begin to present symptoms at any age, teenagers are also encouraged to seek medical attention if they experience any of these symptoms.

John Sampson coined the term "endometriosis" in the 1920's. Sampson's theory for its causation, still widely accepted, is termed retrograde menstruation. Also called menstrual backup, this theory proposes that the backing up of some menstrual flow into the Fallopian tubes, and then into the abdominal cavity, forms the endometrial implants. Evidence supporting this theory, according to many physicians, is the fact that such backup is common. Others point out, however, that the backup is often found in women who do not have the disease. A surgical experiment was performed on female monkeys to test this theory. Their uteri were turned upside down so that the menstrual flow would spill into the abdominal cavity. Sixty percent of the animals developed endometriosis postoperatively—an inconclusive result.

Complicating the issue is the fact that implants are also found in tissues (such as in the lung) that cannot be reached by menstrual backup. It has been theorized that the presence of these implants results from the entry of endometrial cells into the lymphatic system, which returns body fluid to the blood and protects the body from many other diseases. This transplantation theory is supported by the occurrence of endometriosis in various portions of the lymphatic system and in tissues that could not otherwise become sites of endometriosis.

A third theory explaining the growth of implants is the iatrogenic, or nosocomial, transmission of endometrial tissue. These terms both indicate an accidental creation of the disease through the actions of physicians. Such implant formation is viewed as occurring most often after cesarean delivery of a baby when passage through the birth canal would otherwise be fatal to mother and/or child. Another proposed cause is episiotomy—widening of the birth canal by an incision between the anus and vagina—to ease births.

Any surgical procedure that allows the spread of endometrial tissue can be implicated, including surgical procedures carried out to correct existing endometriosis, because of the ease with which endometrial tissue implants itself anywhere in the body. Abnormal endometrial tissue growth, called adenomyosis, can also occur in the uterus and is viewed as a separate disease entity.

Other theories regarding the genesis of endometriosis include an immunologic theory, which proposes that women who develop endometriosis are lacking in antibodies that normally cause the destruction of endometrial tissue at sites where it does not belong, and a hormonal theory, which

suggests the existence of large imbalances in hormones such as the prostaglandins that serve as the body's messengers in controlling biological processes. Several of these theories—retrograde menstruation, the transplantation theory, and iatrogenic transmission—all have support, but none has been proved unequivocally. Future evidence will identify whether one cause is dominant, whether they all interact to produce the disease, or whether endometriosis is actually a group of diseases that simply resemble one another in the eyes of contemporary medical science.

TREATMENT AND THERAPY

Laparoscopic examination most often identifies endometriosis as chocolate-colored lumps (chocolate cysts) ranging from the size of a pinhead to several inches across or as filmy coverings over parts of abdominal organs and ligaments. Once a diagnosis of the disease is confirmed by laparoscopy, endometriosis is treated by chemotherapy, surgery, or a combination of both methods. The only permanent, contemporary cure for endometriosis, however, is the onset of the biological menopause at the end of a woman's childbearing years. As long as menstruation continues, implant development is likely to recur, regardless of its cause. Nevertheless, a temporary cure of endometriosis is better than no cure at all.

The chemotherapy that many physicians use to treat mild cases of endometriosis (and for prelaparoscopy periods) is analgesic painkillers, including aspirin, acetaminophen, and ibuprofen. The analgesics inhibit the body's production of prostaglandins, and the symptoms of the disease are merely covered up. Therefore, analgesics are of quite limited value except during a prelaparoscopy diagnostic period or with mild cases of endometriosis. In addition, the long-term administration of aspirin will often produce gastrointestinal bleeding, and excess use of acetaminophen can lead to severe liver damage. In some cases of very severe endometriosis pain, narcotic painkillers are given, such as codeine, Percodan (oxycodone and aspirin), or morphine. Narcotics are addicting and should be avoided unless absolutely necessary.

More effective for long-term management of the disease is hormone therapy. Such therapy is designed to prevent the monthly occurrence of menstruation—that is, to freeze the body in a sort of chemical menopause. The hormone types used, made by pharmaceutical companies, are chemical cousins of female hormones (estrogens and progestins), male hormones (androgens), and a brain hormone that controls ovulation (gonadotropin-releasing hormone, or GnRH). Appropriate hormone therapy is often useful for years, although each hormone class produces disadvantageous side effects in many patients.

The use of estrogens stops ovulation and menstruation, freeing many women with endometriosis from painful symptoms. Numerous estrogen preparations have been prescribed, including the birth control pills that contain them.

Drawbacks of estrogen use can include weight gain, nausea, breast soreness, depression, blood clotting abnormalities, and elevated risk of vaginal cancer. In addition, estrogen administration may cause endometrial implants to enlarge.

The use of progestins arose from the discovery that pregnancy—which is maintained by high levels of a natural progestin called progesterone—reversed the symptoms of many suffering from endometriosis. This realization led to the utilization of synthetic progestins to cause prolonged false pregnancy. The rationale is that all endometrial implants will die off and be reabsorbed during the prolonged absence of menstruation. The method works in most patients, and pain-free periods of up to five years are often observed. In some cases, however, side effects include nausea, depression, insomnia, and a very slow resumption of normal menstruation (such as lags of up to a year) when the therapy is stopped. In addition, progestins are ineffective in treating large implants; in fact, their use in such cases can lead to severe complications.

In the 1970's, studies showing the potential for heart attacks, high blood pressure, and strokes in patients receiving long-term female hormone therapy led to a search for more advantageous hormone medications. An alternative developed was the synthetic male hormone danazol (Danocrine), which is very effective. One of its advantages over female hormones is the ability to shrink large implants and restore fertility to those patients whose problems arise from nonfunctional ovaries or Fallopian tubes. Danazol has become the drug of choice for treating millions of endometriosis sufferers. Problems associated with danazol use, however, can include weight gain, masculinization (decreased bust size, facial hair growth, and deepened voice), fatigue, depression, and baldness. Those women contemplating danazol use should be aware that it can also complicate pregnancy.

Because of the side effects of these hormones, other chemotherapy was sought. Another valuable drug that has become available is GnRH, which suppresses the function of the ovaries in a fashion equivalent to surgical oophorectomy (removal of the ovaries). This hormone produces none of the side effects of the sex hormones, such as weight gain, depression, or masculinization, but some evidence indicates that it may lead to osteoporosis.

Thus, despite the fact that hormone therapy may relieve or reduce pain for years, contemporary chemotherapy is flawed by many undesirable side effects. Perhaps more serious, however, is the high recurrence rate of endometriosis that is observed after the therapy is stopped. Consequently, it appears that the best treatment of endometriosis combines chemotherapy with surgery.

The extent of the surgery carried out to combat endometriosis is variable and depends on the observations made during laparoscopy. In cases of relatively mild endometriosis, conservative laparotomy surgery removes endometriosis implants, adhesions, and lesions. This type of procedure attempts to relieve endometriosis pain, to minimize the chances of postoperative recurrence of the disease, and to allow the patient to have children. Even in the most severe cases of this type, the uterus, an ovary, and its associated Fallopian tube are retained. Such surgery will often include removal of the appendix, whether diseased or not, because it is very likely to develop implants. The surgical techniques performed are the conventional excision of diseased tissue or the use of lasers to vaporize it. Many physicians prefer lasers because it is believed that they decrease the chances of recurrent endometriosis resulting from retained implant tissue or iatrogenic causes.

In more serious cases, hysterectomy is carried out. All visible implants, adhesions, and lesions are removed from the abdominal organs, as in conservative surgery. In addition, the uterus and cervix are taken out, but one or both ovaries are retained. This allows female hormone production to continue normally until the menopause. Uterine removal makes it impossible to have children, however, and may lead to profound psychological problems that require psychiatric help. Women planning to elect for hysterectomy to treat endometriosis should be aware of such potential difficulties. In many cases of conservative surgery or hysterectomy, danazol is used, both preoperatively and postoperatively, to minimize implant size.

The most extensive surgery carried out on the women afflicted with endometriosis is radical hysterectomy, also called definitive surgery, in which the ovaries and/or the vagina are also removed. The resultant symptoms are menopausal and may include vaginal bleeding atrophy (when the vagina is retained), increased risk of heart disease, and the development of osteoporosis. To counter the occurrence of these symptoms, replacement therapy with female hormones is suggested. Paradoxically, this hormone therapy can lead to the return of endometriosis by stimulating the growth of residual implant tissue.

PERSPECTIVE AND PROSPECTS

Modern treatment of endometriosis is viewed by many physicians as beginning in the 1950's. A landmark development in this field was the accurate diagnosis of endometriosis via the laparoscope, which was invented in Europe and introduced into the United States in the 1960's. Medical science has progressed greatly since that time. Physicians and researchers have recognized the wide occurrence of the disease and accepted its symptoms as valid; realized that hysterectomy will not necessarily put an end to the disease; utilized chemotherapeutic tools, including hormones and painkillers, as treatments and as adjuncts to surgery; developed laser surgery and other techniques that decrease the occurrence of formerly ignored iatrogenic endometriosis; and understood that the disease can ravage teenagers as well and that these young women should be examined as early as possible.

As pointed out by Niels H. Lauersen and Constance De-Swaan in *The Endometriosis Answer Book* (1988), more research than ever is "exploring the intricacies of the disease." Moreover, the efforts and information base of the proactive American Endometriosis Association, founded in 1980, have been very valuable. As a result, a potentially or presently afflicted woman is much more aware of the problems associated with the disease. In addition, she has a source for obtaining objective information on topics including state-of-the-art treatment, physician and hospital choice, and both physical and psychological outcomes of treatment.

Many potentially viable avenues for better endometriosis diagnosis and treatment have become the objects of intense investigation. These include the use of ultrasonography and radiology techniques for the predictive, nonsurgical examination of the course of growth or the chemotherapeutic destruction of implants; the design of new drugs to be utilized in the battle against endometriosis; endeavors aimed at the development of diagnostic tests for the disease that will stop it before symptoms develop; and the design of dietary treatments to soften its effects.

Regrettably, because of the insidious nature of endometriosis—which has the ability to strike almost anywhere in the body—some confusion about the disease still exists. New drugs, surgical techniques, and other aids are expected to be helpful in clarifying many of these issues. Particular value is being placed on the study of the immunologic aspects of endometriosis. Scientists hope to explain why the disease strikes some women and not others, to uncover its etiologic basis, and to solve the widespread problems of iatrogenic implant formation and other types of endometriosis recurrence.   —*Sanford S. Singer*

See also Amenorrhea; Cervical, ovarian, and uterine cancers; Childbirth, complications of; Dysmenorrhea; Female genital disorders; Infertility in females; Menorrhagia; Menstruation; Pregnancy and gestation.

FOR FURTHER INFORMATION:

Barnhart, Edward R., ed. *The Physician's Desk Reference*. 45th ed. Oradell, N.J.: Medical Economics, 1991. This atlas of prescription drugs includes the drugs used against endometriosis, the companies that produce them, their useful dose ranges, their effects on metabolism and toxicology, and their contraindications. A useful reference work for physicians and patients that is found in most public libraries.

Breitkopf, Lyle J., and Marion Gordon Bakoulis. *Coping with Endometriosis*. New York: Prentice Hall, 1988. This book explores how patients cope with endometriosis in a clear manner. Topical coverage includes an overview of endometriosis, interactions between afflicted patients and physicians, causation theories, severity classification, treatment, infertility, and the management of endometriosis. Contains a glossary and a bibliography.

Lauersen, Niels H., and Constance DeSwaan. *The Endometriosis Answer Book: New Hope, New Help*. New York: Rawson Associates, 1988. This detailed book covers endometriosis well. Some of the main subdivisions are an explanation of the disease, the choice of a physician, medical and surgical treatment, and support groups. An extensive bibliography is included.

Older, Julia. *Endometriosis*. New York: Charles Scribner's Sons, 1984. Discusses endometriosis causation theories, diagnosis of the disease, its medical and surgical treatment, possible complications, racial and age relatedness, and prevention of the disease. The glossary and bibliography are also very useful.

Sherwood, Lauralee. *Human Physiology: From Cells to Systems*. St. Paul, Minn.: West, 1989. This college text contains much useful biological information. Included are details about the menstrual cycle, hormones, the endometrium, and many helpful definitions. Valuable diagrams and glossary terms also abound. Clearly written, the book is a mine of information for interested readers.

Weinstein, Kate. *Living with Endometriosis*. Reading, Mass.: Addison-Wesley, 1987. The main divisions of this handy book are medical aspects, treatments and outcomes, emotional problems, and pain and psychiatric problems. Highlights include the complete description of the female reproductive system and menstruation, the glossary, and appendices on organizations, literature, and pain management centers.

Wigfall-Williams, Wanda. *Hysterectomy: Learning the Facts, Coping with the Feelings, and Facing the Future*. New York: Michael Kesend, 1986. Explains clearly the reasons that hysterectomy may be necessary, including the presence of endometriosis. Gives solid guidelines for physician and surgery choice. Also explores the depression that may follow this procedure and how to deal with it, hormone replacement therapy, and alterations in sexual function. A glossary and many references are included.

ENURESIS. *See* BED-WETTING.

ENVIRONMENTAL DISEASES

SYSTEMS AFFECTED: All

SPECIALISTS: Environmental medicine physicians, epidemiologists, occupational medicine physicians, public health specialists, toxicologists

DEFINITION: A wide variety of conditions and diseases resulting from largely human-mediated hazards in both the natural and human-made (for example, home and workplace) environments; an area of special concern given rapid environmental degradation during the twentieth century.

KEY TERMS:

emphysema: the overinflation of bronchial tubes and alveoli with air, resulting in reduced lung function *environment:* the biological, physical, cultural, and mental factors that influence health; anything external to an individual

food chain: a sequence—plant, herbivore, primary carnivore, and secondary and tertiary carnivore—in which each level depends on the stored energy from the lower level and often concentrates contaminants in the process

mutagen: a substance or event that effects a permanent, inheritable change in the genetic makeup of an organism

organic compound or waste: a chemical compound based on carbon, with or without hydrogen and other elements—in the context of environmental disease, usually a manufactured product

risk factor: a factor that increases the chances of an effect

teratogen: a substance or event that causes malformation in a developing fetus

Causes and Symptoms

Environmental health explores the influence of external factors on human health and disease. Technically, almost any condition except those of purely genetic origin could be considered as environmentally caused or having an environmental component, but the term "environmental disease" is usually applied to the effects of human alterations in the physical environment and excludes transmissible disease caused by pathogenic organisms, except in cases where human alteration of the environment is an important factor in epidemiology. Health hazards generally classed as environmental include air and water (including groundwater) pollution, toxic wastes, lead, asbestos, pesticides and herbicides, ionizing and nonionizing radiation, noise, and light.

In the United States, the Clean Air Act of 1970 established maximum levels for sulfur and nitrogen dioxide, particulates, hydrocarbons, ozone, and carbon monoxide—the most common air pollutants of concern in urban environments. Even with increasingly stringent controls on emissions from automobiles and industry, air quality in urban areas frequently does not meet minimum standards. Carbon monoxide lowers the oxygen-carrying capacity of the blood, nitrogen and sulfur dioxide react with water to form acids which damage lung tissue, ozone damages tissue directly, and particulates may accumulate in the lungs. The result is decreased lung capacity and function. Cigarette smoking increases susceptibility to other forms of lung damage.

Indoor air quality poses additional concerns. Emphasis on energy efficiency in building design decreases air exchange. Carpets and furniture release organic compounds, and cleaning solvents leave a volatile residue. Formaldehyde from foam stuffing and insulation inhibits liver function and is a suspected carcinogen. Breathing in an enclosed space decreases atmospheric oxygen and increases carbon dioxide. In some areas, radioactive radon gas released by the soil becomes concentrated in buildings. A ventilation system which draws its air from a polluted outdoor environment, such as a loading dock, will fail to perform its function. Secondhand cigarette smoke poses the same hazards of emphysema and lung cancer to people chronically exposed to it in an enclosed environment as to the smokers themselves. The phenomenon known as "sick building syndrome," in which large numbers of people in one building complain of respiratory illness, headaches, and impaired concentration, results from a combination of these factors.

Lead additives in gasoline were once a significant source of atmospheric lead, but they are being phased out; unfortunately, they leave a permanent residue in soils of high-traffic areas. Levels of 20 micrograms per deciliter of lead in the blood inhibit hemoglobin production, slow the transmission of nerve impulses, and are suspected of causing cognitive impairment in children; higher levels cause anemia, weakness, stomach pains, and nervous system impairment. Even levels below 5 micrograms may be hazardous to children. Because of lead in the paint and plumbing in old houses and soil contamination, blood lead levels high enough to cause developmental impairment in children occur frequently in older parts of cities; low-income residents are most likely to be at risk. Mercury, another metallic neurotoxin, is introduced into water in small amounts through industrial effluent but becomes concentrated in the food chain, where it poses a hazard to people who eat large quantities of fish. Any waterborne pollutant that is not rapidly degraded has the potential for being concentrated in the food chain. Shellfish, which filter nutrients from seawater, can concentrate toxins. The most notorious cause of shellfish poisoning is a naturally occurring neurotoxic alga, but polychlorinated biphenyls (PCBs) and pesticides have also been implicated. Some metals, including lead, arsenic, and mercury, remain toxic indefinitely and are exceedingly difficult to remove from an environment into which they have been introduced.

Inhalation of asbestos fibers carries a high risk of developing lung cancer after an interval of twenty or thirty years, a connection first established among shipyard workers. Between 1940 and 1970, asbestos was used extensively in public buildings as insulation. It is estimated that three to five million workers in the United States were exposed to unacceptably high levels of airborne fibers during this period, and millions of people continue to be exposed when building materials deteriorate. Asbestos abatement adds considerably to the cost of renovating old public buildings.

Urban drinking water in industrialized countries is monitored for hazardous contaminants; there is some question as to whether chlorine and fluoride, added for legitimate health reasons, are completely without negative effects. Well water in irrigated agricultural areas may have high levels of nitrates, which decrease blood oxygen and have been implicated in miscarriages and birth defects.

Organic chemical compounds make up 60 percent of the hazardous wastes generated by industry. This category

Asbestosis

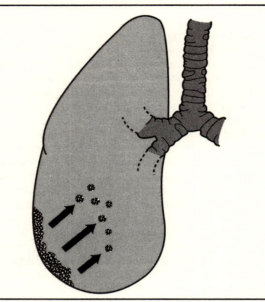

Asbestosis—the progressive destruction of respiratory tissues via inhalation of dust-sized asbestos fibers that attach to the walls of the lung and then spread outward—is often the result of prolonged exposure to asbestos-containing materials (in shipyards, office buildings, manufacturing plants); it is one of a wide variety of environmental diseases.

includes PCBs (including dioxin), chlorofluorocarbons, phthalate esters, chlorinated benzenes, and chloromethanes, solvents (such as benzene and carbon tetrachloride), plasticizers, fire retardants, pesticides, and herbicides. Many are acutely toxic—dioxin is one of the most potent toxins known—and require elaborate precautions to prevent worker exposure or accidental contamination of foodstuffs. PCBs, which are used in a wide variety of manufacturing processes, have been shown to cause cancer and reproductive disorders in laboratory animals and have been linked to these conditions in humans. The herbicide 2,4,5-T, the defoliant "Agent Orange" used during the Vietnam War, is the subject of continuing claims against the manufacturer and the Veterans Administration by soldiers who later developed neurological symptoms, immune disorders, or cancer or who had children with birth defects.

The burial of toxic by-products of manufacturing processes in landfills has created an ongoing environmental health crisis as containers rupture and chemicals leach into the surrounding soil. Underground fuel storage tanks pose a similar problem. Toxins leached from a waste dump eventually enter streams and become disseminated or, if volatile, enter the atmosphere. Residents of the infamous Love Canal

site in New York State were made ill by fumes from contaminated soil and groundwater.

High energy from X-ray sources and radioactive materials is termed "ionizing" because such radiation can cause chemical changes in molecules, including genetic material. Chronic exposure to ionizing radiation poses a high risk of cancer, inheritable mutations, and fetal malformation. Exposure may be occupational, as with workers in the nuclear power industry or hospital radiology laboratories. Some radioactive by-products of nuclear weapons testing and reactor accidents (such as strontium 90 or carbon 14) are exceptionally hazardous because they are structurally incorporated into living tissue and become concentrated in the food chain. The by-products of the nuclear reactor accident in Chernobyl, Ukraine, in 1987 were disseminated across international boundaries and will continue to endanger the health of millions of people in Belarus, Ukraine, and Eastern Europe. Whether widespread atmospheric testing of nuclear weapons in the 1950's caused radiation damage in the population at large is unknown; military personnel involved in the testing and inhabitants of the regions near test sites report increased rates of suspected radiation-induced illness.

Hazards of nonionizing radiation (visible, ultraviolet, infrared, or microwave) are less well established. Intense visible light can damage vision. Artificial lighting is known to disrupt reproductive cycles in plants and invertebrates and could have subtle effects on human biology. That the level of microwave radiation to which the public at large is inadvertently exposed is well below levels known to produce adverse effects is not completely reassuring. Ultraviolet light, principally from sunlight, is a factor in skin cancer, which is increasing both because of the popularity of sunbathing and because ozone depletion increases ultraviolet exposure.

A category of severe lung disease affects workers in environments with a high concentration of particulate matter in the air: black lung disease, from coal dust in coal mines; silicosis, from fine rock powder in mines; and byssinosis, from textile fibers in spinning and weaving mills. The result of long-term breathing of particulates is obstruction and emphysema, which may be fatal.

Electromagnetic fields produced by power lines and electrical devices are an area of increasing controversy as electricity becomes more ubiquitous. One study found a higher-than-average rate of childhood leukemia near high-tension power lines; other studies have failed to confirm this finding. Women who work constantly at video display terminals have somewhat higher miscarriage rates than other office workers.

Exposure to industrial solvents has been a significant source of workplace illness. Among the most dangerous solvents are benzene, used in a variety of processes and produced as a by-product in the coking industry; vinyl chloride, used in plastics manufacture; and formaldehyde. All of these chemicals are carcinogenic.

Repetitive-motion injuries are an increasing occupational hazard. Any body part subject to constant, selective hard use, especially where tasks and workstations are poorly designed, may develop problems. The most common compensation claims arise from damage to the spinal column from lifting heavy objects and damage to nerves in the hand and forearm from repetitive, rapid hand movements (such as carpal tunnel syndrome).

SOCIETAL INTERVENTION

In order to improve environmental health, health professionals and regulatory agencies must anticipate and minimize future hazards, identify existing health problems that may have an environmental component and attempt to determine whether a connection exists, and redress the mistakes of the past. It is notoriously difficult to prove that an illness has an environmental cause. Suspicion arises when epidemiological statistics on reportable illnesses show that some condition known to be influenced by environmental factors—such as cancer, endocrine disorders, reproductive disorders, or immunodeficiency—occurs at an unusually high frequency in some subset of the population, occurs in a restricted geographical area, or is increasing throughout the general population. Even then, the cause may not be environmental; the acquired immunodeficiency syndrome (AIDS) epidemic was thought by some to be an environmental effect until the causative organism was identified.

The time interval between exposure and illness can be as long as twenty or thirty years, during which the exposed population may have dispersed and may no longer be readily identifiable. Subtle effects such as mild immunosuppression or cognitive impairment may escape detection or be dismissed as psychosomatic. Multiple environmental, behavioral, and even genetic factors are often involved, confounding efforts to pinpoint a cause. In the United States and Western Europe, high rates of exposure to pollutants are correlated with poverty and thus with higher-than-normal rates of malnutrition, alcohol and drug abuse, and inadequate access to health care. Tobacco smoking is a common confounding behavioral factor in environmental diagnosis. Where liability is involved, there are powerful financial incentives on the side of disproving the environmental or occupational linkage.

When a new technology or chemical is introduced, regulations in most countries require an assessment of health impact, which includes experimentation with animal models and risk assessment to determine the probable impact on the human population. Animal experimentation is most effective at demonstrating short-term and acute effects of toxic materials, but it is poor at demonstrating effects of long-term, low-level exposure. Risk assessment must take into consideration unusually susceptible individuals (pregnant women, for example), deliberate or accidental overexposure, and synergistic effects. In the realm of environmental legislation, risk assessment is also influenced by psychology; people are more willing to accept familiar risks over which they have personal control.

PERSPECTIVE AND PROSPECTS

Concern for occupational health begins with the Industrial Revolution in the early nineteenth century, finding some of its earliest expression in the recognition that some industrial jobs were inappropriate for children. Although many occupations in preindustrial societies carried a high risk trauma, only a few involved chronic exposure to toxic substances. The combined effects of heavy physical labor and malnutrition are not infrequently seen in skeletons from archeological excavations, but injury caused by repetitive motion under assembly-line conditions is a modern phenomenon.

Concerns about the effects of pollution and toxic wastes on the general population are of even more recent origin. Sanitarians in the first half of the twentieth century directed their attention toward reducing transmissible disease through the prevention of water and food supply contamination and the control of insect vectors. Several factors increased public awareness of environmental health problems in the United States and led to creation of agencies and legislation to address the problem, beginning in 1970: Urban-industrial air pollution contributed to hundreds of deaths from respiratory disease in Pennsylvania (1948) and London (1952); there was much publicity surrounding the dangers of pesticides to wildlife in the 1960's; a variety of health problems, including increased cancer risk, were found in Love Canal, a housing development in New York State built on a toxic waste dump; and it was demonstrated that urban lead levels were high enough to impair psychomotor development in children.

The increase in the proportion of morbidity and mortality attributable to environmental factors in the late twentieth century is the result of not only the exponential increase in energy use and the output of complex synthetic chemicals but also of changing demographics. Effects of low-level exposure to toxins may take decades to produce disease and may never become apparent in populations with a low life expectancy. In developing countries, where environmental protection is rudimentary and life expectancies are increasing rapidly, the adverse health effects of environmental degradation are particularly visible.

In the United States, specific legislation addresses compensation for miners, asbestos workers, and other specific victims of exposure to hazardous materials. On a worldwide basis, monitoring of hazardous substances is a prime concern of the World Health Organization. As incidents such as the accidental release of cyanide from a fertilizer plant in Bhopal, India, indicate, provisions for industrial safety and for separating residential and industrial areas in the developing world are unsatisfactory. The former Soviet Union represents what in many ways is a worst-case scenario combing rapid, concentrated industrialization with poor environmental controls. Some of the earliest signs that the Communist regime was weakening came from the environmental movement in its agitation for better protection for human and natural resources. Safeguarding environmental health and addressing existing hazards and environmentally caused illnesses requires a major expenditure of funds and effort, which is likely to continue growing as the delayed effects of industrial practices introduced since World War II continue to become apparent.

—*Martha Sherwood-Pike*

See also Asthma; Bronchitis; Cancer; Emphysema; Food poisoning; Lead poisoning; Lung cancer; Poisoning; Pulmonary diseases; Radiation sickness; Skin cancer.

FOR FURTHER INFORMATION:

Congressional Quarterly Inc. *Environment and Health.* Washington, D.C.: Author, 1981. The focus of this report is legislation introduced between 1970 and 1980 in Congress to address environmental health problems, including the background that led to the introduction of such legislation. The table "The Regulatory Maze: Agencies Involved in Environmental and Occupational Health" and the chronology of legislation by year and type of problem are clear and informative.

Cooper, M. G., ed. *Risk: Man-Made Hazards to Man.* Oxford, England: Clarendon Press, 1985. A book about how people perceive and assess risks, factors that affect environmental legislation. In addition to a discussion of statistics and the effects of publicity, this British publication adopts a conservative view that hazards are often overstated.

Cralley, Lester V., Lewis J. Cralley, George D. Clayton, and John Jurgiel. *Industrial Environmental Health: The Worker and the Community.* New York: Academic Press, 1972. Part of the Environmental Science Interdisciplinary Monograph Series from Academic Press. A detailed catalog of known workplace hazards, including toxic materials, radiation, and noise. The emphasis is on monitoring techniques and a thorough survey of the literature. The text is rather technical.

Greenberg, Michael R., ed. *Public Health and the Environment: The United States Experience.* New York: Guilford Press, 1987. This text explores modern environmental problems from the point of view of public health. Part 1, a survey of the contribution of the environment to disease, includes sections on worker health and lifestyle as a factor in chronic disease.

Journal of Environmental Health, 1963-   . This journal published by the National Environmental Health Association offers articles on a wide variety of environmental and occupational health issues. Topics covered in 1992-1993 included sanitation aspects of flooding on the Mississippi River in 1993, hazardous consumer products, medical waste, the hazards of illegal drug laboratories, and studies attempting to link radon with cancer. The journal also acts as a forum for concerns of environmental health professionals and sanitarians.

National Research Council. Committee on Environmental Epidemiology. *Public Health and Hazardous Wastes.* Vol. 1 in *Environmental Epidemiology.* Washington, D.C.: National Academy Press, 1991. The report of a committee assigned to investigate the question of whether the federal hazardous waste programs in the United States actually protect human health. Reviews agencies and the methodologies of exposure assessment, the extent of the problem in the United States, and specific examples of hazardous wastes in air, groundwater, soil, and food. Includes charts and maps summarizing data and extensive bibliographies. A lengthy glossary is provided. A good factual reference on many aspects of environmental health.

Rom, William N., ed. *Environmental and Occupational Medicine.* Boston: Little, Brown, 1983. The emphasis in this textbook is on industrial occupational safety, with approximately a third of the work devoted to the diagnosis and pathology of occupational lung diseases, including byssinosis and black lung disease. The effects of acute and chronic exposure to heavy metals, solvents, and other toxic substances are organized by agent. Intended as a guide for medical practitioners treating patients with environmental illnesses and as a guide to the prevention of exposure for professionals concerned with workplace safety.

EPILEPSY

SYSTEMS AFFECTED: Brain, nervous

SPECIALISTS: Neurologists, neurosurgeons

DEFINITION: A serious neurologic disease characterized by seizures, which may involve convulsions and loss of consciousness.

KEY TERMS:

anticonvulsant: a therapeutic drug that prevents or diminishes convulsions

aura: a sensory symptom or group of such symptoms that precedes a grand mal seizure

clonic phase: the portion of an epileptic seizure that is characterized by convulsions

electroencephalogram (EEG): a graphic recording of the electrical activity of the brain, as recorded by an electroencephalograph

grand mal: a type of epileptic seizure characterized by severe convulsions, body stiffening, and loss of consciousness during which victims fall down; also called tonic-clonic seizure

idiopathic disease: a disease of unknown origin

petit mal: a mild type of epileptic seizure characterized by a very short lapse of consciousness, usually without convulsions; the epileptic does not fall down

seizure: a sudden convulsive attack of epilepsy that can involve loss of consciousness and falling down

seizure discharges: characteristic brain waves seen in the EEGs of epileptics; their strength and frequency depend upon whether a seizure is occurring and its type

status epilepticus: a rare, life-threatening condition in which many sequential seizures occur without recovery between them

tonic-clonic seizure: another term for a grand mal seizure

tonic phase: the portion of an epileptic seizure characterized by loss of consciousness and body stiffness

CAUSES AND SYMPTOMS

Epilepsy is characterized by seizures, commonly called fits, which may involve convulsions and the loss or consciousness. It was called the "falling disease" or "sacred disease" in antiquity and was mentioned in 2080 B.C. in the laws of the famous Babylonian king Hamurabi. Epilepsy is a serious neurologic disease that usually appears between the ages of two and fourteen. It does not affect intelligence, as shown by the fact that the range of intelligence quotients (IQs) for epileptics is quite similar to that of the general population. In addition, many epileptics have achieved fame, such as Alexander the Great, Saint Paul, English poet Lord Byron, Julius Caesar, Russian novelist Fyodor Dostoevski, and Dutch artist Vincent Van Gogh.

In 400 B.C., Hippocates of Cos proposed that epilepsy arose from physical problems in the brain. This origin of the disease is now known to be unequivocally true. Despite many centuries of exhaustive study and effort, however, only a small percentage (20 percent) of cases of epilepsy caused by brain injuries, brain tumors, and other diseases are curable. This type of epilepsy is called symptomatic epilepsy. In contrast, 80 percent of epileptics can be treated to control the occurrence of seizures but cannot be cured of the disease, which is therefore a lifelong affliction. In these cases, the basis of the epilepsy is not known, although the suspected cause is genetically programmed brain damage that still evades discovery. Most epilepsy is, therefore, an idiopathic disease (one of unknown origin), and such epileptics are thus said to suffer from idiopathic epilepsy.

A common denominator in idiopathic epilepsy, and also in symptomatic epilepsy, is that it is evidenced by unusual electrical discharges, brain waves, seen in the electroencephalograms (EEGs) of epileptics. These brain waves are called seizure discharges. They vary in both their strength and their frequency, depending on whether an epileptic is having a seizure and what type of seizure is occurring. Seizure discharges are almost always present and recognizable in the EEGs of epileptics, even during sleep.

There are four types of common epileptic seizures. Two of these are partial (local) seizures called focal motor and temporal lobe seizures, respectively. The others, grand mal and petit mal, are generalized and may involve the entire body. A focal motor seizure is characterized by rhythmic jerking of the facial muscles, an arm, or a leg. As with other epileptic seizures, it is caused by abnormal electrical discharges in the portion of the brain that controls normal movement in the body part that is affected. This abnormal electrical activity is always seen as seizure discharges in the EEG of the affected part of the brain.

In contrast, temporal lobe seizures, again characterized by seizure discharges in a distinct portion of the cerebrum of the brain, are characterized by sensory hallucinations and other types of consciousness alteration, a meaningless physical action, or even a babble of some incomprehensible language. Thus, for example, temporal lobe seizures may explain some cases of people "speaking in tongues" in religious experiences or in the days of the Delphic oracles of ancient Greece.

The term "grand mal" refers to the most severe type of epileptic seizure. Also called tonic-clonic seizures, grand mal attacks are characterized by very severe EEG seizure discharges throughout the entire brain. A grand mal seizure is usually preceded by sensory symptoms called an aura (probably related to temporal lobe seizures), which warn an epileptic of an impending attack. The aura is quickly followed by the grand mal seizure itself, which involves the loss of consciousness, localized or widespread jerking and convulsions, and severe body stiffness.

Epileptics suffering a grand mal seizure usually fall to the ground, may foam at the mouth, and often bite their tongues or the inside of their cheeks unless something is placed in the mouth before they lose consciousness. In a few cases, the victim will loose bladder or bowel control. In untreated epileptics, grand mal seizures can occur weekly. Most of these attacks last for only a minute or two, followed quickly by full recovery after a brief sense of disorientation and feelings of severe exhaustion. In some cases, however, grand mal seizures may last for up to five minutes and lead to temporary amnesia or to other mental deficits of a longer duration. In rare cases, the life-threatening condition of status epilepticus occurs, in which many sequential tonic-clonic seizures occur over several hours without recovery between them.

The fourth type of epileptic seizure is petit mal, which is often called generalized nonconvulsive seizure or, more simply, absence. A petit mal seizure consists of a brief period of loss of consciousness (ten to forty seconds) without the epileptic falling down. The epileptic usually appears to be daydreaming (absent) and shows no other symptoms. Often a victim of a petit mal seizure is not even aware that the event has occurred. In some cases, a petit mal seizure is accompanied by mild jerking of hands, head, or facial features and/or rapid blinking of the eyes. Petit mal attacks can be quite dangerous if they occur while an epileptic is driving a motor vehicle.

Diagnosing epilepsy usually requires a patient history, a careful physical examination, blood tests, and a neurologic examination. The patient history is most valuable when it includes eyewitness accounts of the symptoms, the frequency of occurrence, and the usual duration range of the seizures observed. In addition, documentation of any preceding severe trauma, infection, or episodes of addictive drug exposure provides useful information that will often differentiate between idiopathic and symptomatic epilepsy.

Evidence of trauma is quite important, as head injuries that caused unconsciousness are often the basis for later symptomatic epilepsy. Similarly, infectious diseases of the brain, including meningitis and encephalitis, can cause this type of epilepsy. Finally, excess use of alcohol or other psychoactive drugs can also be causative agents for symptomatic epilepsy.

Blood tests for serum glucose and calcium, electroencephalography, and computed tomography (CT) scanning are also useful diagnostic tools. The EEG will nearly always show seizure discharges in epileptics, and the location of the discharges in the brain may localize problem areas associated with the disease. CT scanning is most useful for identifying tumors and other serious brain damage that may cause symptomatic epilepsy. When all tests are negative except for abnormal EEGs, the epilepsy is considered idiopathic.

It is thought that the generation of epileptic symptoms occurs because of a malfunction in nerve impulse transport in some of the billions of nerve cells (neurons) that make up the brain and link it to the body organs that it innervates. This nerve impulse transport is an electrochemical process caused by the ability of the neurons to retain substances (including potassium) and to excrete substances (including sodium). This ability generates the weak electrical current that makes up a nerve impulse and that is registered by electroencephalography.

A nerve impulse leaves a given neuron via an outgoing extension (or axon), passes across a tiny synaptic gap that separates the axon from the next neuron in line, and enters an incoming extension (or dendrite) of that cell. The process is repeated until the impulse is transmitted to its site of action. The cell bodies of neurons make up the gray matter of the brain, and axons and dendrites (white matter) may be viewed as connecting wires.

Passage across synaptic gaps between neurons is mediated by chemicals called neurotransmitters, and it is now believed that epilepsy results when unknown materials cause abnormal electrical impulses by altering neurotransmitter production rates and/or the ability of sodium, potassium, and related substances to enter or leave neurons. The various nervous impulse abnormalities that cause epilepsy can be shown to occur in the portions of the gray matter of the cerebrum that control high-brain functions. For example, the frontal lobe—which controls speech, body movement, and eye movements—is associated with temporal lobe seizures.

Treatment and Therapy

Idiopathic epilepsy is viewed as the expression of a large group of different diseases, all of which present themselves clinically as seizures. This is extrapolated from the various types of symptomatic epilepsy observed, which have causes that include faulty biochemical processes (such as inappropriate calcium levels), brain tumors or severe brain injury, infectious diseases (such as encephalitis), and the chronic overuse of addictive drugs. As to why idiopathic epilepsy causes are not identifiable, the general biomedical wisdom states that present technology is too imprecise to detect its causes.

Symptomatic epilepsy is treated with medication and either by the extirpation of the tumor or other causative brain tissue abnormality that was engendered by trauma or disease or by the correction of the metabolic disorder involved. The more common, incurable idiopathic disease is usually treated entirely with medication that relieves symptoms. This treatment is essential because without it most epileptics cannot attend school successfully, maintain continued employment, or drive a motor vehicle safely.

A large number of anticonvulsant drugs are presently available for epilepsy management. It must, however, be made clear that no one therapeutic drug will control all types of seizures. In addition, some patients require several such drugs for effective therapy, and the natural history of a given case of epilepsy may often require periodic changes from drug to drug as the disease evolves. Furthermore, every therapeutic antiepilepsy drug has dangerous side effects that may occur when it is present in the body above certain levels or after it is used beyond some given time period. Therefore, each epileptic patient must be monitored at frequent intervals to ascertain that no dangerous physical symptoms are developing and that the drug levels in the body (monitored by the measurement of drug content in blood samples) are within a tolerable range.

More than twenty antiepilepsy drugs are widely used. Phenytoin (Dilantin) is very effective for grand mal seizures. Because of its slow metabolism, phenytoin can be administered relatively infrequently, but this slow metabolism also requires seven to ten days before its anticonvulsant effects occur. Side effects include cosmetically unpleasant hair overgrowth, swelling of the gums, and skin rash. These symptoms are particularly common in epileptic children. More serious are central nervous effects including ataxia (unsteadiness in walking), drowsiness, anemia, and marked thyroid deficiency. Most such symptoms are reversed by decreasing the drug doses or by discontinuing it. Phenytoin is often given, together with other antiepilepsy drugs, to produce optimum seizure prevention. In those cases, great care must be taken to prevent dangerous synergistic drug effects from occurring. High phenytoin doses also produce blood levels of the drug that are very close to toxic 25 micrograms per milliliter values.

Carbamazepine (Tegretol) is another frequently used antiepileptic drug. Chemically related to the drugs used as antidepressants, it is useful against both psychomotor epilepsy and grand mal seizures. Common carbamazepine side effects are ataxia, drowsiness, and double vision. A more dangerous, and fortunately less common, side effect is the inability of bone marrow to produce blood cells. Again, very serious and unexpected complications occur in mixed-drug therapy that includes carbamazepine, and at high doses toxic blood levels of the drug may be exceeded.

Phenobarbital, a sedative hypnotic also used as a tranquilizer by nonepileptics, is a standby for treating epilepsy. It too can have serious side effects, including a lowered attention span, hyperactivity, and learning difficulties. In addition, when given with phenytoin, phenobarbital will speed up the excretion of that drug, lowering its effective levels.

Four major lessons can be learned from these three drugs. First, individual antiepilepsy drugs have many different side effects. Second, there are concrete reasons that epileptics taking therapeutic drugs must be monitored carefully for physical symptoms. Third, at high antiepileptic drug doses, the blood levels attained may closely approximate and even exceed toxic values. Fourth, drug interactions in mixed drug therapy can be counterproductive.

About 20 percent of idiopathic epileptics do not achieve adequate seizure control after prolonged and varied drug therapy. Another option for some—but not all—such people is brain surgery. This type of brain surgery is usually elected after two conditions are met. First, often-repeated EEGs must show that most or all of the portion of the brain in which the seizures develop is very localized. Second, these affected areas must be in a brain region that the patient can lose without significant mental loss (often in the prefrontal or temporal cerebral lobes). When such surgery is carried out, it is reported that 50-75% of the patients who are treated and given chronic, postoperative antiepilepsy drugs become able to achieve seizure control.

The most frequent antiepilepsy surgery is temporal lobectomy. The brain has two temporal lobes, one of which is dominant in the control of language, memory, and thought expression. A temporal lobectomy is carried out by removing the nondominant temporal lobe, when it is the site of epilepsy. About 6 percent of temporal lobectomies lead to a partial loss of temporal lobe functions, which may include impaired vision, movement, memory, and speech.

Another common type of antiepilepsy surgery is called corpus callosotomy. This procedure involves partially disconnecting the two cerebral hemispheres by severing some of the nerves in the corpus callosum that links them. This surgery is performed when an epileptic has frequent, uncontrollable grand mal attacks that cause many dangerous falls. The procedure usually results in reduced numbers of seizures and decreases in their severity.

Physicians now believe that many cases of epilepsy may be prevented by methods aimed at avoiding head injury (especially in children) and the use of techniques such as amniocentesis to identify potential epileptics and treat them before birth. Furthermore, the prophylactic administration of antiepilepsy drugs to nonepileptic people who are afflicted with encephalitis and other diseases known to produce epilepsy is viewed as wise.

PERSPECTIVE AND PROSPECTS

A great number of advances have occurred in the treatment of epilepsy via therapeutic drugs and surgical techniques. With the exception of symptomatic epilepsy, drug therapy has been the method of choice because it is less drastic than surgery, easier to manage, and rarely has the potential for irreversible damage to patients that can be caused by the removal of a portion of the brain. The main antiepileptic drugs are phenytoin, carbamazepine, and phenobarbital, but a tremendous variety of other chemical therapies has been investigated and utilized successfully.

Such treatments include high doses of vitamins, injections of muscle relaxants, and changes in diet. The variety is unsurprising, considering the vast number of disease issues that can cause seizures. For example, the rare genetic disease phenylketonuria (PKU) can cause epilepsy. Phenylketonuric epilepsy is often treated by use of a ketogenic diet rich in fats; the clear value of this treatment is unexplained. Readers are encouraged to investigate the many epilepsy treatments that have not been noted. Such an examination may be quite valuable because there are about a million epileptics in the United States alone, and some estimates indicate that four of every thousand humans are likely to develop some epileptic symptoms during their lifetime.

Modern surgical treatment of epilepsy reportedly began in 1828, with the efforts of Benjamin Dudley, who removed epilepsy-causing blood clots and skull fragments from five patients, who all survived despite primitive and nonsterile operating rooms. The next landmark in such surgery was the removal of a brain tumor by the German physician R. J. Godlee, in 1884, without the benefit of X rays or EEG techniques, which did not then exist.

By the 1950's EEGs were used to locate epileptic brain foci, and physicians such as the Canadians Wilder Penfield and Herbert Jasper pioneered its use to locate brain regions to remove for epilepsy remission without damaging vital functions. After considerable evolution over the course of forty years, antiepilepsy surgery by the 1990's had become widespread, commonplace, and relatively safe.

Nevertheless, because of the imperfections of all available methodologies, 5 to 8 percent of epileptics cannot achieve seizure control by any method or method combination and even the "well-managed" epilepsy treatment regimen has its flaws. There is still much to be learned about curing epilepsy. It is hoped that the efforts of ongoing biomedical research, both in basic science and in clinical settings, will eliminate epilepsy through the development of new therapeutic drugs and sophisticated advances in surgery and other nondrug methods. —*Sanford S. Singer*

See also Brain disorders; Seizures; Unconsciousness.

FOR FURTHER INFORMATION:

Barnhart, Edward R., ed. *The Physician's Desk Reference.* 45th ed. Oradell, N.J.: Medical Economics, 1991. An atlas of all the prescription drugs available in the United States. Includes a listing of the drugs used against epilepsy, their producers, their useful dose ranges, their metabolism and toxicology, and their contraindications. Found in most public libraries, it is a valuable reference for physicians and patients.

Berkow, Robert, and Andrew J. Fletcher, eds. *The Merck Manual of Diagnosis and Therapy.* 15th ed. Rahway, N.J.: Merck Sharp & Dohm Research Labs, 1987. Contains a compendium of data on the characteristics, etiology, diagnosis, and treatment of adult epilepsy. Also discusses seizure disorders of children and newborns. Designed for physicians, the material is also useful to less specialized readers.

Gumnit, Robert J., ed. *Living Well with Epilepsy.* New York: Demos, 1990. Designed to give people with epilepsy the outlook necessary to live successfully with the disease. Among the topics covered are causes and treatment, high-quality care, medical and surgical options, the problems of epileptic children, sexuality and pregnancy, the workplace, rights, and resources.

Hopkins, Anthony. *Epilepsy: The Facts.* New York: Oxford University Press, 1981. The author wishes to eliminate misunderstanding about epilepsy and educate people about it. This is done nicely by clear coverage of topics including explanation of epilepsy, seizure types and causes, epilepsy treatment methods, and information on living with the disease.

Nogen, Alan G. *Epilepsy: A Medical Handbook for Physicians, Nurses, Teachers, and Parents.* Dallas, Tex.: Taylor, 1980. This comprehensive handbook provides a valuable overview for physicians, nurses, teachers, and parents of epileptics. Topical coverage includes history, epilepsy types, diagnosis and causes, treatments, life with epilepsy, and community resources for epileptics. Also contains an excellent glossary.

Scott, Donald. *About Epilepsy.* New York: International Universities Press, 1973. This book "aims to inform a wide range of people about epilepsy." Included are causation, types and diagnosis, treatment, medication, the history of epilepsy, famous and infamous epileptics, and care and familial aspects. Contains a bibliography and a glossary.

EPSTEIN-BARR VIRUS. *See* **CHRONIC FATIGUE SYNDROME; MONONUCLEOSIS.**

EYE DISORDERS. *See* **CATARACTS; GLAUCOMA; VISUAL DISORDERS.**

MAGILL'S MEDICAL GUIDE

HEALTH
AND
ILLNESS

ALPHABETICAL LIST OF CONTENTS

Entries by Medical Specialization

AEROSPACE PHYSICIANS
Altitude sickness
Motion sickness

ALL
Disease
Iatrogenic disorders

ALLERGISTS
Allergies
Asthma
Bites and stings
Eczema
Itching
Nasopharyngeal disorders
Pulmonary diseases
Rhinitis
Viral infections

ANESTHESIOLOGISTS
Hyperthermia and hypothermia

AUDIOLOGISTS
Aging
Ear infections and disorders
Hearing loss
Ménière's disease
Speech disorders

BURN SPECIALISTS
Burns and scalds
Electrical shock
Inflammation
Radiation sickness
Wounds

CARDIOLOGISTS
Aging
Aneurysms
Angina
Anxiety
Arrhythmias
Atherosclerotic disease
Cholesterol
Congenital heart disease
Dizziness and fainting
Endocarditis
Heart attack
Heart disease
Heart failure
Hypertension
Ischemia

Mitral insufficiency
Palpitations
Rheumatic fever
Thrombosis and thrombus
Varicosis
Venous insufficiency

CHILD PSYCHIATRISTS
Autism
Dyslexia
Speech disorders

COLORECTAL SURGEONS
Abdominal disorders
Colon cancer
Cysts and ganglions
Diverticulitis and diverticulosis
Hemorrhoids
Intestinal disorders
Malignancy and metastasis

DENTISTS
Caries, dental
Dental diseases
Endodontic disease
Gingivitis
Halitosis
Head and neck disorders
Periodontitis
Toothache

DERMATOLOGISTS
Abscesses
Acne
Albinism
Athlete's foot
Carcinoma
Chickenpox
Cysts and ganglions
Dermatitis
Eczema
Fungal infections
Hair loss and baldness
Itching
Keratoses
Lice, mites, and ticks
Lupus erythematosus
Malignancy and metastasis
Pimples
Poisonous plants
Psoriasis
Puberty and adolescence

Rashes
Rosacea
Scabies
Skin cancer
Skin disorders
Warts

DIETITIANS, REGISTERED
Anorexia nervosa
Beriberi
Cholesterol
Malnutrition
Obesity
Vitamin and mineral deficiencies
Weight loss and gain

EMBRYOLOGISTS
Birth defects
Brain disorders
Cerebral palsy
Down syndrome

EMERGENCY PHYSICIANS
Abdominal disorders
Aging
Altitude sickness
Aneurysms
Appendicitis
Asphyxiation
Bites and stings
Bleeding
Botulism
Burns and scalds
Choking
Coma
Concussion
Diphtheria
Dizziness and fainting
Domestic violence
Electrical shock
Fracture and dislocation
Frostbite
Head and neck disorders
Heart attack
Heat exhaustion and heat stroke
Hyperthermia and hypothermia
Intoxication
Meningitis
Peritonitis
Plague
Pneumonia
Poisoning

Radiation sickness
Reye's syndrome
Salmonella
Shock
Snakebites
Spinal disorders
Staphylococcal infections
Streptococcal infections
Strokes and TIAs
Typhoid fever and typhus
Unconsciousness
Wounds

ENDOCRINOLOGISTS
Addison's disease
Anorexia nervosa
Cushing's syndrome
Diabetes mellitus
Dwarfism
Endocrine disorders
Gigantism
Goiter
Growth
Hair loss and baldness
Hyperparathyroidism and
   hypoparathyroidism
Hypertrophy
Hypoglycemia
Infertility in females
Infertility in males
Menopause
Menstruation
Obesity
Osteoporosis
Paget's disease
Pancreatitis
Puberty and adolescence
Sexual dysfunction
Stress
Thyroid disorders
Tumors
Vitamin and mineral deficiencies
Weight loss and gain

ENVIRONMENTAL MEDICINE
   PHYSICIANS
Environmental diseases
Frostbite
Heat exhaustion and heat stroke
Hyperthermia and hypothermia
Lice, mites, and ticks
Lyme disease
Plague
Poisonous plants

Skin cancer
Snakebites

EPIDEMIOLOGISTS
Acquired immunodeficiency
   syndrome (AIDS)
Arthropod-borne diseases
Bacterial infections
Childhood infectious diseases
Cholera
Elephantiasis
Environmental diseases
Food poisoning
Hepatitis
Influenza
Legionnaires' disease
Leprosy
Lice, mites, and ticks
Malaria
Measles, red
Parasitic diseases
Plague
Poisoning
Poliomyelitis
Rabies
Salmonella
Sexually transmitted diseases
Viral infections
Yellow fever
Zoonoses

FAMILY PHYSICIANS
Abdominal disorders
Abscesses
Acne
Acquired immunodeficiency
   syndrome (AIDS)
Alcoholism
Allergies
Alzheimer's disease
Anemia
Angina
Athlete's foot
Bacterial infections
Bed-wetting
Bell's palsy
Beriberi
Bleeding
Bronchitis
Candidiasis
Chickenpox
Childhood infectious diseases
Chlamydia
Cholecystitis

Cholesterol
Chronic fatigue syndrome
Cirrhosis
Cluster headaches
Common cold
Constipation
Coughing
Death and dying
Depression
Diabetes mellitus
Diarrhea and dysentery
Dizziness and fainting
Domestic violence
Factitious disorders
Fatigue
Fever
Fungal infections
Grief and guilt
Halitosis
Headaches
Heart disease
Heartburn
Heat exhaustion and heat stroke
Herpes
Hyperlipidemia
Hypertension
Hypertrophy
Hypoglycemia
Incontinence
Indigestion
Infection
Inflammation
Influenza
Intestinal disorders
Laryngitis
Male genital disorders
Measles, red
Mitral insufficiency
Mononucleosis
Motion sickness
Mumps
Muscle sprains, spasms, and
   disorders
Nasopharyngeal disorders
Obesity
Pain, types of
Parasitic diseases
Pertussis
Pharyngitis
Pimples
Pneumonia
Poisonous plants
Puberty and adolescence
Rashes

Rheumatic fever
Rubella
Rubeola
Scabies
Scarlet fever
Sciatica
Sexuality
Shingles
Shock
Sibling rivalry
Sinusitis
Sore throat
Strep throat
Stress
Tetanus
Tonsillitis
Ulcers
Viral infections
Vitamin and mineral deficiencies
Wounds

GASTROENTEROLOGISTS
Abdominal disorders
Appendicitis
Bulimia
Cholecystitis
Cholera
Colitis
Colon cancer
Constipation
Crohn's disease
Cysts and ganglions
Diarrhea and dysentery
Diverticulitis and diverticulosis
Food poisoning
Gallbladder diseases
Gastrointestinal disorders
Heartburn
Hemorrhoids
Indigestion
Intestinal disorders
Liver cancer
Liver disorders
Nausea and vomiting
Obstruction
Pancreatitis
Poisonous plants
Roundworm
Salmonella
Shigellosis
Stomach, intestinal, and pancreatic cancers
Tapeworm
Trichinosis

Ulcers
Weight loss and gain
Worms

GENETICISTS
Aging
Albinism
Alzheimer's disease
Birth defects
Breast cancer
Breast disorders
Color blindness
Down syndrome
Dwarfism
Genetic diseases
Hemophilia
Immunodeficiency disorders
Mental retardation
Phenylketonuria
Porphyria
Sexuality

GERIATRIC SPECIALISTS
Aging
Alzheimer's disease
Amnesia and memory loss
Bed-wetting
Blindness
Bone disorders
Brain disorders
Death and dying
Dementia
Domestic violence
Fatigue
Hearing loss
Incontinence
Osteoporosis
Parkinsonism
Visual disorders

GYNECOLOGISTS
Amenorrhea
Anorexia nervosa
Breast cancer
Breast disorders
Breast-feeding
Cervical, ovarian, and uterine cancers
Childbirth
Chlamydia
Conception
Cystitis
Cysts and ganglions
Dysmenorrhea

Endometriosis
Female genital disorders
Gonorrhea
Herpes
Incontinence
Infertility in females
Mastitis
Menopause
Menorrhagia
Menstruation
Ovarian cysts
Pelvic inflammatory disease (PID)
Peritonitis
Postpartum depression
Pregnancy and gestation
Premenstrual syndrome (PMS)
Sexual dysfunction
Sexuality
Sexually transmitted diseases
Syphilis
Urethritis
Urinary disorders
Warts

HEMATOLOGISTS
Anemia
Bleeding
Chronic fatigue syndrome
Hemophilia
Hodgkin's disease
Hyperlipidemia
Infection
Jaundice
Leukemia
Lymphadenopathy and lymphoma
Malaria
Septicemia
Sickle-cell anemia
Thalassemia
Thrombosis and thrombus
Toxemia

IMMUNOLOGISTS
Acquired immunodeficiency syndrome (AIDS)
Allergies
Asthma
Autoimmune disorders
Bacterial infections
Bites and stings
Candidiasis
Childhood infectious diseases
Chronic fatigue syndrome
Fungal infections

Human immunodeficiency virus
   (HIV)
Immunodeficiency disorders
Leprosy
Lupus erythematosus
Pulmonary diseases
Stress

INFECTIOUS DISEASE
   PHYSICIANS
Acquired immunodeficiency
   syndrome (AIDS)
Arthropod-borne diseases
Bacterial infections
Candidiasis
Chickenpox
Childhood infectious diseases
Chlamydia
Cholera
Common cold
Conjunctivitis
Cystitis
Diarrhea and dysentery
Diphtheria
Encephalitis
Hepatitis
Infection
Inflammation
Influenza
Legionnaires' disease
Measles, red
Meningitis
Mononucleosis
Parasitic diseases
Pertussis
Pneumonia
Poliomyelitis
Protozoan diseases
Shingles
Sleeping sickness
Staphylococcal infections
Strep throat
Streptococcal infections
Syphilis
Viral infections
Worms
Yellow fever
Zoonoses

INTERNISTS
Abdominal disorders
Acquired immunodeficiency
   syndrome (AIDS)
Addison's disease

Alcoholism
Allergies
Alzheimer's disease
Anemia
Angina
Anorexia nervosa
Anxiety
Arrhythmias
Arthritis
Atherosclerotic disease
Autoimmune disorders
Bacterial infections
Bell's palsy
Beriberi
Bleeding
Bone cancer
Bronchitis
Bursitis
Candidiasis
Carcinoma
Chickenpox
Childhood infectious diseases
Cholecystitis
Cholesterol
Chronic fatigue syndrome
Claudication
Cluster headaches
Colitis
Colon cancer
Constipation
Coughing
Crohn's disease
Cushing's syndrome
Death and dying
Diabetes mellitus
Diarrhea and dysentery
Diverticulitis and diverticulosis
Dizziness and fainting
Domestic violence
Edema
Embolism
Emphysema
Endocarditis
Factitious disorders
Fatigue
Fever
Fungal infections
Gallbladder diseases
Gangrene
Gastrointestinal disorders
Genetic diseases
Glomerulonephritis
Goiter
Gout

Guillain-Barré syndrome (GBS)
Headaches
Heart attack
Heart disease
Heart failure
Heartburn
Heat exhaustion and heat stroke
Hepatitis
Hernia
Herpes
Hodgkin's disease
Human immunodeficiency virus
   (HIV)
Hyperlipidemia
Hypertension
Hyperthermia and hypothermia
Hypertrophy
Hypoglycemia
Incontinence
Indigestion
Infection
Inflammation
Influenza
Intestinal disorders
Ischemia
Itching
Jaundice
Kidney disorders
Legionnaires' disease
Leprosy
Leukemia
Liver cancer
Liver disorders
Lung cancer
Lupus erythematosus
Lyme disease
Lymphadenopathy and lymphoma
Malignancy and metastasis
Mitral insufficiency
Mononucleosis
Motion sickness
Multiple sclerosis
Nephritis
Obesity
Paget's disease
Pain, types of
Palpitations
Palsy
Pancreatitis
Parasitic diseases
Parkinsonism
Peritonitis
Pertussis
Pharyngitis

Phlebitis
Pneumonia
Psoriasis
Puberty and adolescence
Rashes
Renal failure
Reye's syndrome
Rheumatic fever
Rheumatoid arthritis
Rubella
Rubeola
Scabies
Scarlet fever
Schistosomiasis
Sciatica
Scurvy
Septicemia
Sexuality
Sexually transmitted diseases
Shingles
Shock
Sickle-cell anemia
Sinusitis
Sore throat
Staphylococcal infections
Stones
Strep throat
Streptococcal infections
Stress
Strokes and TIAs
Tetanus
Thrombosis and thrombus
Tonsillitis
Toxemia
Tumors
Ulcers
Viral infections
Vitamin and mineral deficiencies
Wounds

MAXILLOFACIAL SURGEONS
Head and neck disorders

MICROBIOLOGISTS
Abscesses
Bacterial infections
Protozoan diseases
Smallpox
Tuberculosis

NEONATOLOGISTS
Childbirth
Childbirth, complications of
Chlamydia

Congenital heart disease
Fetal alcohol syndrome
Hydrocephalus
Jaundice
Premature birth

NEPHROLOGISTS
Cysts and ganglions
Edema
Glomerulonephritis
Hypertension
Kidney disorders
Lupus erythematosus
Nephritis
Renal failure
Stones

NEUROLOGISTS
Aging
Altitude sickness
Alzheimer's disease
Amnesia and memory loss
Aphasia and dysphasia
Apnea
Ataxia
Bell's palsy
Botulism
Brain disorders
Cerebral palsy
Claudication
Cluster headaches
Concussion
Death and dying
Dementia
Dizziness and fainting
Dyslexia
Dystrophy
Ear infections and disorders
Electrical shock
Encephalitis
Epilepsy
Guillain-Barré syndrome (GBS)
Hallucinations
Head and neck disorders
Headaches
Hearing loss
Hemiplegia
Ischemia
Lead poisoning
Learning disabilities
Ménière's disease
Meningitis
Migraine headaches
Motor neuron diseases

Multiple sclerosis
Nausea and vomiting
Neuralgia, neuritis, and neuropathy
Numbness and tingling
Pain, types of
Palsy
Paralysis
Paraplegia
Parkinsonism
Phenylketonuria
Poliomyelitis
Porphyria
Quadriplegia
Rabies
Reye's syndrome
Sciatica
Seizures
Snakebites
Spina bifida
Spinal disorders
Strokes and TIAs
Stuttering
Tetanus
Thrombosis and thrombus
Tics
Trembling and shaking
Tumors
Unconsciousness
Visual disorders

NEUROSURGEONS
Brain disorders
Cysts and ganglions
Epilepsy
Gigantism
Head and neck disorders
Spinal disorders
Tics

OBSTETRICIANS
Birth defects
Breast-feeding
Cervical, ovarian, and uterine
  cancers
Childbirth
Childbirth, complications of
Conception
Down syndrome
Eclampsia
Ectopic pregnancy
Female genital disorders
Fetal alcohol syndrome
Genetic diseases
Gonorrhea

Growth
Incontinence
Menstruation
Miscarriage
Postpartum depression
Pregnancy and gestation
Premature birth
Rubella
Sexuality
Spina bifida
Stillbirth
Toxoplasmosis

OCCUPATIONAL MEDICINE PHYSICIANS

Altitude sickness
Asphyxiation
Environmental diseases
Hearing loss
Interstitial pulmonary fibrosis (IPF)
Lead poisoning
Lung cancer
Nasopharyngeal disorders
Pulmonary diseases
Radiation sickness
Skin disorders
Tendon disorders

ONCOLOGISTS

Aging
Bone cancer
Bone disorders
Breast cancer
Cancer
Carcinoma
Cervical, ovarian, and uterine
  cancers
Colon cancer
Female genital disorders
Hodgkin's disease
Liver cancer
Lung cancer
Lymphadenopathy and lymphoma
Male genital disorders
Malignancy and metastasis
Prostate cancer
Pulmonary diseases
Radiation sickness
Sarcoma
Skin cancer
Stomach, intestinal, and pancreatic
  cancers
Stress
Tumors

OPHTHALMOLOGISTS

Albinism
Astigmatism
Blindness
Cataracts
Color blindness
Conjunctivitis
Dystrophy
Glaucoma
Macular degeneration
Myopia
Visual disorders

ORTHOPEDISTS AND ORTHOPEDIC SURGEONS

Arthritis
Bone cancer
Bone disorders
Cancer
Cerebral palsy
Dwarfism
Foot disorders
Fracture and dislocation
Osteoporosis
Paget's disease
Scoliosis
Slipped disk
Tendon disorders

OTOLARYNGOLOGISTS

Common cold
Ear infections and disorders
Halitosis
Head and neck disorders
Hearing loss
Laryngitis
Ménière's disease
Motion sickness
Nasopharyngeal disorders
Nausea and vomiting
Pharyngitis
Rhinitis
Sinusitis
Sore throat
Strep throat
Tonsillitis
Voice and vocal cord disorders

PATHOLOGISTS

Breast cancer
Inflammation
Malignancy and metastasis

PEDIATRICIANS

Acne
Bed-wetting
Birth defects
Childhood infectious diseases
Cholera
Cleft palate
Cystic fibrosis
Domestic violence
Down syndrome
Fever
Genetic diseases
Growth
Hydrocephalus
Kwashiorkor
Learning disabilities
Measles, red
Menstruation
Multiple sclerosis
Mumps
Muscular dystrophy
Pertussis
Phenylketonuria
Poliomyelitis
Premature birth
Puberty and adolescence
Reye's syndrome
Rheumatic fever
Rickets
Roseola
Rubella
Rubeola
Scarlet fever
Seizures
Sexuality
Sibling rivalry
Sore throat
Stammering
Streptococcal infections
Sudden infant death syndrome
  (SIDS)

PERINATOLOGISTS

Birth defects
Breast-feeding
Childbirth
Fetal alcohol syndrome
Premature birth

PHYSIATRISTS

Muscle sprains, spasms, and
  disorders
Muscular dystrophy
Numbness and tingling

Legionnaires' disease
Leishmaniasis
Leprosy
Lice, mites, and ticks
Lyme disease
Malaria
Malnutrition
Measles, red
Meningitis
Mumps
Parasitic diseases
Pertussis
Plague
Poliomyelitis
Protozoan diseases
Rabies
Radiation sickness
Roundworm
Rubella
Rubeola
Salmonella
Schistosomiasis
Sexually transmitted diseases
Shigellosis
Sleeping sickness
Smallpox
Syphilis
Tetanus
Toxoplasmosis
Trichinosis
Tuberculosis
Typhoid fever and typhus
Worms
Zoonoses

PULMONOLOGISTS
Asthma
Bronchitis
Coughing
Cystic fibrosis
Emphysema
Fungal infections
Interstitial pulmonary fibrosis (IPF)
Lung cancer
Pleurisy
Pneumonia
Pulmonary diseases
Tuberculosis
Tumors

RADIATION ONCOLOGISTS
Cancer
Liver cancer
Lung cancer

Prostate cancer
Radiation sickness
Sarcoma

RADIOLOGISTS
Cancer
Radiation sickness

RHEUMATOLOGISTS
Arthritis
Autoimmune disorders
Bone disorders
Bursitis
Gout
Inflammation
Lyme disease
Osteoarthritis
Rheumatic fever
Rheumatoid arthritis
Spondylitis

SLEEP SPECIALISTS
Apnea
Narcolepsy
Sleep disorders

SPEECH PATHOLOGISTS
Aphasia and dysphasia
Autism
Cerebral palsy
Dyslexia
Speech disorders
Stammering
Stuttering

SPEECH THERAPISTS
Cleft palate
Voice and vocal cord disorders

SPORTS MEDICINE PHYSICIANS
Athlete's foot
Head and neck disorders
Heat exhaustion and heat stroke
Muscle sprains, spasms, and
    disorders
Tendon disorders

SURGEONS, GENERAL
Aging
Appendicitis
Burns and scalds
Cancer
Cholecystitis
Cirrhosis

Colon cancer
Crohn's disease
Diverticulitis and diverticulosis
Ectopic pregnancy
Female genital disorders
Frostbite
Gallbladder diseases
Gangrene
Hernia
Hyperthermia and hypothermia
Intestinal disorders
Malignancy and metastasis
Obstruction
Peritonitis
Phlebitis
Stomach, intestinal, and pancreatic
    cancers
Stones
Tumors
Varicosis
Wounds

THORACIC SURGEONS
Aneurysms
Hyperthermia and hypothermia

TOXICOLOGISTS
Bites and stings
Botulism
Eczema
Environmental diseases
Food poisoning
Hepatitis
Intoxication
Itching
Lead poisoning
Leukemia
Poisoning
Poisonous plants
Rashes
Snakebites
Staphylococcal infections
Streptococcal infections
Toxemia
Toxoplasmosis

TROPICAL MEDICINE
    PHYSICIANS
Arthropod-borne diseases
Cholera
Diarrhea and dysentery
Elephantiasis
Itching
Leishmaniasis

Malaria
Parasitic diseases
Protozoan diseases
Roundworm
Schistosomiasis
Sleeping sickness
Tapeworm
Worms
Yellow fever
Zoonoses

UROLOGISTS
Bed-wetting
Cystitis
Gonorrhea
Incontinence
Infertility in males

Male genital disorders
Prostate cancer
Schistosomiasis
Sexual dysfunction
Sexually transmitted diseases
Syphilis
Urethritis
Urinary disorders
Warts

VASCULAR SURGEONS
Aneurysms
Atherosclerotic disease
Cholesterol
Claudication
Congenital heart disease
Embolism

Endocarditis
Heart failure
Ischemia
Phlebitis
Strokes and TIAs
Thrombosis and thrombus
Varicosis
Venous insufficiency

VETERINARIANS
Rabies
Zoonoses

VIROLOGISTS
Viral infections

Entries by System Affected

ABDOMINAL ORGANS
Peritonitis

ALL
Aging
Autoimmune disorders
Cancer
Carcinoma
Cushing's syndrome
Death and dying
Disease
Domestic violence
Dystrophy
Environmental diseases
Fatigue
Fever
Gangrene
Genetic diseases
Growth
Hyperthermia and hypothermia
Hypertrophy
Hypochondriasis
Iatrogenic disorders
Infection
Inflammation
Intoxication
Ischemia
Malignancy and metastasis
Malnutrition
Pain, types of
Parasitic diseases
Psychosomatic disorders
Puberty and adolescence
Sexually transmitted diseases
Staphylococcal infections
Streptococcal infections
Sudden infant death syndrome
   (SIDS)
Suicide
Tumors
Viral infections
Vitamin and mineral deficiencies
Wounds
Zoonoses

AUDITORY
Dyslexia
Ear infections and disorders
Hearing loss
Ménière's disease
Motion sickness
Speech disorders

BLOOD
Anemia
Arthropod-borne diseases
Bleeding
Candidiasis
Hemophilia
Hyperlipidemia
Hypoglycemia
Ischemia
Jaundice
Leukemia
Malaria
Scurvy
Septicemia
Sickle-cell anemia
Thalassemia
Toxemia
Yellow fever

BRAIN
Addiction
Alcoholism
Altitude sickness
Alzheimer's disease
Amnesia and memory loss
Aphasia and dysphasia
Brain disorders
Cluster headaches
Coma
Concussion
Dementia
Dizziness and fainting
Down syndrome
Dwarfism
Dyslexia
Embolism
Encephalitis
Epilepsy
Fetal alcohol syndrome
Gigantism
Guillain-Barré syndrome (GBS)
Hallucinations
Head and neck disorders
Headaches
Hydrocephalus
Lead poisoning
Learning disabilities
Malaria
Meningitis
Mental retardation
Migraine headaches
Narcolepsy

Nausea and vomiting
Phenylketonuria
Poliomyelitis
Rabies
Reye's syndrome
Seizures
Sleep disorders
Sleeping sickness
Stammering
Strokes and TIAs
Syphilis
Tetanus
Thrombosis and thrombus
Tics
Toxoplasmosis
Trembling and shaking
Unconsciousness
Yellow fever

BREASTS
Breast cancer
Breast disorders
Breast-feeding
Mastitis

CIRCULATORY
Aneurysms
Asphyxiation
Atherosclerotic disease
Bacterial infections
Bleeding
Candidiasis
Childbirth, complications of
Cholesterol
Claudication
Diabetes mellitus
Dizziness and fainting
Eclampsia
Edema
Embolism
Heart disease
Heat exhaustion and heat stroke
Hemorrhoids
Hypertension
Ischemia
Phlebitis
Plague
Protozoan diseases
Radiation sickness
Septicemia
Shock
Sleeping sickness

Nephritis
Renal failure
Reye's syndrome
Stones

LIVER
Alcoholism
Cirrhosis
Edema
Hepatitis
Jaundice
Liver cancer
Liver disorders
Malaria
Reye's syndrome
Schistosomiasis
Yellow fever

LYMPHATIC
Bacterial infections
Breast cancer
Breast disorders
Edema
Elephantiasis
Hodgkin's disease
Lymphadenopathy and lymphoma
Sleeping sickness

MUCOUS MEMBRANES
Chickenpox
Chlamydia
Herpes
Leishmaniasis
Sexually transmitted diseases
Strep throat
Syphilis

MUSCULAR
Ataxia
Bed-wetting
Bell's palsy
Beriberi
Botulism
Cerebral palsy
Childhood infectious diseases
Chronic fatigue syndrome
Claudication
Cysts and ganglions
Depression
Dwarfism
Fetal alcohol syndrome
Foot disorders
Guillain-Barré syndrome (GBS)
Head and neck disorders

Hemiplegia
Motor neuron diseases
Multiple sclerosis
Muscle sprains, spasms, and
    disorders
Muscular dystrophy
Numbness and tingling
Palsy
Paralysis
Paraplegia
Parkinsonism
Poisoning
Poliomyelitis
Quadriplegia
Rabies
Rheumatoid arthritis
Sarcoma
Seizures
Speech disorders
Tendon disorders
Tetanus
Tics
Trembling and shaking
Trichinosis
Weight loss and gain
Yellow fever

NERVOUS
Addiction
Alcoholism
Altitude sickness
Alzheimer's disease
Anxiety
Apnea
Arthropod-borne diseases
Ataxia
Autism
Bell's palsy
Beriberi
Botulism
Cerebral palsy
Claudication
Cysts and ganglions
Diabetes mellitus
Diphtheria
Down syndrome
Eclampsia
Electrical shock
Encephalitis
Epilepsy
Fetal alcohol syndrome
Guillain-Barré syndrome (GBS)
Hallucinations
Head and neck disorders

Hearing loss
Hemiplegia
Lead poisoning
Leprosy
Lyme disease
Meningitis
Motor neuron diseases
Multiple sclerosis
Neuralgia, neuritis, and neuropathy
Numbness and tingling
Paget's disease
Palsy
Paralysis
Paraplegia
Parkinsonism
Poisoning
Poliomyelitis
Porphyria
Premenstrual syndrome (PMS)
Quadriplegia
Sciatica
Seizures
Shingles
Snakebites
Spina bifida
Spinal disorders
Stuttering
Tics

PSYCHIC-EMOTIONAL
Addiction
Aging
Alcoholism
Amnesia and memory loss
Anorexia nervosa
Anxiety
Autism
Brain disorders
Breast cancer
Breast disorders
Bulimia
Childbirth
Chronic fatigue syndrome
Death and dying
Depression
Domestic violence
Dyslexia
Eating disorders
Factitious disorders
Grief and guilt
Hallucinations
Hypochondriasis
Learning disabilities
Manic-depressive disorder

Lice, mites, and ticks
Lupus erythematosus
Lyme disease
Measles, red
Numbness and tingling
Obesity
Pimples
Poisonous plants
Porphyria
Premenstrual syndrome (PMS)
Psoriasis
Radiation sickness
Rashes
Rosacea
Roseola
Rubella
Rubeola
Scabies
Scarlet fever
Scurvy
Shingles
Skin cancer

Skin disorders
Smallpox
Warts

TEETH
Caries, dental
Dental diseases
Endodontic disease
Toothache

TISSUE
Abscesses
Bacterial infections
Birth defects
Burns and scalds
Frostbite

URINARY
Bed-wetting
Candidiasis
Cystitis
Incontinence

Urethritis
Urinary disorders

VISUAL
Albinism
Altitude sickness
Astigmatism
Blindness
Cataracts
Chlamydia
Color blindness
Conjunctivitis
Diabetes mellitus
Dyslexia
Glaucoma
Gonorrhea
Jaundice
Macular degeneration
Myopia
Visual disorders